PEDIATRIC CARE OF THE ICN GRADUATE

ROBERTA A. BALLARD, M.D.

Chief, Department of Pediatrics,
Director, Newborn Services,
Mount Zion Hospital and Medical Center
San Francisco, California

1988

W. B. SAUNDERS COMPANY

Harcourt Brace Jovanovich, Inc.

Philadelphia, London, Toronto, Montreal, Sydney, Tokyo

W. B. SAUNDERS COMPANY
Harcourt Brace Jovanovich, Inc.

The Curtis Center
Independence Square West
Philadelphia, PA 19106

Library of Congress Cataloging-in-Publication Data

Pediatric care of the ICN graduate.

    1. Infants (Newborn)—Diseases—Complications and sequelae.   2. Neonatal intensive care—Longitudinal studies.   3. Sick children—Home care.   I. Ballard, Roberta A.   [DNLM: 1. Follow-Up Studies—in infancy & childhood.   2. Home Care Services.   3. Infant, Low Birth Weight.   4. Infant, Newborn, Diseases.   5. Infant, Premature, Diseases.   6. Primary Health Care. WS 420 P3674]
RJ255.P34   1988   618.92′01   87-24333
ISBN 0-7216-1404-3

Developmental Editor: Debbie Rosenthal
Production Manager: Frank Polizzano
Manuscript Editor: Agnes Kelly
Indexer: Bonnie Boehme

Pediatric Care of the ICN Graduate   ISBN   0-7216-1404-3

Last digit is the print number: 9   8   7   6   5   4   3   2

Dedicated to

My parents, Bert and Charlotte Anderson
My husband, Phil
My sons, Dustin and Christopher

With love and appreciation

CONTRIBUTORS

RONALD L. ARIAGNO, M.D.

Professor of Pediatrics, Stanford University School of Medicine. Associate Director of Nurseries and Associate Director of Premature Research Center, Stanford University Hospital Medical Center, Stanford, California.

Management of Apnea in the ICN Graduate

ANN M. ARVIN, M.D.

Associate Professor of Pediatric Infectious Diseases, Department of Pediatrics, Stanford University School of Medicine, Stanford, California.

Infectious Disease Issues in the Care of ICN Graduate

ROBERTA A. BALLARD, M.D.

Chief, Department of Pediatrics; Director, Newborn Services, Mount Zion Hospital and Medical Center, San Francisco, California.

The Transition from Hospital to Home; Well-Baby Care of the ICN Graduate; Outcome After Neonatal Intensive Care

MADELEINE BOOTH BEHLE, R.N., M.S.

Pediatric Nurse Practitioner, Intensive Care Nursery Follow-up Clinic, Department of Pediatrics, Mount Zion Hospital and Medical Center, San Francisco, California.

The Transition from Hospital to Home

STEPHANIE A. BERMAN, M.S.W.

Social Work Supervisor, Pediatric-Perinatal Social Services, Mount Zion Hospital and Medical Center, San Francisco, California.

Support of the Family Whose Infant Dies

C. MICHAEL BOWMAN, Ph.D., M.D.

Assistant Professor of Pediatrics, University of Southern California School of Medicine. Attending Pulmonologist, Children's Hospital of Los Angeles, Los Angeles, California.

Cystic Fibrosis

JOHN C. CAREY, M.D., M.P.H.

Associate Professor of Pediatrics, University of Utah School of Medicine. Chief, Division of Medical Genetics, Department of Pediatrics, University of Utah Medical Center, Salt Lake City, Utah.

Health Supervision and Anticipatory Guidance for Infants with Congenital Defects

SEYMOUR R. COHEN, M.D.

Clinical Professor of Surgery (Otolaryngology), University of Southern California School of Medicine. Former Head, Division of Pediatric Otolaryngology, Children's Hospital of Los Angeles, Los Angeles, California.

Management of Airways Obstruction and Other Abnormalities Affecting Pulmonary Care; Home Care of Infants with Chronic Lung Disease

SUSAN H. DAY, M.D.

Director of Pediatric Ophthalmology, Pacific Presbyterian Medical Center, San Francisco. Consultant Ophthalmologist, Mount Zion Hospital, San Francisco, and Children's Hospital, Oakland, California.

The Eyes of the ICN Graduate

ALFRED A. DE LORIMIER, M.D.

Professor of Surgery, University of California, San Francisco, School of Medicine. Chief, Pediatric Surgery, University of California, San Francisco, Medical Center, San Francisco, California.

Care of ICN Graduates After Neonatal Surgery

MARJORIE E. DERECHIN, R.N., M.S.

Pediatric Nurse Practitioner, Departments of Neurological Surgery and Pediatrics, University of California, San Francisco, Medical Center, San Francisco, California.

Neurosurgical Problems in the Infant

MURDINA M. DESMOND, M.D.

Professor of Pediatrics, Baylor College of Medicine. Director, Meyer Center for Developmental Pediatrics, Texas Children's Hospital, Houston, Texas.

Historical Perspectives

LILLY M.S. DUBOWITZ, M.D., D.C.H.

Research Lecturer, Hammersmith Hospital, London, England.

Neurologic Assessment

MICHAEL S.B. EDWARDS, M.D.

Associate Professor of Neurosurgery and Pediatrics and Director, Division of Pediatric Neurosurgery, University of California, San Francisco, School of Medicine, San Francisco, California.

Neurosurgical Problems in the Infant

AVROY A. FANAROFF, M.D.

Professor of Pediatrics and Reproductive Biology, Case Western Reserve University School of Medicine; Vice Chairman, Department of Pediatrics. Director of Nurseries, University Hospitals; Director of Neonatology, Rainbow Babies & Children's Hospital of University Hospitals, Cleveland, Ohio.

Growth Patterns in the ICN Graduate

MARTIN A. GOLDSMITH, M.D.

Assistant Clinical Professor, University of California, San Francisco, School of Medicine, San Francisco. Director, Pediatric Endocrinology, Valley Children's Hospital, Fresno, California.

Endocrine Problems in the High-Risk Infant

PETER A. GORSKI, M.D.

Assistant Professor and Director, Behavioral and Developmental Research and Training, Department of Pediatrics, Northwestern University Medical School. Chief, Behavioral and Developmental Pediatrics, The Evanston Hospital, Evanston; Attending Physician, Children's Memorial Hospital, Chicago, Illinois.

Fostering Family Development After Preterm Hospitalization

JOAN GROBSTEIN, M.D.

Neonatologist, Intensive Care Nursery and Attending Pediatrician, Department of Pediatrics, Community Hospital, Santa Rosa, California.

Outcome After Neonatal Intensive Care

MAUREEN HACK, M.B., Ch.B.

Associate Professor, Case Western Reserve University School of Medicine. Neonatologist and Director of High-Risk Follow-up, Rainbow Babies & Children's Hospital of University Hospitals, Cleveland, Ohio.

Growth Patterns in the ICN Graduate

JOSEPH HEADLEE, M.S.W.

Pediatric Social Worker, Pediatric-Perinatal Social Services, Mount Zion Hospital and Medical Center, San Francisco, California.

Community and Agency Resources

LORI J. HOWELL, R.N., M.S.

Assistant Clinical Professor, University of California, San Francisco, School of Nursing. Clinical Nurse Specialist, Pediatric Surgery/Pediatric Critical Care, University of California, San Francisco, Medical Center, San Francisco, California.

Home Ostomy Care

THOMAS G. KEENS, M.D.

Associate Professor of Pediatrics, University of Southern California School of Medicine. Attending Physician, Division of Neonatology and Pediatric Pulmonology, Children's Hospital of Los Angeles, Los Angeles, California.

Ventilatory Management at Home; Home Care of Infants with Chronic Lung Disease; Outcome After Neonatal Intensive Care: Chronic Lung Disease

MARION A. KOERPER, M.D.

Associate Clinical Professor, Department of Pediatrics, University of California, San Francisco, School of Medicine. Director, Hemophilia Treatment Center, University of California, San Francisco, Medical Center, San Francisco, California.

Anemia in the ICN Graduate

MARGARET DEKLE LANG, R.N., P.N.P.

Pediatric Nurse Practitioner, Intensive Care Nursery Follow-up Program, Department of Pediatrics, Mount Zion Hospital and Medical Center, San Francisco, California.

The Transition from Hospital to Home; Well-Baby Care of the ICN Graduate

CAROL H. LEONARD, Ph.D.

Psychologist, Intensive Care Nursery Follow-up Program, Department of Pediatrics, Mount Zion Hospital and Medical Center, San Francisco, California.

High-Risk Infant Follow-up Programs; Developmental and Behavioral Assessment

CHERYL D. LEW, M.D.

Clinical Associate Professor of Pediatrics, University of Southern California School of Medicine. Attending Neonatologist and Pediatric Pulmonologist, Division of Neonatology and Pediatric Pulmonology, Children's Hospital of Los Angeles, Los Angeles, California.

Management of Airways Obstruction and Other Abnormalities Affecting Pulmonary Care; Home Care of Infants with Chronic Lung Disease; Outcome After Neonatal Intensive Care: Chronic Lung Disease

ROBERT PIECUCH, M.D.

Director, Intensive Care Nursery Follow-up Program; Attending Neonatologist, Department of Pediatrics, Mount Zion Hospital and Medical Center, San Francisco, California.

Cosmetics: Skin, Scars, and Residual Traces of the ICN

ARNOLD C.G. PLATZKER, M.D.

Professor, Department of Pediatrics, University of Southern California School of Medicine. Head, Division of Neonatology and Pediatric Pulmonology, Children's Hospital of Los Angeles, Los Angeles, California.

Chronic Lung Disease of Infancy; Management of Airways Obstruction and Other Abnormalities Affecting Pulmonary Care; Home Care of Infants with Chronic Lung Disease

JOELYN RYAN, M.S., C.C.C.

Consultant, Mount Zion Hospital Intensive Care Nursery Follow-up Program, San Francisco, California.

Hearing and Speech Assessment

DAVID TEITEL, M.D.

Assistant Professor of Pediatrics (Cardiology), University of California, San Francisco, School of Medicine. Attending Physician, University of California, San Francisco, Medical Center, San Francisco, California.

Care of the Infant with Heart Disease

VALERIE ANN THOM, M.A., R.P.T.

Assistant Professor of Public Health and Preventive Medicine, Child Development and Rehabilitation Center, Oregon Health Sciences University. Physical Therapy Training Director, University Affiliated Program, Child Development and Rehabilitation Center, Oregon Health Sciences University, Portland, Oregon.

Physical Therapy: Follow-up of the Special-Care Infant

JEROME THOMPSON, M.D.

Assistant Clinical Professor, University of Southern California School of Medicine. Attending Physician, Children's Hospital of Los Angeles, Los Angeles, California.

Management of Airways Obstruction and Other Abnormalities Affecting Pulmonary Care; Home Care of Infants with Chronic Lung Disease

SUSAN D. THURBER, R.P.T.

Adjunct Instructor, Department of Physical Therapy, University of Texas School of Allied Health Science, Galveston; Honorary Faculty Member, School of Physical Therapy, Texas Women's University; Staff Member, Department of Pediatrics, Baylor College of Medicine, Houston. Coordinating Physical Therapist, Meyer Center for Developmental Pediatrics, Texas Children's Hospital, Houston, Texas.

Historical Perspectives

DIANE W. WARA, M.D.

Professor, Department of Pediatrics, University of California, San Francisco, School of Medicine. Director, Division of Pediatric Immunology/Rheumatology; Director, Pediatric Clinical Research Center, University of California, San Francisco, Medical Center, San Francisco, California.

The Newborn and Host Defense

SALLY L. DAVIDSON WARD, M.D.

Assistant Professor of Pediatrics, University of Southern California School of Medicine. Attending Physician, Children's Hospital of Los Angeles, Los Angeles, California.

Ventilatory Management at Home; Home Care of Infants with Chronic Lung Disease

PEGGY S. WEINTRUB, M.D.

Assistant Clinical Professor, University of California, San Francisco, School of Medicine. Attending Physician, University of California, San Francisco, Medical Center, San Francisco, California.

The Newborn and Host Defense

FOREWORD

   The advent of neonatal intensive care and the survival of infants who in former eras would have died have raised the question as to whether there has been an increase in the incidence of long-term disabilities in children. However, childhood problems that originate in the neonatal period are not a new phenomenon. At the beginning of the 18th Century, while 25 per cent of live-born infants in London died in the first month of life, 50 per cent of the survivors were dead before they reached 5 years of age. Much of this staggering mortality was due to a crowded, dirty, sunless environment, which promoted infection, malnutrition and infanticide. By 1850, the chance that an infant would reach school age had increased from 25 to 75 per cent, but survivors still had a high incidence of debilitating malformations, and malnutrition and chronic infections remained common.

   During the first decades of the 20th Century, neonatal mortality was still high; 13 per cent of newborn infants in Massachusetts died in the first month of life, and the long-term outlook for many of the survivors remained grim. At this point, the quest for the source of high neonatal mortality and long-term morbidity began to focus on premature birth, and special units for the care of prematurely born babies were developed. The prematurely born infant was kept in a warm environment, shielded from infectious agents and became better nourished. This and the improved hygiene and feeding practices for all newborn infants was accompanied by another dramatic drop in mortality, from about 15 per cent in 1900 to 8 per cent in 1920 and to 4 per cent in 1940. Thus, over two centuries and long before modern methods of intensive care were available to newborns, chances of their survival increased almost ten-fold. But, with each triumph over mortality, the residues of neonatal disease appeared to climb. By the end of the Second World War, death in the first month of life had become unusual rather than expected. As a consequence, each newborn death was viewed, not unreasonably, as something that could be prevented—if only we understood why the infants died, we could prevent their deaths. The stage was set for a vigorous assault on the causes of the residual mortality.

   By 1950, deaths in the newborn period were primarily due to infection or respiratory failure in prematurely born infants. The introduction of new and more effective antibiotics quickly diminished the threat of death from bacterial infection, leaving respiratory distress as the leading cause of neonatal death. Because pediatricians believed that this problem could also be eliminated, they focused their attention on defining the pathophysiology of respiratory distress and devising methods for its treatment. By the end of the decade, Reid and Tunstall and Donald and Lord in England, Heese in South Africa, Delavoria-Papado-poulos and Swyer in Canada and Stahlman in the United States, among others, were beginning to have success using assisted ventilation in the management of infants with respiratory distress. Subsequently, nurseries, which had been designed for the incubation and feeding of prematurely born infants, rapidly evolved into units designed for the aggressive application of ventilatory and circulatory support for infants with respiratory distress. In less than a decade, the premature nursery became the intensive care nursery and neonatal mortality again dropped, from about 2 per cent in 1970 to less than 1 per cent today.

However, as in previous epochs, the active intervention of the last two decades raised the possibility that intensive care for the newborn infant was increasing the proportion of infants with residual illness living into childhood. Successful treatment of infants with meningitis can cause irreversible central nervous system damage; infants with severe asphyxia who are vigorously and successfully resuscitated may have cerebral palsy. Similarly, the increasing salvage of the very lowest birth weight infants has been accompanied by an increase in intracranial hemorrhage, hydrocephalus, chronic lung disease, visual and auditory impairments and cognitive problems ranging from learning disabilities to mental retardation. Fortunately, despite the concern of critics of neonatology, the percentage of surviving sick newborn infants who have unfavorable outcomes has decreased over the past 30 years. Nonetheless, particularly with the striking increase in survival for the very low birth weight infants, the absolute number of children with residual problems has increased. The continuing care of this group of children and the early recognition and treatment of their problems is a major challenge to society.

Today, intensive care for newborn infants is not restricted to the support of low birth weight infants. About 8 per cent of newborn infants are born prematurely, and as many as half of these require intensive care. Some 4 per cent of infants born at term have infections, asphyxia, congenital anomalies and other problems requiring sophisticated care in the newborn period. Thus, out of an estimated 4 million babies to be born this year in the United States, more than a quarter of a million will require some form of special care in the days following birth. In this book, Dr. Ballard and her colleagues address the important problems presented by this large group of infants. The special and uniquely valuable contribution of these authors is their focus on the critical post-hospital period of convalescence for the recipients of neonatal intensive care. They have given us splendid descriptions of the cardio-pulmonary, neurological, cognitive and social consequences of surviving contemporary newborn care along with guidelines for providing appropriate care.

This publication is extremely timely. As increasing amounts of our health care dollars go to providing sophisticated care for newborn infants, it is essential that the providers of that care attend to the subsequent welfare of these infants with much greater assiduity than in the past. Dr. Ballard and her co-authors point the way with this remarkable volume. *Pediatric Care of the ICN Graduate* should be in the library of all health professionals who provide care for infants and children.

WILLIAM H. TOOLEY, M.D.

Professor of Pediatrics
University of California, San Francisco
School of Medicine

PREFACE

The idea for **Pediatric Care of the ICN Graduate** emerged from a conversation concerning books needed in the field of pediatrics. As the discussion progressed and the ideas were later shared with others, it became clear that there was, indeed, a need for a book to help those who care for the growing number of infants who represent the successes of our advances in neonatal intensive care but who leave the intensive care nursery with very special sets of problems and needs. For the most part, these infants have an excellent eventual outlook for growth and development and can expect full participation in a wide range of activities, both as children and as adults. Their early care, however, provides a tremendous challenge to the professionals who care for them.

This book is for all those who provide care for these special infants, particularly the primary care physicians, whether they are pediatricians, residents in training, or family doctors, who play the central role in providing their medical management, supporting their families, and coordinating the multiple services they may require. The book is also intended to help the multidisciplinary staff who participate in assessing these infants in special follow-up programs. Finally, it is hoped that the book will also be helpful to staff in neonatal intensive care units, enabling them to work better with the families of these infants and to deal realistically with their expectations for care after discharge.

In developing this book, I sought to draw on the expertise of many outstanding specialists in the fields of both developmental and neonatal pediatric medicine and to have them focus their chapters on the particular issues that these infants face, primarily in the first two years after discharge from the intensive care nursery. To help make the material relevant to the family physicians and pediatricians who make up the primary audience of the book, the manuscript was then reviewed by several physicians in office practice for relevance, accuracy, and plain common sense and annotated by them to highlight areas of controversy and points of emphasis.

The objectives of the book were several. First, it is designed to help those who care for intensive care nursery graduates, whether they are prematures or others with special problems, to understand the expected "normal" differences in behavior, growth, development, and medical needs of these infants. Second, it is intended to provide information on "how to" follow-up the infants' growth, development, vision and hearing, and other special needs, as well as to review some published studies outlining expectations of specific groups. Third, the book is intended to provide practical guidelines for both reassurance and "when to worry" about numerous issues that may arise in caring for intensive care nursery graduates. Fourth, the book addresses common medical problems faced by particular groups of graduates, such as those with chronic lung disease, congenital heart disorders, common chromosomal abnormalities, and other problems. Included are practical guidelines for home care of infants with chronic lung disease or those who have had surgery. Finally, the book seeks to emphasize throughout many of the developmental issues that require particular understanding and parental support, beginning with the transition from hospital to home. A separate chapter addresses the support of the family whose infant has died.

This book would not have been possible without the ideas, support, and encouragement of many people. William Tooley, M.D., provided crucial initial enthusiasm for this project, as he has for many aspects of my professional career in neonatology. Arnold Platzker, M.D., shared my concerns about the need for this book, helped to develop its outline, and wrote a significant major section on chronic lung disease. Ronald Clyman, M.D., and Susan Sniderman, M.D., colleagues at Mount Zion Hospital and Medical Center, provided enthusiastic support and invaluable help in outlining the book's contents.

All of the staff involved in the Mount Zion Neonatal Follow-up Program—Carol Leonard, Ph.D., Robert Piecuch, M.D., Margaret Lang, P.N.P., Madeleine Behle, R.N.,M.S., Sally Sehring, M.D., and Carol Miller, M.D.—have been instrumental in the production of this book. Not only have they offered an outstanding service, which provides a model for others who wish to do neonatal follow-up care, but they have been central in helping structure, review, write, and annotate this book.

I sincerely thank all of the contributors who extended themselves to produce a new approach to their various topics focused on these special infants. In addition, my great appreciation goes to Myles Abbott, M.D., Peter Gorski, M.D., Brock Bernsten, M.D., Robert Piecuch, M.D., and Alan Rosen, M.D., for their patience, commitment, and essential contribution in reviewing and annotating the contents and thus providing one of this book's special features, and, I hope, special usefulness to the primary care physician.

My greatest indebtedness is to the two individuals who truly gave of themselves to make it possible for me to complete this work. Phil Ballard, my colleague in this and many other endeavors, provided constant steady support and encouragement, with both intellectual aspects and essential family chores. Finally, Jane Belanger provided extraordinary editorial assistance in the preparation of the manuscript and gave many extra caring hours to guarantee its quality. It has truly been a privilege to work with all of these very gifted people.

ROBERTA A. BALLARD

CONTENTS

SECTION III
BEHAVIORAL, DEVELOPMENTAL AND NEUROLOGIC EVALUATION

SECTION IV
MANAGEMENT OF PULMONARY SEQUELAE AND SUBSPECIALTY PROBLEMS

SECTION V
APPENDICES

SECTION I

INTRODUCTION

1

HISTORICAL PERSPECTIVES

MURDINA M. DESMOND, M.D., and SUSAN D. THURBER, R.P.T.

At the beginning of this century, death rates of parturient women and newly born infants were appallingly high. Clearly, more than observation of the reproductive process was required. Slowly but consistently, medicine and public health began to confront the magnitude of the mortalities, to investigate their causes, and to apply measures for improvement of child bearing and child rearing.

Beginning in the 1910's and early 1920's, the newly created Children's Bureau garnered and distributed statistical information on infant deaths. In 1922 a special and successful nursery for the premature (prematurity being the largest contributor to infant mortality) was opened by Hess in Michael Reese Hospital in Chicago. It is noteworthy that this nursery had a transport system for bringing infants into the nursery, a breast milk supply program, and a follow-up program featuring home and clinic visits as well as longitudinal developmental assessment.[1] During the thirties similar nurseries proliferated, and the emerging specialty of pediatrics assumed medical responsibility. Gradually obstetricians relinquished the care of the healthy term newborn as well as the premature or sick infant to the pediatrician, and more efficient incubators and feeding methods were designed. In the forties the age of technologic advance began with the Chapple incubator, the intravenous catheter, blood banks, and antibiotics. In the fifties babies began to be considered as individuals rather than members of weight groups,

and prenatal influences on the developing newborn were increasingly recognized. With this, the term *high risk* came into being to describe a greater than average risk for neonatal morbidity or disability later in childhood.

With the 1960's, special-care nurseries (intensive, intermediate, transitional) were opened, permitting more precise surveillance of the newly born and the ill. These units served all infants, regardless of birth weight. Pediatricians with special interest and expertise in newborn medicine were termed *neonatologists.* In the seventies, intensive care nurseries were regionalized. They were soon broadened in scope to become perinatal centers serving high-risk mothers as well as high-risk infants.

Spectacular decreases in perinatal and infant mortality followed in the seventies, and the fall continued into the early eighties. In 1984, infant mortality reached the lowest figure in history, i.e., 10.6 per 1000 live births, or at least 10 times below the estimated infant mortality of 1900. During the past decade the highest gains in survival were shown by the very low birth weight groups, i.e., less than 1500 grams. Today 80 per cent of infants weighing 750 to 1000 grams at birth are expected to survive.

Regionalized special perinatal and neonatal care is now successfully established throughout the United States. Although the hospital format generally follows the three-level system begun in 1976, the intake policies and design of individual nurseries tend to conform to local needs.

Some hospitals offer level III (intensive care) and II (intermediate care); others, level I (normal newborn care); still others, all three. Level III units may be architecturally combined with level II so that a single unit serves a sick infant throughout acute and convalescent phases of transitional disease. Thus, within a given locale or region, all levels of care are generally available, although populations served in individual units may vary within the total system.

Overall, intensive care is provided to 5 to 6 per cent of all live-born infants. In the majority of nurseries the very small premature infant (who comprises only 1 per cent of births) is the predominant patient—because of the high level of medical and technologic expertise required in the immediate neonatal period and the longer nursery stay. Low birth weight infants (2500 grams or less) comprise 50 to 60 per cent of intensive care nursery (ICN) admissions, while the very low birth weight infants, i.e., those under 1500 grams, comprise 25 per cent.[2] Because of their prolonged hospitalizations, the proportion of very low birth weight infants is high in the daily census.

And what of the baby after discharge from the nursery? In the early years of regionalized intensive care, a great discontinuity existed between the high quality of care and family support offered within the level III units and the care available to child and family after discharge.[3]

The pathways taken by the infant after discharge from the nursery back to the local primary health care system may be as diverse as the pathways into the ICN. Follow-up care may be geographically distant from the ICN. The family is fortunate if the primary care physician is already known to them, has been in communication with the intensive care nursery, and receives a discharge summary. Frequently, however, the physician is new to the family, or the infant enters a public clinic system. Under these circumstances the physician is unaware of the prior prenatal and nursery course and the cumulative anxieties of the parents and is at great disadvantage in understanding the base from which post-nursery development will proceed.[3]

The well-child routines of earlier years have proven inadequate to serve the demands and needs of the post–intensive care population, particularly the very low birth weight infant. Many ICN follow-up programs were designed to provide rapid feedback information to ICN's subsidized by federal or state funds. However, with increasing understanding of the post-nur-sery course, family stresses, infant vulnerabilities, and the timetable for emergence of handicap, more complex networking follow-up systems have evolved. Today, follow-up may be viewed as a natural forward extension of perinatal and neonatal intensive care. Present programs are characterized by closer communication among the ICN, the primary care physician, the child developmentalist, and community resources for education and habilitation.

INFANTS TO BE SERVED IN INTENSIVE CARE FOLLOW-UP

Which infants require the most closely monitored pediatric care and developmental surveillance? Such a selection implies an estimation of future developmental risk. This estimation is not simple, since continuing complex biologic and environmental factors act to mold growing organisms, and predictions may be fallible.

However, infants from level III and level II units have already encountered transitional morbidity and thus began extrauterine life suboptimally. They may be considered as carrying some degree of developmental risk, moderate to high.

High-risk status would include infants of very low birth weight, those both preterm and undergrown; those with prior central nervous system symptomatology (infection, seizure, hemorrhage), chronic respiratory disease, or significant congenital or recurrent infections; and those making unusually slow progress in reaching milestones appropriate for postconceptional age. Moderate-risk status would include infants who were born following adverse perinatal circumstances and those with illness who nevertheless made good physiologic progress prior to discharge. Infants born at great psychosocial disadvantage would also fit into this category.

The follow-up plan for infants with congenital malformations is usually individualized in accordance with the particular constellation of problems presented (see Chapter 24).

In practical terms the physician can work out a flexible post-nursery care plan that considers present health and progress while providing developmental surveillance at key ages.

APPROACH TO DEVELOPMENTAL ASSESSMENT

Developmental assessment may be defined as a measurement of the integrity of the central nervous system, in terms of the infant's or child's ability to *function* within his or her age and milieu. Assessment encompasses more than evaluation of cognitive function, since it includes the ability to *do,* i.e., carry out tasks appropriate for the age.

Screening differs from overall assessment, but serves an extremely useful purpose for the physician. A screening examination is a preliminary and necessarily limited list of yes-no questions or a check list of "can do it, cannot do it" tasks. It is not designed to make a diagnosis, but rather to guide the physician toward more definitive professional evaluation if the child's abilities are discrepant, of poor quality, or below age expectation. Present pediatric policy recommends that all children be screened at regular intervals. For high-risk children, including those who have required intensive care, regular screening followed by multidisciplinary professional assessment when indicated is more urgent and is considered optimal only when it extends through age of school entrance.

Over the past decade, developmental assessments have been carried out by a variety of professionals in many settings. The present consensus within the field indicates that the principles given below are generally held and followed.

Developmental assessment should:

1. Be preceded by the gathering of relevant information, including the history of the prenatal and nursery course, developmental status on nursery discharge, and present health.

2. Provide a profile of developing skills related to postconceptional age within the following areas: gross motor, fine motor, language, and social and adaptive (or mental) performances. The battery chosen and the length of the evaluation should be appropriate for the child's medical stability.

3. Allow for optimal performance through sensitivity of the assessing professionals to signs of fatigue, overstimulation, or vasomotor change in the child.

4. Be interdisciplinary or transdisciplinary, with all examiners exchanging findings in conference and approaching consensus, followed by unified diagnoses and recommendations according to priority.

5. Provide developmental information that is useful for either home management or intervention programs and, in both written and spoken form, is clearly understandable to parents.

EVOLUTION OF FOLLOW-UP PROGRAMS WITH SPECIAL REFERENCE TO LOW BIRTH WEIGHT INFANTS

Follow-up assessment of the infant with prior perinatal morbidity is an old custom, not a new phenomenon. Outcome studies comprise a vast and fascinating literature that dates from mid nineteenth century Europe. This literature concerns mainly the prematurely born subject. Not only is it massive, but it is fraught with conflicting opinions and differing perceptions regarding the definitions of successful vs unsatisfactory outcome. This diversity is probably a result of the numerous epidemiologic, environmental, and medical variables involved; the problems of sampling; definitions of prematurity; continuing changes in nursery care technology; impact of post-nursery events; terminology of morbidity and handicap; and the characteristics of test instruments available at the period of study. Change in the field has been so rapid that it is difficult to relate one decade to another even in the same geographic area or hospital. An unwritten but probably important factor in the conflicting conclusions of past studies relates to individual nursery policies for the use, or withdrawal, of resuscitation and other life support systems in "previable" infants or in those with overt major central nervous system damage.

The extreme differences of opinion concerning the outcome of the premature baby may be illustrated by quotations from two highly respected investigators.

> The fate of immature children is not enviable; almost half die during the first year of life. Of those that remain alive, the majority are physically as well as mentally underdeveloped. Some of them show a later mental development; others show a condition of psychic infantilism, while others show permanent and severe mental diseases. When they are passed in review, one is surprised at the variety and amount of abnormality encountered.
>
> *Capper (1928)[4]*

> The majority of premature infants born after the 32nd week into a proper environment without birth injuries undergo a normal mental development, progressing more slowly than the full-term infant during the first years. They average walking and talking about six months later, and are somewhat slower in learning to coordinate, as evidenced by clumsiness and ease of falling, slight speech defects, etc. All of these are, however, usually temporary manifestations and are followed by normal progress.
>
> *Hess, J.H., quoted by Gesell (1933)[5]*

Formal assessment utilizing objective testing was introduced in the late twenties and early thirties by Sunde (utilizing the Binet-Simon-Stanford instrument) and by Gesell and Hess with the Gesell instrument.[5,6] In 1930, Mohr and Barthelme, utilizing Gesell schedules, introduced the concept of evaluating prematurely born infants from the reference point of post-conceptional rather than chronologic age.[7] Gesell in his writings emphasized that prematurity did not, of itself, markedly distort, hasten, or retard the course of development when development was reckoned from date of conception. Complications of prematurity did, however, alter the developmental course. Many authors considered the importance of home and social environment in outcome, but their significance for later development was firmly established through the studies of Drillien and Blegen.[8,9]

By 1950, although views on outcome were still divergent, the consensus seemed to be that premature infants as a group had higher infant and childhood death rates, a higher incidence of central nervous system disturbances, and more disorders of vision, hearing, behavior, attention, speech, and reading than did term infants at comparable ages. Prematurely born infants tended to develop slowly during their first two years, but after surviving early childhood the majority did well.[10]

By the mid 1950's, the widespread movement to provide pediatric specialty care for the very small or very sick infant was firmly established in the United States. Specialized techniques, e.g., gavage feeding, intravenous fluids, blood transfusions, efficient incubators, and antibiotics, were available. The early withholding of feeding was widely practiced. However, subsequent studies reported that the outcome of very small low birth weight infants born during this decade was disappointing overall and was characterized by a high incidence of neurologic handicap, visual impairment, and mental defect. These unfavorable findings were unexpected. Although some later authors ascribe the cause to the practice of early withholding of feedings, this setback has not yet been fully explained.

In the sixties, in level III and II units, rapid progress was made toward providing respiratory, nutritional, and metabolic support. Progress was reflected in gains in both the survival and quality of survival over the previous decade. Outcomes in the fifties and sixties for the first time were related to the infant's growth status at birth (appropriate, small, or large for gestational age), as well as to presence or absence of specific newborn neonatal complications, such as respiratory distress syndrome, seizures, and sepsis.

During the 1970's, perinatal mortality, particularly that of the very low birth weight infant, dropped dramatically as fetal monitoring, techniques of assisted ventilation, and precise monitoring of thermal and metabolic status became available in perinatal centers. But at the same time, retrolental fibroplasia began to reappear. With the new computed tomography, intracerebral hemorrhage was diagnosed during life in a high proportion of early-gestation infants. The focus of neonatal research shifted quickly to investigate not only respiratory physiology but also the neurologic problems of intracranial hemorrhage, cerebral blood flow, and the effects of transport and handling on the infant.

In the current decade, the eighties, awareness of a need for more careful follow-up of infants experiencing intensive care has spread widely throughout this country. As indicated previously, early follow-up assessment programs were established to provide feedback information to intensive care units. However, although important, this was no longer the only priority. The infant was the first priority. An increasing population of intensive care survivors required not only meticulous medical care and assessment, but the continuing guidance of a knowledgeable primary care physician and parental understanding of the many first-year medical problems and high-risk developmental status. Society is providing, through federal, state, and local support, many opportunities for the education and habilitation of young infants and children with particular needs. It is only through early identification of developmental aberrations that the child and family can utilize such opportunities.

The ultimate outcome for vulnerable infants will be greatly influenced by postnatal events, parental perceptions of the child, the nurture provided in the home, and the quality of the health care environment after discharge from the neonatal intensive care nursery. The role of the primary care physician here is paramount, since he or she is in the key position to provide anticipatory care and guidance to the family.

VULNERABILITIES AND HANDICAPS

Although the health monitoring of post-intensive care infants, in its basics, is similar to the monitoring of infants whose perinatal course was exemplary, certain differences do exist. These differences involve the parents or home environment and the infant.

The parents have passed through a difficult time and may be emotionally and financially stressed as well as socially isolated. They often assume that major problems are behind them because the baby lived. They may be remarkably unprepared for the realities of home care. The baby in its first months is often demanding —crying a great deal, feeding slowly, and sleeping little. Crying and restlessness are behaviors of less moment to nursery personnel (who are concerned with survival and work on shifts) than they are to parents who carry 7-day, 24-hour care. The ICN baby began adaptation to extrauterine life in the environment of intensive care and intermediate care nurseries, areas tending to be brightly lighted and full of sound and motion. Here a diversity of sleeping and crying behaviors is acceptable. At home such behaviors are disruptive. The baby may take weeks to months to adapt to predictable sleep-awake day-night patterns that permit formulation of practical family schedules. At the same time the parents must come down from the emotional peaks of complicated birth and sequential crises onto the plateau of day-to-day living. For these reasons, support by the physician is extremely important to the parent during early infancy, and frequent visits and telephone consultations are desirable and often necessary.

The growing post–intensive care infant, particularly the immaturely born, is an interesting, often intricate, pediatric patient requiring close medical monitoring throughout infancy and preschool and early school years. The major reasons for monitoring encompass the early health vulnerabilities, the risk of emerging handicap, the often uneven development of the preschool years, and the academic problems encountered on school entrance. These are summarized in Table 1–1 and will be discussed in greater detail in later chapters. Both temporary and static problems follow an age-related timetable, emerging with increasing age and cerebral maturation. The totality of static handicap may not be evident in the preschool years (Fig. 1–1).

The majority of present-day parents are well aware that severe prolonged perinatal morbidity places the infant at greater risk for disability in later years. They tend to welcome with relief a definite plan that proposes to follow developmental progress.

In outlining the later handicaps of infants re-

TABLE 1–1. Vulnerabilities of Very Low Birth Weight Infants*

1. **Infections (particularly first year)**
   Lower respiratory infections
   Otitis media—and retention of middle ear fluid
   Gastroenteritis
2. **Sudden death in infancy**
3. **Neurologic and neurodevelopmental disorders**
   Transient tone and movement abnormalities
   Unevenness of maturation
   Hyper-responsivity to sound
   Cerebral diplegia and other forms of cerebral palsy
   Cerebral dysfunction or minimal cerebral dysfunction
   Mental retardation or low average intelligence
   Epilepsy
   Hydrocephalus
4. **Organically based behavior disorders**
   Poor neural integration
   Disturbed sleep-awake patterns
   Excessive crying
   Short attention span
   Hyperkinesis or inactivity
   Impulsiveness
   Perseveration
   Low frustration threshold
5. **Vision**
   Retrolental fibroplasia
   Myopia
   Strabismus
   Refractive errors
6. **Speech and language**
   Conductive hearing impairment (secondary to middle ear disorder)
   Neurosensory hearing loss
   Speech and articulation disorders
   Receptive and expressive language deficits
7. **Academic**
   Marginal school readiness
   Learning disabilities
8. **Sociomedical disorders**
   Child abuse
   Child neglect
   Failure to thrive

* From Desmond MM, Wilson GS, Alt EJ, Fisher ES: The very low birth weight infant after discharge from intensive care: Anticipatory health care and developmental course. Current Problems in Pediatrics. Chicago, Year Book Medical Publishers, Inc., April 1980, pp 3–59. Reproduced with permission.)

---

quiring intensive care because of immaturity and its complications or because of infection, hemorrhage, malformation, or perinatal asphyxia, it is practical to consider three aspects —the severity of the handicap, its frequency, and its natural history, i.e., the age of emergence or identification. (At the outset, it cannot be assumed that by monitoring post–intensive care infants *only* one will identify all handicapped children, since many handicaps are of prenatal origin and associated with smooth transition to extrauterine life.)

THE DIAGNOSIS OF DELAY OR DISABILITY BY AGE

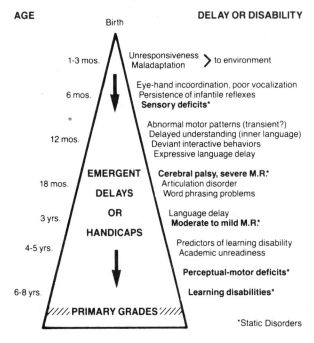

AGE   **DELAY OR DISABILITY**

Birth

1-3 mos.   Unresponsiveness   ⟩ to environment
           Maladaptation

6 mos.   Eye-hand incoordination, poor vocalization
         Persistence of infantile reflexes
         Sensory deficits*

12 mos.   Abnormal motor patterns (transient?)
         Delayed understanding (inner language)
         Deviant interactive behaviors
         Expressive language delay

EMERGENT   **Cerebral palsy, severe M.R.***
18 mos.   Articulation disorder
DELAYS   Word phrasing problems

OR   Language delay
3 yrs.   **Moderate to mild M.R.***

HANDICAPS

4-5 yrs.   Predictors of learning disability
         Academic unreadiness

         Perceptual-motor deficits*

6-8 yrs.   **Learning disabilities***

///// **PRIMARY GRADES** /////

*Static Disorders

FIGURE 1–1. The emerging totality of handicap in very high-risk infants, related to the postconceptional ages at which the diagnosis is most commonly made. (From Desmond MM, Wilson GS, Alt EJ, Fisher ES: The very low birth weight infant after discharge from intensive care: Anticipatory health care and developmental course. Current Problems in Pediatrics. Chicago, Year Book Medical Publishers, Inc., April 1980, pp 3–59. Reproduced with permission.)

SEVERITY OF HANDICAP

Major handicaps include neurosensory impairments (blindness, deafness), cerebral palsy, and mental retardation. Each type occurs within a spectrum of severity, and multiple impairments are not uncommon. Handicaps generally considered *mild* comprise lesser degrees of neurosensory impairment, motor disability (clumsiness, fine motor incoordination, balance) in ambulatory children, speech-language disorders, disturbances in behavior (short attention span, sleep-wakefulness, hyperactivity, impulse control), and central processing disorders. The last include problems of spatial relations and specific learning disability defined as a discrepancy between the child's measured intelligence and ability to master basic skills (reading, writing, spelling, and counting) in the classroom.

The categorization of a child as "mildly" or "severely" handicapped is often misleading, since many children manifest more than one handicap at school age. The presence of more than one mild handicap (e.g., fine motor incoordination and learning disability) may in the sum become overwhelming to the child. An organically based behavior disorder, either alone or superimposed upon another handicap, may determine educability regardless of intellectual level.

FREQUENCY OF HANDICAP

The incidence and prevalence figures for handicap in high-risk and post–intensive care infants have been variously reported. In those reports the definitions of major vs minor handicap differ as does the age of the child at time of identification. Here the child's overall history may provide clues to the prior causative insult or combination of insults.

For the low birth weight infant, the rate of later handicap interfering with functioning appears to increase as the birth weight decreases, largely because the very immature baby tends to have a more complicated neonatal course. The rate of major involvements ranges from one in ten to one in five as birth weight and gestational age decline (see Appendix D).

In estimation of risks in larger infants as well as in low birth weight infants with intrauterine growth retardation, the etiology is important. Children with congenital rubella, cytomegaloviral disease, or neonatal meningitis demonstrate a wide spectrum of neurologic sequelae as well as a high incidence of hearing loss. For congenital illness of viral origin, the hearing loss may not be evident in early infancy but appear later on in childhood and progress in severity with age. For infants suffering bacterial meningitis the hearing loss tends to appear early in the disease and is more stable in degree.

The major handicap rate in children with difficult to control neonatal seizures approximates one in four to one in five. However, if the child has hemiplegic cerebral palsy seizures are more common and tend to appear later on in childhood. Thus the total course of the infant, from prenatal life onward, must be considered before totality of risk can begin to be approximated.

Handicaps are largely expressed in *rates* or percentage by physicians, and comparisons over time periods are made on this basis. However, to educators or agencies concerned with services to the handicapped, only the absolute *numbers* of handicapped persons are meaningful. The number to be served determines the size of the budget necessary for provision of services. Numbers of handicapped translate directly into numbers of classrooms, numbers of teachers and therapists, and numbers receiving SSI, Medicaid, and the like. This difference in reference point often leads to poor communication between physicians and either educators or governmental agencies. As the total number of surviving infants increases, the number of handicapped children will increase if the rate of handicap *does not drop over the same period as the increase in survival.* Thus, a 10 per cent handicap rate will yield 10 handicapped children if 100 survive, but 20 if 200 children survive. The number of normal children surviving neonatal intensive care is the focus of the neonatologist, while normal children are not visible to agencies serving special-needs children.

TYPES OF HANDICAP

Temporary. Infants who have been systemically ill for weeks to months and who have a developmental aberration may present the physician with a bewildering array of possible diagnoses during infancy. Is this delay, discrepancy, malposition, neurologic aberration, or behavior a manifestation of the infant's recovery process, the maturation process, a lingering drug or medication effect, or a true residuum? This question is often difficult to answer, and caution must be exercised.

Infants who were hypotonic in the ICN on the basis of immaturity or disease, or those immobilized for long periods, tend to show nursery-acquired malpositions (see Chapters 9 and 10). These asymmetries or unusual postures tend to be temporary. If they are identified as such, guided home care programs can reinforce the natural tendency toward improvement seen in the vigorous baby.

Transient motor abnormalities noted during the first year have been reported by many authors, e.g., imbalance of extensor-flexor movements, fluctuating hypertonicity, and subtle asymmetries. However, in those children with transitory abnormalities, the major precursors of cerebral palsy, i.e., persistence of infantile reflexes, poverty of movement, and abnormal involuntary movements, tend to be absent or minimal (see Chapters 9 and 10).

Static. The most severe handicaps characteristically appear relatively early. In the majority of instances, significant visual and hearing impairments, mental retardation (global delay), and cerebral palsy are identifiable before 18 months of age. The recognition of speech-language problems and borderline to low average intelligence must await ages at which language and the use of symbols can be assessed with some degree of confidence.

Thus it is appropriate for the physician, at the beginning, to assure parents that developmental surveillance and monitoring will continue on into the school years. It is clearly not enough to rejoice that the child has escaped major handicap by 18 months, or that cognitive abilities fall within the normal range at the age of three years. The more subtle problems of central processing and the behaviors they engender are more frequent than major handicaps in very high risk populations. Unexpected school failure in a child of normal intelligence is a shocking experience for all concerned, and the effects on the child's life are long lasting. For the physician the most realistic approach to the development of the post–intensive care infant is to keep in mind the age-related emergence of handicap as the child matures while taking a positive approach to current developmental status.

REWARDS—THE POSITIVES

Although premature and other infants in intensive care units begin life precariously and require unusual health and developmental monitoring during the early years, the majority tend to do well in supportive nonpressuring home environments. Even the most frequently encountered deterrent to achievement, i.e., difficulty in acquiring basic skills, can be anticipated and managed to some degree prospectively before the child fails and self-esteem plummets in the classroom.

Shirley, an early student of premature behavior, noted that the sensitivity of prematures to sound and color is a source of enjoyment to them as children and underlies their tendency to

---

TABLE 1–2. High-Risk Infants Famed in Later Life

Birth Asphyxia (considered stillborn)
  Samuel Johnson
  Pablo Picasso
  Thomas Hardy
  Johann Wolfgang Goethe
  Franklin Delano Roosevelt
Prematurely Born
  Isaac Newton
  Charles Wesley
  Charles Darwin
  Winston Churchill
  Jean Jacques Rousseau
  François Marie Arouet Voltaire
  Anna Pavlova
  Victor Hugo
  Napoleon Bonaparte
  Willie Shoemaker
  Joey Bishop
  Elisabeth Kübler-Ross
  Johannes Kepler

---

seek out artistic pursuits in later life.[10] Former premature infants have made great additions to the knowledge and diversity of the human experience.[3] And even infants reported to have had severe birth asphyxia may contribute significantly to society (Table 1–2). Sharing the list with parents is enjoyable for them and assistive in fostering an attitude of supportive realism, an attitude necessary for the parent to maintain equanimity over the long haul. Many of those listed had extraordinary difficulty during the preschool and school-age years, but nevertheless rose to eminence. For a weary parent, such information may brighten the long day.

Winston Churchill, for example, was almost singular in his school difficulties. His biography suggests an excellent visual memory but poor auditory processing, leading to difficulty with the learning of any language other than English. In the classroom he was disruptive and possibly hyperkinetic. His great joy as a child was a collection of lead soldiers that he arranged and rearranged in battle formation for long periods —a type of solitary activity known to child care specialists as self-quieting. His sleep-awake patterns were always unusual.

Among contemporary well-known persons who were premature are Joey Bishop, the entertainer and comedian, and Willie Shoemaker, the champion jockey. For parents struggling with a child's speech, it may be heartening to recall Bishop's fluent delivery as a comedian and master of ceremonies and his three-pound birth weight. "In kindergarten," he states, "I flunked sand pile." Willie Shoemaker was both premature and intrauterine growth retarded and passed his neonatal period in an open oven in a shoebox. He discovered a vocation for which being small (4 feet $11\frac{1}{2}$ inches, 100 pounds) was an asset, riding on to fame and fortune.

Drs. R.S. and C.M. Illingworth, pediatricians, in published studies of the early life of famed men and women and the patterns of their development concluded:

> . . . the stories were fascinating. They provide many important precepts for parents and teachers. They indicate the great difficulty and virtual impossibility of forecasting achievement, the difficulty of detecting a child's potential, and the difficulty of determining the best home and scholastic background for enabling a child to develop his potential to the full.

We would like to feel that this will help parents and teachers to be more tolerant of their charges. Children may reach fame in spite of, or because of, the unusual and perhaps difficult features of their personality. The child who is backward today (unless he is mentally subnormal) may be the genius of tomorrow. Whether he will reach eminence or not, he certainly deserves sympathy, encouragement and help to make the most of what he has.[11]

For investigators and educators the search for early predictors of future outcome and academic achievement is endless and serves useful purposes. For the parent, however, expressed predictions are not always a blessing. Not knowing the future clearly leaves room for hope in the present. As stated by Stevenson, "to travel hopefully is a better thing than to arrive."

SUMMARY

Despite intensive research, the data available concerning the long-term effects of perinatal morbidity on the development of the child have not led to clear-cut findings. Previous research does indicate that the infant is "at risk" through school age and that the parents' perception of the child and the harmony between the child and his or her environment are powerful determinants of outcome.

The implications for medical care are clear. The developing high-risk infant is best served by close medical supervision, particularly during the turbulent early years. Health care should include ongoing screening and developmental assessment at least through school entrance so that emerging vulnerabilities or deficits may be addressed as early as possible, thus impeding developmental progress minimally.

An optimal care plan includes active partnership with the parents in detection of weaknesses, reinforcement of strengths, and formulation of recommendations for behavioral and educational management. For the physician this will require clinical acumen, an understanding of the child within the context of his or her environment, an attitude of supportive realism, and a long view. It is an opportunity to practice preventive pediatrics in one of its most productive forms.

References

1. Hess JH, Mohr GJ, Barthelme PT: The Physical and Mental Growth of Prematurely Born Children. Chicago, University of Chicago Press, 1934.
2. Adams J: Statistics of Texas Children's Hospital, Neonatal Intensive Care Unit.
3. Desmond MM, Wilson GS, Alt ES, et al.: The very low birth weight infant after discharge from intensive care: Anticipatory health care and development course. Curr Probl Pediatr 10:5 (April), 1980.
4. Capper A: The fate and development of the immature and the premature child. Am J Dis Child 35:262, 443, 1928.
5. Gesell A: The mental growth of prematurely born infants. J Pediatr 2:676, 1933.
6. Sunde A: Die Prognose der Frühgebornen und de Profylaxe des Geburtstraumas. Acta Obstet Gynaecol Scand 9:477, 1930.
7. Mohr G, Barthelme P: Mental and physical development of children prematurely born. Am J Dis Child 40:1000, 1930.
8. Drillien CM: The Growth and Development of the Prematurely Born Infant. Baltimore, Williams & Wilkins Company, 1964.
9. Blegen SD: The premature child. Acta Paediatr Scand 42: suppl 88, 1953.
10. Shirley M: A behavior syndrome characterizing prematurely born children. Child Dev 10:115, 1939.
11. Illingworth RS, Illingworth CM: Lessons from Childhood—Some Aspects of the Early Life of Unusual Men and Women. Baltimore, Williams & Wilkins Company, 1960, pp. 348–350.

Recommended Reading

Apley J (ed.): Care of the Handicapped Child. Clinics in Developmental Medicine no. 67. Philadelphia, J.B. Lippincott Company, 1978.

Christopherson ER (ed.): Developmental and behavioral issues in perinatology. Clin Perinatol 12: no. 2, 1985.

Hurt H (ed.): Continuing Care of the High Risk Infant. Clin Perinatol 11: no. 1, 1984.

Oliver TK, Kirschbaum TK (eds.): Low birth weight infants. Semin Perinatol 6: no. 4, 1982.

Schwartz JL, Schwartz LH (eds.): Vulnerable Infants. A Psychosocial Dilemma. New York, McGraw-Hill Book Company, 1977.

Shosenberg N, Minde K, Swyer PR, et al.: The Premature Infant. A Handbook for Parents. Toronto, The Hospital for Sick Children, 1980.

Thurber SD, Armstrong LB: Developmental Support of Low Birth Weight Infants: Parents' Guide, Nurses' Guide, 2nd ed. Houston, Office of Educational Resources, Texas Children's Hospital, 1982.

2

THE TRANSITION FROM HOSPITAL TO HOME

MARGARET DEKLE LANG, R.N., P.N.P., MADELEINE BOOTH BEHLE, R.N., M.S., and ROBERTA A. BALLARD, M.D.

The hospitalization of a sick premature or term newborn may last from a few days to five or six months. A tiny premature's survival may be precarious and dependent for a protracted period upon sophisticated equipment and skilled personnel, and his or her family may be subjected to many alternating periods of optimism and discouragement. Obviously the intensity of the impact of the hospitalization upon the developing child and the family will vary widely with the nature of their experience. However, it cannot be assumed that the infant who is born at term or is a good-sized premature, and thus separated from the family for a shorter time than a very small premature, will have an easier adjustment to the home environment. Parental and physician perceptions of the baby's state of health may not coincide. Sensitivity to the parents' views of their infant's illness is important in identifying early fears and behaviors that may lead to later parenting difficulties. Much can be done in the hospital prior to discharge to help ease the transition to the home and to identify special needs and problems.

Since the care of an ICN graduate will, at the very least, differ from the parents' original expectations, it is helpful to all those involved to establish communication early during the hospitalization concerning the infant's condition and progress, and his or her personality and behaviors.

PARENT PARTICIPATION DURING THE HOSPITALIZATION

Communication. In any crisis situation, careful, complete, and supportive communication helps, not only in dealing with the crisis but with the later transition to home.

Visiting. Parents should be encouraged to visit their infant in the intensive care nursery (ICN) as often as possible and at different times of the day, so that they become familiar with the baby's daily patterns. It is helpful for them to assist with the infant's care as much as they are able. With the guidance of the staff, they can learn to recognize their infant's particular responses to daily events. How does the infant behave when hungry and when full? Does he or she sometimes become overstimulated and cry excessively? Infants may respond to environmental overstimulation by becoming pale or slightly dusky, having apneic episodes, spitting up, or averting their gaze. If these behaviors are observed the parents can learn ways to diminish sensory input, e.g., by slowing down their movements and talking to the baby in more quiet tones; holding *or* rocking *or* talking may be

12

helpful, but not all simultaneously, as may feeding the infant in a quiet place away from distractions. With support from the ICN staff they can thus gain confidence and practical skills that will reduce their anxiety in caring for their baby at home.

Feeding. In the regionalized system of perinatal care, parents and infants are often separated by great distances. The family may find that one of the few parenting tasks available to them is to provide breast milk. Although the advantages of involving the family in the care of their infant are recognized,[1] the establishment and maintenance of the mother's milk supply by artificial means over a lengthy hospitalization may also create additional stress for the parents. The support and guidance of the infant's primary physician, whose relationship with the family has already been established through prenatal visits or care of siblings, can provide insight into this important facet of care during the infant's hospitalization.

The mother of a premature who wishes to breast-feed her infant needs support in three major areas: (1) initial assistance in establishing a milk supply, (2) continuing encouragement over the long months of hospitalization, and (3) help in making the transition to actual breast-feeding later. Once the mother's health is stabilized after her infant's birth and early during the hospitalization, realistic goals can be set, and she can begin establishing her milk supply with a breast pump. The physician can assist by periodically discussing her progress with her and assuring appropriate attention to rest, diet, and general health maintenance. Acknowledgment of the infant's weight gain from her milk and including the infant's father in the interactions are important to success.

The following are suggestions for supporting successful breast-feeding prior to the infant's discharge from the hospital and in preparing for the transition to the home.

1. Most special-care nurseries give the infant's first nipple feeding from a bottle. However, if it is possible for the infant to go directly from gavage to breast-feeding, the confusion many infants encounter in switching from an artificial nipple to the mother's breast may be avoided.

2. Encouraging the parents to be available for the first nipple feeding and having the mother breast-feed the baby provide an important message to both parents and staff that breast-feeding will eventually be the infant's primary source of nutrition.

3. Increasing the use of the breast pump to eight times per day, including once during the night, for seven to ten days before the baby's discharge from the hospital will help increase the mother's milk supply. If possible, the mother should try to nurse the baby once or twice a day prior to discharge to gain confidence with breast-feeding techniques and her infant's feeding behaviors.

4. Appropriate and realistic expectations should be discussed with the parents at discharge. Although some premature infants can be totally breast-fed, most parents cannot visit often enough to establish complete nutrition with breast-feeding and will need to provide some supplementation as well.

5. Temporary use of Lactaid may help encourage a reluctant nurser to suck. If the baby is sleepy, frequent burping and switching to the opposite breast every five minutes or so may lengthen awake periods and promote efficient sucking.

6. It may be helpful to remind parents that their infant's breast-feeding pattern may be like a term newborn's, i.e., nursing every one and one-half to three hours even though the infant may be two to three months old.

7. To alleviate parents' anxiety whether the baby is "getting enough," it may be helpful to instruct them to observe the infant for signs of contentment following a feeding and to note evidence of adequate intake (six to eight diapers per day) and also to teach them to listen for swallowing during nursing.

8. After the infant's arrival home, initial weight gain may be somewhat slow, or the baby may even lose weight until the mother's milk supply builds and the baby adjusts to breast-feeding. The infant should not lose more than four ounces or more than 10 per cent of discharge weight over the first few days at home and should begin to gain by the end of the first week.

PARENT SUPPORT GROUP

Many neonatal programs have found that developing a group of parents who can provide support for new parents, either with respect to an infant's hospitalization in the ICN or to specific disease entities, has been valuable. The mechanisms for the parent interactions vary from institution to institution, but the added understanding and emotional support can be very helpful during the family's ICN experience and also facilitate the transition from hospital to home.

PRIMARY CARE PHYSICIAN

A recent study[2] of whether primary pediatricians and family physicians feel prepared to provide medical supervision for sick infants after discharge indicated that, although the pediatricians felt less insecure than the family practitioners in assuming this responsibility, only a few felt confident of their ability to supervise their care. The primary physicians were asked to offer suggestions of how care for ICN graduates might be improved. Many responded that it was desirable to be kept well informed about the baby's progress in the ICN, about new diagnostic and therapeutic methods, and about development of mechanisms for continued participation by neonatal staff in the infant's care in conjunction with the primary physician. It is, of course, important not only to the primary physician that communication be maintained but also to the regional center staff, since it will be the pediatrician's responsibility ultimately to assure that discharge plans are carried out and that the infant's care is coordinated (particularly in the case of infants with complex or chronic problems). In addition, obviously, it is important to the infant and the family, since such communication will assure consistency of care and an understanding of the infant's problems in the intensive care nursery and after discharge.

ROLE OF THE FOLLOW-UP TEAM

Most tertiary centers have some arrangements for neonatal follow-up. Both the information and the support provided by the follow-up team can be improved by having the group involved with the infant's care during hospitalization. This can take the form of rounds, so that the team identifies early the infants who are likely to be followed over a long period and begins to become familiar with their problems during the hospitalization. In addition, they should be included in weekly social service conferences, so that they are aware of some of the social issues that are complicating the care of these infants. It is also beneficial to have members of the family meet the team prior to discharge and to establish links with the primary physician as well.

DISCHARGE PLANNING

Careful and complete planning makes an important contribution to a smooth transition from hospital to home for both the infant and the family. The following components should be included in the discharge plan for any baby who has required neonatal intensive care.

1. The expected length of stay will have been discussed with the family almost from the day of admission to the nursery. However, the parents may have lost track of the expected discharge date and should be given at least a week to 10 days' notice of the expected time of discharge, if at all possible.

2. Staff should review important information related to the infant's illness and procedures that need to be done prior to discharge enough in advance to assure their being accomplished in a timely fashion (this includes follow-up x-ray studies, hematocrit, circumcision if indicated, and so on).

3. All plans should be made related to the infant's care after discharge, including initial follow-up appointments with the pediatrician, with specialists, and with any other individuals who may be involved in the care of the child, such as public health department staff.

4. All special screening examinations needed before discharge should be organized and completed in time for any unusual or abnormal findings to be discussed and future follow-up included in the discharge plan. (This includes examination of the eyes for retinopathy of prematurity, as well as screening examinations for hearing.)

5. When at all possible, the family should be encouraged to spend one or two nights rooming in within the hospital, so that they can become acquainted with providing 24-hour caregiving with the "lifeguard" staff still close by.

6. A careful discharge examination should be carried out, including accurate measurements of growth parameters. When possible, this should be done by someone with experience in evaluating infant behavior, and the family should be present, so that they have an opportunity to become familiar with their infant's unique characteristics and responses and to ask questions.

7. A discharge meeting at a site away from the bedside should be arranged with the family and members of the nursing and medical staff who have cared for the infant (and, when possible, with the pediatrician who will be providing care after discharge) to review the infant's course in the hospital, to answer any questions that remain in the parents' minds, to discuss expectations for behavior, feeding, and other problems at home, and to reinforce the dates and times of follow-up examinations.

8. If the pediatrician cannot be present at the discharge meeting, it is important that a

member of the staff call him or her on the day of discharge. Needed information on weight, length, head circumference, hematocrit, other kinds of medically important data, and the discharge recommendations should be written and sent within the next few days.

9. For infants who have particularly complex home care needs related to chronic pulmonary problems, a complete discussion of the check list for discharge planning for infants with pulmonary disease, as well as medications and equipment, is provided in Appendix A.

TRANSITION TO THE HOME

At the time of discharge the family becomes acutely aware that the many support services that they have come to rely upon during the hospitalization are being withdrawn. Making hospital staff available for telephone consultation may be extremely important during this transitional time. One of the support services that is particularly helpful at this time is home visits by a member of the staff whom the family has met during the hospitalization.

HOME VISIT SUPPORT

The home visit is one way of maintaining the relationship between a family and the hospital staff and offers the opportunity to assess the infant's status and parents' problems and coping skills; provide family-specific counseling, education, and moral support; and collect data on outcome between follow-up visits at the tertiary center.

The adjustment period immediately after the ICN graduate's homecoming is critical to the child's and family's well-being. By the time of discharge the family's orientation of their concerns has shifted from the question of their infant's survival to questions related to quality of life (from Will my baby make it? to Will my baby be OK?). They have mixed feelings as they look forward to resuming a normal family routine, but experience anxiety as they assume the full responsibility of caring for their infant. A home visit can reassure them that their infant is doing well in the interval between discharge and formal follow-up; if there are signs of inappropriate parent-child interactions or developmental concerns, early intervention is facilitated.

Poverty, limited education, and lack of transportation account for a loss of up to 70 per cent of high-risk infants from follow-up programs.[3] Three times as many children were lost to fol-

low-up when no home visit was provided as when continuity was maintained by this mechanism. Not only are families who receive home visits more likely to comply with scheduled clinic visits for assessment, but in some cases the home visit may indeed be the only means of obtaining important outcome data for the evaluation of perinatal care.

CONTENT OF A HOME VISIT

Environmental conditions and social supports are probably the strongest influences on the ability of the parents to nurture their child's development. During a home visit, opportunities abound for fostering mother-infant attachment and promoting parenting and coping skills. To be an effective counselor and educator for the family, the home visitor, by experience and training, should be sensitive to cultural and ethnic differences and expectations.

Realistically the home visit requires approximately an hour for a comfortable dialogue to be established and for the visitor to assimilate the environmental, psychological, and medical information requisite to providing pertinent support.

The appropriate technique to encourage verbalization of concerns will vary from family to family, but an expressed observation about the infant's activity at the start of the visit or comments on changes in states of alertness or cry usually open the way for discussion. Time-specific statements, such as "Tell me about the last 24 hours," help the parent focus on a specific topic and usually provide a beginning for a historical review of feeding and sleep behaviors. Confirmation of parent observations, e.g., that *you* hear that sound when the baby breathes, can validate a mother's confidence that she is an accurate historian and foster her trust and enable her to ask questions. Fears of possible abnormalities may dissipate as the home visitor acknowledges such phenomena as fine tremors, a pulsating fontanelle, skin mottling, pseudostrabismus, and other common observations parents make and worry about after they arrive home with the baby. Real perinatal problems that were discussed with the parents by staff from the ICN during the hospitalization may have been incompletely or inaccurately perceived because of the stresses of the time. The home visitor may need to retransmit or clarify this information and assist the parents' comprehension.

Other parts of the care plan, such as when to see the baby next, community referrals, and special needs, should be reviewed within the context of the family's resources to comprehend and to achieve compliance with the plan. The home visit also gives insight into the circumstances of the family that will affect their ability to comply with ongoing care recommendations. The home visitor, recognizing that the family may be unlikely or unable to comply with a plan, can make an important contribution to the ongoing care of the infant by helping to develop a realistic plan in coordination with the family's primary care provider and the perinatal center team.

After the initial home visit, subsequent visits focus more on assessing the infant's growth and development. Growth parameters are recorded and graphed routinely. Later visits provide increasing opportunities to demonstrate even the tiniest baby's progress. When the infant's eyes are shown to follow objects, the parent is reassured that the infant can see. Adolescent or poorly educated mothers often provide low levels of stimulation and often have ill-founded beliefs, e.g., that babies see only in shadows. Such myths discourage interaction and early social development. These mothers benefit from special education and encouragement about their infant's ability to see and from training in how to elicit positive behaviors that help to establish parent-infant attachment.

Verbal stimulation can also be demonstrated effectively by holding and talking to the baby. Parents frequently become more responsive to their infant when these simple assessments of visual and auditory acuity are performed.

The basic schedule of home visits during the first year after discharge from the ICN should be planned to evaluate the infant's maturational sequence, i.e., loss of primitive reflexes, evolution of more integrated voluntary motor skills, and so on. Records of the visits should note the reflexes as present, emerging, diminishing, or absent. Muscle tone and strength, while not predictive, should also be observed. When neuromuscular observations are combined with other developmental evaluations, they are helpful in identifying early developmental lags or other areas of concern, such as asymmetric development.

SUMMARY

The "homecoming" of an infant who has been in an intensive care nursery can be smoothed greatly if the process of planning begins while the infant is still in the nursery. Attention to communication, as well as careful discharge planning, can contribute to making this experience one of excitement and to diminishing some of the natural stress that occurs at this time. If home visiting is possible, it too can provide important support over the first critical months.

References

1. Klaus MH, Kennell JH: Parent-Infant Bonding. St. Louis, CV Mosby Company, 1982.
2. Hurt H (ed.): Continuing Care of the High-Risk Infant. Clin Perinatol II: no. 1, 1984.
3. California State Department of Health Services: Report to State Legislature on High Risk Infant Follow-up Project, 1979–1981; 1982.

Recommended Reading

Bromberger P: Premature infant's nutritional needs: Preterm breast milk. Perinatol Neonatol 6:79, 1982.
Desmond MM, Wilson GS, Alt EJ, et al.: The very low birth weight infant after discharge from intensive care: Anticipatory health care and developmental course. Curr Probl Pediatr 10:5 (April), 1980.
Gross S, David R, Balmaun L, et al.: Nutritional composition of milk produced by mothers delivering preterm. J Pediatr 96:641, 1980.
Meier P: A program to support breastfeeding in the high-risk nursery. Perinatol Neonatol 4:43, 1980.
Pereira G, Schwartz D, Gould P, et al.: Breastfeeding in the neonatal intensive care nursery. Perinatol Neonatol 8:35, 1984.
Richards M, Lang M, McIntire C, et al.: Breastfeeding the VLBW infant. Clin Res 34:124A, 1986.
Sell E: Follow-up of the High-Risk Newborn—A Practical Approach. Springfield, Ill., Charles C Thomas, 1980.
Trause M, Hilliard J, Malek V, et al.: Successful lactation in mothers of preterms. Perinatol Neonatol 5:22, 1985.

3

HIGH-RISK INFANT FOLLOW-UP PROGRAMS

CAROL H. LEONARD, Ph.D.

There are many reasons for the existence of follow-up programs for high-risk infants, but they are primarily for provision of family support after discharge, identification of developmental disabilities, and collection of data to allow assessment of outcome and its relation to nursery practices. The last can be either formal, as in outcome studies, or more informal, as in providing information to nursery personnel about the outcome of infants they have treated.

PARENT SUPPORT

While the infant is in the intensive care nursery, ideally his or her parents, siblings, and extended family are also receiving care. Attention is given to how the family is coping with the infant's hospitalization and to how well prepared the family is to take the infant home. After discharge the follow-up program continues this aspect of care and support by phone calls and by visits into the home. Follow-up staff members often facilitate parent support groups in the local community in addition to introducing parents of current ICN infants to parents whose infants have "graduated" from the ICN.

EARLY IDENTIFICATION OF DISABILITIES

As a complement to the primary medical care the infant is receiving, follow-up programs provide specialized neurodevelopmental assessments for the purpose of identifying developmental disabilities as early as possible. The developmental patterns of high-risk infants vary with the perinatal course of each, and the staff members of follow-up programs that include large numbers of infants may be more familiar with these patterns. There is greater variation in the developmental progress of high-risk infants, and some findings that would be abnormal in a low-risk population are not abnormal in a high-risk population (see Chapters 11 and 12).

OUTCOME DATA COLLECTION

Some follow-up programs function primarily as clinical programs, providing direct services to families, while others have a primary research focus. All programs, however, can function as information-gathering services for the neonatal and obstetric programs they serve. Additionally, smaller research studies, and even anecdotal studies, may make important scientific contributions to the intensive care of high-risk infants and to their pediatric care after leaving the nursery. Although it has been argued that outcome data may not be a useful priority for all follow-up programs, the history of medicine often advances from the single, unusual case study that

---

TABLE 3–1. Infants at High Risk: Staff for Follow-Up Program

Core Team
  Physician
  Nurse
  Social worker
  Psychologist
  Coordinator
Consultants
  Ophthalmologist
  Audiologist
  Speech pathologist
  Physical-occupational therapist
  Neurologist

---

generates a new way of looking at certain problems.

This chapter describes one model of a follow-up program. It is a hospital-based program with clear and definite outreach into the communities it serves. Aspects of this program may be adapted to other follow-up programs. Regional differences, as well as differences in staffing patterns and characteristics and philosophies of neonatal units, will have a substantial effect on how a follow-up program is designed and operates. A minimal level of follow-up is often mandated by state regulations. The program described below is one that has evolved not out of legal necessity (although regulations are sometimes helpful in acquiring the necessary resources to support the program), but it is one that has as a foundation a commitment to parents that does not end with discharge from the intensive care nursery.

The program has been developed in an urban area in a well-populated state with maximum travel distance for staff of about 400 miles (round trip for satellite clinic). Some neonatal units must cover a much wider area, and others are fortunate to cover a more condensed area.

FOLLOW-UP STAFF

Core Team

It is most cost-effective to develop a core team for follow-up and to use special consultants as needed, depending on the number and type of infants served. At the least the core team will usually consist of a medical component (physician and nurse), social worker, allied health professionals who specialize in child development (psychologist, child development specialist), and a coordinator (Table 3–1).

The core staff of this model follow-up program is restricted to professionals likely to be involved with evaluations of every infant or child. The core staff makes weekly rounds in the neonatal unit for infants who will be included in the follow-up program. In the transition to home, home visits are essential for continuity of care; depending on the number of infants residing out of town, much time may be spent in travel, and therefore the nursing component may require more staff than other aspects of the program.

PHYSICIAN

The usual subspecialty interests of the medical director of a follow-up program are neonatology, neurology, or developmental pediatrics. The physician should perform a discharge assessment of the infant prior to the infant's discharge or transfer from the neonatal unit. In addition to assessing the neurodevelopmental status of infants and children in the follow-up program, the physician acts as a consultant to primary care providers for aspects of care that are complex, for example, management of home oxygen or protocols for discontinuing respiratory medications after discharge. Some primary care physicians are comfortable managing all aspects of a high-risk infant's care after discharge; others avail themselves of telephone consultation with the follow-up physician; and still others ask that specific components of care be managed by the follow-up physician.

A formal report of the infant's or child's evaluation in the follow-up program is sent to the primary care provider. When there have been abnormal findings in an infant or child, these should be communicated to the primary care provider directly by telephone as well as by a written report. This communication gives the primary care provider immediate feedback on an infant's status and also allows for coordinated plans to be made if further specialty consultation is needed for the infant.

NURSING

Nursing may be represented in the follow-up program by registered nurses, pediatric nurse practitioners, or public health nurses. Ideally the nurse should have previous nursing experience in the neonatal unit. This allows a good understanding of what the family experiences while in the nursery and also provides a background for the common medical problems of the ICN graduate.

The primary function of the nurse is as liaison between the hospital and the family. This begins with a home visit shortly after discharge and two or three other visits in the first year for infants not coming into clinic to see other team members. The follow-up nurse performs neurodevelopmental screening and reports concerns to the medical director. A report of the home visit is sent to the primary care provider. In many programs, nurses have been trained to administer infant developmental scales. Much of the coordinating of community services may be done by the program nurse.

SOCIAL WORK

The follow-up social worker meets families while the infant is still in the intensive care nursery. She or he may be involved clinically with the families or may meet them only to introduce the idea of follow-up. The social worker may make home visits for psychosocial assessments of infants at high social risk and meet with families when they come into clinic. In our program the social worker edits a parent newsletter and attends parent support group meetings held both at our hospital and in surrounding areas. When the team travels to satellite clinics, the social worker meets with parent support group members in outlying areas. The social worker also arranges parent-to-parent support, by having families with infants of similar perinatal history meet or talk to each other by telephone. The social worker becomes involved with any referrals for child protective services deemed necessary by other team members.

PSYCHOLOGY – CHILD DEVELOPMENT

For programs following infants and children beyond two years, a psychologist is a necessary core staff member if standard intellectual assessments are to be performed. As noted above, many allied health professionals perform developmental assessments of infants. The administration of standard intelligence tests, however, is restricted to trained psychologists. Psychologists may also perform psychosocial assessments and work with families of high-risk infants according to their interest and training. Some psychologists perform Brazelton assessments in the neonatal unit. The psychologist may attend Individual Educational Program meetings for follow-up children.

COORDINATOR

The coordinator for the follow-up program is responsible for record keeping and seeing that appointments are made on a regular schedule. Other duties may include scheduling case reviews and case conferences with core staff and community personnel.

Consultants

High-risk infants may have subtle sensory problems and can show delays in motor development related to difficulties in the perinatal period and the often lengthy hospitalization they may undergo. Differential diagnosis between permanent disability and simple delay that will resolve is important. Specialists in many areas serve as consultants to the follow-up program to assist in this differential diagnosis. Five areas that will usually require specialized assessments are: vision, hearing, speech and language, motor development, and central nervous system functioning.

OPHTHALMOLOGY

Infants receiving oxygen in the intensive care nursery generally receive routine eye examinations while in the nursery, and after discharge they should be scheduled for follow-up eye examinations for retinopathy of prematurity. Ideally these repeat eye examinations can be scheduled by the discharge planner in the nursery before discharge. Families residing locally may choose to continue with the ophthalmologist who has observed the infant in the nursery; families of transported infants will need referral to ophthalmologists in the local community. Follow-up programs should maintain an active referral list of vision specialists for primary care providers and families (see Chapter 13).

SPEECH PATHOLOGY

Speech and language should be assessed routinely in very low birth weight infants (less than 1250 grams) at 18 months. This should be performed by a speech pathologist with pediatric experience. Very premature and other high-risk infants whose language development is of concern should be referred for speech and language evaluation earlier—as soon as the concern is noted. It is useful to have all larger premature infants (1251 to 1500 grams) observed at 2½ years for articulation and other language disorders (see Chapter 12).

AUDIOLOGY

High-risk infants should have a hearing assessment prior to discharge from the nursery. Infants failing this assessment need to have it repeated. Infants with language delay in the first year of life need full audiologic assessment, even if their hearing assessment while in the nursery was satisfactory. Language development for premature infants should be based on their adjusted age, not chronologic age, for at least the first 12 months of life—longer for the extremely premature infant (see Chapter 12).

PHYSICAL THERAPY–OCCUPATIONAL THERAPY

For infants for whom there is concern with motor development, more specialized assessment of gross and fine motor movement patterns may be necessary. In infancy this evaluation may be performed by either physical or occupational therapists. In early childhood, for both diagnosis and treatment, one or the other of the therapists may be more appropriate, depending on the problem (see Chapter 10).

NEUROLOGY

A small number of high-risk infants will require neurologic evaluation. Some follow-up programs have a neurologist as part of the core staff; if this is not the case a neurologist should be a consultant to the program (see Chapter 9).

LOCATION OF PROGRAM

An intensive care nursery often includes infants whose home communities are far from the center where the unit is located. To adequately observe these infants, the staff of the follow-up program must go where the infants are. Compliance with visits is generally much higher when infants are seen in or near their own community. Although some infants will be seen in clinic at the tertiary center, clinics located in the local community hospital or a referring pediatrician's office can serve infants living farther from the hospital.

While it is desirable to see infants at highest risk frequently in the first year, a combination of home visits by nursing personnel and team visits at a satellite clinic may be the most effective way to manage this for infants who live far from the center.

TERTIARY HOSPITAL–BASED CLINIC

In terms of staff time this is the most convenient clinic, since no traveling is involved for follow-up personnel. Location of the clinic on or near hospital grounds means that nursery personnel may be able to come to the clinic to see families of infants they cared for in the nursery. Evaluations of the high-risk infants can also serve as teaching rounds for pediatric and nursery staff. If possible, installation of one-way mirrors facilitates the examination of infants. Core staff can observe each other's assessments so that certain parts of the examinations do not have to be duplicated. (For example, the speech pathologist can observe language behavior during a developmental evaluation by the developmental specialist.) When examinations are also serving as teaching rounds, a staff member can comment on the assessment in the observation room while it is being performed in the examination room.

SATELLITE CLINICS

For families living some distance from the hospital, satellite clinics are useful. Sites used may include public health clinic space, private pediatric offices, or church conference rooms. There is a very high compliance rate with satellite clinic appointments. Families appreciate the outreach by the hospital and, if willing to make an appointment, will generally appear for the appointment. The disadvantage of satellite clinics is that, because large numbers of children need to be seen, there is often little time for lengthy visits with families. For this reason the families of infants or children who are developing abnormally are sometimes asked to come to the hospital-based clinic rather than to a satellite clinic nearer their home.

Another important opportunity is inclusion of community personnel in satellite clinics. Primary care providers, public health nurses, physical and occupational therapists, teachers, and other professionals involved with the children being seen are invited to come to the clinic site and meet with the clinic staff. A list of infants and children being seen at the satellite clinic and their appointment times is sent to primary care providers and public health agencies.

HOME VISITS

Home visits are made by nursing personnel for parent support and developmental screening. In addition, they provide information about the home environment. The content of these visits is described elsewhere. Team home visits may be made when a family is noncompliant or too overwhelmed to make clinic appointments but will accept a follow-up visit at home. Team home visits may also be made for assessments of chronically ill infants or extremely shy infants whose development has been a matter of concern. The familiarity of the home setting may elicit better performance.

FOLLOW-UP POPULATION

To parents, any birth resulting in the infant's being in the intensive care nursery may be traumatic. Although there are "routine" admissions to the special care nursery, for example, term infants admitted for observation, intensive care is never routine to parents, and the parents' and professionals' perceptions of the survival of the infant's illness may not match. Following is an example:

A mother requested that a report of her daughter's $2\frac{1}{2}$-year-old assessment be sent to a psychologist friend of the family who had seen the child periodically. When the psychologist was told that the child had scored in the superior range of intelligence on the Stanford-Binet Intelligence Scale, she expressed amazement that a 500-gram premature infant had done so well. The follow-up psychologist, on the other hand, was amazed that the family thought their child had weighed 500 grams at birth because the child had actually weighed 1500 grams and was not considered at great risk for developmental problems. The parents had asked the family friend to see their child periodically because she was "so tiny and so premature." Even though the child had been seen on home visits during the first year of life the misconception about her birth weight had never surfaced.

Health professionals certainly view the element of risk very differently from parents. Some populations of infants are observed because they are part of new research protocols or because they are in groups already known to be at risk for developmental disability. A clinical population for follow-up may vary from nursery to nursery. There is most likely to be agreement about the following groups:

Birth weight less than 1500 grams
Significantly small for gestational age (more than two standard deviations outside range)
Seizures in the newborn period
Intracranial hemorrhage in any infant regardless of weight
Chronic medical problems
Bronchopulmonary dysplasia
Short-bowel syndrome
Special problems of term infants
Metabolic disease
Persistent pulmonary hypertension
Infectious disease: herpes
Asphyxia in term infants

Some nurseries will follow infants with congenital anomalies. When support groups exist and referral for special services is made directly from the nursery before discharge, as in Down syndrome, follow-up services may duplicate services already being provided by others. Infants with other problems, such as fetal alcohol syndrome, may or may not receive referral for special services prior to discharge, since there is a continuum of problems associated with the syndrome. For infants whose congenital anomalies or syndromes have been diagnosed before discharge and who have been referred for intervention services, a general guideline is to provide follow-up services if parents wish, but not to knowingly duplicate assessments unless parents have requested assessment from the follow-up program as an independent evaluation of their child's progress.

SCHEDULE OF ASSESSMENTS

As a general guideline, high-risk infants should be seen four to five times in the first year of life and less frequently thereafter. Suggested visits after 12 months are at $2\frac{1}{2}$ and $4\frac{1}{2}$ years. In addition, very premature infants and term infants with significant perinatal problems should also be seen at 18 months and should be followed until school age. Many subtle problems will not be apparent until the formal learning process begins in school (see Chapter 11).

A triage system can be followed, with infants at lower risk for developmental problems (such as premature infants greater than 1250 grams) being screened at home by nurse practitioners in the first year of life. A recommended schedule of visits for infants is found in Tables 3–2 and 3–3.

This protocol works well for infants who are developing normally. Infants showing deviation from a normal pattern of development that is significant and of concern should be seen more frequently and may require specialty consultations.

Infants with chronic health problems, such as

TABLE 3–2. Infants at Highest Risk: Schedule for Follow-Up Visits

---

Home Visit by Nurse
   Shortly after infant's discharge
Clinic Visit for Team Assessment
   6 weeks*
   3 months
   5 months
   8 months
   12 months
   18 months†
   2½ years
   4½ years
   7 years

---

* Age adjusted for premature infants (<1250 grams) until the second birthday.

† Speech and language evaluation at this and following visits.

bronchopulmonary dysplasia, may also be seen more frequently. Weekly phone calls by follow-up nursing personnel to families who have infants at home receiving oxygen have been found useful for parent support.

INTERFACE BETWEEN FOLLOW-UP PROGRAM AND NEONATAL UNIT

One of the functions of a follow-up program is to provide feedback to the neonatal staff. It is important that various treatment protocols be continually evaluated. A crucial variable in these treatment protocols is the outcome of the infants. After the infant is discharged, follow-up staff may maintain contact with families over a period of years for long-term follow-up, but

---

TABLE 3–3. Infants at Lower Risk: Schedule for Follow-Up Visits

---

Home Visit by Nurse
   Shortly after infant's discharge
   6 weeks*
   3–5 months
   7–9 months
Clinic Visit for Team Assessment
   12 months
   2½ years†
   4½ years

---

* Age adjusted for premature infants (>1250 grams) until the second birthday.

† Speech and language evaluation at this and following visit.

issues of confidentiality may arise for particular infants and families.

Formal presentations to the ICN staff by the follow-up staff may focus on group outcomes for infants meeting common criteria. Informal follow-up log books or notebooks with minimal information on individual infants may be kept in the unit during the first year of life to communicate developmental progress to the nursing staff. Pictures taken at follow-up visits may, with the family's consent, be posted in the unit with minimal information (name, birth weight, and age). If primary nurses are concerned about specific infants, information about single infants may be conveyed privately. A consent for follow-up visits and permission to relay information back to the neonatal unit should be obtained at the first follow-up visit. Even with this consent, however, discretion should be practiced and the privacy of the family respected.

INTERFACE BETWEEN FOLLOW-UP PROGRAM AND COMMUNITY

Hospital-based follow-up programs need an interface with the local community at many different levels. The first level is with the infant's primary care provider. A second level is with programs concerned with health maintainence, such as public health nursing, social services, and child protective services. A third level is with programs providing special educational services, such as infant intervention programs, the Variety Club, and public schools that have preschool and school-age special services for children with developmental disabilities. The hospital-based program is primarily diagnostic; rehabilitation services the infant may require should be located in his or her local community.

Currently many states have funded community-based follow-up programs. These may be incorporated into public health nursing units, into units already providing rehabilitation services to children, or into public schools mandated to serve significantly handicapped children beginning at the age of three years.

Hospital-based programs will continue to follow certain infants. These will usually be defined by standards of perinatal care or by research protocols. Inevitably there will be overlap with the criteria for high-risk infants being observed in community-based programs. There are important differences between hospital- and community-based programs, and they address different needs.

Hospital-based follow-up programs are more familiar with the experience of the family while the infant was in the intensive care nursery. The first home visit of the follow-up nurse is often a time of many questions from the family about events and procedures that occurred in the neonatal unit. Hospital-based programs generally will follow infants for a longer time than community-based programs. At a community level, children may pass from one agency to another as determined by their ages or their special needs. Children may move from one community to another; however, their relationship with the hospital where they received their newborn care can remain constant. Although follow-up should be available to all infants in intensive care nurseries, infants at highest medical risk are likely to receive the most extensive and intensive services.

Community-based programs are likely to have better access to many families. An area heavily populated with Spanish-speaking persons, for example, may have many bilingual community health workers as well as translators. Often families identified as being at high social risk while their infant is in the neonatal unit are quite well known in their local communities and may already be involved with social agencies.

There are many benefits from coordinating care between hospital-based and community-based follow-up programs. The first and most obvious is avoiding duplication of services. Assisting each other in finding lost children is another important benefit. Making occasional joint home or clinic visits is useful for families to see how hospital care and community care are meshing, as well as being a time of skill sharing among professionals. In many cases, visits by hospital and community personnel have different goals, and it is helpful to see what each program is doing. Since communities have direct services to offer families, alternating visits between hospital-based and community-based programs is a valuable way for the hospital-based program to maintain contact with families for long-term follow-up but to reserve more time for families with greater needs.

Community personnel can be helpful in locating space for satellite clinics, communicating with families who have no phones, translating for non-English–speaking families, and at times providing transportation for families who lack it. All these are direct services to families of high-risk infants by community personnel cooperating with and coordinating care with a hospital-based follow-up program.

A final benefit of follow-up team–community interface is that it allows families choice in the aftercare of their high-risk infant. Some families will decline community contacts, except for primary care, preferring follow-up only from the hospital-based program. The opposite may also occur, a family wishing no further contact with the hospital after discharge of the infant. Particularly in situations in which the family is already at high social risk, often only one agency or program will be admitted by the family into the home, or even onto the doorstep. This fragile relationship must be supported by everyone so that at least one contact is available to support the family and serve as advocate for the child.

SUMMARY

A hospital-based follow-up program can operate effectively with a small core staff and use of specialty consultations. To follow high-risk children effectively the program must be versatile, combining home visits, satellite clinics, and clinics at the hospital site. Because of late-appearing problems, infants at highest risk should be followed into school age. A hospital-based program must coordinate care with the primary health care provider and with social or health agencies in the community who may be involved with the high-risk infant and his or her family.

Recommended Reading

ACCESS to Developmental Services for NICU Graduates. A State-of-the-Art Paper of New England. Project Access, Boston, Wheelock College, 1985.

Desmond MM, Wilson GS, Alt EJ, et al.: The very low birth weight infant after discharge from intensive care: Anticipatory health care and developmental course. Curr Probl Pediatr 10:5 (April), 1980.

Hunt J: Longitudinal research: A method for studying development of high-risk pre-term infants. In Field T (ed.): Infants Born at Risk. New York, Spectrum Publications, 1979, pp 443–460.

Parmelee AH, Cohen SE: Neonatal follow-up services for infants at risk. In Harel KS, Anastasiow NJ (eds.): The At-Risk Infant: Psycho/Socio/Medical Aspects. Baltimore, Paul H. Brooks, 1985, p. 269.

SECTION II

PRIMARY CARE MANAGEMENT

4

FOSTERING FAMILY DEVELOPMENT AFTER PRETERM HOSPITALIZATION

PETER A. GORSKI, M.D.

I finally had my baby home with me. I couldn't believe how tiny she was. She needed me for everything — she had to learn about me, about our family, and home. After all our planning and expectation, I felt totally unprepared to become her parent. That first week at home I went in to check her sleep every few hours to make sure she was breathing. I tried to prevent her from crying — yet she seemed to cry all the time she was awake. She fed every couple of hours at first, and we both had to learn how to use my breasts for feeding. I had so many questions about what to do with and for my baby. I felt constantly exhausted, worried and nervous. But she was mine, I had worked hard to have her home with me, and I felt so happy and proud.

These words were spoken to me by a first-time mother who had recently given birth to a healthy full-term baby girl. The physical circumstances during pregnancy, labor, and delivery proceeded without medical complications, and baby and mother went home from the hospital on the second postnatal day.

I use this quotation to point out how easily our preconceptions can mislead our judgment. And, conversely, I want to demonstrate how little our theoretical understanding teaches us about the practical experience of parenting any infant, much less one born at risk. My aim is to use this chapter to suggest helpful yet cost-effective pediatric interventions that, in the context of clinical practice, can optimally provide support for families with vulnerable infants. Furthermore, I hope to convince the reader that integrating developmental and psychosocial care into office routines will maximize the physician's efficient use of diagnostic time in the office as well as on the telephone.

The best platform from which to offer counsel comes from a good understanding of how families experience premature birth, neonatal hospitalization, and transition to family care at home. The pediatrician with realistic insight into predictable as well as uniquely individual differences between the early experience for families of full-term and premature infants is in a position to predict and support the developmental course of the children and families in his or her practice.

THE PREMATURE PREGNANCY

Let me return to the opening example of the average birth experience. Families continually remind me just how fragile an accomplishment any birth can be. In becoming parents, we invest enormous effort in changing ourselves and our lives on behalf of becoming a family. Pregnancy, in particular, is a remarkable physical and emotional process that over nine months takes parents into a new involvement with life, permanently changing their human attachments and perspectives. This huge developmental shift associated with childbirth therefore justly identifies pregnancy as perhaps the quintessential psychosomatic condition. For, indeed, physical and psychological changes co-occur during pregnancy, and the two influence each other's eventual outcome. Bibring and her colleagues described the characteristic psychological stages of preparation that accompany the physical progress through pregnancy.[1]

Most of the exciting mental turbulence occurs during the last half of pregnancy, beginning in earnest when the woman first feels her fetus move inside her. At that moment the preceding period of nausea and fatigue culminates and passes into the reality of life being created within and still physically part of the mother-to-be. From then on, "expectancy" takes on powerful and complex meaning. As the fetus grows to term inside the mother, both parents use this time to reconsider the value and uncertain course of important relationships they have— to each other, to their own parents, to their work and careers, to friends, and to their accustomed life style. Influenced by these thoughts, parents gradually attribute separate and unique characteristics, physical and behavioral, to the yet unborn child. Only just before the full gestational period climaxes at term do most parents accept, with excited anticipation, the physical separation and emergence of the infant as a person. To the expectant parents this new person is already part of them, yet uniquely individual. This emerging parental capacity to love the other self they created also enables the parents to begin to nurture the child's emerging strengths, even while they protect the child during immature or vulnerable stages of health and development.

Consider now the prenatal experience of parents of premature infants. By definition, they are at a disadvantage for having aborted the psychological stages of pregnancy along with the physical. The infant born at 26 to 34 weeks of gestation is out in the world before the mother becomes physically overburdened enough to eagerly wish the child out. At this final stage, too, parents tend to feel imbued with the sense of connectedness existent in the relationship to the baby. The time of much preparatory individuation has not yet grown prominent. When birth occurs prematurely, few parents have yet created a nursery at home for their infant to have his or her "own" place to live. Not surprisingly then, parents interviewed after losing a baby born so early use words that express the death as a loss or amputation of a part of their bodies, of themselves.

Not only are the parents underprepared to react to the birth of the infant, but their families and friends also are often at a loss to organize the much relied-on support needed by all new parents. The birth of a high-risk premature infant often immobilizes other people's responses to the family. There is no place for the ritual support of celebrations such as baby showers.

The experience itself of hospitalization of a preterm infant begins as a forceful confirmation to parents of their parental inadequacies and helplessness. Instead of enjoying the anxious fulfillment of bringing home a healthy newborn, parents of premature infants have to learn to adapt to a neonatal intensive care unit. With that comes much awesome equipment, dozens of professional care givers attending to their baby, no privacy or clear role for parents, and constant vigilance and anticipation of life-threatening possibilities. ICN staffs strive hard and well as they help move parents from such initial distress toward eventual establishment of faith in themselves as parents and in their child as bound for a promising future. But infants usually leave ICN's before complete health or catch-up growth has recovered. The family's pediatrician then becomes the pivotal support and guide on the parents' road to emotional stability, competence, and reward.

PREMATURE INFANT BEHAVIOR

DIFFERENCES BETWEEN PREMATURE AND TERM INFANTS' BEHAVIOR

Just as many other complaints brought to the attention of pediatricians are not due to parental dysfunction, so it is with many of the developmental and behavioral problems of premature infants following discharge home from hospital. Many premature infants are difficult babies for months after homecoming. The preterm infant is born prior to the extensive organization of the central nervous system, which permits infants born at term much more relative control of sleep, arousal, alerting, attention, fussing, feeding, and activity. What's more, the still imper-

TABLE 4–1. Patterns of Behavior of Preterm Infants (as Compared with Full-Term Infants) in Their First Months at Home

Spend less time awake
When awake, less alert and responsive
Less active but more fussy
Shorter sleep-wake cycles
Rouse with fussing more frequently at night
Weaker when sucking, and therefore
  Demand to be fed more often
  Delayed in motor self-help skills, such as sitting without
    support

fect environment of the ICN cannot provide the organizing envelope for infants to acquire neurobehavioral self-regulatory controls comparable to their full-term peers by the time they go home.

Premature infants, as a general rule, behave in unexpected and often frustrating patterns for the first three to six months after arriving home. Compared with full-term infants of similar age, even healthy premature infants have more demanding patterns of sleep, activity, and feeding (Table 4–1). While many of these differences can be overcome by six months or so, the interval is typically one of behavioral disorganization for the infant and challenge for the parents. Even the most stable, fortunate parents would be heavily burdened by the level of behavioral immaturity common to prematures. If you consider the added psychological load weighing upon parents whose baby was delivered early and who endured intensive care hospitalization along with their baby, you might readily appreciate the need and benefit of a concerted approach to developmental and psychosocial care by the pediatrician.

PARENT-INFANT INTERACTION

The pediatric and developmental literature is replete with warnings about the increased incidence of parenting failures in the form of nonorganic failure to thrive, child neglect, and abuse of premature infants. Causal hypotheses incriminate, among others, prolonged parent-infant separation during hospitalization, with resultant failure to "bond," unresponsive and therefore unrewarding infant behavior, and parental emotional or financial stress.

Qualitative analyses of parent-infant interaction do indeed highlight differences between premature infant-parent interaction during the first 3 to 6 months (corrected age). Most obvious differences regard the finding that mothers of premature infants are much more active in initiating social interactions with their infants than are mothers of full-term infants. Mothers of full-term infants tend to follow the lead of their infants. Intervention studies with prematures during face-to-face interactions claim increased infant gaze toward mother is achieved when mothers consciously diminish their natural engagement efforts and, instead, wait to respond to the infant's eliciting signals.

These interesting results begin to point directions for professionals to support the cause of social synchrony between infants born at risk and their parents. Moreover, such studies indicate the strong hope for most parent-infant relationships to achieve a sense of harmony and success during the first long year after discharge from the ICN. Most parent-infant relationships can and do succeed, despite challenging beginnings. We professionals should be well beyond belief in the false magic of bonding, which misled parents to worry that the first few hours of life with their newborn determined the quality of their lifelong emotional tie to the child. The landmark contribution from Klaus and Kennell and their co-workers instead focused our attention on new opportunities for institutional environments and clinical practices to facilitate, from the start, the enduring effort of developing an intimate attachment between parent and child.[2] The process of emotional attachment continues over years, with sensitive periods recurring at touch points throughout the life of any close relationship. Therefore, instead of expecting failure, we must actively support parents of hospitalized newborns in the knowledge and hope that their love for their child can overcome the initial period of physical separation and emotional ambivalence.

OPPORTUNITIES FOR SUPPORTING THE FAMILY

The challenge for the pediatrician is to support and guide the family as they recover from their early experience. I have some recommendations for offering anticipatory guidance about infant behavior and development, for promoting parental autonomy and preventing overdependence and overuse of the pediatrician, and most importantly, for protecting the child from imagining and behaving as though he or she were overly fragile or vulnerable.

We all feel more secure when we know what to expect. The trouble is that what pediatricians advise parents to look forward to with full-term infants does not, at least initially, apply to those born prematurely. Educating (or reminding) the family of the concept of corrected age is useful and helpful, and periodic reinforcement may be needed.

There are, however, differences beyond those explained by corrected age. The most vital differences concern the development of patterns of sleep, wakefulness, fussing, and feeding. These behaviors also happen to be the ones through which babies dominate entire households for the first four to six months of life.

Sleep. We expect full-term infants to be able to sustain an eight-hour sleep period at night by the age of four months. Premature infants, probably because of neurologic immaturity, nutritional demands, and metabolic differences, wake frequently from sleep. It is common, in fact, for such babies to rouse and fuss every two hours until 3 to 4 months of age (corrected) and only extend restful sleep to its expected duration by six to eight months. This demands enormous patience and sacrifice from tired parents who do not rest well anyway at this stage, still worried for the child's healthy survival; but if they are informed from the outset of this immature sleep organization, they can more easily keep from attributing the infant's behavior to distress, disease, or desperate parents.

Conversely, premature infants' awake states emerge during the daytime hours in atypical fashion. Parents should be guided to anticipate qualitative changes before quantitative differences in alerting and attention. Ten to 15 minutes of sustained eye opening is expected at two weeks *or* two months past term conceptual age. However, within that brief interval of alerting, parents can take great pride, reward, and relief from observing their infant's expanding capacity to raise the eyelids to full open position and to focus the gaze without glassing over. After two months the duration of sustained alert responsiveness increases sharply and obviously to all parents.

Crying. While pediatricians ought to be advising parents of all newborns to expect the amount of fussing to increase to a maximum of two to four hours per day at six weeks, parents of prematures can anticipate the amount and intensity of crying to rise to a peak at three to four months of age (corrected). This undoubtedly reflects the lag in neuromaturation of the premature's central nervous system as well as overall strength and energy. Crying and sleep organization emerge side by side in all infants, which explains why the baby who continues to be diffi-cult to console will not yet be likely to sleep through the night.

One very important added consideration about both crying and sleep: Many prematurely born infants appear to be hypersensitive to the sights and sounds normally abundant in a baby's life. Whereas most full-term infants can sleep through any distraction and remain alert in the face of several grandparents, siblings, and pets, busy environments commonly overwhelm the sensory nervous system capacities of premature infants during the first four months or so of cortical behavioral organization, described above. Parents of such hypersensitive infants can be advised about initially protecting their child from more than a couple of simultaneous sensory stimuli. When simply removed from a room full of people, a busy supermarket, or even a climactic soap opera on television, these children may quiet, and become brightly alert, or sleep soundly.

> However, for some infants, the lights and hustle-bustle of the ICN are so much a part of their experience that they must be withdrawn gradually. Parents may report that their infants quiet in response to music or the vacuum cleaner.
>
> *Editor*

Feeding. Feeding the prematurely born infant is often more "demanding" than feeding the term baby. Recommendations must include not only feeding techniques but also methods of protecting the young infant's energy reserves from being used on everything except sucking. The infant's mouth is small, oral musculature is weak, and sucking mechanisms are still organizing a coordinated effort. Individual premature infants may benefit from any or all of the following interventions: frequent, small-volume feedings; soft bottle nipples; supporting the head, neck, and hips in slight flexion; minimal talking during eye contact; and a quiet, even darkened, room. Parents should be supported into recognizing that the volume ingested at each feeding is less important than the mutual pleasure, comfort, and relaxation experienced by parent and infant.

Parent Needs. An important part of understanding and supporting parents through the stresses of caring for a premature infant during the first few months is encouraging them to maintain time for themselves. Even though these times may be short, some amount of privacy and recreation for the parents is essential if they are to meet successfully the challenge of caring for their infant.

SCHEDULING OFFICE VISITS

I trust I have made a point of the unique characteristics of premature infant behavior and development during the first half year at home. These first six months etch a deep impression into the sense of reward and competence from parenting any child. The early adjustment period to families of premature infants adds psychological and behavioral challenges to the ones regularly experienced by all new parents.

The pediatrician has a pivotal opportunity, then, to help parents build on their initially fragile hopes for success. Perhaps paradoxically, the best way to guarantee parental security and autonomy from the physician is to first foster a more dependent than usual relationship. The first visit should occur within one week of discharge, with enough time allowed to review the pregnancy and neonatal course as well as the current status of the infant. Asking the parents to review a typical 24-hour period will allow insight into the family's scheduling of daily events, the baby's individual characteristics, and the interactions of family members. Weekly or biweekly office visits during this precarious transition period from hospital to parental care allow the parents to count on some regular time when their questions can be asked and progress can be measured. Given this regular opportunity during the first two to four months, parents do not need to resort to the emergency phone calls or office visits that are predictable when anxiety peaks at a time far from the next scheduled checkup. While weight checks can serve as a rationale for frequent appointments, they should not dominate the content of the visit. This can easily misdirect parents to exert undue concern, effort, or control of this one dimension of their relationship with the child. Instead, office visits can highlight observations about behavioral changes in activity, strength, attention, crying, vocalizing, sleep, and emerging personality.

THE VULNERABLE CHILD SYNDROME

The preceding discussion was intended to offer practitioners insights that can maximize our position of influence and support during pediatric visits with infants newly home from premature birth and hospitalization. The hope we share with families is for optimal growth and development with minimal problems or complications. Thanks to advances in neonatal intensive care, prospects are indeed excellent for most infants born too soon. Yet there exists an understandable anxiety among parents of these initially vulnerable infants that sometimes diminishes their expectation of a future free of significant problems. In fact, I am convinced that premature graduates these days are more prone to psychological limitations than physical disabilities or dysfunction. The primary care pediatrician is the best person to help prevent parents from labeling their formerly fragile child as forever vulnerable to physical or emotional stress.

More than 20 years ago, Green and Solnit described a syndrome of imagined vulnerability among their pediatric patient population.[3] Despite healthy findings on examination, parents insisted these children (now school age or older) were fragile and sickly. The physician realized that the parents needed to view their child as more vulnerable than was actually the case. For reasons they were not able to specify, these parents overprotected their child from participation in sports, from high academic expectations, or from social experiences with peers. As a result, the healthy, mentally normal children had grown to perceive themselves as fragile and psychosocially handicapped.

The most common presenting signs included:

1. Prolonged separation anxiety exhibited well beyond early childhood
2. Prolonged infantile behavior in the form of tantrums, biting, hitting, and poor impulse control
3. Psychosomatic disorders—perhaps in an attempt to focus the general parental anxiety to one organ system and free the rest of the child's experience
4. Underachievement at school—likely due to spending so much energy just to separate from vigilant parents and go to school that attention once at school was an impossible extra demand

Green and Solnit discovered that many of these children had been truly medically vulnerable early in life. Prematurity, apnea, bradycardia, and failure to thrive occurred disproportionately often in these children's medical histories. Reversing the pathology, when still possible, was achieved by asking parents to identify and then recall in minute, vivid detail the circumstances that took place years earlier when the child was indeed very ill or fragile. Only then could parents stop generalizing their concern for their child and separate the anxious beginning from the healthy present state of the child's health and development.

Our greatest opportunity and challenge as pediatricians to families of premature infants lies in *preventing* the syndrome from permanently establishing itself. All parents will feel insecure and anxious about their child's health or their parenting skills during the first weeks and months of having the premature infant at home. This is natural following a period in hospital when the infant was identified as at risk and when a full professional staff substituted for the untrained, helpless parents. Frequently it is impossible for the family pediatrician to visit the infant during the period of intensive care. How can parents fully trust this doctor, then, to know how the child looks and when he or she might again destabilize and perhaps die? With the intensive care hospital out of reach and the community resources perceived as naive about the child's worst threats, parents all too easily assume total responsibility for securing the protection of their child's health — and thus is born this pernicious syndrome of parental overprotection and functional limitations.

Physicians can help avert the syndrome of imagined vulnerability with several well-timed interventions, none of which appreciably adds to time spent in patient care. These include:

1. Participating as an associate member of the neonatal team during the hospitalization, if at all possible. Brief weekly visits to the hospitalized infant throughout the nursery course establishes the physician as a trusted observer of the child's condition. If this is not possible, telephone communication with the parents and ICN staff may help demonstrate interest and knowledge of the infant's course.

2. Seeing the infant in the office within the first week home from the hospital. This clearly tells the family that the doctor is continuing the comprehensive support received from the nursery staff. The first days home are bound to provoke new questions and fears that can be nipped in the bud.

3. Weekly office visits are deemed helpful during the first month, or longer if needed. In addition to the advantages already mentioned, this practice serves to wean the family more gradually and therefore reassuringly from the hospital's intensive care setting.

4. Review of areas of physical and behavioral progress from each visit to the next. This also provides a measure of how completely the parents accept and respond to the child as recovering normal health.

5. Referral of the child and family to whatever early intervention support programs are appropriate and available in their region. Such programs vary considerably in content and quality, and referral in any given situation should be based on the individual family's needs and the available program's ability to meet them.

SUMMARY

Premature birth, neonatal intensive care, and the transition to raising an immaturely developed child at home all contribute to the unique challenges experienced by families whose babies are born too soon. Perhaps through mastering these very stresses, parents can also feel an extraordinarily deep pride and devotion toward these special children. This blend of adversity, commitment, and profound fulfillment epitomizes both the potential experience for families of premature infants and the soulful satisfaction we can feel from our medical careers.

References

1. Bibring GL: Some considerations of the psychological processes in pregnancy. Psychoanal Study Child 14:113, 1959.
2. Klaus MH, Kennell JH: Parent-Infant Bonding. St. Louis, C.V. Mosby Company, 1982.
3. Green M, Solnit A.: Reactions to the threatened loss of a child: A vulnerable child syndrome. Pediatrics 34:58, 1964.

Recommended Reading

Aylward GP: Forty-week full-term and preterm neurologic differences. In Lipsitt LP, Field TM (eds.): Infant Behavior and Development: Perinatal Risk and Newborn Behavior. Norwood, New Jersey, Ablex Publishing Corporation, 1982.

Brown JV, Bakeman R: Relationships of human mothers with their infants during the first year of life: Effects of prematurity. In Bell RW, Smotherman WF (eds.): Maternal Influence and Early Behavior. Jamaica, NY, Spectrum Publications, 1980.

Field TM: Effects of early separation, interactive deficits and experimental manipulations on infant-mother face-to-face interaction. Child Dev 48:763, 1977.

Goldberg S: Premature birth: Consequences for the parent-infant relationship. Am Sci 67:214, 1979.

Gorski PA: Experience following premature birth: Stresses and opportunities for infants, parents and professionals. In Call J, Galenson E, Tyson, R (eds.): Frontiers of Infant Psychiatry. New York, Basic Books, 1984, Vol 2.

Gottfried A, Gaiter J (eds.): Infant Stress under Intensive Care. Baltimore, University Park Press, 1985.

5

GROWTH PATTERNS IN THE ICN GRADUATE

MAUREEN HACK, M.B., Ch.B., and AVROY A. FANAROFF, M.D.

For the pediatrician, measurements of growth provide one of the simplest, as well as one of the best, tests of the general well-being of infants. Subtle changes in growth can be sensitive indicators of problems of both a physical and social nature. Physical growth and ultimate body size, although strongly influenced by parental stature, provide a highly sensitive index of the effect of early illness and environmental events on the developing child. Any deviation from normal growth patterns provides an easily documented, accurate, and important outcome measure. The purpose of this chapter is to review expected growth patterns, causes of deviation, and the subsequent outcome of infants who began their lives in an ICN, whether because they were of very low birth weight, were intrauterine growth retarded (or both), or suffered from some other neonatal problem.

In the evaluation of growth of premature ICN graduates on pediatric growth charts, it is extremely important that measurements are plotted for the corrected age (adjusted for prematurity) of the infant. In general, this practice should be continued until the child is two and one half to three years of age. Although there have been some charts devised specifically for monitoring growth of low birth weight infants, it is perhaps less cumbersome to use standardized growth charts with the knowledge that deviations are

"normal." This has the secondary benefit of giving the pediatrician the opportunity to familiarize himself better with the characteristics of growth of prematures and to recognize aberrations of growth in this subset of the population.

GROWTH PATTERNS FOUND AMONG ICN GRADUATES

Intrauterine Growth Retardation

The onset of a growth disorder in infants with intrauterine growth retardation obviously occurs prior to their arrival in the ICN, and in many cases the disorder has an effect on both their course in the ICN and their growth potential after discharge.

Definition. A variety of definitions have been used to classify infants as subnormal in growth at birth, including intrauterine growth retardation (IUGR) and small for gestational age (SGA). Some writers have included all infants whose birth weight falls below the 10th percentile, whereas others include only those below the third percentile (more than two standard deviations below the mean). Whereas the 10th percentile cutoff is important as a screen for neonatal problems, it is those infants below the third percentile in weight, length, or head circumference at birth who are the most severely deprived, and, consequently, at the highest risk for permanent growth retardation and other long-term sequelae. These infants therefore need to be most closely observed and followed after discharge from the ICN.

Pathogenesis. The three major causes of IUGR are (1) intrauterine infection, which may result from a variety of organisms; (2) congenital anomalies, including chromosomal abnormalities or syndromes; and (3) placental insufficiency secondary to hypertension-proteinuria syndromes (placental insufficiency), multiple gestation, or, frequently, unknown causes. In infants with syndromes or significant congenital infection, growth failure begins during the first trimester and therefore affects cell number and tends to be symmetric; i.e., weight, length, and head circumference are all reduced. Growth retardation due to placental insufficiency that occurs during the latter part of the second trimester or during the third trimester may spare growth of the head and/or length at the expense of weight. If the placental insufficiency is severe or prolonged, however, all of the basic growth parameters will be affected; again, symmetric growth retardation will occur. However, in this group of infants the majority are less severely affected and demonstrate the "brain-sparing" type of growth retardation. It is evident that, in any evaluation of expected outcome in these infants, the pathogenesis of the growth retardation must be considered. Thus, the infant with a syndrome or other congenital abnormality has different expectations from the infant with asymmetric growth retardation secondary to maternal pre-eclampsia.

Expected Growth Patterns. The growth patterns of infants who are symmetrically growth retarded secondary to intrauterine infection or congenital anomalies and syndromes vary with the specific problem, and they will be discussed in the chapters dealing with these entities. For IUGR infants who are also preterm at birth, it is rare that complete catch-up growth will occur during the neonatal period, since, in addition to the causes of their intrauterine growth failure, these infants usually have a variety of neonatal problems that further affect growth in the ICN. Hack et al. have reported that 91 per cent of infants who are both of very low birth weight and SGA at birth will be subnormal in weight at 40 weeks postconceptual age, i.e., expected term date.[1] In contrast, only 46 per cent of infants who are of very low birth weight but average for gestational age (AGA) will be subnormal at this time.

The poor neonatal growth among low birth weight, SGA infants is undoubtedly due to a number of factors, including inadequate nutrition during the acute phase of neonatal disease; increased caloric requirements in the infant with chronic illness; poor feeding; neurologically impaired or very ill children; and the less than optimal environment for growth that occurs in the ICN. The most severe neonatal growth failures tend to occur in the infants with the lowest birth weights, who have been most seriously ill and have required the longest hospital stays. As these conditions resolve, and when an optimal environment is provided, catch-up growth may occur. The period of most rapid growth and/or catch-up body growth in SGA infants occurs between 40 weeks (corrected age) and one year of age. In the study of Hack et al., 49 per cent of SGA infants were still growth retarded at eight months of age, and there was no significant change in relative growth achievement in this population when the infants were re-evaluated at three years of age (46 per cent). There is little evidence in the literature to suggest any potential for further catch-up growth in later years. Therefore the prognosis for growth in these infants is quite guarded. In this area, as well as in others to be discussed later, it is important to remember, however, that the child's ultimate growth will be influenced strongly by genetic potential and parental size.

The determinants of poor catch-up growth in the SGA population are not well understood. In experimental animals the potential for catch-up growth depends upon the timing, duration, and severity of growth failure. In humans this concept is supported by the findings of poor catch-up growth in the SGA infants who suffered from the most profound, early, and severe intrauterine growth failure.

Head Growth. Fifty per cent of SGA infants are born with subnormal head circumference, and at 40 weeks' gestational age, 38 per cent still have subnormal head size. Brain growth, critical for later development, may occur for the first six to eight months; however, very little catch-up growth occurs thereafter, for either SGA or AGA infants. The impact of growth failure on ultimate neurodevelopmental outcome will be discussed later in this chapter.

The Very Low Birth Weight Infant Who Is Normal

The following section describes the expected growth of the preterm infant whose course in the

ICN was generally benign. These infants are typically discharged between 38 and 42 weeks' corrected age. Infants who remain in the ICN after their due dates should be viewed with some increased concern by the pediatrician, since this is almost always an indication that the child had a complicated neonatal course. Normal preterm infants generally weigh between $4\frac{1}{2}$ and 5 pounds at discharge, and therefore have some degree of growth failure at that time.

Expected Growth Patterns. Data from AGA infants of very low birth weight, born between 1977 and 1978 at Rainbow Babies and Children's Hospital in Cleveland, demonstrate that the percentage of infants with subnormal growth in this group falls from 46 to 27 per cent at age eight months and to 17 per cent by three years of age, after which the percentage appears to stabilize. There are a variety of patterns that seem to appear for catch-up growth. In preterm infants born closer to term (32 to 36 weeks' gestation) a single catch-up period generally occurs within the first three months after term, with the infant achieving full genetic growth potential early in the first year. The very low birth weight infant may have numerous, sporadic episodes of accelerated growth velocity during the first year of life. Although it is difficult to predict when these episodes of rapid growth will occur, if they are totally absent, particularly between 4 and 12 months (corrected age), the pattern is abnormal, and some underlying disorder should be considered (e.g., borderline hypoxia or inadequate caloric intake).

In very low birth weight infants during the first year of life, a period of rapid weight gain ordinarily slightly precedes a gain in length, but the two curves generally increase together. It should be possible to predict (to the same extent as for a term infant) the ultimate predisposition for height by the end of the second year of life. (See Fig. 5–1 for a comparison of growth curves of AGA and SGA infants.)

Head Growth. Head circumference of very low birth weight infants should be monitored very closely. It is important for the pediatrician to recognize that when catch-up growth occurs it will affect head circumference first, and therefore head growth should be measured during early office visits. Even though the infant's height and weight measurements continue to fall below the third percentile, the head circumference may be in much higher percentile ranges (sometimes as high as the 95th percentile). One reason for this is that most of these infants have a fairly significant degree of scaphocephaly, and, thus, for a given volume of brain tissue the cir-

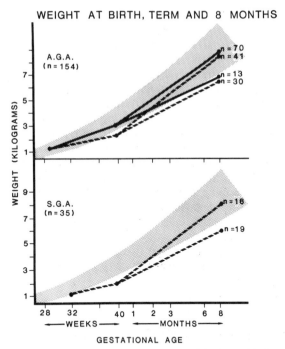

FIGURE 5–1. Varying growth patterns of AGA and SGA very low birth weight infants.

cumference of the head is greater than if the skull were spherical. However, the most important factor contributing to an increasing head size is accelerated velocity of brain growth. Even during the ICN course, once the infant has achieved positive nutritional balance, dramatic changes in head circumference are observed. Many very low birth weight infants may show increases in head circumference of as much as 1.5 to 1.7 cm per week during the first 6 weeks, with widely split skull sutures. These infants do not have evidence of hydrocephalus, but simply delayed calcification of the skull, which lags behind the rest of their rapid growth. Obviously, it is important in following these infants that the pediatrician be aware of whether or not the infant was reported to have had any evidence of intracranial hemorrhage during the neonatal course. Intracranial hemorrhage in sick neonates is discussed below, under specific problems associated with poor growth.

Although the first three months after term is the period when head growth most dramatically exceeds relative weight and length, measurements of head circumference may continue to fall along the 90th to 98th percentile throughout the first year of life, and, indeed, in many of these children this observation may continue through the fourth or fifth year of life. This can be considered normal only if the configuration of the growth curve is normal.

In fact, early postnatal head growth is a very important indicator of the impact of the infant's perinatal course on the ultimate potential for both growth and neurodevelopment. Ordinarily the pediatrician should begin to see signs of catch-up growth in head circumference by six weeks (corrected age) in a preterm infant in good nutritional balance. Certainly if no increase in the head circumference, as compared to height and weight, has occurred by five to eight months, the implications for eventual outcome are grave. Similarly, if head circumference measurements have been increasing appropriately, and then begin to wane at five or six months (corrected age), this is an extremely ominous sign for eventual neurodevelopmental outcome.

The Very Low Birth Weight Infant Who Is Sick

For very low birth weight infants whose neonatal course has been complicated by any combination of disorders likely to affect these infants (e.g., respiratory distress syndrome, patent ductus arteriosus, necrotizing enterocolitis, infection), it is clear that positive nutritional balance will be achieved at a later point; in addition, these infants will have sustained increased caloric requirements during much of their stay in the ICN and probably following discharge.

Expected Growth Patterns. The growth patterns of very low birth weight, AGA infants with more complicated courses in the ICN will have some similarities with those of "healthy," AGA, very low birth weight infants, but there will be a delay in the timing of growth acceleration as well as damping impact on their growth curves. A general rule of thumb is that their residual illness should be managed aggressively, with the goal of attaining at least some weight gain. In some infants, such as those with chronic lung disease, this may be as little as 1 to 2 ounces per month initially. In general, in this group of infants it should be expected that if both medical and nutritional needs are optimally managed within the first year of life, the child should have achieved the fifth percentile or greater on the growth curve by one year of age (corrected). If not, it is no longer appropriate to attribute the retarded growth to the child's low birth weight or initial illness, and the infant should be considered to have failure to thrive, which should be

TABLE 5–1. Factors Affecting Growth

Past History
  Gestational age at birth
  Head circumference, weight, and length at birth
  Length of growth delay
    Days necessary to regain birth weight
    Measurements at term date
  Head circumference, weight, and length at discharge

Medical Complications

  Risk Factors for Generalized Postnatal Growth Retardation
    Bronchopulmonary dysplasia
    Short-bowel syndrome
    Inadequate home environment
    Neurologic damage
    Anemia
    Cholestatic jaundice
    Patent ductus arteriosus
    Other congenital heart disease
    Renal disease
    Subglottic stenosis

  Risk Factors for Aberrant Head Growth
    1. Increased Growth
      Intracranial hemorrhage
        Subarachnoid hemorrhage
        Intraventricular hemorrhage
        Subdural hemorrhage
      Intracranial infection
    2. Decreased growth
      Hypoxia
      Hypotension
      Hypoglycemia
      Seizures
      Intracranial infection

  Risk Factors for Diminished Length
    Short-bowel syndrome
    Cholestatic jaundice
    Inadequate intake of calcium, phosphorus, or vitamin D

Present Assessment
  Status of previous medical complications
  Infant's dietary intake: content and amount
  Family acceptance and comprehension of infant's needs

* From Manser JI: Growth in the high-risk infant. Clin Perinatol 11:19, 1984.

investigated accordingly (Table 5–1). The primary evaluation is a reassessment of the factors that can contribute to poor growth in these infants: environmental influences, chronic pulmonary disease, gastrointestinal factors, and renal factors. If the child continues to fail to thrive once these areas have been completely investigated, a secondary evaluation similar to that for a term infant should be undertaken. This includes evaluation for congenital heart disease or endocrine, immunologic, or metabolic disease. When an evaluation of this nature is conducted it should be noted that bone age studies are not reliable in infants who are receiving long-term diuretic therapy for chronic lung disease.

Conditions Associated with Poor Growth

Chronic Lung Disease. From 10 to 40 per cent of very low birth weight infants who have suffered from respiratory distress syndrome will progress to develop some degree of chronic pulmonary insufficiency. (See Chapter 14 for full discussion of management of these infants.) Energy expenditure is very high in these infants, secondary to increased metabolic rate, which is only partially due to increased work of breathing. Since infants with chronic lung disease (CLD) must have restricted fluid intake, management of adequate nutritional intake can be extremely difficult. The course of CLD infants is also complicated by their tendency to be irritable and to put additional stress on their families. If the family situation is already borderline, the failure of these infants to grow results from the combination of increased oxygen requirements, decreased nutritional intake, and stressful home existence. Ordinarily at the time of discharge from the ICN, infants with CLD evidence failure of growth in weight, length, and head circumference. Head circumference, however, usually falls in a much higher percentile than weight and height, unless the infant has also suffered some brain ischemia. If it is possible to maintain enough positive nutritional status to sustain even minimal weight gain, the infants frequently are observed to have growth spurts that mimic those of the typical low birth weight infant. These growth spurts usually begin some time after the 6th month of life and often continue into the second or third year of life, with each growth spurt becoming more impressive as the child's pulmonary status improves. Such infants can be expected to achieve their full genetic growth potential. Infants who do not demonstrate this type of growth pattern deserve a more in-depth evaluation of the management of their pulmonary disease to determine whether they might require oxygen at home or adjustments in nutritional intake (i.e., do they need additional caloric supplementation? See Table 14–7.) In these infants a small head circumference at 8 to 12 months of age is a poor prognostic sign for their eventual growth and neurodevelopmental outcome.

Environmental Compromise. It is well known that the incidence of preterm birth is higher among families of low socioeconomic status. These families are also usually least able to cope with the problems of caring for an ICN graduate. In spite of the involvement of agencies that provide support for families of premature infants, the underlying problems of poor nutrition and unstable family environment will continue and be exacerbated by the addition of the high-risk infant to the home. In this setting the incidence of child abuse and neglect also increases, and the infants are frequently referred to child protective services. When adequate nutritional and emotional support is provided to infants from such homes, customary patterns of catch-up growth are observed. If aggressive intervention is maintained, most of these infants will achieve normal growth.

Malabsorption. Infants who have had necrotizing enterocolitis or who have required bowel resection for other problems may suffer from malabsorption. The severity of malabsorption depends upon the amount and integrity of the remaining bowel. Infants with malabsorption may also have vitamin deficiencies and electrolyte abnormalities secondary to the short bowel, and these imbalances may also interfere with growth. Again, if these infants do not show some signs of growth, a more vigorous evaluation and consideration of parenteral nutrition for some period are indicated.

Intracranial Hemorrhage. It is important that the pediatrician be aware of whether or not an infant had any signs of intracranial hemorrhage during hospitalization and, if so, whether it was considered to be severe. In general, it is believed that most ventriculomegaly following intracranial hemorrhage occurs approximately two weeks after the insult. Therefore if an infant sustains intracranial hemorrhage early during the neonatal course, and if ventricular size has been stable for several weeks prior to discharge, it is highly unlikely that hydrocephalus will develop later. Infants with more severe forms of intracranial hemorrhage tend to have also sustained other serious problems during the neonatal course, and their growth may be affected by these other factors as well. Evaluation of head circumference in infants who have had intracranial hemorrhage can be truly challenging, since a rapid increase in head circumference may be a positive indicator of adequate nutritional status or a negative indicator of developing hydrocephalus. Fortunately the availability of ultrasound evaluation, both in the hospital and for follow-up of these infants, makes this task easier now than formerly.

When in doubt about the significance of head growth, the pediatrician should request a repeat ultrasound study for comparison with previous studies done in the hospital. As with other very low birth weight infants, if the head circumference does not increase by 1.1 to 1.5 cm per week, the pediatrician should have a high index of suspicion of damage to the central nervous system.

Congenital Anomalies. A number of congenital anomalies, particularly congenital heart conditions, may be associated with growth failure. In infants with cyanotic congenital heart disease, the issues of oxygenation, adequate circulating red blood cells, and adequate nutrition are, again, very important (see Chapter 22).

GROWTH AS A PREDICTOR OF OUTCOME

The following general observations can be made to parents, based on current information about growth patterns:

1. Some growth needs to occur in weight, length, and circumference of the head during the first six months after discharge from the ICN if eventual growth potential and neurodevelopment are to be good.

2. In SGA infants, catch-up growth that is likely to occur will generally be in the first year of life; after that time it is unlikely that further catch-up growth will occur.

3. In very low birth weight infants, catch-up growth is likely to occur in intermittent spurts and may continue to be observed up to the age of two and one half or three years.

4. For all groups of preterm infants, increase in head circumference should be dramatically higher on the growth charts than increase in weight and length.

5. Head growth at 8 months of age is one of the best predictors of eventual growth for the infant, as well as for eventual neurodevelopmental outcome (but nothing is absolute).

6. A slowing of head growth at five to six months of age is an ominous sign.

WHEN TO WORRY

The pediatrician should become concerned and consider further evaluation or referral under the following circumstances:

1. If an infant fails to gain weight altogether or has lost more than 10 per cent of body weight following discharge

2. If an infant's head circumference is not growing faster than weight and length

3. If a preterm infant has not had impressive growth spurts by the end of the first year of life (corrected age)

4. If an infant has not entered onto the growth curve (fifth percentile or greater) by the end of the first year of life

5. If an infant's head circumference is growing at a rate greater than 1.75 cm per week (Repeat evaluation of ventricular size is indicated.)

6. If an infant's head growth levels off at five to six months of age

SUMMARY

Measurement of growth of ICN graduates remains a powerful tool for assessment of both the adequacy of the medical treatment and the social situation, and it also has value as a predictor of eventual outcome. Although it was previously believed that a high proportion of very low birth weight infants remained stunted in growth, modern approaches in care have improved the prognosis for outcome, so that it can now be expected that only 17 per cent of AGA infants will remain subnormal in weight by the third year of life. On the other hand, 46 per cent of SGA infants will remain subnormal in weight after three years of age. (For a complete bibliography, see Appendix D.) Although we continue to struggle to optimize the outcome for very low birth weight infants, the ideal solution remains prevention of preterm birth and early detection of intrauterine growth failure so that optimal management can be provided.

Reference

1. Hack M, Merkatz IR, McGrath SK, et al.: Catch-up growth in very-low-birthweight infants. Am J Dis Child 138:370, 1984.

Recommended Reading

Babson SG, Benda GI: Growth graphs for the clinical assessment of infants at varying gestational age. J Pediatr 89:814, 1976.
Davies DP: Growth of "small for dates" babies. Early Hum Dev 5: 95, 1981.
Fancourt R, Campbell S, Harvey D, et al.: Follow-up study of small-for-dates babies. Br Med J 1:1435, 1976.
Georgieff MK, Hoffman JS, Pereira GR, et al.: Effect of

neonatal caloric deprivation on head growth and 1-year developmental status in preterm infants. J Pediatr 107:581, 1985.

Hack M, Breslau N: Very low birth weight infants: Effects of brain growth during infancy on intelligence quotient at 3 years of age. Pediatrics 77:196, 1986.

Hack M, Rivers A, Fanaroff AA: The very low birthweight infant: The broader spectrum of morbidity during infancy and early childhood. J Dev Behav Pediatr 4:343, 1983.

Hurt H (ed.): Continuing Care of the High-Risk Infant. Clin Perinatol, 11: no. 1, 1984.

Ross G, Krauss AN, Auld PAM: Growth achievement in low-birth-weight premature infants: Relationship to neurobehavioral outcome at one year. J Pediatr 103:105, 1983.

Sann L, Darre E, Lasne U, et al.: Effects of prematurity and dysmaturity on growth at age 5 years. J Pediatr 109:681, 1986.

Villar J, Smeriglio V, Martorell R, et al.: Heterogeneous growth and mental development of intrauterine growth-retarded infants during the first 3 years of life. Pediatrics 74:783, 1984.

6

WELL-BABY CARE OF THE ICN GRADUATE

MARGARET DEKLE LANG, P.N.P., and ROBERTA A. BALLARD, M.D.

For the primary physician, care of a high-risk infant and the family presents the challenge of establishing a sense of normality after the baby's discharge home, while still encouraging the parents to voice concerns that their child is or will be "different." Their fears may resurface with any serious illness, as well as during times of normal developmental crises (i.e., mastery of new motor skills, increasing independence and separation, toilet training, and the like).

The family's first visit to the primary physician is often most productive if it is made within the first week after discharge and if sufficient time is planned to review the pregnancy, neonatal course, and current status of the infant with the parents. This coalesces the historical information and provides a common base of understanding for both the parents and the physician.

> I suggest that the physician consider either an office visit with the parents or telephone consultation prior to the infant's discharge or transfer back to the community hospital.
>
> *A. Rosen*

During the baby's first office visit, review of a typical 24-hour period for the infant-family will allow insight into the family's scheduling of daily events, the baby's individual characteristics, and the interactions among family members. Frequent office visits (as often as every one to two weeks) during the early post-discharge period will enable frequent weight checks and health assessments, as well as provide an opportunity to gauge the family's adjustment to the infant's homecoming and to provide emotional support and anticipatory guidance. (See Chapter 4.)

The family physician's role and availability should be discussed within the structure of the follow-up plan for the infant. The plan will include more frequent visits during infancy than is usual for well term newborns and progress to the standard well-child schedule as the child matures and progresses. Most parents of ICN graduates are aware of their infant's "at-risk" status and will find it reassuring that the physician is providing a plan for appropriate screening visits (i.e., developmental, hearing, vision, language) as needed. If the infant is being followed by perinatal center consultants, as well as by the primary physician, the parents should understand the mechanism for coordination of care and communication among the participants.

> Encourage the family to be linked up with *one* pediatrician within a group practice, rather than seeing a different doctor each time.
>
> *A. Rosen*

In addition to well-child visits with the primary care provider, most neonatal centers rec-

40

ommend follow-up ophthalmologic examinations for infants at risk for retinopathy of prematurity. The discharge summary from the center should include this recommendation if ophthalmologic follow-up is indicated (see Chapter 13 for guidelines); if it does not, the family pediatrician or general physician should query the neonatal center staff. Additional subspecialty follow-up consultations may be recommended when the infant is discharged (e.g., neurologic, genetic, orthopedic, cardiac). The primary care provider plays a central role in coordinating the consultations, in interpreting the information for parents, and in integrating the findings into the overall plan for the child's care.

INFANT BEHAVIORS AND PARENTAL ACTIVITIES

The pediatrician or primary physician can be most supportive to the parents by helping them remember to "correct" the age of their baby to adjust for prematurity, so that their expectations are related to the infant's "real" age, and they understand that their 32-week premature will not exhibit the development of a 2-month term infant until he/she is at least 4 or 5 months old. The primary physician also has both the opportunity and responsibility to assist the family in understanding and managing areas in which the behavior and care of ICN graduates differ from those of normal term infants, e.g., feeding, sleeping, and crying. If the parents become discouraged or experience feelings of failure and frustration, there may be adverse effects on the long-term parent-child relationships. The different expectations for prematures and family support approaches are discussed in Chapter 4.

DAILY CARE

The daily care at home of the ICN graduate who does not have any residual chronic disease requires little alteration from customary well-baby care, within the constraints of common sense regarding the weather and infant's general health. The premature infant should be dressed similarly to other infants, with consideration given to seasonally appropriate clothing and to the premature infant's less mature thermoregulatory mechanisms. The indoor temperature in the home should be comfortable for other family members and should be at least 65° to 68° F.

The baby can be dressed accordingly, with a cap and coverings for hands and feet if necessary.

> I advise parents to dress their babies similarly to themselves, i.e., the number of layers of clothes, sweaters, caps, etc. (Also, I remind them that the Eskimos' babies do well.)
>
> A. Rosen

Daily bathing is not necessary, and for the first few weeks, cleaning only the face, hands, and diaper area is probably sufficient. If bath time is upsetting to the infant, keeping his tee shirt on during the bath may have a quieting effect.

Prematurely born babies may seem to sleep a great deal initially, although they may wake frequently for feeding. Especially at night, this behavior may cause the parents to feel that they have been up all night. The adjustment to the home environment from the brightly lit, noisy special care nursery is difficult for some babies, and soothing music from a radio and gradually dimming lights may be helpful in establishing night sleeping behavior. Some infants seem to prefer sleeping against a firm surface, and many parents use a small bassinet or cradle when the baby first comes home. (See also Chapter 4.)

"COLIC"

It is not uncommon for parents of prematures to perceive their infant as crying for long periods and therefore to have "colic." Their ability to quiet the crying infant is an important parenting task, and parental confidence may be undermined by their infant's lack of response to comforting overtures. It is probably less important to determine whether the infant actually has colic than to help the parents read the baby's behavioral cues and respond appropriately to the distress signals before crying becomes paroxysmal. The following suggestions for parent-child interactions, which can be begun in the intensive care nursery (ICN), may help parents become familiar with their baby's behavior and increase their repertoire of care-giving skills.

When the parents visit the ICN they should be encouraged to get to know their baby and appreciate his or her unique personality and behaviors. If the staff members point out specific behaviors and responses, such as how the baby signals hungry and full, parental enjoyment of the baby will be increased and their confidence bolstered. Learning when the infant is full is a trial-and-error process, and the baby's signals change as he or she grows. The physician's guidance may be needed after the baby comes home

---

TABLE 6–1. Techniques for Quieting a Crying Infant

---

1. Place your hands on the baby's abdomen or hold his or her arms close to the body. Talk in a soothing voice. If the baby is jumpy, slow your movements.
2. Help the infant to bring a hand to the mouth to suck on it.
3. Try a change of the baby's position to the tummy or side.
4. Pick up the baby if he or she is still upset, trying a variety of rhythmic movements.
5. Hold the infant across your lap on his or her tummy, massage the back. Burp the baby again.
6. Check the clothing. The baby may be too hot or too cold.
7. Try swaddling the infant. Try a pacifier.
8. Walk with the infant. Try a Snuggli.
9. Try a wind-up swing, but only if this does not make the baby more jumpy (increase or cause tremors or startles).
10. Try soft music or turn on TV.
11. Turn on a monotonous sound, e.g., a vacuum cleaner or hair dryer.
12. Put the baby back in the crib for 15 minutes, then hold him or her for 15 minutes.
13. Take a ride in the car or walk with the stroller.
14. Try to relax yourself with breathing or other relaxation techniques.
15. In the end, remember that parents may need to "spell" each other, taking turns with the baby.

---

to assure adequate nutrition and also to prevent overfeeding. Suggestions for supporting breast-feeding mothers are offered in Chapter 2, and Table 6–1 gives some suggested techniques for quieting a crying infant.

During the first few weeks at home, as the parents listen to the baby's cries, and as the baby matures, they will learn to differentiate between signals of hunger, discomfort, and need for touching. Since the signals may not be readily interpreted at first, the parent can help clarify communication by playing with the baby when the baby is fully awake, feeding promptly when hungry, and allowing undisturbed sleep.

"SPOILING"

Some parents feel compelled to make up to the baby for the premature birth and separation and to become "superparents." They may need guidance to assure them that being "good enough" parents will enable them to meet better their infant's physical and emotional needs. However, they may simultaneously wonder if they are overdoing their caring. Concern over spoiling this special child may be expressed by

questions about whether they are holding the baby too much, and they may need to hear from the doctor that consistent responses to their infant's cries by cuddling, talking, and offering a feeding when the baby might reasonably be hungry are ways of reestablishing the communication system that was interrupted by the hospitalization. As with any child, helping parents set appropriate and consistent limits is an important aspect of the child's care. However, parents of prematures may need more than usual support to become secure in their ability to determine limits, especially later when they may have difficulty disciplining a child they continue to see as vulnerable. The counseling offered by the pediatrician can play a very important role in preventing the parents from labeling their child as forever fragile and thereby inhibiting his or her ability to achieve full potential. (The vulnerable child syndrome is discussed in Chapter 4.)

TRAVEL

The premature ICN graduate tolerates trips away from home just as any young infant; obviously the family should avoid taking the baby into large crowds or groups of children with potential for infectious exposure, as they would any newborn. After an initial adjustment period at home, long-distance travel is not contraindicated unless the baby continues to show evidence of chronic lung disease. Air travel generally is well tolerated.

Automobile Travel. The pediatric community is well aware that traffic fatalities contribute heavily to childhood death rates. Indeed, it is clear that infants held in their mothers' arms are at the greatest risk for serious injury and that the youngest infants are the most vulnerable. Thus, health professionals have felt it mandatory that infants, including low birth weight babies, use car seats from the time of discharge from the hospital. Two fairly recent articles have attempted to address the issues of safe car seats for preterm infants.[1,2] Bull and Strope point out that head and trunk support of both premature and term infants are improved by the addition of a blanket roll on both sides of the baby, inside the car seat. They stress that the infant should always face the rear of the car to decrease impact on the infant's head, neck, and back in the event of an accident. They also point out that car seats with a lap pad or shield are *not* adaptable for an infant who weighs less than 5 pounds. Willett et al.,[2] however, raise the issue of possible hypoventilation in preterm infants while positioned in car seats. They found that a significant percentage of preterm infants will demonstrate some evidence of decreased oxygen saturation while placed in a car seat. They suggest that if this problem is severe (especially for infants with residual pulmonary disease), some type of apnea or oxygen saturation monitoring should be used while the infant is traveling in an automobile.

It is very important, however, that parents not be convinced by well-intentioned friends or relatives that the baby is "too small" for a car seat.

A. Rosen

There is obviously a need for further study of design of car seats for preterm infants. At present when it is necessary for a preterm infant to ride in a car, it is important that the infant be in a car seat with an adult sitting in a manner that permits watching the baby for any signs of distress. In addition, if infants with residual pulmonary disease must travel a long distance, it may be appropriate to recommend monitoring and/or supplemental oxygen.

Air Travel. The major risk of air travel is potential arterial hypoxemia, which an infant may experience at reduced cabin air pressure. Although commercial airliner cabins are pressurized, the pressure may drop to the equivalent of 5000 to 8000 feet above sea level (equal to breathing 15 to 16 per cent oxygen). This decrease in ambient oxygen may produce a drop in arterial oxygen saturation in infants with residual pulmonary disease. The following guidelines may be helpful for predicting how infants will tolerate travel.

1. If the infant's resting arterial PaO_2 is normally greater than 80 mm Hg, the infant would not be expected to have any significant difficulty.

2. If the infant has an arterial PaO_2 somewhat less than 80 mm Hg, but a normal or low $PaCO_2$, indicating that residual pulmonary disease is not interfering with minute ventilation, the infant probably will not experience difficulty; however, since supplemental oxygen might be needed, it would be appropriate to test the infant prior to travel with an inspired gas of 15 per cent oxygen.

3. If an infant has an arterial PaO_2 less than 60 mm Hg in room air, he or she will require continuous oxygen during air travel. If, in addition, the baby has an elevated $PaCO_2$, it probably would be most appropriate to discourage permitting the infant to travel by commercial airliner, if at all possible.

GENERAL HEALTH ISSUES

Nutrition

BREAST-FEEDING AND FORMULA

Prior to the 1940's, premature infants who survived were given human milk. After it was observed that low birth weight infants grew faster when receiving higher-protein feedings, breast milk was largely replaced in special-care nurseries by artificial formulas. In recent years, however, breast-feeding has gained in popularity among mothers, and professional concern has grown about possible side effects of casein-predominant formulas. Breast milk has again become an important source of nutrition for premature infants. Its special properties of digestibility, unique protein composition, low renal-solute load, and immunologic characteristics have contributed to a reevaluation of ICN nutrition protocols. Although the debate on the advantages and limitations of breast milk for premature infants continues, many neonatal units have undertaken to resolve the issues by adding vitamin, mineral, and/or special supplements to mother's milk.

Most ICN graduates are generally discharged on a regimen of formula supplements, even if they are being breast-fed. High calorie special care formulas, however, are no longer necessary for adequate weight gain (20 to 30 grams per day) unless the infant has some residual chronic illness. For infants over 1800 grams, demand feeding allows the baby to establish appropriate sleep-awake cycles and fosters contingent care giving patterns at home. (See section on feeding in Chapter 2.) For the sleepy baby, regular waking and feeding at least every four hours during the first weeks at home will establish adequate nutritional intake.

SOLID FOODS

Solid foods can be introduced into the diet of a premature infant according to American Academy of Pediatrics guidelines, beginning about 4 to 6 months of age. The infant's developmental stage is the best guide to readiness. Solid foods seem to be tolerated best when the baby displays an interest in foods, is able to maintain head control and trunk support in a supported sitting position, and is able to coordinate muscular control for chewing action, rather than sucking. As with most infants, switching to cow's milk is tolerated best after 1 year of age.

Parents of prematures frequently voice concerns about "constipation." Questioning usually reveals that the difficulty is not constipation per se, but rather excessive grunting and straining when passing stool. This situation appears to improve as the child matures, and the parents should be reassured in this regard.

VITAMINS

Standard multivitamins are recommended for the first year of life, and an iron supplement is usually provided at the time of discharge from the hospital. Premature infants require iron supplements earlier than normal term infants, because they are deficient in the initial iron stores accumulated during the third trimester of gestation. (See Chapter 7.)

Immunizations

The American Academy of Pediatrics recommends that preterm infants be immunized with full-dose DPT (0.5 ml) and OPV vaccine at the routine intervals appropriate for full-term infants, i.e., 2, 4, and 6 months of age. Bernbaum et al.[3] studied initial immune responses in a group of 25 preterm infants with an average birth weight of 1200 grams and gestation of 31 weeks. These infants were given full-dose immunizations at chronologic ages of 2, 4, and 6 months. Prior to the first immunization, it was noted that 84 per cent of preterm infants showed evidence of transplacental transfer of maternal antibodies to diphtheria and tetanus antigens, compared with 100 per cent among term infants used as controls. Following the first immunization, 86 and 82 per cent of the preterm infants showed adequate antibody response to diphtheria and tetanus, respectively, compared to 100 per cent of the control infants. Following the second immunization, 100 per cent of the preterm infants showed protective levels of antibodies.

Only 16 per cent of the premature group showed evidence of transplacental transfer of antibody for pertussis, versus 85 per cent of the term group used as controls. Results after the first immunization were similar, and it was not until after the second immunization that protective antibody levels against pertussis were developed in 90 per cent of the preterm infants.

In light of recent controversy concerning the sequelae of DPT immunizations, the question arises whether the premature or sick newborn is at greater risk of adverse reaction. There is no evidence of increased untoward effects of full-dose immunizations in this population. In fact, Bernbaum et al.[3] noted fewer febrile or local reactions among their preterm infants than among term infants. There were no differences between the groups in behavioral responses, i.e., crying, irritability, or change in appetite, and no episodes of apnea or neurologic complications were reported.

> In fact, most pediatricians would probably wait until the baby obtains a weight of about 10 pounds, although there is no good reason for this. Although most babies receive their immunizations in a timely fashion, I doubt that 50 per cent are within two weeks of the recommended schedule for the first three immunizations.
>
> *A. Rosen*

Because of the high morbidity due to pertussis vaccine, there has been much interest in whether the current dosage schedule is optimal. Barkin et al.[4] reported that, in term infants, a reduced dose of 0.25 ml was effective in producing adequate protective antibody titers and that the incidence of febrile reactions and behavioral changes was also reduced.

For infants who remain hospitalized at the time of the usual initial immunizations, DPT vaccine may be given, but immunization with OPV live virus should be postponed until after discharge.[4] In the infant with a normal electroencephalogram after early onset of seizures, the standard regimen is probably suitable; however, consultation is suggested with the neurologist who is familiar with the baby.

SPECIAL PROBLEMS OF ICN GRADUATES

It has been well documented that ICN graduates are at increased risk for numerous problems, many of which are discussed within this book. In addition, there are some that might ordinarily fall within the general practice of pediatrics.

INGUINAL HERNIA

The incidence of demonstrable inguinal hernia is known to be higher in low birth weight infants than in term babies. Indeed, low birth weight infants are also at higher risk for bowel incarceration and vascular compromise of bowel and gonadal tissue. Peevy et al.[5] recently demonstrated that the highest incidence of inguinal hernia occurs in infants less than 32 weeks of gestation or less than 1250 grams at birth. Intrauterine growth retardation also increases the risk for development of inguinal hernias, particularly in male infants. Since low birth weight infants are also at risk for recurrent apnea, anesthesia morbidity, and increased postoperative complications, it is important that the hernia be repaired at the earliest possible date by a surgeon with skill and frequent experience in dealing with this very delicate operation, and that the infant's care be provided at a medical center where the nursing and medical staff are skilled in managing respiratory problems of very small infants.

DENTITION

It is important that parents understand that the onset of dentition is related to conceptual age; however, infants who were very immature or who have had prolonged illnesses during the neonatal period may have some enamel hypoplasia. These infants may also have an increased incidence of malocclusion. There is no evidence, however, that dental caries are related to prematurity.

INFECTIONS

As discussed in Chapter 21, ICN graduates have increased susceptibility to infections for a variety of reasons. The pediatrician may find that there is an increased incidence of otitis media, bronchiolitis, and gastroenteritis and that they more frequently require hospitalization in the neonatal period than term infants with these problems.

SUMMARY

Care of ICN graduates after discharge from the hospital poses a challenge to the primary care provider who desires to meet the special needs of these infants while promoting normal family relationships. Fortunately, most of these babies require usual, although initially more frequent, well-child care, as indicated by their age adjusted for the degree of prematurity. Much of the effort of the primary physician goes into reassuring, educating, and guiding the parents in making a smooth transition to the home environment and to helping them learn their infant's individual cues.

Whenever the responsibility for an infant's care is transferred from the neonatal intensive care unit to the primary physician, the perinatal center should provide at least a discharge summary and recommendations; ideally the primary care provider will have been kept apprised of the infant's progress and problems throughout the hospitalization and be well informed about the medical and psychosocial implications for ongoing care. If the center provides home visit support, the home visitor should communicate with the physician concerning assessment findings and observations. If an infant falls into a high-risk group being followed by the perinatal center, follow-up assessments will be helpful to the physician in monitoring the child's progress and coordinating community resources and in providing anticipatory guidance for the family. When infants return home with residual chronic conditions, the perinatal center should provide specific recommendations for care and subspecialty consultants. For children with complex, multiple problems, the primary care provider is the best person to coordinate the overall plan of care, clarify information for the parents, and support the family.

References

1. Bull MJ, Strope KB: Premature infants in car seats. Pediatrics 75:336, 1985.
2. Willett LD, Leuschen MP, Nelson LS, et al.: Risk of hypoventilation in premature infants in car seats. J Pediatr 109:245, 1986.
3. Bernbaum J, Borian F, Anolik R, et al.: Immune response of preterm infants to diphtheria, pertussis and tetanus toxoid (DPT). Pediatr Res 17:223A, 1983.
4. Barkin RM, Samuelson JS, Gotlin LP: DTP reactions and serologic response with a reduced dose schedule. J Pediatr 105:189, 1984.
5. Peevy KJ, Speed RA, Hoff CJ: Epidemiology of inguinal hernia in preterm neonates. Pediatrics 77:246, 1986.

Recommended Reading

Bull MJ, Bryson CQ, Schreiner RL, et al.: Follow-up of infants after intensive care. Perinatol Neonatol 6:23, (Jan-Feb), 1986.

California Thoracic Society: Safe Flying for Patients with Lung Disease. Oakland, American Lung Association of California.

Corner B: Prematurity: The Diagnosis, Care and Disorders of the Premature Infant. Springfield, Ill., Charles C Thomas, 1960.

Desmond MM, Wilson GS, Alt EJ, et al.: The very low birth weight infant after discharge from intensive care: Anticipatory health care and developmental course. Curr Probl Pediatr 10:5 (April), 1980.

McCormick MC, Shapiro A, Starfield BH: Rehospitalization in the first year of life for high-risk survivors. Pediatrics 66:991, 1980.

Report of the Committee on Infectious Diseases, Elk Grove Village, Ill., American Academy of Pediatrics, ed 9. 1982, p. 20.

7

ANEMIA IN THE ICN GRADUATE

MARION A. KOERPER, M.D.

It is normal for preterm infants to experience a decrease in hemoglobin, hematocrit, erythrocyte count, and mean corpuscular volume in the first two to three months of life. This occurs even in infants receiving supplemental iron and has therefore been called the physiologic anemia of prematurity. The reason or reasons for the failure of a "normal" hemoglobin value to be maintained are not completely understood, but are known to involve the regulation of erythropoietin secretion.

NORMAL RED CELL VALUES

It is important to take into account the normal, expected changes in red blood cell parameters in assessing whether a premature infant is pathologically anemic. Table 7–1 lists lower limits for red cell values during the first year of life, derived from a group of premature infants who received iron supplementation from birth.

It is clear that most premature infants have a remarkable capacity to compensate for these "low" values, including increasing cardiac output, improving oxygen unloading capacity, redistributing blood flow, and greater oxygen extraction. The challenge to the pediatrician, therefore, is not just to detect a measurement that falls below the norm, but to determine when the infant is actually symptomatic secondary to anemia. The symptoms will actually reflect less than appropriate "available oxygen" and may include poor feeding, tachycardia, tachypnea, lethargy, and less than normal weight gain.

Causes of Anemia

The cause of anemia in preterm infants is often multifactorial. Their hemoglobin concentration will be affected by iron stores laid down prior to birth, erythropoietin levels, nutritional factors, oxygen requirements, dilutional factors associated with growth, developmental changes that occur in preterm infants, and, last but not least, iatrogenic variables.

NUTRITIONAL CAUSES OF ANEMIA

Iron Deficiency. Iron deficiency is the most common anemia seen in the premature infant. Ordinarily the fetus receives the majority of its iron stores in the third trimester, and it can be calculated that for each month of prematurity the baby fails to attain 20 to 25 per cent of the expected neonatal iron supply. Further, even the healthy premature exhausts neonatal iron stores by rapid growth. For the sick infant these problems are compounded by the frequent blood sampling necessary for care. In addition, milk, the normal food of the neonate, is a poor source of iron, containing only about 0.5 to 1 mg/liter. Breast milk iron is more bioavailable, however, than the iron in cow's milk, and therefore breast-feeding should be encouraged for the

46

TABLE 7–1. Red Cell Values in Prematures with Iron Supplements

	AGE IN MONTHS							
	0.5	1	2	3	4	5	6	8
Hgb	10.7	8.1	7.2	8.6	9.7	10.4	11.3	11.1
Hct	31	23	21	25	29	29	31	32
MCV	91	87	75	72	68	67	68	71
Retic	0.7	0.6	1.4	0.6	0.5	0.6	0.5	0.5

first year of life, if possible. When this is not possible, the infant should receive an iron-containing formula. The preterm infant, whether breast or bottle fed, should receive iron supplementation in the form of ferrous sulfate drops, 2 mg/kg per day, from 8 weeks of age until the age of 4 months and then 4 mg/kg per day until the age of 12 months. By 1 year of age the infant should be taking iron-rich solid foods well. The hematocrit should be checked monthly until the infant is 6 months old and then every 2 months through the first year of life.

Folic Acid Deficiency. Folic acid deficiency may result in megaloblastic anemia, with mean corpuscular volume above the upper limit of normal for age in the absence of reticulocytosis. In folic acid deficiency the red blood cells not only are large, they are also oval. Another clue to the presence of folate deficiency may be the finding of hypersegmented polymorphonuclear cells. A low red cell–folate level will confirm the diagnosis.

While breast milk and infant formulas contain adequate folate for the full-term infant, they may not meet the increased need of the rapidly growing preterm infant. Therefore the preterm infant should receive a multivitamin supplement containing 50 μg of folate daily for the first eight months of life. Infants with recurrent infection or diarrhea, undergoing Dilantin therapy, or receiving a goat's milk diet are at particularly high risk and should be monitored for signs of folic acid deficiency.

Vitamin E Deficiency. Vitamin E deficiency in the infant not receiving supplements occurs as a normocytic anemia with elevated reticulocyte and platelet counts. Additional findings in the full-blown syndrome include periorbital and labial or scrotal edema. The diagnosis is confirmed by finding a serum vitamin E level below 5 IU/dl. Treatment consists of prescribing vitamin E 25 IU per day.

Because vitamin E is fat soluble, it is poorly absorbed by the preterm infant's intestine, resulting in normocytic hemolytic anemia. Premature infants should receive routine supplements with an aqueous form of vitamin E while they are in the ICN. After discharge they may continue to need the vitamin at a dose of 20 IU per day for an additional month if they weigh less than 2500 grams. After that the intestine should have matured sufficiently to be able to absorb an adequate supply of the fat-soluble vitamin found in breast milk and infant formulas.

Copper Deficiency. Copper deficiency has been observed in preterm infants who were not receiving adequate supplementation, in those with protracted diarrhea, and in those receiving parenteral nutrition without proper supplements. Copper deficiency results in a microcytic, hypochromic anemia that is not responsive to iron therapy and may also be associated with neutropenia. The term infant ordinarily has ample copper stores at the time of birth; however, the premature infant's copper stores are marginal, and supplementation is required in the second and third months of life. The diagnosis of copper deficiency is established if the serum copper level is less than 40 μ/dl in early infancy and if serum copper is less than 70 μ/dl after 6 months of age. It is believed that daily dietary intake of 80 μg of copper should prevent deficiency. Once copper deficiency is diagnosed, it will respond to administration of 500 μg daily. It should be noted that while cord blood copper levels of premature infants are not significantly different from the levels obtained in term infants, small for gestational age (SGA) infants have a much reduced plasma copper level at the time of birth. This may be related to decreased hepatic synthesis of ceruloplasmin in these infants. Attention to provision of adequate copper stores for the very low birth weight, SGA infant is therefore particularly important.

HEMOLYTIC ANEMIA

Infants who had ABO or Rh incompatibility in the newborn period should be followed after discharge with weekly hematocrit checks until the hematocrit begins to rise. Delayed anemia due to hemolysis will be normocytic; the reticulocyte count will be elevated, but the Coombs test may be negative. Diagnosis may be difficult in a preterm infant who may suffer other nutritional deficiencies as well. Transfusion may be necessary if the hematocrit falls low enough for the infant to become symptomatic.

TABLE 7–2. Laboratory Evaluation of Anemia in the High-Risk Infant

	NEUTRO-PHILS	PLATE-LETS	PEROXIDE HEMOLYSIS	RETICULO-CYTE LEVEL	MEAN RED CELL VOL	PERIPHERAL BLOOD SMEAR
Iron deficiency	N	N	N	↓	↓	Hypochromia; microcytosis
Folate deficiency	N or ↓	N or ↓	N	↓	N	Macrocytosis; hypersegmented neutrophils
Copper deficiency	↓	N	N	N or ↓	N	Hypochromia
Vitamin E deficiency	N	↑	↑	↑	N or ↑	Anisopoikilocytosis; polychromatophilia
Physiologic anemia	N	N	N	↓	N	
Recovery phase of physiologic anemia	N	N	N	↑	N	

From Sabio H: Anemia in the High-Risk Infant, Clin Perinatol 11:59, 1984.
N = Normal; ↑ = increased; ↓ = decreased

Anemia in Infants with Erythroblastosis Fetalis. A special group of infants with anemia are those who have erythroblastosis fetalis, particularly those who have experienced an intrauterine transfusion. The following considerations are important.

1. Because of phototherapy, most of these infants will not have had an exchange transfusion, and therefore will *not* have had their sensitized cells "washed out."

2. These infants will therefore continue to have hemolysis of affected cells and may develop an anemia that becomes symptomatic and requires transfusion.

3. For infants who have received intrauterine transfusions, the presence of adult cells with different levels of 2,3-diphosphoglycerate will cause the infant to have a slightly higher mixed venous PaO_2. Since a low mixed venous PaO_2 is one of the stimuli necessary to "turn on" new red cell production, hematocrit in these infants frequently falls to the low 20's, and they become symptomatic.

4. When these infants finally do begin to produce red cells, they are often Coombs positive because of residual antibody.

LABORATORY EVALUATION OF ANEMIA

Table 7–2 presents an appropriate laboratory evaluation of anemia and the expected findings. Evaluation is indicated for an infant in whom there is clinical suspicion of anemia or in whom values are lower than those expected.

WHEN TO WORRY

1. If the infant develops clinical symptoms that might be related to anemia, including difficulty in feeding, tachycardia, tachypnea, dyspnea, decreased activity, pallor, and poor weight gain

2. If the infant's hemoglobin level has not begun to rise by 4 months corrected age

3. If red cell indices are abnormal

4. If there is a continued fall in the hemoglobin level after 4 months of age, in spite of iron, folic acid, vitamin E, and copper therapy

5. If the infant has other residual illness, including chronic lung disease, ostomy following intestinal surgery, or residual renal disease

WHEN TO TRANSFUSE

When to perform transfusion is undoubtedly the most difficult question to answer, since the concerns about the possible problems with transfusion are very real and likely to be of great concern to the parents. Stockman has recently reviewed this topic.[1] He points out that the infant's ability to make oxygen available to the tissues in response to a specific demand is almost as dependent upon modifiers of oxygen uptake and release as upon the hemoglobin concentration itself. Since these modifiers are constantly changing, usually unpredictably, the most important aspect of determining whether or not an infant requires transfusion is the assessment of the capability of providing oxygen to the tissues, relative to need. Certainly, in infants in whom chronic lung disease has produced poor ability to deliver oxygen to the blood, it would seem appropriate to attempt to keep the hemoglobin at an optimal level. However, for the infant for whom, in spite of chronic lung disease or other residual illness, weight gain is still adequate, it is probably not appropriate to consider transfusion. It is clear that in spite of our current knowledge about the premature and the causes of anemia and our understanding of the principles of physiology as applied to these infants, the indications for transfusion are less than completely scientific.

Reference

1. Stockman JA III: Anemia of prematurity: Current concepts in the issue of when to transfuse. Pediatr Clin North Am 33:111, 1986.

Recommended Reading

Barness L: Nutrition in the tiny baby. Update and Problems. Clin Perinatol 4:377, 1977.

Blank J, Sheagren TC, Vajara J, et al.: The role of RBC transfusion in the premature infant. Am J Dis Child 138:831, 1984.

Brown MS, Garcia JF, Phibbs RH, et al.: Decreased response of plasma immunoreactive erythropoietin to "available oxygen" in anemia of prematurity. J Pediatr 105:793, 1984.

Committee on Nutrition: Iron supplementation for infants. Pediatrics 58:765, 1977.

Gellis SS: How long is the exclusively breast-fed infant protected against iron deficiency? Pediatr Notes 9:101, 1985.

Meberg A: Hemoglobin concentrations and erythropoietin levels in appropriate and small for gestational age infants. Scand J Haematol 24:162, 1980.

Meberg S, Jackobsen E, Halvorsen K: Humoral regulation of erythropoiesis and thrombopoiesis in appropriate and small for gestational age infants. Acta Paediatr Scand 71:769, 1982.

Oski FA, Naiman JL: Hematologic Problems in the Newborn, 3rd ed. Philadelphia, W.B. Saunders Company, 1982.

Sabio H: Anemia in the high-risk infant. Clin Perinatol 11:59, 1984.

Simes MA, Jarvenpaa A-L: Prevention of anemia and iron deficiency in very low birth weight infants. J Pediatr 101:277, 1982.

Victorin LH, Olegard R: Iron in the preterm infant: A pilot study comparing Fe^{2+} and FE^{3+} tolerance and effect. J Pediatr 105:151, 1984.

Wardrop CAJ, Holland BM, Veale KEA, et al.: Non-physiological anemia of prematurity. Arch Dis Child 53:855, 1978.

Zipursky A, Broth EJ, Watts J, et al.: Oral vitamin E supplementation for the prevention of anemia in premature infants: A controlled trial. Pediatrics 79:61, 1987.

8

COSMETICS:
Skin, Scars, and Residual Traces of the ICN

ROBERT PIECUCH, M.D.

Although advances in perinatal care have contributed greatly to increased survival of very low birth weight infants, as well as improved outcome, it is not without aggressive treatment that these success stories exist. These infants battle their way through very unstable periods, suffering multiple complications, not only from their disease but from the mechanics involved in treating their problems. The use of catheters and deep lines, endotracheal tubes, and chest tubes and the occasional need for surgical procedures may leave the child with battle scars reminiscent of a war almost lost.

Even if the child has not been exposed to a very rocky neonatal course, our good-natured attempts to imitate the in utero environment are usually fairly unsuccessful. We place the child in positions unnatural for the "fetus," and the mattress of an isolette is very unlike the free-floating environment of amniotic fluid. Our attempts to provide good nutrition fall short of what the mother would provide during this time. Weight gain may actually be in the form of fatty jowels rather than the laying down of muscle mass, and deficiencies in mineral supplements may result in soft bony structures and

contribute to misshaped heads. All of this may make our nursery graduates appear far different from the typical smiling Gerber baby.

Although these problems may sound like minor complications that could not be avoided in an attempt to save a young infant's life, as pediatricians we do bear a responsibility to that child in the future. Long after a child has been discharged and is termed a well child, these supposedly mild residua of the nursery experience are often reminders of a very vulnerable period, and some scars may still be visible well into the adolescent years, interfering perhaps with the child's self-concept as a healthy individual.

Although some permanent residua may occur, the majority can be avoided when care is taken with procedures in the nursery, and even when lesions are noted in follow-up, dermatologic care may actually minimize their appearance. Even the most obvious lesions can be repaired at a much later date with plastic surgery procedures. In this chapter I shall review the most common lesions noted after discharge from the nursery, how many of them can be prevented or treated, and how to counsel family members as to long-term outcome.

DEFORMITIES OF THE HEAD

Scaphocephaly. One of the most prevalent stigmas of prematurity is head shape. The most common presentation is that of scaphocephaly, which typically involves an elongated fronto-occipital distance, very flattened parietal areas, and an egg-shaped occipital area. This is probably caused by a combination of factors. The skull is made up of a number of bone plates, ideally suited for re-formation and molding during the birth process. Unfortunately, in the premature infant this already very malleable structure is further softened by decreased calcification of bone due to nutritional deficiency and often complicated by the use of diuretics and xanthines for treatment of respiratory complications. This situation is coupled with positioning of the head on an isolette mattress for long periods, resulting in prominent parietal flattening. Even if the full-term infant had been faced with a similar situation, molding would not be obvious, since the child developmentally is able to right the head and freely turn from side to side.

In the intensive care nursery (ICN), scaphocephaly may be reduced by the use of water beds—even if an infant requires mechanical ventilation—to imitate the free-floating environment of the amniotic sac. However, once an infant's developmental stage is equivalent to a gestational age of 34 to 35 weeks, use of water *pillows* has been encouraged to enhance development of proprioceptive senses. Some nurseries have implemented the use of air doughnuts or foam and bean-bag pillows, which allow the head to be in a midline position when the infant is lying supine. Scaphocephaly may continue to evolve after discharge from the hospital, and such pillows can be used at home until adequate head control is achieved.

Although these methods do indeed help to lessen deformation of the skull, caution must be exercised in using them. Water pillows and air doughnuts, if overfilled, can cause excessive forward flexion of the head, thus crimping the trachea and reducing air flow to the lungs. Use of water beds may paradoxically increase the frequency of episodes of apnea and bradycardia; and nursing staff find it very difficult to care for a very sick infant on a water bed, especially if a respirator, chest tubes, or arterial lines are needed.

Except for its appearance, rarely is scaphocephaly a worrisome finding. There have been no reported complications other than craniosynostosis. Unlike skull molding in the term infant, scaphocephaly is not reversible. Little can be done to reshape the skull, yet efforts should be taken to prevent worsening of the problem. Infants who suffer from conditions that can interfere with bone mineralization, (e.g., short-bowel syndrome, chronic lung disease, or blood pressure abnormalities treated with diuretics) probably benefit from calcium supplementation. Frail infants with poor head control may benefit from frequent position changes, infant seats, and regular use of water or air pillows.

Other unusual head shapes may result from behavioral patterns. For example, occipital flattening may appear in infants who are accustomed to lying in a supine position, and occasionally, flattening of the top of the skull may result from a "game" in which the infant scoots on the mattress until his head presses against the headboard of the crib.

These forms of head molding may be subtle and become unnoticeable when hair growth helps round out the head shape. The changes may persist, however, and the skull measurements of an adolescent who was born prematurely may show increased fronto-occipital distance and shortening of the biparietal measurements, compared to other family members.

Craniosynostosis. Premature birth is also associated with a somewhat higher incidence of craniosynostosis than is term birth, and there is some concern that the repeated apposition of skull plates might impede later brain growth. Occasionally, fusion of some of the minor sutures has been observed, but although this may create a cosmetic problem, it usually does not interfere with brain growth. In our experience, craniosynostosis has been a rare complication, and the usual pattern is one of accelerated brain growth during the first few months after term. The presence of craniosynostosis is probably an ominous sign that the infant has suffered some kind of extensive brain damage that has caused inadequate brain growth.

Craniotabes. An area of craniotabes may occasionally be noted, secondary to poor bone mineralization. Typically this lesion is seen in infants who have received long-term diuretic treatment. Anecdotally, I have also observed a discrete area of craniotabes in one infant with a substantial porencephalic lesion. It is my impression that the craniotabes resulted from pressure from the porencephalic area.

Split Sutures. The pediatrician should be aware that during the first few post-term weeks when brain growth is accelerated (see Chapter

5), the sutures are usually widely separated and the anterior fontanelle is typically much larger than that seen in the full-term infant of comparable age. This is no cause for alarm unless growth is too rapid.

Hair. Hair growth may have low priority as an area of concern for the pediatrician, but parental concern about hair growth may be second only to their concern about the infant's survival. If multiple areas of the head have been shaved for placement of intravenous apparatus, it might be suggested that the entire head be shaved to present a much more uniform pattern of scalp hair. We also suggest that the pediatrician carefully examine the hair of infants who required long periods of parenteral alimentation. Scant patches of hair or areas of very white or silver hair may signal mineral deficiencies (e.g., copper, zinc).

The use of assisted ventilation is perhaps the single most important factor associated with improved survival in premature infants. However, some intubation techniques can result in cosmetic problems.

> I have noticed that most parents cope with the "premie head shape" and "ICN haircut" with affection and a certain amount of pride, as if they were a statement that says, "I survived the ICN Prematurity/Run-for-Your-Life Marathon."
>
> *A. Rosen*

DEFORMITIES RELATED TO INTUBATION

Deviation of the Nasal Septum. In the past, nasotracheal intubation was used frequently in conjunction with assisted ventilation. This method has been largely abandoned because of associated technical difficulties, as well as cosmetic complications. A number of nasal deformities may occur in children in whom this technique was used, the most subtle of which is septal deviation. Despite attempts to alternate the nares when this technique is used, septal deviation may occur in a very short time, the deviated septum impinging on the nonintubated nares and prohibiting alternation. If the period of intubation is very brief, the resulting septal deviation may resolve gradually; however, with lengthy intubation, more serious complications occur. These include stenosis of the nares and even nasoseptal erosion. Erosion of the outlet of the nares can result from taping procedures if an infant is very active.

If nasal prongs are used to provide continuous positive airway pressure for extended periods, necrosis of the nasal inlets and septum may result. This is exaggerated if the prongs are applied tightly and upward pressure exerted when a harness is placed to keep the prongs in place. Usually these deformities are mild and resolve without treatment, yet in some instances, reconstructive surgery may be necessary later.

Injury to the Palate. Prolonged orotracheal intubation may cause a very highly arched palate and/or a deep palatal groove. In mild cases this deformity resolves within the first year of life; even in the severe cases it does not appear that this palatal groove creates a communication between the oral and nasal cavities. In very severe cases, despite improvement during the first few years, a highly arched palate may persist. In our population we have found no correlation between the presence of a highly arched palate and groove and abnormal speech development.

Dentition. The influence of long-term orotracheal intubation on future dentition is still unknown. We have observed abnormally shaped central incisors with notching in a few infants who were intubated for a long time. Although parents may be convinced that this is related to orotracheal intubation, we have found that once other teeth begin to erupt the same deformities may appear in teeth other than the central incisors. Typically, infants who have undergone long-term intubation are those with severe bronchopulmonary dysplasia. These babies have experienced nutritional deficiencies and received diuretics and/or xanthines for long periods. Although dental eruption is usually mildly delayed in premature infants (even allowing for corrected age), greater delays are common in chronically ill infants. Tooth structure often appears to be abnormal, but we are finding that older children who had these conditions as infants now have normal secondary tooth eruption.

Trauma to Trachea and Vocal Cords. Infants who have been intubated are also at risk for tracheal and vocal cord trauma. Typically, only the most severe of these problems are observed during the nursery stay. The trachea and vocal cords usually are not examined prior to discharge, and even if minor abnormalities are known to be present, these may not become problematic until later. Complications that require treatment usually become apparent during the first year of life, sometimes when a minor stenotic area is enlarged by edema secondary to laryngotracheal bronchitis or other viral syndrome. At this time the upper respiratory obstructive disease may become apparent and require aggressive treatment.

The infants at greatest risk for upper airway

obstruction are those described as having "noisy" or "rattly" breathing while at rest, which becomes exaggerated when they are excited. These infants need to be observed closely, and liberal use of mist-aerosols is recommended during episodes of respiratory infections. Early evaluation with bronchoscopy is useful in some cases. Laser therapy and/or tracheostomy may be necessary in a few cases.

BURNS AND SCARS

Although in the past we counseled parents that scars would get smaller as the child grew, we now know that initially scars grow with the child and become more apparent rather than less so. Later, over the first two to three years of life, as the skin matures, they become less obvious. It is only at this point, when the full maturation of a scar or burn can be appreciated, that corrective surgery should be entertained.

No matter how unsightly some scars are, almost all of them can be improved in appearance. There are, of course, some patients who are keloid formers or who have such extensive scarring that simple repair may not be possible; yet even in such instances, some improvement usually can be achieved. If repeated surgical procedures are necessary, these should be delayed until the child is old enough to understand why they are being performed. We suggest that surgical repairs be done within that window of time prior to the development of body awareness but not during delicate periods of the child's psychic development. The optimal time for surgery will depend on each individual child's level of maturity.

> To minimize the emotional trauma of this (or any) surgery, remember that a parent should be with the child during hospitalization.
>
> *M. Abbott*

PREVENTION OF RESIDUAL TRACES

Scars can be minimized in the ICN if basic surgical principles are adhered to. As in adults, any necessary incisions should follow skin lines so that they become less obvious during healing. Puncture wounds and incisions that might dimple should not be made in prominent areas (e.g., chest tubes should not be placed in areas of breast tissue). Nursing personnel should minimize placement of tape and other adhesive appliances on the skin and must be very cautious when removing them. If areas of scarring do occur, good skin care with emollients (e.g., vitamin E cream, lanolin, zinc acetate creams) and

gentle massage may help avoid adhesions, which make a scar more prominent.

The most common scars and burns are caused by:

1. Insertion of subclavian or jugular venous lines
2. Surgical repair of patent ductus arteriosus
3. Chest tube placement
4. Abdominal surgery
5. Removal of tape, monitor leads, and transcutaneous monitor probes
6. Intravenous infiltrates

> Feedback to the ICN staff, in the form of pictures, can be very helpful in reinforcing their awareness of the need for careful attention to details that can minimize or prevent scars or burns.
>
> *Editor*

Sites of Subclavian and Jugular Venous Lines. These sites usually do not become major cosmetic problems. If the incision is made at the base of the neck and along skin lines, this type of scar becomes less and less obvious over the first two years of life. Cosmetic problems are most frequently caused by the paraphernalia surrounding the incision sites. Occasionally a line is secured with sutures that originate some distance from the incision itself, and these suture sites may later adhere to lower fascial sheets and dimple quite prominently. Adherence to the fascial sheets can usually be avoided if these areas are well cared for. Massage of the area will soften the scars, and the prominent dimpling may not occur. If dimpling cannot be prevented, a fairly simple plastic surgical procedure later can remedy the problem. However, this should be done before school age, when the child may become self-conscious of the scars because they mimic the appearance of so-called vampire bites.

Surgical Correction of Patent Ductus Arteriosus. Although fewer infants now require surgical correction of patent ductus arteriosus, occasional infants still do not respond to medical treatment. Although the scar from this incision is fairly large, the incision should follow skin lines; if it is superficially closed with Steri-Strips the incision line will eventually be very faint. Occasionally, scars are more prominent in infants who have severe respiratory distress for a long period after repair of the ductus. If the child has intercostal retractions for even a short time, the incision may separate, and a much larger scar may form. In spite of this concern, we have discouraged the use of suture closure of the incision, since the puncture wounds of suture placement become much more difficult to repair cosmetically. If a gaping scar does form, this area can be excised easily and complete correction of the defect obtained after the chest wall is more stable.

Scars from Chest Tubes. Placement of chest tubes is fairly common in the ICN. Frequently the situation is so emergent that little thought is given to later cosmetic problems. Chest tubes should be placed as far laterally as possible, with care to avoid areas that will eventually have breast tissue, if at all possible. Residual pneumothoraces occur frequently in the anterior portion of the lung, where evacuation with laterally placed tubes is difficult. Some centers have recommended anterior and superior placement of chest tubes to alleviate this problem.

We encourage careful placement of chest tubes no matter how emergent the situation. Initial needle aspiration through an anterior site, with a butterfly attached to a stopcock and syringe, is very effective in evacuating free air and allows stabilization of the infant without any skin marks. Once the chest tube is removed and the scar has formed, gentle massage decreases the likelihood of adhesion formation, which would result in dimpling. If these maneuvers are unsuccessful, surgical release of adhesions at a much later date will improve the appearance.

Abdominal Scars. Infants who require abdominal surgery are frequently prematures who have suffered from necrotizing enterocolitis. Unfortunately they generally have linear scars that traverse the largest and most prominent aspect of the abdomen, as well as puncture scars resulting from gastrostomy or colostomy placement. These usually are very prominent, even as the child grows older. Virtually all of these extensive abdominal scars eventually require cosmetic surgery.

Burn Scars. Burns result from the use of adhesive tapes and fixation of monitor leads and probes to the skin. In removal of the tape, one or more layers of very delicate skin may also be removed. Some infants therefore have scar patterns over their entire bodies well into the first year of life, such as an H-type pattern from tape used to secure umbilical arterial lines or round discolored areas the exact size of monitor leads that can be traced back to tape used to hold subclavian lines in place. Once the skin matures during the second year of life, most of these areas will become less apparent. Unfortunately, in darker-skinned children and in lighter-skinned children who tan, these areas become obvious as lighter patches of skin. The lesion left by a transcutaneous monitor probe can be most ominous, presenting as concentric rings with a bull's-eye appearance. There is no effective treatment for these after the infant's discharge from the ICN, but they rarely remain as significant lesions.

Sites of Infiltration of Intravenous Fluid. Peripheral veins used for hydration and parenteral hyperalimentation in infants are tiny and tenuous, so that infiltration of the infusion into the surrounding tissues is common. Although solutions containing only dextrose may not be a major hazard when this occurs, skin sloughing can result if a large enough quantity of fluid leaks into the tissues. When extravasation does occur, early treatment of the site with hyaluronidase and elevation may lessen the severity of the problem. When infiltration occurs during administration of hypertonic hyperalimentation solutions, especially those with calcium, sloughing is common and may lead to a major area of disfigurement; consultation with a plastic surgeon while the child is still in the ICN is recommended.

If areas of sloughing occur over joints the problems become much more complicated. Scarring of deeper fascial sheets can cause contractures that will interfere with joint movement. Splinting and physical therapy manipulations may be necessary during the neonatal hospital stay, and after discharge frequent evaluation by a plastic surgeon may be desirable. Massage is helpful in softening scars, and passive exercises will probably be necessary. The areas should be watched closely; although skin grafting for cosmetic reasons may be deferred until later in childhood, scars that interfere with joint function may require aggressive intervention during the first year of life.

Complications Related to Arterial Lines. The use of arterial lines has become standard practice in both tertiary and secondary level nurseries. *Umbilical* arterial catheters have been used most widely, but recently *radial* arterial catheters have also been used.

Umbilical Artery Catheters. Although hemorrhage resulting from vessel perforation has been reported, the most common complications are vasospasm (blanch) and cyanosis ("blue toes") from thromboembolism. A small percentage of infants with leg blanches or cyanosis develop major long-term complications.

Usually complications from arterial catheters will present dramatically during the hospitalization. Although infrequent (less than 1 percent), leg foreshortening may be the only late complication. Even in infants whose leg measurements are monitored closely, discrepancies in leg length may not be noted until late in the first year of life. Many infants will "toe-ambulate" in an attempt to achieve balance. This is often mistaken for mild cerebral palsy with toeing secondary to tight heel cords. If a discrepancy in leg length is present, orthopedic intervention will be necessary. Depending on the severity of the foreshortening, shoe adjustments and/or bracing may be necessary throughout life.

Radial Artery Catheters. When first instituted, it was hoped that the use of radial artery catheters would decrease the number of complications from arterial catheterization. Unfortunately, both spasm and thromboembolism can occur, and ischemic necrosis of the digits has been reported. Although the last is rare, its long-term sequelae can be disastrous. Asymmetry in hand size and function should be watched for closely during the first year of life. Subtle presentations, including early hand preference, may be a worrisome sign. Therapeutic measures may or may not be helpful, depending on the level of involvement. Severe abnormalities may require surgical intervention to reestablish function.

THE EXTREMITIES: LUMPS, BUMPS, AND OUT-TURNING

Virtually all infants who weigh less than 1250 grams at birth are found on follow-up to have some out-turning of both legs. On close examination this appears to involve components of external rotation of the femurs, with resultant external rotation of the rest of the leg distally. In premature infants who have poor mineralization, and especially in those who have received long-term therapy with diuretics and xanthines, softening of the pelvic bones may occur, similar to the situation that results in molding of the skull. Since most sick infants (especially those with catheters in place) spend almost all of their early time in a supine position, the pelvic joints may be unduly relaxed, with subsequent external rotation of the lower extremities. No aggressive manipulation (splinting, physical therapy) has been indicated, and we have not noted any significant pathologic sequelae in the hips associated with this syndrome. In all of our cases the infants have been found to correct this stance once ambulation is well established (three to four months of independent walking). We have also noted some overcorrection that results in temporary in-toeing of either one or both feet. This tends to be frustrating to care givers and parents, yet appears to be self-resolving. (See also Chapters 9 and 10.)

Another almost universal finding among infants who have been in an ICN is nodular heel lesions caused by multiple heel-stick procedures for blood sampling. Although the more severe nodules are generally noted in infants who have

had large numbers of heel-stick procedures, very small nodules can be detected in infants who have had very few procedures. The nodules can be noted by the time of discharge and are found, like other scars in this population, to grow along with the infant for a time. Initially they may be felt to be deeper in the skin, and then gradually, as they enlarge, they migrate closer to the surface of the skin. The consistency may also change from that of a pinpoint, hard nodule to an almost cystic-appearing, round, smooth nodule with the consistency of a tapioca pearl. These lesions do not appear to be painful, and in our experience most children have not seemed to be aware that the nodules even exist; ambulation does not seem to be hampered by their presence. Radiographs of the lesions show homogeneous calcium deposits. Aspiration of the nodules during the "cystic" phase will yield sterile fluid. We do not suggest that this be done, since aspirating the lesion re-creates the initial insult and causes the nodule to enlarge. Although Sell and associates have reported that these lesions disappear when the infant is 18 to 30 months of age, we have found some of them to persist to school age.[1]

WHEN TO WORRY

1. When head deformities present at discharge from the ICN appear to be accentuated by lack of adequate positioning at home
2. When scars are attached to deep fascial planes or involve joints and cause restriction of movement
3. When "premature posturing" interferes with development of midline skills
4. When leg growth is unequal as the child approaches walking
5. When scars interfere with the child's socialization, impairing self-image
6. When an infant who customarily has noisy breathing or hoarseness develops an upper respiratory infection

SUMMARY

The various factors that contribute to making premature infants look like the "typical premature" are reviewed. Although some scars and deformities might be preventable, most are not. The pediatrician may find the following rules of thumb helpful in counseling parents:

1. Some situations are not reversible, yet measures after discharge from the ICN can pre-

vent worsening of the condition, e.g., use of water or air pillows to avoid scaphocephaly.

2. Bony deformities are usually accentuated by poor mineralization. Adequate nutritional supplementation will be helpful, especially if a child is receiving long-term diuretic treatment.

3. Although worrisome, many deformities will resolve without intervention (e.g., foot out-turning).

4. Initially, scars continue to enlarge as the child grows, yet most will become less apparent as the skin matures.

5. Massaging most scars *lightly* will help soften them and prevent adhesion formation and dimpling.

6. Plastic surgery can improve the appearance of virtually every scar, but the appropriateness and timing of such procedures vary greatly.

7. Although cosmetic considerations are important, lesions that hamper function should be monitored and corrected early (within first year of life).

8. Cosmetic surgery should be scheduled when the child is older and can understand the need for the procedure.

Reference

1. Sell EJ, Hansen RC, et al.: Calcified nodules on the heel: A complication of neonatal intensive care. J Pediatr 96:473, 1980.

Recommended Reading

Allen R, Jung A, Lester P: Effectiveness of chest tube evacuation of pneumothorax in neonates. J Pediatr 99:629, 1981.

Barrett J, Brooksbank M, Simpson D: Scaphocephaly: Aesthetic and Psycholosocial Considerations. Dev Med Child Neurol 23:183, 1981.

Brown A, Hoelzer D, Percy S: Skin necrosis from extravasation of intravenous fluids in children. Plast Reconstr Surg 64:145, 1979.

Cochran W: Umbilical arterial catherization. In 69th Ross Conference on Pediatric Research: Iatrogenic Problems in Neonatal Intensive Care. Columbus, Ross Laboratories, 1976, pp 28–32.

Erenberg A, Nowak AJ: Palatal groove formation in the orotracheal intubated infant. Pediatr Res 18:320A, 1984.

Fergus M, Maylan M, Seldin E, et al.: Defective primary dentition in survivors of neonatal mechanical ventilation. J Pediatr 96:106, 1980.

Golden S: Skin craters: A complication of transcutaneous oxygen monitoring. Pediatrics 67:514, 1981.

Hilliard J, Schiener R, Prest J: Hemiperitoneum associated with exchange transfusion through an umbilical arterial catheter. Am J Dis Child 133:216, 1979.

Jung AL, Thomas GK: Structure of the nasal vestibule: A complication of nasotracheal intubation in newborn infants. J Pediatr 86:412, 1974.

Pettett G, Merenstein GB: Nasal erosion with nasotracheal intubation. J Pediatr 87:149, 1975.

Pimlott J, Fitzhardinge P, et al.: Dentition in the low-birth-weight infant. Pediatr Res 18:111A, 1984.

Saunders BS, et al.: Acquired palatal groove in neonates. J Pediatr 89:988, 1976.

Schwartzman J: Hyaluronidase: A review of its therapeutic use in pediatrics. J Pediatr 39:491, 1951.

Sell E (ed.): Follow-up of High-Risk Newborns—A Practical Approach. Springfield, Ill., Charles C Thomas, 1980.

SECTION III

BEHAVIORAL, DEVELOPMENTAL AND NEUROLOGICAL EVALUATION

9

NEUROLOGIC ASSESSMENT

LILLY M.S. DUBOWITZ, M.D., D.C.H.

Management of the high-risk infants who are now surviving intensive care gives rise to new problems for the pediatricians who look after them in early infancy. There will obviously be a wide range of differences in the behavior and development of these infants, compared to more normal term ones, as well as in parental attitudes toward them.

FACTORS INFLUENCING BEHAVIOR AND MANAGEMENT

ENVIRONMENT

In approaching the care of these infants it is essential to recognize that there are many factors other than disease or prematurity that will influence the development and behavior of intensive care nursery (ICN) graduates. The environment in which these infants often spend weeks or months is very different from what nature intended. The normal full-term infant usually spends his or her time in relatively quiet surroundings in a crib, often swaddled and tightly tucked in. The stimuli received are pleasurable ones, mainly aimed at satisfying needs. The fetus normally spends its time in a flexed posture in a dark, fluid environment. As it grows, its movements are limited and modified by the elasticity of the uterine wall, and by kicking against it the fetus receives continual sensory input. The situation of the prematurely born

infant is a very different one. Instead of the weightlessness of the fluid uterine environment, the infant is fully stretched out on his or her back, with movements often restrained so that the precious lifesaving intravenous drips are not dislodged; or, at best, lying prone on a flat mattress where his or her own weight prevents movement. There are a continuous bright light shining in the eyes and strange noises and needle pricks to disturb sleep. It is thus to be expected that there will be physiologic adjustments to these situations and that the development of tone, movement, and visual and auditory function in these infants will be different.

PARENTAL ATTITUDES

The attitude of the mother toward her infant will also be very different from that with a healthy full-term infant. In these infants, the normal relationships important for attachment are, at least to some degree, disrupted. Often the mother can barely touch the infant; and even if she can, because of the fear that she might yet lose the baby, she will often put an unconscious brake on her emotional attachment. The circumstances also do not allow the infant to recognize the mother as its main care giver. A normal full-term infant, for instance, recognizes very early his or her own mother's voice and the smell of her breast milk and learns to respond to them. This feedback mechanism and the cues from infant to mother are almost completely lacking during the period of intensive care. Attachment may be further disturbed by maternal anxiety, often due to conflicting opinions and advice or to excessive and often misinterpreted medical knowledge. Understimulation of the infant due to lack of attachment and overprotection due to anxiety about handling the baby will further accentuate any neurologic deficit.

> However, a sensitive, responsive parent does not always provide "more stimulation" to the infant, but rather tends to offer contingent care, timed and weighted in accordance with the baby's calls for activity or rest.
>
> *P. Gorski*

PHYSICIAN-PATIENT RELATIONSHIP

The relationship between the primary care physician and the young patient will also start off on a completely different footing. Instead of getting to know mother and infant soon after the delivery, the physician may be introduced to them when the infant is already several weeks old. Often much has happened in those preceding weeks, much of which comes to him as second-hand information. Unfortunately, neonatal summaries will give all the details about the laboratory investigations, but often contain very little information about the clinical state and responsiveness of the infant. Also, the exact information the mother was given about the nature of her infant's illness and her interpretation of it usually are not mentioned. The physician often will have to make judgments and give support and guidance with little background information, yet the expected hazards for abnormal development and emotional disturbance are certainly greater in this population than in normal full-term infants. A full appraisal of the whole situation will be essential at the first visit.

The aim of this chapter is to present a personal view of (1) the methods that are most suitable to evaluate the status of these infants, (2) the physical signs that would be considered abnormal in infants reared under normal circumstances but that are of little or no significance in this population, and (3) abnormal signs that are significant and should put physicians on guard.

APPROACHES TO DEVELOPMENTAL ASSESSMENT

INITIAL ASSESSMENT

For *premature infants* 40 weeks' postmenstrual age (PMA) (i.e., gestational age plus post-natal age) is probably the ideal time for an initial assessment. Although it is increasingly evident that premature infants do not necessarily behave the same way as full-term infants in many of their neurologic functions,[1-3] and that their neurologic profile will depend not only on their conceptional age but also on the time spent outside the uterus, an examination at this time has various advantages. As most infants are discharged from the hospital by this age, a number of workers have examined their premature infants at this age, and thus a certain amount of normative data is available. An examination at this stage also takes into account a recovery period, as it is performed in ill infants a few weeks after the insult has taken place.

Full-term infants are best assessed between 3 and 4 weeks of age, as this too allows for a period of recovery.

Review of All Neonatal Data. Results of all investigations and treatment given so far should be known to the physician before the patient is seen. The physician also should be familiar with what information the parents have been given so far. In particular, are any neurologic abnormalities suspected? If so, on what grounds? Has there been any suggestion about any intervention program?

Interview with the Mother. It is most important to find out at this stage what the mother thought about her infant's illness, any particular problems the infant had, and how he or she has progressed. One wants to know what her feelings were about having her infant in the special care unit and what effect she thought this might have had on her or her infant. One wants to know if she has handled the baby and how much, and if she has not, whether this was due to her feeling that the infant was too fragile to touch. The mother should be asked to recount what happened to the infant while in the unit. Her account may be at considerable variance with that given in the report by the hospital. These discrepancies may serve to highlight lack of information, genuine misinterpretations of medical information, or false beliefs that may give rise to additional anxiety. For example, some parents have been told that their baby had intracranial bleeding or perhaps that "part of the baby's brain is missing." Although they might have been reassured that the outcome for an individual child cannot necessarily be predicted from ultrasound imaging or computed tomography (CT), in their minds a hemorrhage, however small, may very well be equated with an adult stroke and its prognosis.

The mother's narrative should then be directed toward her baby's present behavior and any changes noted since discharge. Particular attention should be paid to her description of her infant's "temperament." Is this an irritable baby who is difficult to pacify? Is this an infant who is difficult to feed, or tends to throw himself or herself back and stiffen up?

Another account might describe an infant who is an "extremely good baby," who never cries, not even for his or her feeding. The mother might comment that the baby is often difficult to hold and tends to slip through her hands. Feeding might take a very long time, as the baby tends to fall asleep during it. When this last type of behavior is described, a check should always be made that the infant is not receiving barbiturates or other anticonvulsants. In general, the abnormal behavior described by the mother is often more apt to be indicative of neurologic deficit, because it occurs repeatedly, than abnormalities observed by the physician during a brief period of examination when the infant might just be hungry or sleepy.

Neurologic Examination. During the past two decades, several reports have shown the value of the neonatal neurologic examination in predicting future prognosis.[4-7] The initial reports were based on a modification of the classic neurologic examination evolved for older children. The examination of Paine and Oppe[8] used in the National Perinatal Project is one of these. In more recent years, examinations more specific to neonates and with better predictive value have been employed.

METHODS OF EVALUATION

The original impetus for a standardized examination suitable for newborn infants came from Andre-Thomas[9] and Dargassies[10] who mapped out the maturation of tone and primitive reflexes in the preterm and full-term infant, as well as from Prechtl,[11] in Holland, who carefully defined the neurophysiologic behavior of the normal full-term infant. Parmelee and Michaelis[12] and co-workers developed a simplified quantitative system based mainly on the French work and Prechtl's criteria. Brazelton[13] developed an examination that is intended as a behavioral rather than neurologic examination. Its main importance has been that it has drawn attention to the fact that the newborn has a complex behavior pattern, some of which can be assessed objectively. The examination allows evaluation of the infant's ability to hear and see and is also a gauge of how quickly a given infant

will become irritable or will quiet with intervention.

All these examinations have various advantages and shortcomings. The French examination was limited to tone and reflexes and did not take changes of state during the examination into account. Prechtl drew attention to the state of the infant as an important variable affecting neurologic signs. His examination, however, was geared and standardized only for full-term infants. It assumes that a premature infant, if normal, will behave similarly at 40 weeks' PMA to a newly born, full-term infant.

Parmelee tried to combine some elements from the French examination with those of Prechtl and to use an objective scoring system with the aid of diagrams. The examination was again geared for 40 weeks' PMA. Its greatest shortcoming, however, was that it aimed for a total score. As neurologic abnormality might result in an increased score in some items and decreased in others, neurologically abnormal infants often ended up with a normal total score.

We felt that there was a need for an examination that can be recorded simply and objectively without any special expertise in neonatal neurology and that can be used for preterm and term infants alike, thus allowing for sequential examinations.

We therefore developed an examination consisting of a group of items that test response (habituation), movement, and tone and a number of primitive reflexes and neurobehavioral items.[14] The items employed are listed in Table 9–1. We found that speed and accuracy of the recording were greatly increased by using a single sheet with instructions of how to elicit the items printed on the left-hand side of the chart and with the recording of the response carried out by circling one of five preselected possible responses, usually illustrated with a diagram (Fig. 9–1). Because many neurologic items are influenced by state, they have to be recorded when the infant is in the optimal state. This is best achieved by examining the infant between feedings and ensuring that a set sequence is followed, such as that in Figure 9–1, so that the items requiring the infant to be asleep are tested first, while those requiring a fully alert state are done last.

One is able to get a good visual impression of the neurologic profile of the infants from these proforma items, and, in addition, changes in a given infant are easily monitored with sequential examinations. The individual items can also be grouped together, so that irritability, neck and trunk tone, limb tone, motility, primitive

Text continued on page 66

FIGURE 9–1. Proforma used for scoring neurological examination. (From Dubowitz LMS, Dubowitz V: The Neurological Assessment of the Preterm and Full-Term Newborn Infant. Clinics in Developmental Medicine no. 79. Philadelphia, J.B. Lippincott Company, 1981.)

Popliteal angle Infant supine. Approximate knee and thigh to abdomen; extend leg by gentle pressure with index finger behind ankle.	180-160° R L	150-140° R L	130-120° R L	110-90° R L	<90° R L
Head control, post. neck m. Grasp infant by shoulders and raise to sitting position; allow head to fall forward; wait 30 sec.	No attempt to raise head	Unsuccessful attempt to raise head upright	Head raised smoothly to upright in 30 sec. but not maintained.	Head raised smoothly to upright in 30 sec. and maintained	Head cannot be flexed forward
Head control, ant. neck m. Allow head to fall backward as you hold shoulders; wait 30 sec.	Grading as above	Grading as above	Grading as above	Grading as above	
Head lag * Pull infant toward sitting posture by traction on both wrists. Also note arm flexion.					
Ventral suspension * Hold infant in ventral suspension; observe curvature of back, flexion of limbs and relation of head to trunk.					
Head raising, prone Infant in prone position with head in midline.	No response	Rolls head to one side	Weak effort to raise head and turns raised head to one side	Infant lifts head, nose and chin off	Strong prolonged head lifting
Arm release, prone Head in midline. Infant in prone position; arms extended alongside body with palms up.	No effort	Some effort and wriggling	Flexion effort but neither wrist brought to nipple level	One or both wrists brought at least to nipple level without excessive body movement	Strong body movement with both wrists brought to face or 'press-ups'
Spont. body movement If no spont. movement try to elicit by cutaneous stim.	None or minimal	A. Sluggish. B. Random, incoordinated. C. Mainly stretching.	Smooth movements alternating with random, stretching, athetoid or jerky.	Smooth alternating movements of arms and legs with medium speed and intensity	Mainly: A. Jerky movement. B. Athetoid movement. C. Other abnormal movement.
Mark: 1 / 2					
Tremors Fast (>6/sec) or Slow (<6/sec) Mark:	No tremor	Tremors only in state 5-6	Tremors only in sleep or after Moro and startles	Some tremors in state 4	Tremulousness in all states
Startles	No startles	Startles to sudden noise, Moro, bang on table only	Occasional spontaneous startle	2-5 spontaneous startles	6+ spontaneous startles
Abnormal movement or posture	No abnormal movement	A. Hands clenched but open intermittently. B. Hands do not open with Moro.	A. Some mouthing movement. B. Intermittent adducted thumb.	A. Persistently adducted thumb. B. Hands clenched all the time.	A. Continuous mouthing movement. B. Convulsive movements.

Figure 9-1. *Continued*

Illustration continued on following page

63

Reflexes

	Absent	Present	Exaggerated	Clonus	State	Comment	Asymmetry
Tendon reflexes Biceps jerk Knee jerk Ankle jerk	Absent	Present	Exaggerated	Clonus			
Palmar grasp Head in midline. Put index finger from ulnar side into hand and gently press palmar surface. Never touch dorsal side of hand.	Absent	Short, weak flexion	Medium strength and sustained flexion for several secs.	Strong flexion; contraction spreads to forearm.	Very strong; infant easily lifts off couch			
Rooting Infant supine, head midline. Touch each corner of the mouth in turn (stroke laterally).	No response	A. Partial weak head turn but no mouth opening. B. Mouth opening, no head turn.	Mouth opening on stimulated side with partial head turning.	Full head turning, with or without mouth opening.	Mouth opening with very jerky head turning			
Sucking Infant supine; place index finger (pad towards palate) in infant's mouth; judge power of sucking movement after 5 sec.	No attempt	Weak sucking movement: A. Regular. B. Irregular.	Strong sucking movement, poor stripping: A. Regular. B. Irregular.	Strong regular sucking movement with continuing sequence of 5 movements. Good stripping.	Clenching but no regular sucking.			
Walking Hold infant upright, feet touching bed, neck held straight with fingers.	Absent	Some effort but not continuous with both legs.	At least 2 steps with both legs.	A. Stork posture; no movement. B. Automatic walking.				
Moro One hand supports infant's head in midline, the other the back. Raise infant to 45° and when infant is relaxed let his head fall through 10°. Note if jerky. Repeat 3 times.	No response, or opening of hands only.	Full abduction at the shoulder and extension of the arm.	Full abduction but only delayed or partial adduction.	Partial abduction at shoulder and extension of arms followed by smooth adduction. A. Abd>Add B. Abd=Add C. Abd<Add	A. No abduction or adduction; extension only. B. Marked adduction only.		J S	

Neurobehavioural items

					State	Comment	Asymmetry
Eye appearances Sunset sign Nerve palsy	Transient nystagmus. Strabismus. Some roving eye movement.	Does not open eyes.	Normal conjugate eye movement.	A. Persistent nystagmus. B. Frequent roving movement. C. Frequent rapid blinks.			
Auditory orientation To rattle. (Note presence of startle.)	A. No reaction. B. Auditory startle but no true orientation.	Brightens and stills; Alerting and shifting of eyes; head may or may not turn to source.	Alerting; prolonged head turns to stimulus; search with eyes.	Turning and alerting to stimulus each time on both sides.		S	

Figure 9–1. *Continued*

64

Visual orientation To red woollen ball	Does not focus or follow stimulus	Stills; focuses on stimulus; may follow 30° jerkily; does not find stimulus again spontaneously.	Follows 30–60° horizontally; may lose stimulus but finds it again. Brief vertical glance.	Follows with eyes and head horizontally and to some extent vertically, with frowning.	Sustained fixation; follows vertically, horizontally, and in circle.
Alertness	Inattentive; rarely or never responds to direct stimulation	When alert, periods rather brief; rather variable response to orientation.	When alert, alertness moderately sustained; may use stimulus to come to alert state.	Sustained alertness; orientation frequent, reliable to visual but not auditory stimuli	Continuous alertness, which does not seem to tire, to both auditory and visual stimuli
Defensive reaction A cloth or hand is placed over the infant's face to partially occlude the nasal airway.	No response.	A. General quietening. B. Non-specific activity with long latency.	Rooting; lateral neck turning; possibly neck stretching.	Swipes with arm	Swipes with arm with rather violent body movement
Peak of excitement	Low level arousal to all stimuli; never > state 3	Infant reaches state 4–5 briefly but predominantly in lower states.	Infant predominantly state 4 or 5; may reach state 6 after stimulation but returns spontaneously to lower state.	Infant reaches state 6 but can be consoled relatively easily	A. Mainly state 6. Difficult to console, if at all. B. Mainly state 4–5 but if reaches state 6 cannot be consoled.
Irritability Aversive stimuli: Uncover Ventral susp. Undress Moro Pull to sit Walking reflex Prone	No irritable crying to any of the stimuli	Cries to 1–2 stimuli	Cries to 3–4 stimuli	Cries to 5–6 stimuli	Cries to all stimuli
Consolability	Never above state 5 during examination. therefore not needed.	Consoling not needed. Consoles spontaneously.	Consoled by talking, hand on belly or wrapping up.	Consoled by picking up and holding; may need finger in mouth.	Not consolable
Cry	No cry at all	Only whimpering cry.	Cries to stimuli but normal pitch.	Lusty cry to offensive stimuli; normal pitch.	High-pitched cry, often continuous

Notes

* If asymmetrical or atypical, draw in on nearest figure
Record any abnormal signs (e.g. facial palsy, contractures, etc.). Draw if possible.

Record time after feed:

Examiner:

Figure 9–1. *Continued*

TABLE 9–1. Neurologic Signs Used for Assessment

RESPONSE DECREMENT (HABITUATION)	MOVEMENT AND TONE	REFLEXES	NEUROBEHAVIOR
Light (flashlight)	Posture	Tendon reflexes	Eye appearance
Auditory (rattle)	Arm recoil	Palmar grasp	Auditory orientation
	Arm traction	Rooting	Visual orientation
	Leg recoil	Sucking	Alertness
	Popliteal angle	Moro	Peak of excitement
	Head lag		Irritability
	Ventral suspension		Consolability
	Head control		Cry
	(posterior neck muscle)		
	(anterior neck muscle)		
	Arm release		
	Body movement		
	Tremor		
	Startle		

reflexes, orientation, state control, and abnormal signs can be assessed separately.

The proforma also allows easy comparison between the neurologic profiles of different infants as well as those obtained by repeated examination of the same infant. One is thus able to compare the preterm infant examined at 40 weeks' PMA and the newly born full-term infant (Figs. 9–2 and 9–3). While in some respects they are similar, there are a number of items on which they differ.

FOLLOW-UP ASSESSMENTS

In office practice, the Denver Developmental Screening Test (DDST)[15] is probably the most commonly employed screening test for developmental delay. While it is highly suitable for the screening of full-term infants, it is of limited use in picking up early abnormalities in preterm infants. Although, as with other testing methods, correction should be made for prematurity, more recent data suggest that the DDST at 6 months of age does not accurately identify the infant with later neurologic abnormalities or handicaps.[16] This implies that the test does not identify neurologic abnormalities until they are handicapping enough to affect development. Because intervention is most successful when initiated early, a more sensitive tool is needed for the preterm infant.

In formal neonatal follow-up programs, both developmental tests and neurologic examinations usually are employed. A wide choice of both types of tests is available, with various merits claimed by those employing them. Un-

fortunately, few have been compared in the same infants, and it is therefore difficult to state in absolute terms which are the best.

Several neurologic examinations have been successfully used for detailed assessment of high-risk infants. Some are based primarily on the assessment of active and passive tone[17]; others, on coordinated reactions and movement[18,19] or on primitive reflex profiles.[20] There are again no comparative studies available of these various examinations on the same infant, and it is thus difficult to assess objectively their various merits.

In our follow-up program, we have used a combination of a neurologic examination and a developmental one. The neurologic examination has been developed from the French examination and a modification of Touwen's examination. The developmental examination is the Griffiths scale,[21] which is a Gesell-based test. This system is obviously too complicated for an office examination, but we have found from experience with these tests that there are a number of abnormalities (the ages are given for chronologic age, uncorrected for prematurity) that require attention during the first year of life.

NEUROLOGIC VARIATIONS IN NEWBORN INFANTS

NORMAL VARIATION

On the whole, even healthy preterm infants with a completely uneventful neonatal course will tend to have less marked flexor tone and

Text continued on page 75

Name

HOSP.	NO.	D.O.B./TIME	WEIGHT	E.D.D. L.N.M.P.	E.D.D. U/snd.
RACE	SEX	DATE OF EXAM	HEIGHT	GESTATIONAL	SCORE WEEKS
		AGE **2D**	HEAD CIRC.	ASSESSMENT	**40**

STATES
1. Deep sleep, no movement, regular breathing.
2. Light sleep, eyes shut, some movement.
3. Dozing, eyes opening and closing.
4. Awake, eyes open, minimal movement.
5. Wide awake, vigorous movement.
6. Crying.

Right-hand columns: **State** | **Comment** | **Asymmetry**

Habituation (≤ state 3)

Light — Repetitive flashlight stimuli (10) with 5 sec. gap. Shutdown = 2 consecutive negative responses

					State
No response	A. Blink response to first stimulus. B. Tonic blink response. C. Variable response.	A. Shutdown of movement but blink persists 2–5 stimuli. B. Complete shutdown 2–5 stimuli.	A. Shutdown of movement but blink persists 6–10 stimuli. B. Complete shutdown 6–10 stimuli.	A. Equal response to 10 stimuli. B. Infant comes to fully alert state. C. Startles + major responses throughout.	**2**

Rattle — Repetitive stimuli (10) with 5 sec gap.

No response	A. Slight movement to first stimulus. B. Variable response	Startle or movement 2–5 stimuli, then shutdown	Startle or movement 6–10 stimuli, then shutdown	A. B. C.] Grading as above

Movement & tone
Undress infant

Posture * (At rest – predominant)

| | | | (hips adducted) | (hips adducted) | Abnormal postures: A. Opisthotonus. B. Unusual leg extension. C. Asymm. tonic neck reflex |

Arm recoil — Infant supine. Take both hands, extend parallel to the body; hold approx. 2 secs. and release.

| No flexion within 5 sec. | Partial flexion at elbow >100° within 4–5 sec. | Arms flex at elbow to <100° within 2–3 sec. | Sudden jerky flexion at elbow immediately after release to <60° | Difficult to extend; arm snaps back forcefully |

Arm traction — Infant supine; head midline; grasp wrist, slowly pull arm to vertical. Angle of arm scored and resistance noted at moment infant is initially lifted off and watched until shoulder off mattress. Do other arm.

| Arm remains fully extended | Weak flexion maintained only momentarily | Arm flexed at elbow to 140° maintained 5 sec. | Arm flexed at approx. 100° and maintained | Strong flexion of arm <100° and maintained | State **4·5** |

Leg recoil — First flex hips for 5 secs, then extend both legs of infant by traction on ankles; hold down on the bed for 2 secs and release.

| No flexion within 5 sec. | Incomplete flexion of hips within 5 sec. | Complete flexion within 5 sec. | Instantaneous complete flexion | Legs cannot be extended; snap back forcefully |

Leg traction — Infant supine. Grasp leg near ankle and slowly pull toward vertical until buttocks 1–2" off. Note resistance at knee and score angle. Do other leg.

| No flexion | Partial flexion, rapidly lost | Knee flexion 140–160° and maintained | Knee flexion 100–140° and maintained | Strong resistance; flexion <100° | State **4·5** |

FIGURE 9–2. Proforma illustrating examination of a full-term infant examined at two days of age.

Illustration continued on following page

67

Item	Technique					
Popliteal angle	Infant supine. Approximate knee and thigh to abdomen; extend leg by gentle pressure with index finger behind ankle.	180-160° R L	150-140° R L	130-120° R L	110-90° R L	<90° R L
Head control, post. neck m.	Grasp infant by shoulders and raise to sitting position; allow head to fall forward; wait 30 sec.	No attempt to raise head	Unsuccessful attempt to raise head upright	Head raised smoothly to upright in 30 sec. but not maintained.	Head raised smoothly to upright in 30 sec. and maintained (4-5)	Head cannot be flexed forward
Head control, ant. neck m.	Allow head to fall backward as you hold shoulders; wait 30 sec.	Grading as above	Grading as above	Grading as above	Grading as above	
Head lag *	Pull infant toward sitting posture by traction on both wrists. Also note arm flexion.					
Ventral suspension *	Hold infant in ventral suspension; observe curvature of back, flexion of limbs and relation of head to trunk.					
Head raising, prone	Infant in prone position with head in midline.	No response	Rolls head to one side	Weak effort to raise head and turns raised head to one side	Infant lifts head, nose and chin off	Strong prolonged head lifting
Arm release, prone	Head in midline. Infant in prone position; arms extended alongside body with palms up.	No effort	Some effort and wriggling	Flexion effort but neither wrist brought to nipple level	One or both wrists brought at least to nipple level without excessive body movement	Strong body movement with both wrists brought to face or 'press-ups'
Spont. body movement	If no spont. movement try to elicit by cutaneous stim.	None or minimal	A. Sluggish. B. Random, incoordinated. C. Mainly stretching.	Smooth movements alternating with random, stretching, athetoid or jerky	Smooth alternating movements of arms and legs with medium speed and intensity	Mainly: A. Jerky movement (1). B. Athetoid movement (2). C. Other abnormal movement.
Tremors Mark: Fast (>6/sec) or Slow (<6/sec)		No tremor	Tremors only in state 5-6	Tremors only in sleep or after Moro and startles	Some tremors in state 4	Tremulousness in all states
Startles		No startles	Startles to sudden noise, Moro, bang on table only	Occasional spontaneous startle	2-5 spontaneous startles	6+ spontaneous startles
Abnormal movement or posture		No abnormal movement	A. Hands clenched but open intermittently. B. Hands do not open with Moro.	A. Some mouthing movement. B. Intermittent adducted thumb	A. Persistently adducted thumb. B. Hands clenched all the time.	A. Continuous mouthing movement. B. Convulsive movements.

Figure 9-2. *Continued*

Reflexes

Tendon reflexes

Biceps jerk
Knee jerk
Ankle jerk

	Absent	Present	Exaggerated	Clonus	State	Comment	Asymmetry
	Absent						

Palmar grasp

Head in midline. Put index finger from ulnar side into hand and gently press palmar surface. Never touch dorsal side of hand.

| Absent | Short, weak flexion | Medium strength and sustained flexion for several secs. | Strong flexion; contraction spreads to forearm. | Very strong; infant easily lifts off couch | 4 - 5 | | |

Rooting

Infant supine, head midline. Touch each corner of the mouth in turn (stroke laterally).

| No response | A. Partial weak head turn but no mouth opening. B. Mouth opening, no head turn. | Mouth opening on stimulated side with partial head turning. | Full head turning, with or without mouth opening. | Mouth opening with very jerky head turning | | | |

Sucking

Infant supine; place index finger (pad towards palate) in infant's mouth; judge power of sucking movement after 5 sec.

| No attempt | Weak sucking movement: A. Regular. B. Irregular. | Strong sucking movement, poor stripping: A. Regular. B. Irregular. | Strong regular sucking movement with continuing sequence of 5 movements. Good stripping. | Clenching but no regular sucking. | 4 - 5 | | |

Walking

Hold infant upright, feet touching bed, neck held straight with fingers.

| Absent | Some effort but not continuous with both legs. | At least 2 steps with both legs. | A. Stork posture; no movement. B. Automatic walking. | | | | |

Moro

One hand supports infant's head in midline, the other the back. Raise infant to 45° and when infant is relaxed let his head fall through 10°. Note if jerky. Repeat 3 times.

| No response, or opening of hands only. | Full abduction at the shoulder and extension of the arm. partial adduction. | Partial abduction at shoulder and extension of arms followed by smooth adduction. A. Abd>Add B. Abd=Add C. Abd<Add | A. No abduction or adduction; extension only. B. Marked adduction only. | | J | | |

Neurobehavioural items

Eye appearances

Sunset sign
Nerve palsy

| Transient nystagmus. Strabismus. Some roving eye movement. | Does not open eyes. | Normal conjugate eye movement. | A. Persistent nystagmus. B. Frequent roving movement. C. Frequent rapid blinks. | S | | |

Auditory orientation

To rattle. (Note presence of startle.)

| A. No reaction. B. Auditory startle but no true orientation. | Brightens and stills; Alerting and shifting of eyes; head may or may not turn to source. | Alerting; prolonged stimuli with eyes closed. | Turning and alerting to stimulus each time on both sides. | S | | |

Figure 9–2. Continued

Illustration continued on following page

Visual orientation
To red woollen ball

Defensive reaction
A cloth or hand is placed over the infant's face to partially occlude the nasal airway.

Irritability
Aversive stimuli:
Uncover   Ventral susp.
Undress   Moro
Pull to sit   Walking reflex
Prone

	1	2	3	4	5	Score
Visual orientation	Does not focus or follow stimulus	Stills; focuses on stimulus; may follow 30° jerkily; does not find stimulus again spontaneously.	Follows 30-60° horizontally; may lose stimulus but finds it again. Brief vertical glance.	Follows with eyes and head horizontally and to some extent vertically, with frowning.	Sustained fixation; follows vertically, horizontally, and in circle.	**4 - 5**
Alertness	Inattentive; rarely or never responds to direct stimulation	When alert, periods rather brief; rather variable response to orientation.	When alert, alertness moderately sustained; may use stimulus to come to alert state.	Sustained alertness; orientation frequent, reliable to visual but not auditory stimuli.	Continuous alertness, which does not seem to tire, to both auditory and visual stimuli.	
Defensive reaction	No response.	A. General quietening B. Non-specific activity with long latency.	Rooting; lateral neck turning; possibly neck stretching.	Swipes with arm	Swipes with arm with rather violent body movement	
Peak of excitement	Low level arousal to all stimuli; never > state 3	Infant reaches state 4-5 briefly but predominantly in lower states.	Infant predominantly state 4 or 5; may reach state 6 after stimulation but returns spontaneously to lower state.	Infant reaches state 6 but can be consoled relatively easily.	A. Mainly state 6. Difficult to console, if at all. B. Mainly state 4-5 but if reaches state 6 cannot be consoled.	**4 - 5**
Irritability	No irritable crying to any of the stimuli	Cries to 1-2 stimuli	Cries to 3-4 stimuli	Cries to 5-6 stimuli	Cries to all stimuli	
Consolability	Never above state 5 during examination, therefore not needed.	Consoling not needed. Consoles spontaneously.	Consoled by talking, hand on belly or wrapping up.	Consoled by picking up and holding; may need finger in mouth.	Not consolable	
Cry	No cry at all.	Only whimpering cry.	Cries to stimuli but normal pitch.	Lusty cry to offensive stimuli; normal pitch.	High-pitched cry, often continuous.	

Notes   * If asymmetrical or atypical, draw in on nearest figure

Record any abnormal signs (e.g. facial palsy, contractures, etc.). Draw if possible.

Record time after feed:

Examiner:

Figure 9-2. *Continued*

70

Name

WEIGHT

HEIGHT

HEAD CIRC.

E.D.D.
L.N.M.P.

GESTATIONAL
ASSESSMENT

E.D.D.
U/snd.

SCORE   WEEKS
32

STATES

1. Deep sleep, no movement, regular breathing.
2. Light sleep, eyes shut, some movement.
3. Dozing, eyes opening and closing.
4. Awake, eyes open, minimal movement.
5. Wide awake, vigorous movement.
6. Crying.

Habituation (≤ state 3)

| | No response | A. Shutdown of movement but blink persists 6-10 stimuli. | A. Equal response to 10 stimuli. | State **2** | Comment | Asymmetry |

Light
Repetitive flashlight stimuli (10) with 5 sec. gap.
Shutdown = 2 consecutive negative responses

A. Blink response to first stimulus.
B. Tonic blink response.
C. Variable response.

A. Shutdown of movement but blink persists 2-5 stimuli.
B. Complete shutdown 2-5 stimuli.

A. Shutdown of movement but blink persists 6-10 stimuli.
B. Complete shutdown 6-10 stimuli.

A. Equal response to 10 stimuli.
B. Infant comes to fully alert state.
C. Startles + major responses throughout.

Rattle
Repetitive stimuli (10) with 5 sec. gap.

No response

A. Slight movement to first stimulus.
B. Variable response

Startle or movement 2-5 stimuli, then shutdown

Startle or movement 6-10 stimuli, then shutdown

A.
B. } Grading as above
C.

Movement & tone

Posture *
(At rest - predominant)

Undress infant

Abnormal postures:
A. Opisthotonus.
B. Unusual leg extension.
C. Asymm. tonic neck reflex

State **4-5**

Arm recoil
Infant supine. Take both hands, extend parallel to the body; hold approx. 2 secs. and release.

No flexion within 5 sec.

Partial flexion at elbow >100° within 4-5 sec.

Arms flex at elbow to <100° within 2-3 sec.

Sudden jerky flexion at elbow immediately after release to <60°

Difficult to extend; arm snaps back forcefully

Arm traction
Infant supine; head midline; grasp wrist, slowly pull arm to vertical. Angle of arm scored and resistance noted at moment infant is initially lifted off and watched until shoulder off mattress. Do other arm.

Arm remains fully extended

Weak flexion maintained only momentarily

Arm flexed at elbow to 140° and maintained 5 sec.

Arm flexed at elbow at approx. 100° and maintained

Strong flexion of arm <100° and maintained

State **4-5**

Leg recoil
First flex hips for 5 secs, then extend both legs of infant by traction on ankles; hold down on the bed for 2 secs and release.

No flexion within 5 sec.

Incomplete flexion of hips within 5 sec.

Complete flexion within 5 sec.

Instantaneous complete flexion

Legs cannot be extended; snap back forcefully

Leg traction
Infant supine. Grasp leg near ankle and slowly pull toward vertical until buttocks 1-2" off. Note resistance at knee and score angle. Do other leg.

No flexion

Partial flexion, rapidly lost

Knee flexion 140-160° and maintained

Knee flexion 100-140° and maintained

Strong resistance: flexion <100°

FIGURE 9-3. Proforma illustrating examination of preterm infant born at 32 weeks' gestation, examined at 8 weeks (40 weeks' PMA). Note differences in posture and flexion in ventral suspension in the legs and the better alertness, compared to a full-term infant at the same postmenstrual age.

Illustration continued on following page

Popliteal angle
Infant supine. Approximate knee and thigh to abdomen; extend leg by gentle pressure with index finger behind ankle.

180-160°	150-140°	130-120°	110-90°	<90°

Head control, post. neck m.
Grasp infant by shoulders and raise to sitting position; allow head to fall forward; wait 30 sec.

No attempt to raise head	Unsuccessful attempt to raise head upright	Head raised smoothly to upright in 30 sec. but not maintained.	Head raised smoothly to upright in 30 sec. and maintained	Head cannot be flexed forward

Head control, ant. neck m.
Allow head to fall backward as you hold shoulders; wait 30 sec.

Grading as above	Grading as above	Grading as above	Grading as above	

Head lag *
Pull infant toward sitting posture by traction on both wrists. Also note arm flexion.

Ventral suspension *
Hold infant in ventral suspension; observe curvature of back, flexion of limbs and relation of head to trunk.

Head raising, prone
Infant in prone position with head in midline.

No response	Rolls head to one side	Weak effort to raise head and turns raised head to one side	Infant lifts head, nose and chin off	Strong prolonged head lifting

Arm release, prone
Head in midline. Infant in prone position; arms extended alongside body with palms up.

No effort	Some effort and wriggling	Flexion effort but neither wrist brought to nipple level	One or both wrists brought at least to nipple level without excessive body movement	Strong body movement with both wrists brought to face or 'press-ups'

Spont. body movement
If no spont. movement try to elicit by cutaneous stim.

None or minimal	A: Sluggish. B: Random, incoordinated. C: Mainly stretching.	Smooth movements alternating with random, stretching, athetoid or jerky	Smooth alternating movements of arms and legs with medium speed and intensity	Mainly: A: Jerky movement. B: Athetoid movement. C: Other abnormal movement.

Tremors
Mark: Fast (>6/sec) or Slow (<6/sec)

No tremor	Tremors only in state 5-6	Tremors only in sleep or after Moro and startles	Some tremors in state 4	Tremulousness in all states

Startles

No startles	Startles to sudden noise, Moro, bang on table only	Occasional spontaneous startle	2-5 spontaneous startles	6+ spontaneous startles

Abnormal movement or posture

No abnormal movement	A: Hands clenched but open intermittently. B: Hands do not open with Moro.	A: Some mouthing movement. B: Intermittent adducted thumb	A: Persistently adducted thumb. B: Hands clenched all the time.	A: Continuous mouthing movement. B: Convulsive movements.

Figure 9-3. *Continued*

Reflexes

	Absent	Present	Exaggerated	Clonus	State	Comment	Asymmetry
Tendon reflexes Biceps jerk, Knee jerk, Ankle jerk	Absent						
Palmar grasp Head in midline. Put index finger from ulnar side into hand and gently press palmar surface. Never touch dorsal side of hand.	Absent / Short, weak flexion	Medium strength and sustained flexion for several secs.	Strong flexion; contraction spreads to forearm.	Very strong; infant easily lifts off couch			
Rooting Infant supine, head midline. Touch each corner of the mouth in turn (stroke laterally).	No response / A. Partial weak head turn but no mouth opening. B. Mouth opening, no head turn.	Mouth opening on stimulated side with partial head turning	Full head turning, with or without mouth opening.	Mouth opening with very jerky head turning			
Sucking Infant supine; place index finger (pad towards palate) in infant's mouth; judge power of sucking movement after 5 sec.	No attempt / Weak sucking movement: A. Regular. B. Irregular.	Strong sucking movement, poor stripping: A. Regular. B. Irregular.	Strong regular sucking movement with continuing sequence of 5 movements. Good stripping.	Clenching but no regular sucking.	4 – 5		
Walking Hold infant upright, feet touching bed, neck held straight with fingers.	Absent	Some effort but not continuous with both legs.	At least 2 steps with both legs.	A. Stork posture; no movement. B. Automatic walking.			
Moro One hand supports infant's head in midline, the other the back. Raise infant to 45° and when infant is relaxed let his head fall through 10°. Note if jerky. Repeat 3 times.	No response, or opening of hands only.	Full abduction at the shoulder and extension of the arm	Full abduction but only delayed or partial adduction.	Partial abduction at shoulder and extension of arms followed by smooth adduction. A. Abd>Add B. Abd=Add C. Abd<Add	A. No abduction or adduction; extension only. B. Marked adduction only.	J S	

Neurobehavioural items

	Absent	Present	Exaggerated	Clonus	State	Comment	Asymmetry
Eye appearances Sunset sign, Nerve palsy	Transient nystagmus. Strabismus. Some roving eye movement.	Does not open eyes.	Normal conjugate eye movement.	A. Persistent nystagmus. B. Frequent roving movement. C. Frequent rapid blinks.			
Auditory orientation To rattle. (Note presence of startle.)	A. No reaction. B. Auditory startle but no true orientation.	Brightens and stills; Alerting and shifting of eyes; head may or may not turn to source.	Alerting; prolonged head turns to stimulus each time on both sides	Turning and alerting to stimulus; search with eyes.	S		

Figure 9–3. Continued

Illustration continued on following page

73

Figure 9–3. *Continued*

Item				4	5
Visual orientation To red woollen ball	Does not focus or follow stimulus	Stills; focuses on stimulus; may follow 30° jerkily; does not find stimulus again spontaneously.	Follows 30-60° horizontally; may lose stimulus but finds it again. Brief vertical glance.	Follows with eyes and head horizontally and to some extent vertically, with frowning.	Sustained fixation; follows vertically, horizontally, and in circle.
Alertness	Inattentive; rarely or never responds to direct stimulation	When alert, periods rather brief; rather variable response to orientation.	When alert, alertness moderately sustained; may use stimulus to come to alert state.	Sustained alertness; orientation frequent, reliable to visual but not auditory stimuli.	Continuous alertness, which does not seem to tire, to both auditory and visual stimuli.
Defensive reaction A cloth or hand is placed over the infant's face to partially occlude the nasal airway.	No response.	A. General quietening. B. Non-specific activity with long latency.	Rooting; lateral neck turning; possibly neck stretching.	Swipes with arm	Swipes with arm with rather violent body movement
Peak of excitement	Low level arousal to all stimuli; never > state 3	Infant reaches state 4-5 briefly but predominantly in lower states.	Infant predominantly state 4 or 5; may reach state 6 after stimulation but returns spontaneously to lower state.	Infant reaches state 6 but can be consoled relatively easily.	A. Mainly state 6. Difficult to console, if at all. B. Mainly state 4-5 but if reaches state 6 cannot be consoled.
Irritability Aversive stimuli: Uncover Ventral susp. Undress Moro Pull to sit Walking reflex Prone	No irritable crying to any of the stimuli	Cries to 1-2 stimuli	Cries to 3-4 stimuli	Cries to 5-6 stimuli	Cries to all stimuli
Consolability	Never above state 5 during examination. therefore not needed.	Consoling not needed. Consoles spontaneously.	Consoled by talking, hand on belly or wrapping up.	Consoled by picking up and holding; may need finger in mouth.	Not consolable
Cry	No cry at all.	Only whimpering cry.	Cries to stimuli but normal pitch.	Lusty cry to offensive stimuli; normal pitch.	High-pitched cry, often continuous.

Notes * If asymmetrical or atypical, draw in on nearest figure

Record any abnormal signs (e.g. facial palsy, contractures, etc.). Draw if possible.

Record time after feed:

Examiner:

poorer arm tone, but better trunk tone and head control, and a rather different posture in ventral suspension (Fig. 9–4) than full-term newborn infants. To some extent the development of this tone pattern is dependent on the infant's position in the incubator and may thus vary with nursery practices, depending whether the infant spent most time in the supine, prone, or side position (Figs. 9–5 and 9–6). Premature infants who had the optimal experience of spending most of their growing-up time in an environment with low ambient light, allowing for visual exploration, and in a low-noise environment, allowing for sound discrimination, actually show better visual and auditory responses than full-term infants. This, however, is not so if environmental conditions are unfavorable, i.e.,

overbright or noisy, and there has been little opportunity for them to practice these skills.

These patterns demonstrate the adaptability of the normal preterm infant: The lesser flexor tone does not imply delayed development, nor does better visual function necessarily imply acceleration. They simply show that these infants often follow a different path of development, modified through environmental influences. It is important to remember that these factors make the establishment of universally applicable, absolute norms for tone and motility extremely difficult.

It is possible that this apparent maturity of visual and auditory responses of premature infants at term is something of a false illusion. In our experience with

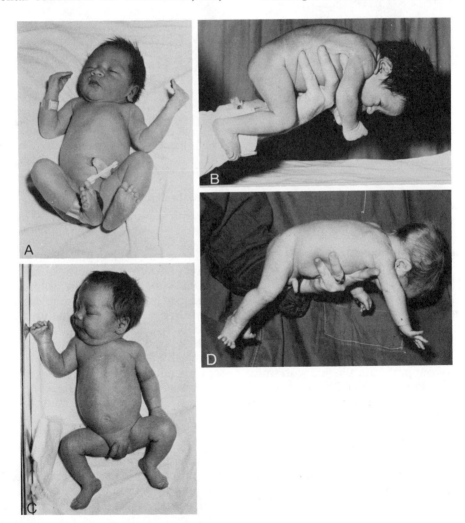

FIGURE 9–4. Comparison of full-term infant in *(A)* supine and *(B)* ventral suspension and preterm infant of 29 weeks' gestation at 11 weeks of age (40 weeks' PMA), *C* and *D*, respectively. Note differences in the posture, with less flexion and adduction of the hips and less flexion of the arms in the preterm infant in the supine and also extension of arms and legs ("spastic") in ventral suspension.

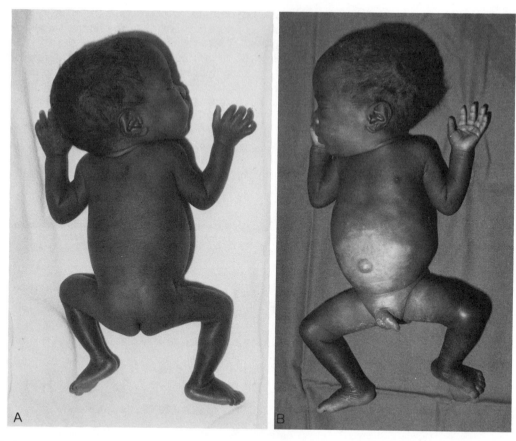

FIGURE 9-5. Premature infant born at 27 weeks' gestation managed in the prone position for eight weeks *(A)*. Note how this produces abduction of the hips and external rotation of the legs.

behavioral examinations (Brazelton, Modified for Prematures), we find that the quality of their visual and auditory pursuit tends to be automatic, somewhat unmodulated in intensity, and often performed only at some cost to regulation of motor tonus (especially face and upper trunk), skin color, integrity, and respiratory control.

P. Gorski

The use of our proforma allows one to study changes in the same infant and has highlighted the importance of repeated examinations. Infants who are initially hypotonic may become hypertonic; if only a single examination were performed, one might examine the infant in a transitional phase when he or she might incorrectly appear either abnormal or normal. By repeated examinations, the speed of resolution of abnormal signs can also be studied.

ABNORMAL FINDINGS IN PREMATURE INFANTS

Premature infants who are very ill during their neonatal period will have an even greater likelihood for a deviant pattern of development, not only because they may have suffered a cerebral insult, but because they will have been exposed to at least some undesirable environmental influences. The more premature they are, the more likely it is that they will have disturbances in physiologic function requiring intervention.

Basically we have been able to recognize two separate patterns of deviant development:

General Delayed Development. The infant may not exhibit any specific abnormal signs, yet development is clearly delayed. When this is most severe, it affects all fields: tone, motility, and orientation. When less severe, limb tone and orientation may be normal, but the development of head and trunk control is delayed, and motility is immature.

Abnormal Signs. The infant, on the other hand, may exhibit a single or combination of deviant signs (Table 9-2), which may be associated with either normal or delayed development. A single "abnormal" sign is not infrequently observed in a completely normal infant; usually this is transient and of no significance.

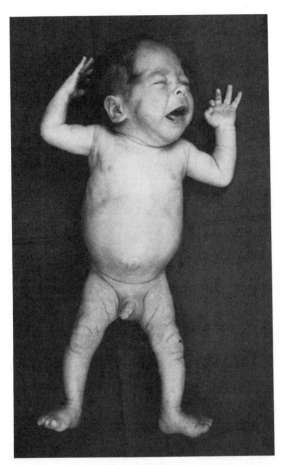

FIGURE 9–6. Abnormal tone pattern in preterm infant born at 30 weeks' gestation. Examination at 11 weeks of age. Note increased flexor tone in the arms with extended legs and arching back. (Compare to Figure 9–4*A*.)

However, the presence of four or more of these abnormal signs on more than one examination is associated with a high risk of abnormal neurologic signs persisting throughout infancy.[7]

PROGNOSTIC SIGNIFICANCE OF ABNORMAL NEUROLOGIC SIGNS IN PREMATURE INFANTS

Any neonatal neurologic examination has a high false-positive rate. This is both understandable and predictable if one takes into account the plasticity of the nervous system.[22] It has been our experience that premature infants born at 34 weeks' gestation or less when found to be normal on our examination at 40 weeks' PMA had more than a 90 per cent chance of being completely normal at 1 year of age, irrespective of any neonatal insults they may have suffered.[6,7] It would appear that if there is the capacity for normalization by this age, the chances for any permanent handicap are small. Infants

TABLE 9–2. Abnormal Neurologic Signs at 40 Weeks' PMA
Arm flexor tone greater than leg flexor tone
Head control abnormal: poor, differential
Increased tremors plus startles
Persistently adducted thumb
Absence of palmar or plantar grasp
Absence of placing
Abnormal Moro reflex (extension only)
Poor orientation (in state 4) (visual or auditory)
Irritability
Asymmetry > 2 points in one limb, 1 point in all limbs

who showed only poor tone (or delayed development) but no other abnormal signs rarely showed any major handicap at follow-up. On the other hand, 65 per cent of infants who had four or more abnormal signs in the neonatal period had abnormal neurologic signs at follow-up, often with functional disability. Although the neurologic examination was able to identify the infants with possible later abnormalities, the nature of the abnormality in the neonatal period bore no relation to the type of deficit observed at 1 year of age.

The chances for normal outcome were better for neurologically abnormal infants *without* evidence of periventricular-intraventricular hemorrhage on ultrasonography in the neonatal period than for those with evidence. Prediction from imaging shows that there is a statistical correlation[23] between the presence and size of the lesion on ultrasonography in the neonatal period and later outcome, but there is no way of predicting the outcome for the individual infant.[24] The absence of any lesion on ultrasonography does not preclude any child from later major handicap, nor does the presence of abnormality preclude normal development. The neonatal brain has incredible plasticity for recovery. On the whole, the presence or absence of small hemorrhages has no relation to outcome, while large parenchymal hemorrhages tend to produce sensory or motor lesions, but not invariably. Mild periventricular leukomalacia when associated with small cyst formation usually produces no sequelae, but extensive cyst formation is associated with a high risk of cerebral palsy and visual abnormalities. (See Appendix D for review of studies of outcomes after intracranial hemorrhage.)

There have been some claims for the predictive value of the neonatal EEG and of evoked potential studies. There are, however, no published comparisons between these investigations and neonatal neurologic assessments. It has been our experience that in infants in whom clinical normalization occurs, normalization of neurophysiologic parameters also occurs. In infants who remain neurologically abnormal with persistent abnormal neurophysiologic findings, the prognosis is poor. However, normalization of the EEG and evoked potentials in a neurologically abnormal infant does not necessarily improve the outlook.

ABNORMAL SIGNS IN TERM INFANTS

The neurologic proforma is equally applicable to the full-term infant; the abnormalities observed are similar, but the significance of the various signs is probably different.

Prognostic Significance. Hypotonia with poor responsiveness in a full-term infant is not due to delayed development, but is an abnormal function and is thus of equal significance to all the abnormalities listed in Table 9–2. The neurologic proforma signs again allow for easy comparison of repeated examinations. In our experience, it is not any individual sign, or even the initial severity of the symptoms, but the speed of recovery that is the best guide to prognosis.

WHEN TO WORRY

Head Circumference Crossing Percentile Lines. (See also Chapter 5.) Often head growth is more rapid than increase in weight or length around 40 weeks' PMA as catch-up growth occurs. This growth, however, rarely crosses more than one percentile line. Head circumference crossing more than two percentile lines needs investigation to exclude progressive ventricular dilatation or subdural effusion, particularly if the infant is known to have had a traumatic delivery or an intracranial hemorrhage in the neonatal period.

Absence of Auditory Response. Newborn infants from 30 weeks' PMA onward are able to orient to a rattle. An infant's repeated failure to respond to a rattle usually means a 60 dB hearing loss. The fact that the infant is said to have previously passed a hearing screening test in the intensive care unit does not necessarily exclude diminished hearing. If the test was done too early, the intensity for screening might have been above this level. An infant with relatively mild sensory loss might have become impaired later because of superimposed conductive hearing loss, to which these infants are prone. Also, hearing loss due to viral infection, such as cyto-

megalovirus, might not become manifest until later in infancy. Signs of abnormal auditory response and vocalization include (1) not localizing a high-pitched rattle at 6 months, or (2) absence of two-syllable babble at 9 months. (See Chapter 12 for further information on assessment of hearing.)

Absence of Visual Responses to a Red Ball. Under optimal conditions and in an optimal state, full-term infants and preterm infants reaching 40 weeks' PMA should be able to track a red ball horizontally and vertically (Fig. 9–1). The absence of this response may indicate inattentiveness, fragility secondary to continued illness, or the presence of disease in the visual pathway. On the other hand, the presence of this response *does not exclude* future abnormalities. Infants who are cortically blind can often track at this age, although they lose the ability at 2 to 3 months of age. Those with significant retrolental fibroplasia can also track, but the quality of the response is often poor.

> The symmetry of tracking to either side of midline should be regarded as seriously as the quality of attention itself. Asymmetric following responses should direct a search for unilateral structural central nervous system damage.
>
> *P. Gorski*

Abnormal Tone Pattern. When abnormal tone patterns are observed, we reassess the infant, and if the findings persist, we refer the patient to a physical therapist.

Head lag associated with marked fisting, increased flexor tone in the arms, and increased extensor tone in the trunk and legs with or without increased adductor tone is the most common pattern in infants who later develop cerebral palsy. If this pattern is seen the infant should be reassessed, and if these findings persist even when the infant is quiet, we would advocate early referral to a physical therapist. Other specific findings include adductor spasm, limitation of the popliteal angle to less than 90 degrees, and limitation of dorsiflexion of the angle to 90 degrees. However, it should be emphasized that by no means do all of these infants develop cerebral palsy (Figs. 9–7 and 9–8).

Marked asymmetry of tone or reflexes, if persistent on two or more consecutive examinations and particularly if associated with deviation of the head to one side, is an indication for referral of the infant to a physical therapist for further evaluation, since these may be the early signs of hemiplegia. Abnormal postural reactions are also of concern, specifically, no forward or sideway protective reflex at 9 months

Text continued on page 83

Name GCI

HOSP.	NO.	D.O.B./TIME	WEIGHT	HEIGHT	E.D.D. L.N.M.P.	E.D.D. U/snd.
RACE	SEX	DATE OF EXAM AGE **11w**	HEAD CIRC.			

GESTATIONAL ASSESSMENT   SCORE   WEEKS **30·5**

STATES
1. Deep sleep, no movement, regular breathing.
2. Light sleep, eyes shut, some movement.
3. Dozing, eyes opening and closing.
4. Awake, eyes open, minimal movement.
5. Wide awake, vigorous movement.
6. Crying.

(Right-hand columns: State · Comment · Asymmetry) State value: **4–6**

Habituation (≤ state 3)

awake

Light
Repetitive flashlight stimuli (10) with 5 sec. gap.
Shutdown = 2 consecutive negative responses

- No response
- A. Blink response to first stimuli. B. Tonic blink response. C. Variable response.
- A. Shutdown of movement but blink persists 2-5 stimuli. B. Complete shutdown 2-5 stimuli.
- A. Shutdown of movement but blink persists 6-10 stimuli. B. Complete shutdown 6-10 stimuli.
- A. Equal response to 10 stimuli. B. Infant comes to fully alert state. C. Startles + major responses throughout.

Rattle
Repetitive stimulus (10) with 5 sec gap.

- No response
- A. Slight movement to first stimulus. B. Variable response
- Startle or movement 2-5 stimuli, then shutdown
- Startle or movement 6-10 stimuli, then shutdown
- A. B. C.] Grading as above

Movement & tone

Posture * (At rest – predominant)
Undress infant

Abnormal postures:
A. Opisthotonus.
B. Unusual leg extension.
C. Asymm.tonic neck reflex

(hips abducted) ... (hips abducted) ... (hips adducted)

Arm recoil
Infant supine. Take both hands, extend parallel to the body; hold approx. 2 secs. and release.

- No flexion within 5 sec.
- Partial flexion at elbow >100° within 4-5 sec.
- Arms flex at elbow to <100° within 2-3 sec.
- Sudden jerky flexion at elbow immediately after release to <60°
- Difficult to extend; arm snaps back forcefully

Arm traction
Infant supine; head midline; grasp wrist, slowly pull arm to vertical. Angle of arm scored and resistance noted at moment infant is initially lifted off and watched until shoulder off mattress. Do other arm.

- Arm remains fully extended
- Weak flexion maintained only momentarily
- Arm flexed at elbow to 140° and maintained 5 sec.
- Arm flexed at approx. 100° and maintained
- Strong flexion of arm <100° and maintained

Leg recoil
First flex hips for 5 secs, then extend both legs of infant by traction on ankles; hold down on the bed for 2 secs and release.

- No flexion within 5 sec.
- Incomplete flexion of hips within 5 sec.
- Complete flexion within 5 sec.
- Instantaneous complete flexion
- Legs cannot be extended; snap back forcefully

Leg traction
Infant supine. Grasp leg near ankle and slowly pull toward vertical until buttocks 1-2" off. Note resistance at knee and score angle. Do other leg.

- No flexion
- Partial flexion, rapidly lost
- Knee flexion 140-160° and maintained
- Knee flexion 100-140° and maintained
- Strong resistance; flexion <100°

FIGURE 9–7. Proforma of the infant in Figure 9–6. Note abnormal posture. Arm recoil greater than leg recoil. Poor head control. Excessive tremors and startles. Absent placing. Absent Moro. (Compare to Figure 9–3.) Abnormal eye movement but good oriculation. This infant at follow-up had spastic quadriparesis that caused developmental delay and cortical blindness.

Illustration continued on following page

Popliteal angle

Infant supine. Approximate knee and thigh to abdomen; extend leg by gentle pressure with index finger behind ankle.

	180-160° R L	150-140° R L	130-120° R L	110-90° R L	<90° R L

Head control, post. neck m.

Grasp infant by shoulders and raise to sitting position; allow head to fall forward; wait 30 sec.

No attempt to raise head	Unsuccessful attempt to raise head upright	Head raised smoothly to upright in 30 sec. but not maintained.	Head raised smoothly to upright in 30 sec. and maintained	Head cannot be flexed forward *

Head control, ant. neck m.

Allow head to fall backward as you hold shoulders; wait 30 sec.

Grading as above	Grading as above	Grading as above	Grading as above	

Head lag

Pull infant toward sitting posture by traction on both wrists. Also note arm flexion. *

Ventral suspension *

Hold infant in ventral suspension; observe curvature of back, flexion of limbs and relation of head to trunk.

Head raising, prone

Infant in prone position with head in midline.

No response	Rolls head to one side	Weak effort to raise head and turns raised head to one side	Infant lifts head, nose and chin off	Strong prolonged head lifting

Arm release, prone

Head in midline. Infant in prone position; arms extended alongside body with palms up.

No effort	Some effort and wriggling	Flexion effort but neither wrist brought to nipple level	One or both wrists brought at least to nipple level without excessive body movement	strong body movement with both wrists brought to face or 'press-ups'

Spont. body movement

If no spont. movement try to elicit by cutaneous stim.

None or minimal	A. Sluggish. B. Random, incoordinated. C. Mainly stretching.	Smooth movements alternating with random, stretching, athetoid or jerky	Smooth alternating movements of arms and legs with medium speed and intensity	Mainly: A. Jerky movement. B. Athetoid movement. C. Other abnormal movement.

Tremors

Mark: Fast (>6/sec) or Slow (<6/sec)

No tremor	Tremors only in state 5-6	Tremors only in sleep or after Moro and startles	Some tremors in state 4	tremulousness in all states

Startles

No startles	Startles to sudden noise, Moro, bang on table only	Occasional spontaneous startle	2-5 spontaneous startles	6+ spontaneous startles

Abnormal movement or posture

No abnormal movement	A. Hands clenched but open intermittently. B. Hands do not open with Moro.	A. Some mouthing movement. B. Intermittent adducted thumb	A. Persistently adducted thumb. B. Hands clenched	A. Continuous mouthing movement. B. Convulsive movements.

4-6

1
2

Figure 9–7. Continued

Reflexes

Tendon reflexes
Biceps jerk
Knee jerk
Ankle jerk

Palmar grasp
Head in midline. Put index finger from ulnar side into hand and gently press palmar surface. **Never** touch dorsal side of hand.

Rooting
Infant supine, head midline. Touch each corner of the mouth in turn (stroke laterally).

Sucking
Infant supine; place index finger (pad towards palate) in infant's mouth; judge power of sucking movement after 5 sec.

Walking
Hold infant upright, feet touching bed, neck held straight with fingers. **no placing no wt. support**

Moro
One hand supports infant's head in midline, the other the back. Raise infant to 45° and when infant is relaxed let his head fall through 10°. Note if jerky. Repeat 3 times.

Neurobehavioural items

Eye appearances
Nerve palsy   ?6th

Auditory orientation
To rattle. (Note presence of startle.)

	Absent	Present	Exaggerated	Clonus	State	Comment	Asymmetry
Tendon reflexes	Absent	Present	Exaggerated	Clonus			
Palmar grasp	Absent	Medium strength and sustained flexion for several secs.	Strong flexion; contraction spreads to forearm.	Very strong; infant easily lifts off couch			
Rooting	No response	A. Partial weak head turn but no mouth opening. B. Mouth opening, no head turn.	Full head turning, with or without mouth opening.	Mouth opening with very jerky head turning			
Sucking	No attempt	Weak sucking movement: A. Regular. B. Irregular.	Strong sucking movement, poor stripping: A. Regular. B. Irregular.	Strong regular sucking movement with continuing sequence of 5 movements. Good stripping.	Clenching but no regular sucking.		
Walking	Absent	Some effort but not continuous with both legs.	At least 2 steps with both legs.	A. Stork posture; no movement. B. Automatic walking.			
Moro	No response, or opening of hands only.	Full abduction but only delayed or partial adduction.	Partial abduction at shoulder and extension of arms followed by smooth adduction. A. Abd>Add B. Abd=Add C. Abd<Add	A. No abduction or adduction; extension only.		**	
Eye appearances	Strabismus. Some roving eye movement.	Does not open eyes.	Normal conjugate eye movement.	A. Persistent nystagmus. B. Frequent roving movement. C. Frequent rapid blinks.		S	
Auditory orientation	A. No reaction. B. Auditory startle but no true orientation.	Brightens and stills; Alerting and shifting of eyes; head may or may not turn to source.	Alerting; prolonged head turns to stimulus with eyes closed.	Turning and alerting to stimulus each time on both sides		S	

Figure 9-7. *Continued*

Illustration continued on following page

Visual orientation To red woollen ball	Does not focus or follow stimulus	Stills; focuses on stimulus; may follow 30° jerkily; does not find stimulus again spontaneously.	Follows 30-60° horizontally; may lose stimulus but finds it again.Brief vertical glance.	Follows with eyes and head horizontally and to some extent vertically, with frowning	Sustained fixation; follows vertically, horizontally, and in circle.
Alertness	Inattentive; rarely or never responds to direct stimulation	When alert, periods rather brief; rather variable response to orientation.	When alert, alertness moderately sustained may use stimulus to come to alert state.	Sustained alertness; orientation frequent, reliable to visual but not auditory stimuli	Continuous alertness, which does not seem to tire, to both auditory and visual stimuli
Defensive reaction A cloth or hand is placed over the infant's face to partially occlude the nasal airway.	No response.	A.General quietening. B.Non-specific activity with long latency.	Rooting; lateral neck turning; possibly neck stretching.	Swipes with arm	Swipes with arm with rather violent body movement
Peak of excitement	Low level arousal to all stimuli; never > state 3	Infant reaches state 4-5 briefly but predominantly in lower states.	Infant predominantly state 4 or 5; may reach state 6 after stimulation but returns spontaneously to lower state.	Infant reaches state 6 but can be consoled relatively easily.	A. Mainly state 6. Difficult to console, if at all. B. Mainly state 4-5 but if reaches state 6 cannot be consoled.
Irritability Aversive stimuli: Uncover Ventral susp. Undress Moro Pull to sit Walking reflex Prone	No irritable crying to any of the stimuli	Cries to 1-2 stimuli	Cries to 3-4 stimuli	Cries to 5-6 stimuli	Cries to all stimuli
Consolability	Never above state 5 during examination, therefore not needed.	Consoling not needed. Consoles spontaneously.	Consoled by talking, hand on belly or wrapping up.	Consoled by picking up and holding; may need finger in mouth.	Not consolable
Cry	No cry at all.	Only whimpering cry.	Cries to stimuli but normal pitch.	Lusty cry to offensive stimuli; normal pitch.	High-pitched cry, often continuous.

Notes * If asymmetrical or atypical, draw in on nearest figure

Record any abnormal signs (e.g. facial palsy, contractures, etc.). Draw if possible.

Acuity½ only no pattern diff.
*retracted shoulders in sitting
**minimal abd+add of moro

Record time after feed:

Examiner:

Figure 9–7. Continued

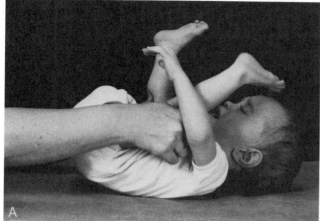
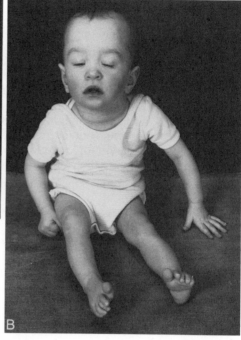

FIGURE 9–8. Asymmetrically tight popliteal angle (right tighter than left) in premature infant born at 28 weeks' gestation, examined at 10 months of age *(A)*. The infant has hemiplegia *(B)*. Note abnormal posture of right hand and right foot.

or on lateral tilting (head below spine) at 9 months.

Asymmetry of placing reaction and asymmetry of plantar grasp, if persistent, are often the only asymmetries observed in the neonatal period in infants with unilateral parenchymal lesions involving the parietal areas. They probably represent sensory impairment, and thus the infant would benefit by additional sensory stimulation on the affected side to minimize abnormal posture.

Marked Irritability, Tremors, Startles, and Poor Feeding. Although there is probably little that can be done about the cause, the presence of these symptoms produces maternal anxiety. Counseling the mother how to handle and feed her infant may help to intercept the vicious circle leading to abnormal attachment.[25]

> Ask the mother to demonstrate her feeding technique. Particular attention should be directed toward positioning of the infant's head and neck and support for shoulders and hips during nippling. Slight (15 degrees) flexion of head and neck, support for internal rotation of shoulders, and flexion at the base of the trunk are essential to facilitate coordinated suck and swallow.
>
> *P. Gorski*

Maternal Concern. The physician should always worry when the mother is concerned or comments that:

"It's difficult to part the infant's legs to put a diaper on."
"When I try to sit him down or carry him around, he always goes stiff."
"It is difficult to wash under his arms."
"It's hard to straighten his arms out to push them through the sleeves."
"When I bounce him on my knees, he goes onto his toes and makes his legs stiff."

Abnormal Milestones. Concern should arise if the following milestones are not normal for corrected age, i.e., if the infant is:

Not grasping at 6 months
Not rolling from side to side at 6 months
Not transferring objects at 9 months or showing other signs of midline activity
Not securing a dangling ring at 9 months
Not crawling at 1 year

Infants who appear to be at the greatest risk of future motor handicap are, in particular, (1) those showing marked hemisyndromes in association with functional deficit and developmental delay; and (2) those with persistent head lag beyond 6 months of age, in association with marked fisting, variable tone in arms, poor trunk control, and popliteal angles that are tight at 90 degrees or less. These infants usually have overt cerebral palsy by 1 year of age.

WHEN TO REASSURE

In many high-risk infants who show some persistent abnormal signs in early infancy there is a tendency to normalization during the second year of life. This is particularly so in infants with mild hemisyndromes who exhibit extensor hypertonia and shoulder retraction. The latter abnormality is most common in neurologically compromised infants and prematures; if present by itself it is not a marker for later motor handicap.[26] Times to reassure the parents include:

1. When there is mild or transient asymmetry in tone
2. When isolated or less than four "abnormal" neurologic signs are present
3. When there is mild to moderate hypotonia in a premature infant
4. When there is apparently spastic posture in ventral suspension in a premature infant (Fig. 9–4)
5. When any of the following is an *isolated* finding:
   a. A tendency to tiptoe
   b. Retracted shoulders
   c. Everted feet
   d. Tight popliteal angle of 100 degrees
   e. Mild hypotonia

WHEN TO INTERVENE

In the following circumstances, however, intervention is indicated:

1. When several of the items listed under When to Worry are present
2. When any of the When to Worry situations persists (Referral to a neurologist or physical therapist is appropriate.)
3. In infants with excessive hypertonia and shoulder retraction. Although normalization occurs in infants with shoulder retraction, the incidence of problems at school age is much greater.[27] Although this abnormality does not seem to interfere with gross motor development, it does prevent midline activity and thus interferes with bimanual manipulation. Therefore, it is felt that this is an area for early intervention by a physical therapist, who teaches the mother optimum handling and manipulation.

SUMMARY

The goal of the physician is to recognize at the earliest possible time sensory neural handicap and developmental delay in these infants, so that by early intervention the severity of the deficit can be managed. It is thus an advantage if early examinations err toward overestimating rather than underestimating the possibility of such an abnormality. This, however, also has its dangers and may give rise to other hazards. Communication of the physician's concern to the mother may increase her anxiety and further disturb the already fragile attachment, leading to behavioral problems and further handicapping the infant's development. We thus feel that while the presence of early abnormalities should keep the physician alerted, it is more important to communicate the need of *appropriate* sensory input in all these infants than the presence of abnormal signs, and their possible implications, as they may yet be transient. Proper counseling and guidance of the mother will help to alleviate her anxiety, thus also reducing the effect of these less appreciated hazards on these vulnerable infants.

References

1. Howard J, Parmelee AH Jr, Kopp, CB, et al.: A neurologic comparison of pre-term and full-term infants at term conceptional age. J Pediatr 88:995, 1976.
2. Kurtzberg D, Vaughan HG Jr, Daum C, et al.: Neurobehavioral performance of low-birthweight infants at 40 weeks' conceptional age: Comparison with normal full-term infants. Dev Med Child Neurol 21:590, 1979.
3. Palmer P, Dubowitz LMS, Verghote M, et al.: Neurological and neurobehavioural differences between preterm infants at term and full term newborn infants. Neuropediatrics 13:183, 1982.
4. Brown JK, Purvis JR, Forfar JO, et al.: Neurological aspects of perinatal asphyzia. Dev Med Child Neurol 16:567, 1974.
5. Nelson KB, Ellenberg JH: Neonatal signs as predictors of cerebral palsy. Pediatrics 64:225, 1979.
6. Bierman-vanEedenburg MEC, Jurgens-Van der Zee AD, Olinga AA, et al.: Predictive value of neonatal neurological examination: A follow-up at 18 months. Dev Med Child Neurol 23:296, 1981.
7. Dubowitz LMS, Dubowitz V, Palmer PG, et al.: Correlation of neurologic assessment in the preterm newborn infant with outcome at one year. J Pediatr 105:452, 1984.
8. Paine R, Oppe T: Neurological Examinations of Infants and Children. Clinics in Developmental Medicine no. 20/21. Philadelphia, J.B. Lippincott Company, 1966.
9. Andre-Thomas de Ajuriaguerra J: Etude Semiologique du Tonus Musculaire. Paris, Editions Medicales Flammarion, 1949.
10. Dargassies SS: Neurological Development in Full-Term and Premature Neonates. Amsterdam, Elsevier/North Holland/Excerpta Medica, 1977.
11. Prechtl H: The Neurological Examination of the Full-Term Newborn Infant. Clinics in Developmental Medicine no. 63. Philadelphia, J.B. Lippincott Company, 1977.

12. Parmelee AH, Michaelis MD: Neurological Examination of the Newborn. In Hellmuth J (ed.): *Exceptional Infant.* New York, Brunner/Mazel, 1971, Vol 2, pp 3–23.
13. Brazelton TB: Neonatal Behavioral Assessment Scale. Clinics in Developmental Medicine no. 50. Philadelphia, J.B. Lippincott Company, 1973.
14. Dubowitz LMS, Dubowitz V: The Neurological Assessment of the Preterm and Full-Term Newborn Infant. Clinics in Developmental Medicine no. 79. Philadelphia, J.B. Lippincott Company, 1981.
15. Frankenberg W, Dobbs J: The Denver Developmental Screening Test. J Pediatr 71:181, 1967.
16. Elliman AM, Bryan EM, Elliman AD, et al.: Denver Developmental Screening Test and preterm infants. Arch Dis Child 60:20, 1985.
17. Amiel-Tilson C: A method for neurological evaluation within the first year of life. Curr Probl Pediatr 7:1, 1976.
18. Milani-Comparetti A, Gidoni EA: Routine developmental examination in normal and retarded children. Dev Med Child Neurol 9:631, 1967.
19. Touwen BCL: Examination of the Child with Minor Neurological Dysfunction, 2nd ed. Clinics in Developmental Medicine no. 71. Philadelphia, J.B. Lippincott Company, 1979.
20. Capute AJ, Accardo PJ, Vinind EPG, et al.: Primitive Reflex Profile. Baltimore, University Park Press, 1978.
21. Griffiths R: The Abilities of Babies. London, University of London Press, 1954.
22. Prechtl HFR: The study of neural development as a perspective of clinical problems. In Connolly KJ, Prechtl HFR (eds.): Maturation and Development: Biological and Physiological Perspectives. Clinics in Developmental Medicine no. 77/78. Philadelphia, J.B. Lippincott Company, 1981.
23. Shankaran S, Slovis TL, Bedard MP, et al.: Sonographic classification of intracranial hemorrhage: A prognostic indicator of mortality, morbidity, and short-term neurologic outcome. J Pediatr 100:469, 1982.
24. Fawer C-L, Levene MI, Dubowitz LMS: Intraventricular hemorrhage in a preterm neonate: Discordance between clinical course and ultrasound scan. Neuropediatr 14:242, 1983.
25. Finnie, NR: Handling the Young Cerebral Palsied Child at Home, 2nd ed. London, Heinmann, 1981.
26. Touwen, BCL, Hadders-Algra M: Hyperextension of neck and trunk and shoulder retraction in infancy— A prognostic study. Neuropediatr 14:202, 1983.
27. Drillien CM: Abnormal neurological signs in the first year of life in low-birthweight infants: Possible prognostic significance. Dev Med Child Neurol 14:705, 1972.

Recommended Reading

Brazelton TB: Neonatal Behavioral Assessment Scale. Clinics in Developmental Medicine no. 50. Philadelphia, J.B. Lippincott Company, 1973.

Dubowitz LMS, Dubowitz V, Palmer PG, et al: Correlation of neurologic assessment in the preterm newborn infant with outcome at one year. J Pediatr 105:452, 1984.

Howard J, Parmelee AH Jr, Kopp CB, et al.: A neurologic comparison of pre-term and full-term infants at term conceptional age. J Pediatr 88:995, 1976.

Palmer P, Dubowitz LMS, Verghote M, et al.: Neurological and neurobehavioural differences between preterm infants at term and full-term newborn infants. Neuropediatrics 13:183, 1982.

Parmelee AH, Michaelis MD: Neurological examination of the newborn. In Hellmuth J (ed.): Exceptional Infant. New York, Brunner/Mazel, 1971, Vol 2, pp 3–23.

Prechtl H: The Neurological Examination of the Full-Term Newborn Infant. Clinics in Developmental Medicine no. 63. Philadelphia, J.B. Lippincott Company, 1977.

10

PHYSICAL THERAPY:
Follow-Up of the Special-Care Infant

VALERIE ANN THOM, M.A., R.P.T.

The assessment and management of sensorimotor development overlaps with the child's total development and has the most potential to be helpful when testing and treatment are approached in that context. The complexity of predicting outcome is well known; even with a specific diagnosis, one can seldom say exactly how an individual child will progress in fulfillment of his or her developmental potential, because this depends on so many variables. This section discusses the integration of sensorimotor findings into the context of the medical history and family and cultural setting to assist the pediatrician in making practical decisions concerning the indications for further motor assessment and therapy.

Applying the concept that there is a continuum of neurologic problems from the extreme (e.g., severe cerebral palsy) to more subtle neurointegrative dysfunctions of the central nervous system, we will focus the discussion here on the assessment and management of motor dysfunction or delay during the first two years of life. It is beyond the scope of this book to address the school-aged child with soft neurologic signs and/or behavioral and learning difficulties, although concern exists that these more subtle

neurologic deficits may be over-represented in this population.

> They may be perhaps even more handicapping than the gross motor deficits with respect to intellectual, social, and psychological outcome!
>
> *P. Gorski*

SENSORIMOTOR DEVELOPMENT IN PRETERM INFANTS

DIFFERENCES BETWEEN PRETERM AND TERM INFANTS

As every pediatrician knows, the first question parents of at-risk infants ask after "Will my baby survive?" is "Will my baby be normal?" The practicing clinician knows that for the preterm infant *different* from full-term infant development does not necessarily mean *abnormal*. What is normal or optimal for the developing preterm infant may vary considerably from what is optimal for the full-term infant. As Pape and Wigglesworth state, "There are greater (anatomical) differences between the brain of a 28-week-gestation infant and that of a 36-week-gestation infant than there are between the brains of a 3-month-old baby and an adult."[1]

There is also evidence that the effects of a specific brain lesion on sensorimotor development in very low birth weight infants differ significantly from those in full-term infants. In addition, there are important differences in developmental rates and capabilities of preterm infants with normal as well as abnormal outcomes, both during and after the immediate neonatal period, since various developmental functions, such as active and passive tone, mature at different rates and take different times to "catch up."

Although the rapid advances in the field of neonatology have greatly improved survival and outcome for premature infants, too often these babies are discussed as a homogeneous group. However, just as with full-term infants, differences in age, birth weight, number and type of medical complications and illnesses, and individual characteristics all influence developmental parameters.

In particular, motor development of preterm infants is influenced by the degree of prematurity, as well as by associated medical conditions during the prenatal, postnatal, and later infancy stages. Postnatal illness has a substantial impact on motor and interactive skills.

However, within these medical risk groups, the organizing capacity of the family probably has the greatest influence on high vs low functioning and developmental outcome.

P. Gorski

"Normal" Findings in Preterm Infants. Table 10–1 summarizes several "normal" sensorimotor findings in preterm infants that are commonly observed at follow-up visits during the first six months of life. (See also Chapter 9.)

MUSCLE TONE. Differences in muscle tone between preterm and full-term infants are found frequently. Drillien[2] reported that approximately 50 per cent of infants of birth weight less than 1500 gm whom she examined had atypical, "stiff" muscle tone and jitteriness in the first few months and that in the majority of cases the stiffness resolved. Clinically, preterm infants may appear advanced in their head control and extensor tone during the first three to four months. Perhaps this is due to their having had more time to practice these skills outside the constraints of the womb, along with decreased need to overcome the physiologic flexor tone and tightness the term infant must deal with.

TABLE 10–1. Common "Normal" Sensorimotor Behavior in Preterm Infants: First Six Months

SENSORIMOTOR COMPONENT	SENSORIMOTOR BEHAVIOR
Muscle Tone	Tendency toward relative dominance of extensor tone over flexor tone (neck, trunk, legs)
	May arch neck and upper trunk into extension with associated shoulder elevation and scapular retraction
	Usually less flexor tone development in the arms than full-term age-mate
	May have "jittery" quality to movements (especially during first 3 months of life)
Movement	Tendency toward decreased midline movements of arms (but not obligate or dominant)
	Less frequent antigravity movement of legs than full-term infant
	Wide range of movements of arms and legs
	May achieve some milestones early (e.g., rolling from prone to supine; advanced head control)
	More likely to stand on tiptoe in supported stance (but range of motion should be within normal limits)
Primitive Reflexes	May have retention of primitive reflexes beyond those expected in full-term age-mate

MOVEMENT PATTERNS. These infants also have notable differences in movement patterns, and their greater extensor than flexor tone may express itself qualitatively as neck arched into extension, elevated and retracted shoulders, retracted scapulae, extended with a relatively immobile pelvis (but occasionally vs continually present), decreased midline movements of arms (not to be confused with persistent head-arm asymmetry to one side), infrequent antigravity movement of the legs, weight bearing on the toes in supported standing (but full passive heel-cord range of motion). A 2-month-old (corrected age) infant might roll from prone to supine, whereas this advanced extensor tone would be of concern in a 2-month-old infant born at term. Primitive reflexes may also persist longer in preterm infants than is normal in full-term infants. (See also Chapter 9.)

Because of these differences, developmental testing of preterm infants often results in motor scores that are more affected than mental scores.

GUIDELINES FOR PEDIATRIC EVALUATION

The following guidelines may be helpful in evaluating management needs of high-risk infants:

1. *Make careful and frequent serial examinations* during early infancy to identify concerns and determine whether abnormal findings persist or signs of developmental delay become apparent. In infants in whom motor disability is not already obvious during the neonatal period, motor deficits can usually be diagnosed by age 6 to 9 months in term infants and within the first year in preterm infants.

> This recommendation for careful motor assessment at 3 to 6 months of age is extremely important, since neonatal neurologic evaluations often may fail to identify infants with abnormal developmental courses.
>
> *P. Gorski*

2. *Consider whether or not the infant's observed behavior* (for corrected age in preterm infants) *is interfering with the developmental tasks* the child should presently be practicing and enjoying. Of equal importance, is it interfering with the parents' ability to enjoy their child's progress? For example, it is common for the preterm infant to show preference for increased trunk and neck extension associated with elevated shoulders and retracted scapulae (the elbows are often also flexed with this pattern) during the first four months of life. If the pediatrician finds on serial examination that the child cannot reverse this pattern (children should, at all ages, be able to reverse to normal a preferential pattern or posture of movement) or that by six months the baby still shows a predominance of this pattern, then concern should begin. At this age, this pattern interferes with normal beginning eye-hand coordination activities, as well as with early swiping and reaching activities. Fairly simple suggestions for handling and positioning may help reverse the dominance of such a pattern and thus foster desired development. Suggestions to the parents might include having the infant lie on the side (with the head aligned with the trunk by a small blanket roll). This position (as opposed to lying supine) helps decrease scapular retraction and elbow flexion and takes advantage of gravity, so that the arms can come together. In this position the baby can see more easily and explore his or her hands. In the side-lying position, or as the parents hold the baby in their arms with the baby's scapulae protracted and the arms together, gentle stroking of the back of the hands will encourage hand opening. An open, moving hand is more interesting to a baby, and therefore it is more likely to catch the infant's visual attention and facilitate eye-hand coordination.

3. *Listen carefully to the parent's concerns* and observe the baby closely in response to the parent's observations. Parents are most often the first to know something is wrong. Common early comments of parents and corresponding findings on examination are listed in Table 10–2.

> When parents recite concerns about development of the ICN graduate, the burden is on the primary care physician to establish that the child is normal.
>
> *M. Abbott*

4. *Look for a combination of signs of concern* rather than a single sign. (See also Chapter 9.) Remember that the full-term asphyxiated newborn may first have proximal muscle weakness and later show a picture of muscular hypertonicity. The full-term baby is more vulnerable to spastic quadriplegic or hemiplegic forms of cerebral palsy and less commonly to the athetoid form. In contrast, the most common form of cerebral palsy in low birth weight infants is spastic diplegia in which the lower extremities and trunk are more involved than the upper extremities.

REFERRAL TO PHYSICAL THERAPY

DECIDING TO REFER

Whether or not to refer for further assessment and/or treatment is an easier decision to make when the parents share or initiate the concern than when the parent is one whom the pediatrician senses would be more burdened than relieved by the suggestion that a problem might be possible.

> Easier, but no more helpful than when the pediatrician initiates concern or first airs unspoken parental concerns.
>
> *P. Gorski*

As Brazelton has so aptly stated: "No longer can we hide behind our wish that parents don't know if you don't tell them when a baby is at risk for being impaired. Instead, we can substitute the idea that if we want to and will provide an umbrella for them, they will respond appropriately to a potentially impaired child, and work to alleviate what may be a deficit."[3]

Parmelee[4] suggests that it is helpful to confirm

TABLE 10–2. Signs and Symptoms Alerting Physician to Need for Further Neurobehavioral Assessment

SIGN OR SYMPTOM	CLIN. EXAM	PARENT'S REPORT
Feeding and sucking difficulties and/or excessive gagging		X
Persistent asymmetry in movements and/or postures	X	
Early consistent preference for one hand	X	
Baby feels "stiff" with diaper changes, bathing, holding		X
Baby is not kicking or moving legs	X	X
Early rolling from prone to supine and "stiff" extended legs in stance without normal balance responses	X	X
Consistent toe walking with associated loss of range of motion of heel cord (check shoe wear and bruises on legs, indicating frequent falling)	X	
Child seems "lazy"; able to do gross motor activities, but will not	X	
Full-term infant: Marked resistance to passive flexion of neck when not fussy or crying		X
Full-term infant: Popliteal angle (subtended angle) greater than 10° after 9 months (tested with hips flexed to 90°)*	X	
Full-term infant: High degree of flexor tone in arms (after 3 months) and/or extensor tone in legs (from birth onward) with little variation in patterns	X	
Difficult to open hands to clean; lint gets caught about neck, arm, and leg creases		X
Sits independently on floor, but has marked tilting posteriorly of pelvis and rounded back; alternately sits between internally rotated hips, but no other on-floor sitting postures available to child; usually associated with limited straight-leg raising	X	
Marked hypotonia with associated paucity of movement	X	
Appears frightened of movement (cries, startles); dislikes having clothes changed, having shirt put over head, bath		X
Postures and movements are inconsistent in various positions (e.g., high degree of developing extension in supine position, but collapses into flexion in supported sitting)	X	

* (See Recommended Reading, Reade E, et al.)

the parents' observations of a lag, rather than to try to assure it away, since the latter produces a credibility gap. Physician and parent can learn to worry together, and, in this way, the physician can help empower the parents to be sensitive observers of their child. Parents can also be told honestly that further assessment and help may provide suggestions to assist the child to enjoy more the activities he or she is ready to be learning.

> Parents have so much hope for their children's future that when the ICN graduate returns home, the memory of the baby's neonatal course can generate considerable fear and anxiety. The physical therapist can often show parents various exercises that both parents and baby will enjoy. Even if the baby is doing exceptionally well, this will give them an opportunity to have a direct effect (real or imagined) on their baby's outcome. It also gives the parents of a handicapped child a clearer understanding of their baby's problems, and therefore they become better historians.
>
> *A. Rosen*

The timing of referral for further motor assessment is also important. Once the parents and physician feel they do indeed have reason for further evaluation, expert definition of the motor impairment at the earliest possible time will allow optimal benefit of medical, developmental, and interactional intervention. The earlier a problem is diagnosed and appropriate intervention begun, the better for the child's development and the parents' adjustment and the easier to remedy the dysfunction.

GUIDELINES FOR REFERRAL

It is clear that differentiating normal motor development from possible deficit is often neither an easy nor a straightforward task. (See also Chapter 9.) However, it is possible to determine when referral to a physical therapist is recommended:

1. *The infant with a definite neuromuscular or skeletal abnormality* (i.e., cerebral palsy, brachial plexus injury, limb deficiencies, arthrogryposis, joint contractures, congenital torticollis, myelomeningocele, marked hypotonia).

2. *The full-term asphyxiated infant who is clinically suspect on follow-up examinations* and has a history of the following associated findings at birth:

a. Early or persistent seizures; persistently abnormal EEG on repeat examination.

b. Abnormal levels of consciousness (stupor or lethargy) for more than five days.

c. Hypotonia lasting more than five days or

changing to extensor tone within the first 24 hours.

d. Delay of more than one minute in onset of respiration or Apgar scores of less than 5 at 5, 10, or 20 minutes.

3. *The full-term or preterm infant with developmental delay* that is beginning to interfere with developmental functioning (e.g., muscle tone is so low that the baby cannot get hands to midline, or the baby is so "stiff" that parents have difficulty with care giving and feeding).

4. *The full-term or preterm infant with persistent asymmetry of tone* on two or three serial examinations.

5. *The very low birth weight infant with a suspect examination,* especially when combined with a clinical history of birth asphyxia, significant intracranial hemorrhage, severe respiratory failure, and/or small size for gestational age.

6. *The preterm or full-term infant with illness requiring repeated hospitalizations during the first year of life, who shows developmental delay.* In this case, very simple suggestions for handling and positioning the baby often enhance development and ease care giving.

ROLE OF THE PHYSICAL THERAPIST

When an obvious neuromuscular or musculoskeletal problem affecting sensorimotor development exists (e.g., severe cerebral palsy, unresolving brachial plexus injury, myelomeningocele), the diagnosis is usually made easily and the infant referred to the care of a therapist. For the more subtly affected child (e.g., mild or moderate cerebral palsy; slowness or clumsiness with mild developmental delay) the therapist may serve as a consultant to the physician.

EXAMINATION BY THE PHYSICAL THERAPIST

To capture both the qualitative and quantitative aspects of motor development, a physical therapist examines specific normal and abnormal movement patterns and postures and carries out some developmental neurologic assessments. This combination of testing capitalizes on the strengths of the various examinations while minimizing the pitfalls associated with any one examination. The information derived is valuable in planning and implementing programs that address the needs of an individual child.

Many therapists presently use Bobath's approach for qualitative sensorimotor assessments.[5] This approach addresses a number of questions: Why do young children move? How is their movement influenced by their sensory input? How are posture and movement influenced by vision and hearing? How do reflexes interface with or interfere with movement patterns or postures? How do movement patterns in various positions, such as prone, supine, sitting, and upright, fit together at a given stage of development?

Although there are few scales specifically designed to evaluate the qualitative aspects of sensorimotor development in infants, the Movement Assessment of Infants Scale being developed by Chandler et al.[6] in Seattle shows promise of being a reliable tool for evaluations during the first 12 months of life. It is presently in the final stages of testing for normative values and validity. If its promise is fulfilled, it will provide a standardized scale for assessing the neurologic and developmental components of motor function and quality of movement, enabling predictive judgments for early identification of cerebral palsy. (See also Chapter 11.)

The results of these assessments, combined with those of other evaluations (such as the Bayley Scales of Infant Development and Manual Muscle Tests), provide baseline information and indications for planning treatment approaches; subsequent testing results can then be used to evaluate the effectiveness of the treatment protocol and the child's development.

EVALUATION AND RECOMMENDATIONS

Following assessment the therapist should provide feedback to both the physician and family in several important areas:

1. Why is sensorimotor performance abnormal? Does the variance appear to be within normal limits, given the baby's history; or might it be due to specific experiences or cultural practices (e.g., an infant who has not been placed in the prone position because of cultural beliefs that this impairs digestion may have delayed performance for prone position motor behaviors); or does the examination indeed suggest the need for specific intervention?

2. Is the observed sensorimotor problem or delay likely to interfere with the child's present or future motor development without intervention?

3. Would specific sensorimotor therapy help the family and other care givers (day care per-

sonnel, teachers) optimize the child's motor development? Early, positive reciprocity between parent and child is very important here, since sensorimotor development is one of the earliest ways for the infant and young child to communicate and to elicit caregiving: *For example,* early difficulties with feeding and handling are common in preterm infants, and even more marked in certain physically handicapped children. This can make it difficult, if not impossible, for the parent and child to get a good start together. The parent who tries repeatedly and unsuccessfully to relate to or help the child may become discouraged and eventually "pull back," not from lack of caring, but from misreading the needs of the child or finding that parenting attempts are unsuccessful.

The therapist integrates the clinical and psychosocial information with test results to establish the basis for specific recommendations concerning the type and frequency of treatment. Recommendations are made to address the child's *specific* problems — the need for and selection of appropriate toys, equipment, or splinting — and how to meet the child's and parents' needs for the emotional encouragement so important to enabling the child to develop and learn. Since the primary physician is the key person to provide support for parents, his or her validation of parental concerns and provision of information, practical suggestions, and supportive therapy may make a major contribution to improving the outcome for a given infant.

PHYSICAL THERAPY MANAGEMENT

GENERAL PRINCIPLES OF TREATMENT

Therapy programs are best built on activities related to the developmental level of the child. Treatment and success-oriented play are inseparable in pediatric therapy. There is no single standardized exercise program applicable to all children; rather, treatment strategies must be individualized to meet the specific needs and tolerances of each child and the child's and family's readiness to respond. In general, once a problem is suspected or identified, immediate referral optimizes the time available to the child, family, and therapist to attenuate or resolve it.

Preventing Abnormal Habits. The therapist should be able to help prevent formation of abnormal habits, since, as in normal development, these habits are more difficult to break and the experience more negative for both child and parent than avoiding their occurrence. The child who is not able to find his or her own ways to progress successfully (because of stiffness, weakness, or both) will soon avoid certain activities and thus fall further behind his or her developmental potential. Like the child with a normal sensorimotor system, the child with a handicap or delay develops best in an environment that provides positive feedback and contingency. Developmental lags initially caused by abnormality, illness, or weakness may soon become complicated by secondary problems, such as abnormal compensation (e.g., sitting independently with marked functional spinal kyphosis because of contracted or spastic hamstring muscles and weak abdominal muscles), deformities, decreased positive feedback, decreased will, and, subsequently, decreased opportunity to optimize function.

The child with brain damage has distorted movements and postures, which may be reinforced and made worse by repetition as musculoskeletal development continues. Although the child may be successful in accomplishing developmental tasks, the abnormal movement patterns and postures may block further developmental progress to more complex skills. For example, a child with hypertonicity in the neck-trunk-pelvis and lower extremities may be able to master the developmental task of rolling from prone to supine position using an abnormal extensor pattern; however, as this abnormal pattern is reinforced, the child may be prevented from learning to sit independently because overdevelopment and overactivity of the extensor muscles (antagonists) have relatively impaired the function of the flexors (prime movers); hence, the child cannot achieve the coordination of the muscle groups necessary to reach the more advanced developmental milestone.

Facilitating the ability of an impaired child to ambulate is also easier and more effective if the therapist can work on developing a functional extension pattern of movement in the trunk, pelvis, and legs before the child begins to use a sitting position. Given the same ambulation potential in a child referred late, after independent sitting is acquired, the therapist must try to counteract the effects of the child's spending most of the day with the legs flexed, and possibly also with early contractures. In addition, there is less time left in which to help the child develop an extension pattern in the legs that will permit functional ambulation at an appropriate point in his or her development.

SUPPORTING PARENT-CHILD ACTIVITIES

In general, therapists working with handicapped children find that early infancy–childhood is the natural time for close parent-infant handling activities to help the child achieve his or her intrinsic physical potential. This period is also the ideal time for maximizing the potential of intervention strategies in certain types of dysfunction, because of the plasticity of the developing nervous system.

Usually parents are given no more than five specific exercises to incorporate into their care at any given time, and to reinforce the desired treatment goals, they are asked to apply only techniques that are being used successfully in therapy. This avoids adding to parent-child frustration by attempting treatment approaches that are too difficult and destined to fail. When a written home program is provided, it should be short and specific, and the parents should feel that the approach is realistic and workable for them. Since skill and training are needed to apply the handling and exercises safely and effectively in a child whose muscle tone and responses are abnormal, parents should not be given a list of exercises that have not been demonstrated and practiced under supervision.

Example: In the stretching of a tight or contracted heel cord, the forefoot should be positioned to protect the normal arches before stretch is applied to the muscle. It is quite possible to tear muscle fibers if attempts to stretch the muscles are made too rapidly, thus compounding the child's pain and problems.

A great deal of treatment must be aimed at education and at providing the child and parents with information and treatment approaches that maximize enjoyment and function, while preventing deformity, further delay, or disability. Effective facilitation of parent-infant participation and interaction is best achieved by recognizing the parents' primary role in fostering their child's development. They are the primary agents of intervention, and any successful intervention program must be consistent with their individual levels of understanding and readiness to assume this responsibility.

FINDING RESOURCES

No single practitioner can meet all the needs of the child with a physically handicapping condition. Therefore it is usually advantageous to consult a team of child development specialists, rather than a single one.

It is not news to the pediatrician that finding the "right" program for a child and family is not always easy. Too often, "Lost, then found: Parents' journey through the community service maze"[7] is all too true. In spite of the many committed, competent, and caring persons working with children with special needs, programs are often organized in ways that are confusing to newcomers. Pediatricians and parents new to the search for appropriate services often do not know how to find those best for them. A phone call to a follow-up clinic, pediatric therapist, or other trusted colleague familiar with working with children with physical and mental handicapping conditions may be of help. (See also Appendix E.)

For the child without an identified, specific disability but still in need of a program to provide intervention and monitor motor development and to offer help and support to the family, private pediatric physical therapists are available in many states. If during the course of treatment it becomes obvious that the child would benefit from more comprehensive assessment and management (i.e., by a pediatric speech pathologist, occupational therapist, orthopedist, neurologist), the therapist should be a valuable resource in identifying appropriate local services and in helping the family to enter the system.

References

1. Pape KE, Wigglesworth JH: Haemorrhage, Ischaemia and the Perinatal Brain. No. 69170, SIMP. London, Heinemann Medical Books, Ltd., 1979.
2. Drillien CM: Abnormal neurological signs in the first year of life in low-birthweight infants: Possible prognostic significance. Dev Med Child Neurol 14:705, 1972.
3. Brazelton TB: Introduction. In Sells EJ (ed.): Follow-Up of the High Risk Newborn: A Practical Approach. Springfield, IL, Charles C Thomas, 1980, p xvi.
4. Parmelee AH: Detection of neurologic disability. In Sell EJ (ed.): Follow-Up of the High Risk Newborn: A Practical Approach. Springfield, IL, Charles C Thomas, 1980, pp 202–212.
5. Bobath B, Bobath K: Motor Development in the Different Types of Cerebral Palsy. London, Heinemann Medical Books, Ltd., 1975.
6. Chandler LS, Andrews MS, Swanson MW: Movement Assessment of Infants: A Manual. PO Box 4631, Rolling Bay, WA 98061, 1980.
7. Rubin S, Quinn-Curran N: Lost, then found: Parents' journey through the community service maze. In Seligman M (ed.): The Family with a Handicapped Child: Understanding and Treatment. New York, Grune & Stratton, 1983, pp 63–94.

Recommended Reading

Als H: Newborn behavioral assessment. In Burns WJ, Lavigne JV (eds.): Progress in Pediatric Psychology. New York, Grune & Stratton, 1984, pp 1–46.

Bobath B, Bobath K: Motor Development in the Different Types of Cerebral Palsy. London, William Heinemann Medical Books, Ltd., 1975.

Campbell SK: Clinical decision making: Management of the neonate with movement dysfunction. In Wolf SL (ed.): Clinical Decision Making in Physical Therapy. Philadelphia, F.A. Davis Company, 1985, pp 295–334.

Campbell SK, Wilhelm IJ: Developmental sequences in infants at high risk for central nervous system dysfunction: The recovery process in the first year of life. In Stack JM (ed.): The Special Infant: An Interdisciplinary Approach to the Optimal Development of Infants. New York, Human Sciences Press, 1982, pp 90–133.

Chandler LS, Andrews MS, Swanson MW: Movement Assessment of Infants: A Manual. PO Box 4631, Rolling Bay, WA 98061, 1980.

Finnie NR: Handling the Young Cerebral Palsied Child at Home, 2nd ed. New York, E.P. Dutton, 1975.

Georgieff MK, Bernbaum JC: Abnormal shoulder girdle muscle tone in premature infants during their first 18 months of life. Pediatrics 77:664–669, 1986.

Georgieff MK, Bernbaum JC, Hoffman-Williamson M, et al.: Abnormal truncal muscle tone as a useful early marker for developmental delay in low birth weight infants. Pediatrics 77:659–663, 1986.

Harrison H, Kositsky A: The Premature Baby Book. New York, St Martin's Press, 1983, p 205.

Palundetto R, Rinaldi P, Mansi G, et al.: Behavioral development of preterm infants. Dev Med Child Neurol 26:347–352, 1984.

Pape KE, Wigglesworth JS: Haemorrhage, Ischaemia and the Perinatal Brain. No. 69170, SIMP. London, William Heinemann Medical Books, Ltd., 1979.

Piper MC, Kunos I, William DM, et al.: Early physical therapy effects on the high-risk infant: A randomized controlled trial. Pediatrics 76:216, 1986.

Parmelee AH: Neurophysiological and behavioral organization of premature infants in the first months of life. Biol Psychiatry 10:501–512, 1975.

Parmelee AH: Detection of neurologic disability. In Sells EJ (ed.): Follow-Up of the High-Risk Newborn: A Practical Approach. Springfield, IL, Charles C Thomas, 1980, pp 202–212.

Reade E, Hom L, Hallum A, Lopopolo R: Changes in popliteal angle measurement in infants up to one year of age. Dev Med Child Neurol 26:774–780, 1984.

Rubin S, Quinn-Curran N: Lost, then found: Parents' journey through the community service maze. In Seligman M (ed.): The Family with a Handicapped Child: Understanding and Treatment. New York, Grune & Stratton, 1983, pp 63–94.

Sells EJ (ed.): Follow-Up of the High-Risk Newborn: A Practical Approach. Springfield, IL, Charles C Thomas, 1980.

Tyler NB, Chandler LS: The developmental therapists: The occupational therapist and physical therapist. In Allen KE, Holms AV, Schiefelbusch RL (eds.): Early intervention—A team approach. Baltimore, University Park Press, 1978, pp 169–196.

11

DEVELOPMENTAL AND BEHAVIORAL ASSESSMENT

CAROL H. LEONARD, Ph.D.

The Premature Infant Station at Sarah Morris Hospital of Michael Reese Hospital, in Chicago, was established in May 1922 as a first special unit for premature babies.[1] These infants were followed after graduation in special clinics for "prophylactic and feeding care." There was interest in both the physical and mental growth of the infants, and, in 1929, a mental hygiene clinic was started. Child development specialists in the mental hygiene clinic assessed infants and children with standardized tests and also interviewed the mother and made direct observations of the behavioral status of the child and his or her sibling(s). There was interest in the personality of the premature infant and in whether premature infants were more prone to "nervous habits."

This early follow-up clinic from Chicago is important for two reasons: First, it is a model for hospital-based follow-up clinics, utilizing specialists in developmental assessment and employing standardized tests. Second, the interest shown in nervous habits of the premature infant was a beginning in systematically attempting to assess behavioral differences in this low birth weight group.

The "after history" of the premature baby, as it was called by Mary Cross, author of a widely printed text on the care of the premature baby, had only six references about later outcome in its first edition in 1945.[2] Today, the after history of the premature infant is a field in its own right, and a review of outcome studies would run to the hundreds of articles. Interest in outcome is not limited to premature infants. The Collaborative Perinatal Project has focused attention on other infants in the intensive care nursery — those infants born at term with perinatal distress.[3] High-risk infants in any pediatric practice may have had a wide range of perinatal problems and are likely to have a wide range of developmental outcomes. They need both well-child care and attention to any immediate sequelae of the perinatal period. They also require vigilance to detect problems that appear late. Intellectual impairment often falls into this category of late-appearing deficits.

This chapter discusses cognitive development in high-risk infants who will be seen in the pediatric office or clinic. This is where the "after history" begins. Mental retardation in general and special problems of particular risk groups are described. Infants with congenital anomalies or known syndromes are not discussed, since their cognitive risks are already established. Most high-risk infants in a pediatric practice will also be followed by hospital- or community-based follow-up programs. Recommendations for developmental assessment in these programs are made at the close of the chapter.

INFANTS AT RISK FOR INTELLECTUAL DEFICIT

Who is at risk for *cognitive* deficit? Although the birth of any premature infant is unsettling to parents, the highest-risk premature infants are those weighing less than 1250 grams (and particularly those under 1000 grams) and/or those premature infants who have had a difficult clinical course in the nursery.[4,5] Certainly infants with complicated intracranial hemorrhage (ventricular dilatation or parenchymal involvement) deserve careful long-term assessment. Infants who are extremely small for gestational age may experience some cognitive difficulty.[6,7] A small number of premature infants develop periventricular leukomalacia. This condition appears to have a strong association with cerebral palsy, possible visual deficit, and likely cognitive impairment.[8,9] Infants at risk for cognitive deficit include those with known sensory impairment and those with chronic illness (Table 11–1).

Term infants with mild or minor problems, such as transient tachypnea of the newborn, would not be expected to have intellectual sequelae of their short nursery stays. However, term infants with perinatal asphyxia are at risk for later developmental problems.[10] Among term infants with perinatal asphyxia, those developing seizures within the first 24 hours and those with prolonged seizures that are difficult

---

TABLE 11–1. Infants at Most Risk for Later Cognitive Impairment

Extremely low birth weight (< 1250 gm)
Preterm infant with intracranial hemorrhage extending to the parenchyma or complicated by moderate ventricular dilatation and/or requiring a shunt
Preterm infant with periventricular leukomalacia
Term infant with significant perinatal asphyxia, with seizures occurring in the first 24 hr after birth, or with seizures difficult to control
Near-term or term infant with significant central nervous system lesion
SGA infant with significant IUGR, particularly that occurring early in pregnancy
Infants with prolonged illness, such as bronchopulmonary dysplasia or short-bowel syndrome
Infants with known or suspected sensory impairment
Infants with social factors contributing to suboptimal environment

---

to control appear to have a higher rate of cognitive impairment, ranging from mild to severe, in long-term follow-up.[11,12] In our experience, infants who develop seizures in the first 24 hours and whose neurodevelopmental examination is abnormal at discharge from the ICN are at extremely high risk for significant neurologic and developmental handicaps later.

Although respiratory distress syndrome (RDS) is often considered a risk factor, this diagnosis can occur across a wide range of birth weights. The degree of respiratory distress and whether or not it is associated with chronic lung disease will have more impact on development than the simple presence or absence of RDS.

There are other illnesses in term infants that are severe and life threatening. Persistent pulmonary hypertension of the newborn (PPHN),[13] metabolic disturbances such as hyperammonemia, and other critical illnesses have varied developmental outcomes. These occur infrequently, and some have only recently been recognized as syndromes, so less long-term follow-up data are available. Preschool age follow-up on PPHN is reviewed in Appendix D.

All of these infants are considered at biologic risk for developmental delay. Some are also at environmental risk for developmental delay. Well-known social factors, such as parental substance abuse, poverty, teen-age parents, and emotional disturbance in one or both parents, may make it difficult for the care-giving environment to support the optimal development of high-risk infants. Since some of these social factors are over-represented in the group of low birth weight infants, there are many infants at both biologic and environmental risk for developmental disability.[14] In office practice, then, if infants are suspected of having cognitive delay, consideration of their environment must be taken into account for its possible part in affecting cognitive development.

The criteria for "high-risk" infants have been selected because there is a greater incidence of developmental disabilities in this group than in the total population. Actually, however, the incidence of infants in the population meeting these criteria is low.[15,16] Therefore, in actual number, high-risk infants do not constitute the majority of children with developmental disabilities. And, most high-risk infants develop normally. A generally accepted morbidity rate for premature infants (birth weight less than 1500 grams) is 10 to 20 per cent, including mild as well as moderate to severe abnormalities. Morbidity for term infants with significant perinatal problems is somewhat higher. (See Appendix D for a summary of reported findings.)

RETARDATION IN HIGH-RISK INFANTS

Several types of cognitive deficits may be seen in high-risk infants (Table 11–2). There may be overall lowering of intelligence and/or isolated deficits in cognitive processing. In most cases there will have been obvious perinatal factors (intracranial hemorrhage, asphyxia) influencing later intellectual development. A high-risk social environment may also be contributory.

PSYCHOSOCIAL RETARDATION

Psychosocial, or environmental, retardation may occur in preterm or ill term infants, just as it occurs in the general population. This usually occurs when there is little stimulation in the home, little responsiveness to the infant's naturally developing mind, and cultural isolation. If the lack of stimulation is severe enough to be considered actual neglect, the infant may also have emotional symptoms. Referral for child protective services may be indicated. If neglect is not an issue, the physician or health practitioner needs to explore with the family whether the parents have any preconceived notions or anxieties that might be preventing them from treating their infant as normal. Assumptions that the child is retarded because of the nursery stay may be preventing them from interacting in an appropriate manner with their child. Finally, some families are socially isolated to such a degree that their infants and children do not experience many of the common activities of the dominant culture. Although not as critical in infancy, this lack of exposure will affect later test scores.

SIMPLE MENTAL RETARDATION – GLOBAL DEVELOPMENTAL DELAY

Mental retardation can occur in sick term or sick premature infants as a result of CNS damage, but is not a frequent outcome by itself. Global developmental delay means mental deficit, accompanied by delayed acquisition of motor skills. Motor skills are delayed but not impaired. The infant acquires adequate, although unrefined, gross and fine motor function at a slower rate; mental growth is slow, and ultimately deficient. Generally, in high-risk infants who later are found to have mental retardation, abnormal motor signs are seen—sometimes transiently.

In the *healthy* premature infant, simple mental retardation is not an expected outcome. Other causes, such as metabolic or organic disease, should be considered. Particularly for premature infants with no vision or hearing deficits, no known or suspected intracranial hemorrhage, and no known or suspected hypoxic events, a full work-up should be done if the infant or child later is found to have simple mental retardation. A referral for genetic counseling may be indicated for the family. Genetic factors or other prenatal events may have predetermined the intellectual outcome for this child, independent of prematurity.

TABLE 11–2. Types of Cognitive Deficit in High-Risk Infants

DEFICIT	COMMENTS
Psychosocial retardation	Related to environmental factors, not biologic risk factors
Simple mental retardation	Rare in healthy preterm infants; seen in some asphyxiated infants
Mental retardation with motor deficit	Difficult to assess cognitive status if motor deficit is severe; with mild or moderate motor deficit, intelligence may be unaffected
Specific cognitive deficit with normal intelligence and no major motor deficit	Seen in some preterm infants with significant intracranial hemorrhage Seen in some infants with hydrocephalus or shunt Seen in some infants with CNS lesion
Cognitive delay	Seen in chronically ill infants; resolves as health is gained. Failure to resolve may indicate involvement by other factors (ICH)

Although global developmental delay, or simple mental retardation, is rare in the high-risk population, it is probably the cognitive deficit easiest to detect, because all milestones are delayed at about the same rate. The infant is likely to walk somewhat later than expected, language development is slower, and general comprehension as evidenced in social and cognitive skills is slower. The practitioner, however, should remember that infants can show wide variations in the ages at which they acquire skills. In addition, some infants will not demonstrate a skill until they can perform it well (walking or talking, for example). If concern arises about general development during examination of a well baby or well child, a return visit can be scheduled shortly thereafter in which development is the main focus. If delayed development is seen across all areas, a referral for formal developmental assessment should be initiated.

MENTAL RETARDATION WITH ASSOCIATED MOTOR DEFICIT

Many high-risk infants have transient mild motor abnormalities, and some have permanent motor impairment. Parents often associate motor deficit with mental retardation. For many children with permanent motor deficit (cerebral palsy), intelligence is unaffected. For others, there may be a degree of mental retardation.

When early motor abnormalities resolve, the same holds true. Intelligence may be unaffected, or there may have been an effect on intelligence that becomes more evident over time. The finding of lowered intelligence when there have been transient motor abnormalities is more likely in asphyxiated term infants than in very premature infants. This is because it is likely that early motor differences in very premature infants are related to CNS maturation factors rather than to CNS damage.

IMPAIRMENT OF SPECIFIC ABILITIES WITH NORMAL INTELLIGENCE

Patterns of specific cognitive deficits in the presence of normal intelligence can be seen in both premature infants[17,18] and ill term infants, primarily in those with CNS insult in the perinatal period. A higher incidence of perceptual-motor problems and difficulties in auditory processing are found in high-risk infants. These may affect learning and academic performance.

TRANSIENT COGNITIVE DELAY

A final type of cognitive delay (not deficit) is that associated with chronic illness following discharge from the ICN. Repeated hospitalizations or general poor health may temporarily depress an infant's level of functioning. This should not be interpreted as permanent to the family.

EXPECTED PATTERNS OF COGNITIVE DEVELOPMENT IN HIGH-RISK GROUPS

This section addresses variations in cognitive development that are specific to particular groups of high-risk infants.

THE EXTREMELY PREMATURE INFANT

The extremely premature infant (birth weight less than 1250 grams) will have had a long hospitalization. During a lengthy hospital stay there may also have been many ups and downs in the infant's health. There is likely to be anxiety and concern from both staff and parents that such a small infant could survive and be normal. As birth weight goes down to less than 1000 grams or less than 800 grams, concern goes up.

The expected intellectual outcome for this infant is normal intelligence.[19,20] (See also Appendix D.) There is, however, an increased incidence of other problems, such as retinopathy of prematurity (ROP) and high-frequency hearing loss. Some of this sensory impairment is subtle and not easily detectable on pediatric clinical examination in the first two years of life. Although ROP may resolve in the nursery, the visual acuity of these children is sometimes decreased. Subtle visual and/or hearing impairment will contribute to lowered developmental test scores. It is important to establish the intactness of the sensory system before ascribing any poor performance to decreased intellectual ability.

In the very premature infant, difficulties in fine motor coordination are not unusual. This may express itself as clumsiness in picking up small objects and as delay in establishing a precise release. Later, drawing skills will be less adept than in age peers. At school age, handwriting may be a troublesome task. For many children, the problem lies in motor execution, not in their ability to analyze visually and reproduce designs or cursive letters; in reproducing designs the elements of the design will be present but poorly drawn. For other children it is both a perceptual and motor difficulty. Visual discrimination tasks may be poorly performed and motor execution as well. These deficits can be mild and often dealt with in a classroom situation. For some high-risk infants, however, either or both components, visual or motor, may be troublesome enough that intervention might be useful at preschool age. Occupational therapy or a sensory-motor integration approach have been found useful.

Difficulty in auditory comprehension is another example of a specific cognitive deficit sometimes seen in the very premature infant. These children process auditory information more slowly and seem to have less cognitive flexibility with verbal material. These are children who need repetition of verbal instructions frequently, in spite of normal hearing. One mother described this as, "I have to tell him everything three times." This should not be confused with the normal inattentiveness of children to parental demands.

PRETERM INFANT WITH INTRACRANIAL HEMORRHAGE

Intracranial hemorrhage in extremely premature infants may range from simple, uncomplicated bleeding in the germinal matrix or ventricles to complicated bleeding into the parenchyma, with ventricular dilatation that may resolve or may require shunting. Little school-age outcome data are available; however, pre-

school-age data suggest the following cognitive outcomes.[21-23] (See also Appendix D.)

The outcome in children with simple germinal matrix hemorrhage or uncomplicated intraventricular hemorrhage is not different from that in infants of similar birth weight without intracranial hemorrhage.

Cognitive deficits may occur in approximately 50 per cent of very premature infants with complicated intracranial hemorrhage. In talking with parents it is important to remember that half of these infants have normal intelligence. Figure 11–1 shows the serial test scores of an 810-gram infant, born at 28 weeks of gestation, who sustained a grade IV intracerebral hemorrhage. This infant had RDS and chronic lung disease, requiring ventilator support for 32 days and supplemental oxygen for 44 days. While in the ICN he was noted to have mild right hemiparesis. Now, at school age, he has no neurologic sequelae and is right-handed. He has consistently scored in the average range for cognitive development. He shows no specific cognitive deficits or "learning disabilities."

In infants who do have intellectual impairment, two patterns are most likely. With bleeding into the cerebellum, some ataxia may be present on neurodevelopmental examination, and borderline or lower intelligence may be found on cognitive assessment. A second pattern may be seen in children with intracranial hemorrhage requiring a shunt. A syndrome including overdeveloped verbal skills, significant impairment in perceptual-motor skills, and decreased ability in concept formation and verbal problem solving occurs in some of these chil-

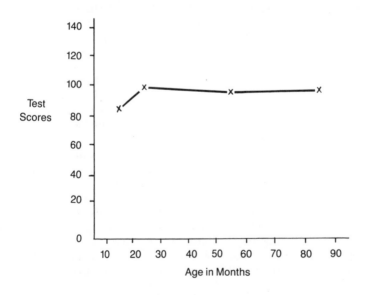

FIGURE 11–1. Developmental test scores of a very low birth weight infant with a significant intracranial hemorrhage. Ages, tests, and test scores indicated by solid line are:

Adjusted Age	19 mos	Bayley MDI = 89
Adjusted Age	25 mos	Bayley MDI = 104
Age	54 mos	McCarthy GCI = 99
Age	84 mos	WISC-R Full Scale IQ = 100

dren. This is a subtle syndrome that would be most apparent by hyperverbalization and poor handwriting skills in the child. A more dramatic version, associated with lowered intelligence, is seen in some children with congenital hydrocephalus or hydrocephalus associated with spina bifida, and has been called the cocktail party syndrome[24] because of the lack of meaningful content in the chatter. It is likely in some cases that there is parental or environmental reinforcement of verbosity in these children and that the hyperverbalization is not necessarily related to CNS dysfunctioning.

SIGNIFICANT PERINATAL ASPHYXIA

Asphyxia in a full-term newborn infant has a wide range of cognitive outcomes. Approximately 50 per cent of asphyxiated infants have no discernible sequelae of their perinatal problems. The other 50 per cent may have subtle or overt difficulties in cognitive development. Since testing of intellectual abilities becomes more elaborate as the child grows, it is not possible to specify in the first two years of life what a child's ultimate range of intelligence will be. When the CNS has had an insult, some reorganization will occur, and a good functional level may be achieved. Long-term follow-up is essential in this group of infants.

Data from the Collaborative Perinatal Project indicate that early and/or prolonged seizures are most related to later cognitive impairment in asphyxiated term infants.[11,12] Some of these infants will have frank neurologic deficit as well. This leads to great difficulty in accurate cognitive assessment, as most tests are constructed for intact infants and children. For children with significant neurologic impairment, diagnosis of cognitive strengths and deficits may not be possible until the infant-child is able to establish a consistent communication system. The infant-child should be treated as having normal intelligence unless it has been established otherwise.

Another pattern of development seen in this group of infants begins with some mild motor involvement that generally resolves, delayed language milestones, and, finally, borderline or mild to moderate mental retardation.[25] Because damage to the brain can be wide ranging, it is important in this group of infants to have specialized audiologic and visual examinations in infancy. Subtle hearing loss and visual field cuts are not uncommon findings in the significantly asphyxiated infant.

The premature brain is different structurally from the brain of a full-term infant. Devastating cognitive damage from perinatal CNS insult is more often seen in full-term than in premature infants. A neurologic diagnosis may be evident early in development, but the full expression of cognitive deficit appears later in development.

Example: A term female infant was born by emergency cesarean section after fetal bradycardia was noted; artificial rupture of membranes revealed thick meconium. Apgar scores were 1 and 5 at one and five minutes, respectively, and seizure activity began at 11 hours of age. The infant was transported to an ICN. Phenobarbital, phenytoin (Dilantin), and paraldehyde drip were required to gain control of the seizures. An EEG obtained on day 3 was abnormal; a follow-up EEG on day 11 was normal. Neurologic examinations throughout the first year of life revealed hypertonicity and declining head circumference percentiles. Developmental assessment at 15 months found that her problem-solving skills were at a 12-month level. At age three years, neurologic diagnosis of mild spastic quadriplegia and microcephaly are consistent with earlier examinations. She has four word approximations and signs two words. Clumsiness and probable visual impairment interfere with completion of nonverbal tasks. She is functionally, if not organically, retarded. Although there is a continuing suggestion of discrepant language and problem-solving abilities, her severe communication handicap interferes with adequate assessment.

SIGNIFICANT CNS LESION IN TERM INFANTS

Term infants can acquire or be born with brain injury that results in circumscribed lesions in the brain. This can occur during an asphyxial process, but it may be related to embolism, stroke, or more specific injury to the brain of the newborn. In some cases the insult to the brain has occurred prenatally. In adults, in whom brain cells have already been committed, specific lesions often result in dramatic, specific deficits. In infants, brain injury affects acquisition of skills, and diffuse impairment is more likely.

It has been only in the last 10 years that technologic developments have made it possible to see lesions or cysts in the brains of surviving infants. While there is much discussion about plasticity of brain function, detailed long-term outcome studies have not been done in this group of infants. In these infants, motor deficit may be present in infancy. More subtle cognitive deficit may be apparent later. Parents can be reassured, however, that frank cognitive deficit, such as significant mental retardation, would be diagnosed early in development and would not appear suddenly at preschool or school age.

INFANTS MARKEDLY SMALL FOR GESTATIONAL AGE

The infant who has markedly low birth weight for gestational age, in the absence of congenital anomalies or intrauterine infection, may be at risk for specific deficits at school age. The presence of neonatal asphyxia increases the chances for intellectual deficit.[7] Infants who are small for gestational age, in whom the slowing of growth has occurred before 26 weeks of gestation (documented by ultrasound examination), have been reported to be within the normal range of intelligence, but to have difficulties with perceptual-motor and other nonverbal tasks.[6] These infants tend to be symmetrically small in height, weight, and head circumference at birth. If slowing of intrauterine growth occurs more toward term, the primary deficits seen later are in physical growth, not mental development. These infants have adequate head circumference and length, but weigh less than expected for their gestational age.

SENSORY IMPAIRMENT

Infants with a diagnosis of significant sensory impairment, such as decreased vision or hearing, prior to discharge from the nursery should have their development followed by a person trained in assessing cognitive development in the presence of these handicaps. For deficits as profound as blindness or deafness, a referral to a regional center should be made prior to discharge from the nursery. In most areas there are infant programs or professional personnel who can visit the home to work with the infant as soon as he or she is home from the hospital. Early intervention for known handicaps is very important in facilitating developmental progress.

Of concern in the general office practice will be infants with significant strabismus or esotropia, which may interfere with the development of good perceptual-motor coordination. Both visual following and coordinated reaching are important in cognitive development. Intermittent hearing loss due to fluid congestion and/or repeated ear infections may affect speech and language development and general auditory comprehension. This, in turn, affects performance of cognitive tasks.

SIGNIFICANT CHRONIC ILLNESS

Infants with bronchopulmonary dysplasia are probably the most difficult to follow in a pediatric practice. The need for medical follow-up of an infant receiving oxygen therapy at home after discharge and the likelihood of rehospitalization for respiratory complications in the first year after discharge often take the emphasis off development. Feeding difficulties are common in this group of infants, and weight gain is often slow.

When development is examined, it can be of great concern. The infant may appear weak, have little energy reserve, and have slow gross motor development secondary to poor growth. Because of limited mobility, due to either slow progress in gross motor movements or limited energy, these infants may have greater opportunity for social and language development. Cognitive development should be appropriate for adjusted age, although less refined fine motor movements and general weakness may make execution of some tasks difficult. On formal tests, such as the Gesell scales or Bayley scales, some delays will be noted in the first two years, and even to 36 months of age. A pattern of slow, gradual progress, as the chronic lung disease improves, is typical.

Figure 11–2 shows an example of this developmental course in a 960-gram infant born at 29 weeks of gestation.

Example: An infant girl had severe hyaline membrane disease, and a ventilator was used for 122 days. She was discharged home at 8 months of age, oxygen being administered by nasal cannula; she remained oxygen dependent until her adjusted age was 14 months (chronologic age 17 months). The infant was significantly delayed in the first 24 months of life. The delays were felt to be consistent with her chronic lung disease and not neurologically based. Her developmental and cognitive test scores reflect the pattern of slow, gradual improvement as her physical health improved. At the age of seven years she is a social and talkative youngster, who is making good progress in first grade. Since her home environment was optimal, she was not referred to an infant development program. In less supportive family circumstances a referral might reasonably be made.

There are conflicting reports of morbidity associated with chronic lung disease.[26-29] Although infants are generally considered to have chronic lung disease if their requirements for additional oxygen persist more than 28 days, some infants need oxygen for more than a year. Some studies that report poor neurologic and intellectual outcome failed to take into account associated encephalopathy or severity of dis-

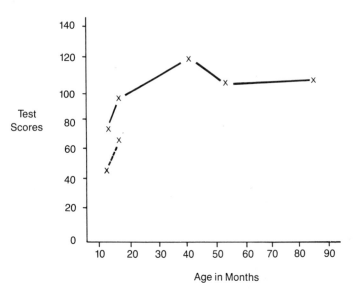

FIGURE 11–2. Developmental test scores of a very low birth weight infant with bronchopulmonary dysplasia. Ages, tests, and test scores indicated by solid line are:
Adjusted age 12 mos Bayley MDI = 76
Adjusted age 15 mos Bayley MDI = 96
Age 40 mos Stanford-Binet
IQ = 123
Age 54 mos McCarthy
GCI = 106
Age 84 mos WISC-R Full Scale
IQ = 108
Dotted line gives Bayley PDI at adjusted ages 12 and 15 mos (50, 62).

ease. Bronchopulmonary dysplasia by itself in an otherwise intact infant is a medical complication that results in chronic illness. When intellectual deficit is found and persists after the illness is over, causal factors other than respiratory illness should be considered. Infants with significant bronchopulmonary dysplasia may have other problems of prematurity, including retinopathy, hearing loss, intracranial hemorrhage, and necrotizing enterocolitis. These other medical problems may contribute to developmental deficit.

Short-bowel syndrome is another medical complication that requires complex medical follow-up and possibly repeated hospitalizations. It may be due to congenital malformation, or it can be a complication of prematurity following necrotizing enterocolitis. Intelligence is generally unaffected if adequate nutrition can be maintained.[30] Repeated hospitalizations may affect developmental progress. Some regression in development is common when infants or toddlers are hospitalized for long periods or have a series of short stays. These regressions are transient and expected.

THE PEDIATRIC DEVELOPMENTAL ASSESSMENT

DEVELOPMENTAL SCREENING

Screening high-risk infants in the pediatric office or clinic setting is not essentially different from screening low-risk or normal-risk infants. An assessment of general development is part of well-baby and well-child examinations. With

high-risk infants, however, special attention should be paid to the integrity of the sensory systems (vision and hearing) and the integration of the sensory systems with motor development. Although cognitive development can proceed in the presence of significant motor deficit, good vision and hearing are essential in helping the infant and young child develop cognitive schemata and problem-solving skills.

Although the child grows as a whole, certain aspects of development are pre-eminent in the first two years of life (Fig. 11–3). Gross motor skills—sitting, crawling, and progress toward independent ambulation—are practiced during this time. Fine motor skills—developing a precision grasp and release and coordinating vision with prehension—evolve and are refined from about 4 months to 18 months of age. Language emerges, so that some intelligible speech is expected of a two-year-old. Problem-solving skills are practiced—looking for lost objects, imitating adults, beginning to perceive cause and effect.

Gross motor integrity and the ability to produce spoken language are well established by the end of toddlerhood. Elaboration and refinement of these basic skills are the tasks of the preschool years. Cognitive development, however, is still in a period of qualitative growth in the preschool years. It is a complex process occupying the rest of childhood and continuing into adolescence.

In the first two years of life, simple problem-solving tasks can often be incorporated into an office examination. Keeping some 1-inch blocks and a couple of small manipulative toys handy is a useful way of engaging the infant and

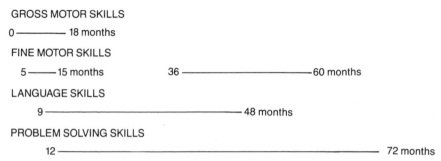

GROSS MOTOR SKILLS

0 ———————— 18 months

FINE MOTOR SKILLS

5 ————15 months   36 ————————————————60 months

LANGUAGE SKILLS

9 ————————————————————— 48 months

PROBLEM SOLVING SKILLS

12 ————————————————————————— 72 months

FIGURE 11–3. Schema for following development. Development occurs continuously across all areas; new skills are constantly attained and refined. This schema reflects general time periods when one area may seem predominant over other areas of development.

allows the examiner to observe the infant's problem-solving skills. The infant's interest in object exploration and manipulation, the quality of the infant's play, and the organization of the play can be sampled.

LOOKING AHEAD—SCHOOL READINESS

Because some of the problems of high-risk infants are more apparent at school age, school readiness is a topic that primary care providers should be able to address with parents.

Readiness implies more than just intellectual readiness for kindergarten. In addition to social maturity, it is important to have a sufficient attention span, to be willing to follow adult instructions, and to be able to inhibit motor activity in the classroom. Facility with fine motor skills is also important as formal handwriting begins.

As the infant moves out of the second year of life, certain questions about his or her development will have been settled. The child may have had a very normal developmental course over the first two years, giving some confidence about the future. By the age of two years, infants with significant deficits should have been identified and rehabilitation efforts begun where possible.

A third group of children is made up of those who have had mild problems or have been of mild concern, for example, the infant who can complete tasks but with poor quality. Short attention span and high activity level are involved in some learning problems; however, they also can be developmental immaturities in some children and not necessarily precursors of learning problems.

Children with late summer or fall birthdays, who are also developmentally immature, may benefit from spending an extra year in preschool before starting kindergarten. If a child has al-

ready spent two years in preschool, a different preschool setting might be considered. Play is the natural setting for maturation of many skills. Preschools that encourage play may assist maturation more efficiently than those that stress rote learning.

The question of beginning kindergarten needs to be discussed at the four-year-old well-child checkup, so parents can begin orienting their child for the next year. If the child has been in preschool and/or in a follow-up program, consulting with the staff in these settings may be useful to parents. Very premature infants (less than 1250 grams) appear to be a high-risk group that benefits from delayed kindergarten entry when low birth weight is combined with a late birthday.

There are some problems that time will not ameliorate. When behavioral concerns about attention span, impulsivity, and activity level are significant, intervention may be indicated. Delaying kindergarten entry is useful only if developmental immaturity is the main concern. No guideline fits every child, and if the high-risk infant appears in all respects "ready" for kindergarten at age five years it is appropriate for him or her to attend.

LOOKING AHEAD—LEARNING PROBLEMS

There are no commonly accepted definitions or diagnostic categories of learning disabilities.[31] True developmental dyslexia, or inability to read, is rare and may have a hereditary component. Many children, regardless of birth status, do have school difficulties. These may be in the area of reading, spelling, or mathematics, or possibly all three. For the child to be considered as having a learning problem, tested intelligence must be in the normal or average range, and formal academic achievement must be significantly discrepant with ability.

True learning problems, then, cannot be documented until the child has had two or three years of formal education and can be shown to be below grade level in achievement. Learning problems may be related to weakness in areas of cognitive functioning, such as attention, concentration, memory, verbal analytic abilities, nonverbal analytic abilities, and visual-motor coordination.

Some high-risk children have weaknesses in one or more of these areas.[32,33] The percentage of premature children (less than 1500 grams) with difficulties may range from 10 to 20 per cent. For term infants with CNS impairment, the percentage is likely to be higher. Learning is a complex interactional process involving an intellectually competent, socially mature, emotionally secure child, a supportive family, and a competent educational system able to deal with individual differences in children. Because of individual variation in development, it is difficult to predict learning problems. Some children learn to compensate for areas of weakness, and other children become very learning-handicapped by the same weakness. The family setting is important in minimizing or maximizing weakness in a child.

There is no simple answer to parents' early questions about learning problems in high-risk infants, because it involves a high degree of prediction in a loosely defined field, where many social or environmental factors can have great effect. When parents do ask, the most helpful direction is to draw attention to the child's present level and quality of performance and to note whether that is consistent or inconsistent with previous evaluations. Early signs such as a high level of distractability and/or fine motor incoordination are not strong predictors by themselves of later learning problems, but they warrant close follow-up.

"NERVOUS HABITS" OF HIGH-RISK INFANTS

The outcome literature on sick *term* infants dwells primarily on the presence or absence of physical or mental handicap. The unexpected early birth and small size of *premature* infants, however, have contributed to psychological distancing and, at time, stereotypical thinking about premature children. The exhibition of premature infants at world fairs and expositions in America during the first half of this century by Martin Cooney may have added to the "sideshow approach" to the development of premature children.[34]

Hess and his colleagues suggested, through their work in the mental hygiene clinic, that nervous habits are more common in premature infants.[1] This idea was further elaborated by Shirley in the late 1930's.[35,36]

Shirley first noted, in 1938, that "a number of peculiar gestures and nervous mannerisms are observable in these premature babies."[35] Hypersensitivity to sound, tension, shyness, noncompliance, and irascibility ("bursting into tears without the slightest provocation") were described as common personality features. Shirley speculated that primiparity and advanced maternal age were important factors in affecting the personalities of the infants. Staff examiners felt that the mothers of prematures were anxious and went to extremes, both overstimulating and understimulating in their care. Shirley clearly related "nervous mannerisms" of premature infants to their immature nervous system and to environmental, caregiving influences.

Today, many aspects of development are viewed from this interactive perspective, emphasizing the role of the caregiver in personality development and behavioral organization, as well as acknowledging aspects of physical and sensory integration that might contribute to variations in the development of some premature or ill term children. A comprehensive review of behavioral effects of prematurity by Minde concludes that, contrary to clinical impression, prematurity, independent of associated cerebral dysfunction, is not related to significant emotional problems.[37] He cautions, however, that long-term follow-up of very low birth weight infants in the modern period of neonatal care, i.e., post-1970, has yet to be carried out.

Variations in personality and in the organization of behavior are seen in both high-risk and low-risk children. Aspects of the physical environment, as well as the social environment, can affect personality and behavioral organization. This is clearly seen in high-risk infants at discharge from the hospital. The "peculiar institution" of the ICN often socializes its longer-term occupants to become more fussy with social interaction, rather than less, and to prefer sleeping with bright lights and a high noise level. These effects of ICN care, however, are usually transient. A home environment with a regular and responsive caregiver can often help an irritable infant smooth out and adapt to his or her new surroundings. A chaotic physical environment and caregiving that is insensitive to the cues of the infant may exacerbate irritability.

When behavioral differences or nervous

habits persist, there may be a delay or subtle deficit in CNS maturation. Even for healthy premature infants, early delivery is a stress to the CNS. State disorganization (going from deep sleep to a full crying state, for example), feeding problems, and little ability for self-consoling may make some high-risk infants difficult for even very competent parents. These behavioral aspects of infant care should be given special attention at pediatric office visits. Each infant may present unique parenting challenges.

DEVELOPMENTAL ASSESSMENT IN FOLLOW-UP PROGRAMS

EVALUATION INSTRUMENTS

A variety of developmental tests are given to infants and children in follow-up programs. The tests vary with the age of the infant or child and with the preferences of each follow-up program. Recommended tests and timing of assessments are listed in Table 11–3. These tests are widely used; a brief description is provided to familiarize health practitioners with them. Authors and publishers of the tests are listed at the end of the chapter.

Bayley Scales of Infant Development. Two scales are utilized in this developmental assessment instrument: the mental development scale and the psychomotor development scale. A third scale, the infant behavior record, is a useful way of recording temperamental and behavioral aspects of an infant's performance. Scores are reported as the mental development index and the psychomotor development index. The mental development index and psychomotor development index are not IQ scores; they represent the infant's developmental performance compared to other infants his or her age.

The mental development scale includes items relating to social, language, and problem-solving skills. Many tasks require adequate fine motor coordination, as well as cognitive skills, to complete. Clumsy infants may score less well on this scale for that reason. The psychomotor development scale includes items regarding the development of gross and fine motor skills.

The Bayley Scales are commonly used in research on high-risk infants because the test is well normed, and numerical scores are easily derived.

Gesell Developmental Schedule. This infant assessment instrument was developed by Arnold Gesell, who had a strong background in child development and education before becoming a physician. It is often administered by physical and occupational therapists, as well as by medical personnel. Most infant tests are derivative from the Gesell Schedules.

Behavior is assessed in five areas: gross motor, fine motor, language, personal-social, and adaptive (problem solving). A summary score can be derived by dividing the age level attained (mental age) by the infant's chronologic age. This method of determining a "developmental quotient" by a ratio of mental age to chronologic age is different from other developmental scores or intelligence quotients, and perhaps for this reason the Gesell Schedule is less used in outcome research than the Bayley Scales as a measure of infant development.

Stanford-Binet Intelligence Scale. The Stanford-Binet Intelligence Scale (third revision) is an intelligence test that covers the age range of 2 to 18 years. A single IQ score is derived. It is recommended for use in follow-up at age $2\frac{1}{2}$

TABLE 11–3. Assessment Protocol for Normally Developing Children

AGE	TEST
0 to 11 mo.*	Formal developmental assessment at 3, 5, and 8 mo. of age, with Bayley Scales of Infant Development or Gesell Developmental Schedules
12 mo.*	Bayley Scales of Infant Development or Gesell Developmental Schedules
18 mo.*	Bayley Scales of Infant Development or Gesell Developmental Schedules
$2\frac{1}{2}$ yr.*	Stanford-Binet Intelligence Scale
$4\frac{1}{2}$ yr.	McCarthy Scales of Children's Abilities
7 yr	Wechsler Intelligence Scale for Children, Revised
12 yr.	Wechsler Intelligence Scale for Children, Revised

* Age adjusted for prematurity, depending on birth weight (see text).

years. At the early age levels of this test there are several tasks (building blocks, drawing, stringing beads) that sample fine motor coordination as well as other cognitive skills. The variety of tasks at early age levels in the Stanford-Binet Scale make it easy to engage even usually shy children. A fourth revision is newly published; some items and materials are substantially different at the early age ranges from the third revision.

McCarthy Scales of Children's Abilities. The McCarthy Scales are designed for children ages $2\frac{1}{2}$ to $8\frac{1}{2}$ years. We recommend their use in follow-up at a mid-age range ($4\frac{1}{2}$ years) as a preschool evaluation instrument. The five scales (verbal, perceptual-performance, quantitative, memory, and motor) are constructed along psychoeducational lines. A child's performance on the individual scales can be analyzed for specific weaknesses that may interfere with formal academic learning. A composite score can be derived from the first three scales and is known as the General Cognitive Index.

Wechsler Intelligence Scale for Children, Revised. The Wechsler Scale, known as the WISC-R, is a standard childhood intelligence test. Ten subtests are commonly given and a verbal IQ, performance IQ, and a full-scale IQ are derived. Patterns of the WISC-R subtest scores are analyzed for strengths and weaknesses in cognitive functioning. Although normed on a representative sample of children, this test, along with most other "intelligence" tests, must be interpreted with caution when administered to minority group children or children from different cultural backgrounds.

BEHAVIORAL ASSESSMENT

There are many ways of sampling and recording the behavior of infants and children. Temperament scales, behavior rating scales, observation of the infant's or child's play, and observation of test-taking behavior are all ways of assessing how a child organizes and interacts with objects and people.

During infancy and preschool years the child is in a process of refining and regulating his or her behavior. There is wide cultural and familial variation in the kinds and quantity of behaviors that parents permit. Mouthing objects, for example, may be actively discouraged by some parents, even though it is a primary behavior pattern at certain ages. Casting, although it is a natural behavior in learning to release objects, is reinforced by some parents, both positively (by laughing and smiling when the infant does it) and negatively (by shouting and frowning). Some parents actively limit their two-year-old's explorations of the examining room, but others do not seem to notice when their toddler is dismantling it. Some infants-toddlers have a high activity level, and others need encouragement to move from one place to another.

The developmental testing situation is a good way to sample appropriateness of behavior. Unlike a play situation, in which there are few demands, the demands of a testing situation are mild but definite. Adequacy of attention span, freedom from distractability, ability to follow instructions, ability to inhibit motor activity, and other behaviors can be sampled. It should be remembered that a child with subtle hearing loss may have a behavior disturbance. This should be addressed when behavior is a problem. Children who have significant difficulty completing an evaluation because of behavioral difficulties may require more extensive psychological evaluation. Follow-up programs may not be equipped to do this, and referral to another source may be necessary.

THE FOLLOW-UP REPORT

The primary care physician or health professional should receive reports of the developmental status of the at-risk infant or child who has been seen at a follow-up visit. In the best of circumstances this physician has regular contact with the patient and family and is perceived by the family as organizing and coordinating care for the child and as interpreting specialty consultations. Although the general results of developmental assessments should have been discussed with parents at the time of the follow-up visit, parents may inquire about the formal report to the physician.

If parents inquire about a child's scores, it is preferable to talk about the range of the child's performance and not specific scores. Scores can vary on repeated testing, and the general performance of the child is more important than any given score. Parents requesting specific scores from a physician should be referred back to the original examiner, so the issue of what the scores mean to the family can be addressed.

The tests administered in follow-up programs vary in content and complexity, but scores are derived from most of them to indicate the child's performance in comparison with age-peers. For the physician or primary health care provider, a general guideline in understanding reports of developmental assessment is that most children will fall within one standard deviation of the mean. A mean or average score is 100, with a standard deviation of 16 (15 on some tests). Scores falling in the range of 84 to 116, then, are considered in the average range.

Children scoring more than one standard deviation above the mean (greater than 116) are performing above average, compared to other children their age. In this circumstance, it is also likely that the home environment is supporting the intellectual development of the child.

Children can score between one and two standard deviations below the mean for a variety of reasons. In this range (68 to 83), factors such as bilingualism, minority status, cultural differences, lack of stimulation, chronic illness, and others can serve to depress the scores of otherwise intact infants and children. Mild visual or auditory impairment may also be affecting performance. Knowledge of the family situation and the medical history of the infant are imperative in interpreting scores in this range and in deciding whether or not any intervention is necessary for the child.

Children scoring greater than two standard deviations below the mean (less than 68) at any time are likely to have true cognitive delay. Again, contributory factors, such as home environment or illness, need to be ruled out before a diagnosis is firmly established. Retesting is also important to rule out situational factors that may have affected the infant's or child's performance on a given day.

ASSESSMENT PROTOCOL FOR NORMALLY DEVELOPING CHILDREN

Follow-up programs may have a research focus, a clinical focus, or both. The selection of tests and when they are given varies widely from program to program. Sometimes this variation is due to differences in staffing patterns. In other cases a research design had determined the protocol, or established clinical practice is being followed. In the setting up of a new program or revision of an older program, consideration should be given to certain factors.

Frequency of Developmental Assessment. Infants receive several different examinations in a follow-up visit. The medical evaluation generally covers neurologic, physical, and medical aspects of the infant's growth and development. General development may or may not be emphasized, depending on the background and interests of the medical examiner. Formal developmental assessments are usually carried out by psychologists or child development specialists.

Highest-risk infants should be seen frequently in the first two years of life and less often thereafter. Healthy premature infants who weighed more than 1250 grams at birth can be seen less intensively in the first two years. (See recommendations in Chapter 9.) Developmental assessment is recommended at 6 weeks and at 3, 5, 8, and 12 months of age. This assessment might consist of a neurodevelopmental examination by a physician or health practitioner (see Chapter 9) or a formal developmental assessment, such as the Bayley Scales, by an allied health professional. In the early months there is little to be gained clinically by submitting a fragile infant to both of these examinations.

For children developing normally in the first year a formal developmental assessment at 12 and 18 months is recommended, in addition to the physician's examination (Table 11–3). Neurodevelopmental and developmental assessments begin to diverge significantly in the kinds of information being obtained from each after the first few months of life. Some follow-up programs begin formal developmental assessments at 8 to 9 months (adjusted age). We recommend 12 months, primarily because of the greater language sample usually obtained at this age. In any case, the 12-month examination should not be omitted.

Assessment of cognitive skills is recommended again at age $2\frac{1}{2}$ years, since at 24 months compliance is often not a priority for the toddler and an age-appropriate high-activity level makes assessments difficult for everyone. The $2\frac{1}{2}$-year-old is more willing to cooperate, and verbal skills can be expected to be relatively better developed. Preschool assessments at $4\frac{1}{2}$ years and school-age assessments at 7 and 12 years of age complete the longitudinal follow-up of high-risk infants.

These ages are selected for two reasons: (1) They represent times when important developmental skills should be acquired. (2) Particularly in clinically based follow-up programs, yearly testing is not "good testing." There is no evidence to suggest that assessing children on their birthday every year is either a good idea or a logical one. Ethical guidelines for the administration of psychological tests should be followed, and children should not be overassessed.

Other assessments may be utilized, depending on the functions of each follow-up program. In infancy and early preschool age, observation of spontaneous play behavior is often useful. The child's ability to organize play is an early index of behavioral adjustment. At preschool age the Developmental Test of Visual-Motor Integration (VMI) is often given. There are drawing tasks on the McCarthy Scales, and the VMI can be given for comparison to those children who lack refinement in perceptual-motor skills. At school age (7 to 8 years), a screening for academic achievement is desirable. The Wide Range Achievement Test, Revised (WRAT-R) is commonly used.

When multiple examinations are planned by the follow-up team, the formal developmental assessment of the infant or child should be accomplished first. The optimal performance of the child is desired, and it is not likely to be obtained if a child has been exhausted or made wary by a physical or neurologic examination. The opportunity for all team members to view different assessments from behind one-way mirrors is ideal for both team discussion and for shortening the actual examination time for the child.

Corrected Age for Prematurity. In the case of premature infants, how long to correct or adjust the age of the infant is a subject of debate.[38-41] Catch-up has been viewed as a unitary phenomenon, although there is some suggestion that, at least in very early infancy, different functions catch up at different rates.[42] For cognitive development, there is evidence that biologic maturity does affect test scores until at least age 2 years in very low birth weight infants, but that by school age differences between premature and term children are not generally related to biologic development. Infants who are small for gestational age should have their age adjusted for their degree of prematurity, if any.

There are different patterns of development among different weight groups of premature infants. Healthy premature infants *more than* 1250 grams at birth tend to catch up over the first 12 months of life. For these infants, age is adjusted at the 12-month examination, but not thereafter.

Premature infants *less than* 1250 grams are significantly more premature. Catch-up is a longer process. Age in this group should be adjusted until the chronologic age of 3 years for developmental test scores. Research literature deals with group means and averages. Some children catch up earlier, and others later. Attention to the individual pattern of each child is most helpful in talking to parents. It should also be remembered that this weight division (less than 1250 grams and more than 1250 grams) is a customary but arbitrary grouping. An infant of 1270 grams is more likely to follow the pattern of an infant less than 1250 grams than that of an infant of 1600 grams.

ASSESSMENT PROTOCOL FOR CHILDREN WITH ATYPICAL DEVELOPMENT

Multidisciplinary Assessment. Children whose development is of concern should be assessed on an as-needed basis by team members appropriate to the areas of concern. For example, abnormal motor development at 5 months of age may be evaluated by the physical therapist and/or neurologist. When slow motor development appears to be part of a global developmental delay, formal developmental assessment should be carried out. Concerns about articulation or language development may be referred to the speech pathologist.

Frequency of Assessment. For cognitive deficit, periodic evaluation is helpful to determine rate of progress. Frequency of assessments is best determined on a case-by-case basis. In the first 18 months, development proceeds rapidly, and as a general rule, serial assessments every three months are useful. These assessments should begin as soon as atypical development is suspected. After 18 months, a general guideline is assessment every six months until stability of cognitive performance is achieved.

Predicting Outcome for Atypical Children. There is little correlation between infant tests and school-age IQ. Infant tests do not assess complex cognitive functioning. The environment also has a powerful impact on a child in shaping "intelligence" as measured by intelligence tests. Socioeconomic status of the family is the most reliable predictor of later measured intelligence, except in the case of the profoundly retarded.

There is no magic age when measured intelligence becomes stable. There is, however, both clinical and research evidence[43] to suggest that at preschool age (4 to 5 years), one can get a fairly good sense about intellectual potential. Experience in preschool or, more precisely, the lack of preschool experience, can affect test scores at this age, however. Some studies suggest that children with either completely normal or always abnormal evaluations in infancy tend toward greater stability in measured intellectual ability than children with borderline evaluations.[32,33] This assumes stability of the environment as well.

Caution must always be applied when considering a diagnosis of mental retardation in a child. This diagnosis can be made only when alternative explanations for test performance have been explored and when the child has been tested in different educational settings to determine actual ability to learn. Diagnosis should be deferred until the child has been given opportunity to demonstrate his or her cognitive level in familiar and comfortable surroundings.

Ability and Disability. Most research on the outcome of high-risk infants has proceeded on a "deficit" model of development. Infants are seen as lacking in abilities rather than as expressing variation in developmental patterns. It has been noted by Kopp and Krakow[3] that assessments of functions shortly after a period of perinatal stress are often assumed to shape development many years later. Deficits in social, cognitive, and perceptual skills and expression of emotions seen in the high-risk infant shortly after discharge from the nursery are regarded as permanent rather than transient differences.

The longitudinal follow-up of high-risk infants brings them under scrutiny that is lacking in low-risk infants, except in a few longitudinal studies of normal growth and development. The disability focus is dominant, as few outcome studies mention or dwell on the many high-risk infants who do well at preschool and school ages. Even in blind studies that attempt to control experimenter bias, the physical appearance of some high-risk children belies their perinatal history.[44]

The role of the family in supporting the optimal development of the child is important. Particularly for healthy premature children the course of development tends toward recovery and normal development.[45] When this tendency is interfered with, often by stresses with the family associated with low socioeconomic status, the natural recovery process falters. Disability should not be confused with perinatal risk factors in some cases in which it may be more strongly related to social risk factors such as poverty, child abuse, and other environmental hazards.

SUMMARY AND GUIDELINES

Important things to be remembered about the mental development of high-risk infants can be summarized as follows for general pediatric care:

1. A significant medical contribution of pediatric care of the high-risk infant is obtaining specialized vision and hearing examinations throughout the first two years of life. By assuring sensory intactness or ascertaining that needed hearing or vision aids are provided as soon as possible, primary pediatric care has provided an important base for further cognitive development.

2. Premature infants with complicated intracranial hemorrhage, with or without a shunt, make up one of the two groups of ICN infants who should have highest priority for detailed, multidisciplinary follow-up. This group and the second—significantly asphyxiated term infants—are made up of the infants with the widest range of outcomes, from completely normal to severely impaired. The role of the pediatrician or health professional is not to assume impairment in every child, but rather to be alert in a particular child for any presenting or evolving signs that call for further assessment. One should remember when talking to parents that many of these children will have normal intelligence.

3. When cognitive deficit occurs, it commonly occurs as overall lowered intelligence in the presence of earlier transient abnormalities or permanent motor deficits. Sometimes it occurs as specific deficits in the presence of normal intelligence ("learning disabilities"). Simple mental retardation is not, by itself, a common outcome of high-risk infants.

4. Although documenting sensory intactness is critically important in the early years, another important task of primary care providers is supporting the family in caring for and nurturing their child. No intervention program or special educator will have the long-term commitment to the child that the family can have if they are supported in their efforts to love and provide for their child, and if they are encouraged to find the appropriate intervention program when needed. The primary care provider has a special relationship to parents that is important in the medical care of the infant or child.

WHEN TO WORRY

The following guidelines are suggested for detecting or confirming cognitive deficit:

1. When parents are worried about mental development, a referral for developmental assessment may be appropriate. Parents may have picked up sutble signs that are worrisome, or they may have general anxiety about the infant's development that can best be addressed by an assessment.

2. When infants score in the borderline range or below (less than 84) on developmental or intellectual assessments, a careful analysis

should be carried out for any medical or environmental factors that might be contributing to low performance. Some intervention may be indicated to facilitate optimal performance for the infant or child.

3. When an infant scores 68 or below on any developmental or intelligence test, testing should be repeated in three months (or sooner, if appropriate), as this may indicate permanent cognitive deficit. When deficit exists, referral to an infant or preschool program is indicated.

4. When behavior interferes consistently with obtaining a formal assessment, it is likely to be interfering with developmental tasks that the child should be mastering. A referral for further evaluation or counseling may be indicated for the child and family.

References

1. Hess JH, Mohr GJ, Bartelme PF: The Physical and Mental Growth of Prematurely Born Children. Chicago, University of Chicago Press, 1934.
2. Cross VM: The Premature Baby. Philadelphia, Blakiston Company, 1945.
3. Kopp CB, Krakow JB: The developmentalist and the study of biological risk: A view of the past with an eye toward the future. Child Dev 54:1086, 1983.
4. Kumar SP, Anday EK, Sacks LM, et al.: Follow-up studies of very low birthweight infants (1250 grams or less) born and treated within a perinatal center. Pediatrics 66:438, 1980.
5. Horwood SP, Boyle MH, Torrance GW, et al.: Mortality and morbidity of 500- to 1,499-gram birth weight infants live-born to residents of a defined geographic region before and after neonatal intensive care. Pediatrics 69:613, 1982.
6. Harvey D, Prince J, Bunton J, et al.: Abilities of children who were small-for-gestational-age babies. Pediatrics 69:296, 1982.
7. Westwood M, Kramer MS, Munz D, et al.: Growth and development of full-term nonasphyxiated small-for-gestational-age newborns: Follow-up through adolescence. Pediatrics 71:376, 1983.
8. Bozynski MEA, Nelson MN, Matalon TAS, et al.: Cavitary periventricular leukomalacia: Incidence and short-term outcome in infants weighing 1200 grams at birth. Dev Med Child Neurol 27:572, 1985.
9. Weindling AM, Rochefort MJ, Calvert SA, et al.: Development of cerebral palsy after ultrasonographic detection of periventricular cysts in the newborn. Dev Med Child Neurol 27:800, 1985.
10. Broman SH: Perinatal anoxia and cognitive development in early childhood. In Field TM (ed.): Infants Born At Risk: Behavior and Development. New York, Spectrum Publications, 1979, pp. 29–52.
11. Holden KR, Mellits ED, Freeman JM: Neonatal seizures. I. Correlation of prenatal and perinatal events with outcomes. Pediatrics 70:165, 1982.
12. Mellits ED, Holden KR, Freeman JM: Neonatal seizures: II. A multivariate analysis of factors associated with outcome. Pediatrics 70:177, 1982.
13. Ballard RB, Leonard CH: Developmental follow-up of infants with persistent pulmonary hypertension of the newborn. Clin Perinatol 11:737, 1984.
14. Escalona SK: Babies at double hazard: Early development of infants at biologic and social risk. Pediatrics 70:670, 1982.
15. Parmelee AH, Cohen SE: Neonatal follow-up services for infants at risk. In Harel KS, Anastasiow, NJ (eds.): The At-Risk Infant: Psycho/Socio/Medical Aspects. Baltimore, Paul H. Brooks, 1985, p. 269.
16. Scott KG, Masi W: The outcome from and utility of registers of risk. In Field TM (ed.): Infants Born At Risk: Behavior and Development. New York, Spectrum Publications, 1979, pp. 485–496.
17. Siegel LS: The prediction of possible learning disabilities in preterm and full-term children. In Field TM, Sostek A (eds.): Infants Born At Risk: Physiological, Perceptual and Cognitive Processes. New York, Grune & Stratton, 1983, pp. 295–315.
18. Klein H, Hack M, Gallagher M, et al.: Preschool performance of children with normal intelligence who were very low-birth-weight-infants. Pediatrics 75:531, 1985.
19. Bennett FC, Robinson NM, Sells CJ: Growth and development of infants weighing less than 800 grams at birth. Pediatrics 71:319, 1983.
20. Hirata T, Epcar JT, Walsh A, et al.: Survival and outcome of infants 501 to 750 gm: A six-year experience. J Pediatr 102:741, 1983.
21. Ment LR, Scott DT, Ehrenkranz RA, et al.: Neonates of < 1250 grams birth weight: Prospective neurodevelopmental evaluation during the first year post-term. Pediatrics 70:292, 1982.
22. Leonard C, Miller C, Piecuch R, et al.: Developmental outcome of 93 infants weighing 1,250 grams or less with and without IVH: Two-year follow-up. Syllabus, Second Special Ross Laboratories Conference on Perinatal Intracranial Hemorrhage. Columbus, Ross Laboratories, 1982, Vol. 2, pp. 1176–1187.
23. Liechty EA, Gilmor RL, Bryson CQ, et al.: Outcome of high-risk neonates with ventriculomegaly. Dev Med Child Neurol 25:162, 1983.
24. Tew B: The "cocktail party syndrome" in children with hydrocephalus and spina bifida. Br J Disorders Commun 14:80, 1979.
25. Nelson KB, Ellenberg JH: Children who "outgrew" cerebral palsy. Pediatrics 69:529, 1982.
26. Vohr BR, Bell EF, Oh W: Infants with bronchopulmonary dysplasia: Growth pattern and neurologic and developmental outcome. Am J Dis Child 136:443, 1982.
27. Goldson E: Bronchopulmonary dysplasia: Its relation to two-year developmental functioning in the very low birth weight infant. In Field TM, Sostek A (eds.): Infants Born At Risk: Physiological, perceptual and cognitive processes. New York, Grune & Stratton, 1983, pp. 243–250.
28. Markestad T, Fitzhardinge PM: Growth and development in children recovering from bronchopulmonary dysplasia. J Pediatr 98:597, 1981.
29. Sauvre RS, Singhal N: Long-term morbidity of infants with bronchopulmonary dysplasia. Pediatrics 76:725, 1985.
30. Dorney SF, Ament ME, Berquist WE, et al.: Improved survival in very short small bowel of infancy with use of long-term parenteral nutrition. J Pediatr 107:521, 1985.
31. Rourke BP: Outstanding issues in research in learning disabilities. In Rutter M (ed.): Developmental Neuropsychiatry. New York, Guilford Press, 1983, pp. 546–574.
32. Vohr, BR, Garcia Coll, CT: Neurodevelopmental and school performance of very-low-birth-weight-infants:

A seven-year longitudinal study. Pediatrics 76:345, 1985.

33. Ross G, Lipper EG, Auld PA: Consistency and change in the development of premature infants weighing less than 1,501 grams at birth. Pediatrics 76:885, 1985.

34. Klaus MH, Kennell JH: Caring for the parents of premature or sick infants. In Klaus MH, Kennell JH: Maternal-Infant Bonding, 2nd ed. St. Louis, C.V. Mosby, 1982, pp. 151–226.

35. Shirley M: Development of immature babies during their first two years. Child Dev 9:347, 1938.

36. Shirley M: A behavior syndrome characterizing prematurely born children. Child Dev 10:115, 1939.

37. Minde KK: The impact of prematurity on the later behavior of children and on their families. Clin Perinatol 11:227, 1984.

38. Parmelee AH, Schulte FJ: Developmental testing of pre-term and small-for-date infants. Pediatrics 45:21, 1970.

39. Hunt JV, Rhodes L: Mental development of preterm infants during the first year. Child Dev 48:204, 1977.

40. Siegel LS: Correction for prematurity and its consequence for the assessment of the very low birth weight infant. Child Dev 54:1176, 1983.

41. Ungerer JA, Sigman M: Developmental lags in preterm infants from one to three years of age. Child Dev 54:1217, 1983.

42. Kraemer HC, Korner AF, Hurwitz S: A model for assessing the development of preterm infants as a function of gestational, conceptional, or chronological age. Dev Psychol 21:806, 1985.

43. Hunt JV: Longitudinal research: A method for studying intellectual development in high-risk pre-term infants. In Field TM (ed.): Infants Born at Risk: Behavior and Development. New York, Spectrum Publications, 1979, pp. 443–460.

44. Goldberg S: The pragmatics and problems of longitudinal research with high-risk infants. In Field TM (ed.): Infants Born at Risk: Behavior and Development. New York, Spectrum Publications, 1979, pp. 427–442.

45. Wilson R: Risk and resilience in early mental development. Dev Psychol 21:795, 1985.

Assessment Instruments

Bayley Scales

Bayley N: Bayley Scales of Infant Development. New York, Psychological Corporation, 1969.

Gesell Schedules

Knobloch HK, Pasamanick B (eds.): Gesell and Amatruda's Developmental Diagnosis, 3rd. ed. Hagerstown, Harper & Row, 1974.

McCarthy Scales

McCarthy M: McCarthy Scales of Children's Abilities. New York, Psychological Corporation, 1972.

Stanford-Binet Scale

Terman LM, Merrill MA: Stanford-Binet Intelligence Scale. Manual for the Third Revision. Form L-M. Boston, Houghton-Mifflin Co., 1973.

Thorndike RL, Hagen EP, Sattler JM: The Stanford-Binet Intelligence Scale, 4th ed. Chicago, Riverside Publishing Company, 1986.

Wechsler Scale

Wechsler D: Wechsler Intelligence Scale for Children, Revised. New York, Psychological Corporation, 1974.

Visual-Motor Integration

Beery KE: Revised Administration, Scoring and Teaching Manual for the Developmental Test of Visual-Motor Integration. Cleveland, Modern Curriculum Press, 1982.

Wide Range Achievement

Jastak S, Wildonson, GS: The Wide Range Achievement Test, Revised. Wilmington, Jastak Associates, 1984.

Recommended Reading

Escalona SK: Babies at double hazard: Early development of infants at biologic and social risk. Pediatrics 70:670, 1982.

Kopp CB, Krakow JB: The developmentalist and the study of biological risk: A view of the past with an eye toward the future. Child Dev 54:1086, 1983.

Minde KK: The impact of prematurity on the later behavior of children and on their families. Clin Perinatol 11:227, 1984.

Nelson KB, Ellenberg JH: Children who "outgrew" cerebral palsy. Pediatrics 69:529, 1982.

Parmelee AH, Cohen SE: Neonatal follow-up services for infants at risk. In Harel KS, Anastasiow NJ (eds.): The At-Risk Infant: Psycho/Socio/Medical Aspects. Baltimore, Paul H. Brooks, 1985, p. 269.

Wilson R: Risk and resilience in early mental development. Dev Psychol 21:795, 1985.

12

HEARING AND SPEECH ASSESSMENT

JOELYN RYAN, M.S., C.C.C.

HEARING

The incidence of deafness in the United States is reported to be about 1 in 1500 births, with hearing loss (including transient losses due to otitis media) occurring in about 5 of every 100 school-aged children. Preterm infants are considered to have an increased risk of hearing loss, with an incidence at birth as great as 1 in 50.

RISK OF HEARING LOSS

The Position Statement (1982) of the American Academy of Pediatrics Joint Committee on Infant Hearing listed the presence of the following factors as identifying those infants who are at risk for having hearing impairment:

1. Family history of childhood hearing impairment
2. Congenital perinatal infection (e.g., cytomegalovirus, rubella, herpes, toxoplasmosis, syphilis)
3. Anatomic malformation involving the head or neck, e.g., dysmorphic appearance, including syndromal and nonsyndromal abnormalities, overt or submucous cleft palate, morphologic abnormalities of the pinna
4. Birth weight less than 1500 grams

5. Hyperbilirubinemia at level exceeding indications for exchange transfusion
6. Bacterial meningitis, especially *Haemophilus influenzae*
7. Severe asphyxia which may include infants with Apgar scores of 0 to 3, or who fail to institute spontaneous respiration by 10 minutes, and those with hypotonia persisting to 2 hours of age.

HEARING ASSESSMENT

The guidelines for perinatal care of the American Academy of Pediatrics and the American Academy of Obstetrics and Gynecology advise the following approach to hearing assessment.

The hearing of infants who manifest any characteristic item on the list of risk criteria should be investigated, preferably under the supervision of an audiologist, and optimally by 3 months of age, but no later than 6 months of age. The initial examination should include observation of behavioral or electrophysiologic response to sound levels. The screening process is considered complete, except when there is a probability of progressive hearing loss, e.g., a family history of delayed onset or degenerative disease, or a history of intrauterine infection. If results of an initial assessment are equivocal, the infant should be referred for diagnostic testing.

Diagnostic hearing evaluation of an infant less than 6 months of age should include a history and general physical examination, encompassing the following:

1. Examination of the head and neck
2. Otoscopy
3. Identification of relevant physical abnormalities
4. Laboratory tests, such as urinalysis and diagnostic test for perinatal infections

Comprehensive audiologic evaluation should include (1) a behavioral history, and (2) behavioral observation audiometry, or (3) testing of auditory evoked potentials, if indicated.

In addition to these known risk factors, infants who do not produce a consistent startle reflex to sudden loud noises, who do not turn toward a sound by 6 months of age, whose verbal output decreases between 6 and 9 months of age, and in particular, infants whose parents are concerned about their child's hearing, should be referred to an audiologist who works with small children. See Table 12–1 for when to worry at various ages.

Early detection and amplification are essential to the optimal speech-oral language development of deaf and hard-of-hearing children. In deaf children, even ability to detect the presence of sound will improve the child's safety, ability to respond to others, and awareness of the environment. Early education is essential for the deaf and the hard-of-hearing child. Guideline B is a list of some do's and don'ts for parents of children with hearing loss.

In common with other children, high-risk infants often develop otitis media and may have transient conductive hearing losses or long-standing losses if the otitis is chronic or if middle ear effusion is untreated.

SPEECH AND LANGUAGE

Language is a complex human skill that requires the coordination of many sensory, motor, and cognitive abilities. By 5 years of age a normally developing child should have essentially mastered native language and should be able to understand and to construct novel sentences that allow exchange of ideas and information with others in his or her environment. It is useful for the pediatrician to be familiar with a few of the many subskills required for successful language learning and usage, their interactions,

and possible deficits resulting from problems common to high-risk infants.

For purposes of this chapter *hearing* is considered a passive system, an area in which the child is or is not physiologically normal. *Listening* is considered a more complex, active process. No clear separation between hearing and listening exists, and an acknowledgment of their overlapping character is assumed. *Articulation* is the movement of orofacial mechanisms to produce *speech* sounds; the rule system upon which these sounds are based is called the *phonologic* system. Articulation may be considered separate from language; the phonologic system is a subsystem of language.

The normal full-term infant is born with or soon acquires the ability to discriminate between vowels and between acoustically similar consonants (e.g., between voiced and unvoiced cognates); he or she has an innate preference for sound in the range of human speech. At birth, or shortly thereafter, the infant is alert and receptive to auditory stimulation.

Sound production through the cooing stage is universal in nature and progresses from front vowels and back consonants to increasingly complex patterns. This process lasts for about the first six months of life for the normal full-term infant and is not dependent on auditory stimulation; profoundly deaf children develop the same pattern of increasingly complex sound production that develops all the sounds of all oral human languages. This stage of sound production is not considered a direct precursor of the phonologic system.

At about 6 months of age the full-term normal infant enters the babbling stage with the purposeful production of syllables, starting with front consonants and back vowels. Babbling is dependent on the auditory stimulation that preceded it and that continues during the babbling stage. Babbling becomes increasingly complex, until it includes all the sounds of the native language produced in appropriate prosodic patterns.

Each child devises a phonologic system on the basis of his or her own experience and ability to hear and to discriminate between sounds. The ability to motor plan and to control speech mechanism affects the output of this system.

Language is a social phenomenon and, as such, there are psychosocial as well as cognitive prerequisites. Caregiver's responsiveness is related to the infant's competence during the first year of life, and the caregiver's responsiveness continues to be an important factor in the infant's development beyond that period. Com-

TABLE 12–1. Indications for Evaluation of Hearing, Speech, and Language

CORRECTED AGE	HEARING	SPEECH	LANGUAGE
Birth	Presence of 1 or more high-risk factors: prematurity (<1500 gm); asphyxia, orofacial anomalies; congenital infection, especially CMV; CNS signs: IVH, meningitis; hyperbilirubinemia; family history of deafness	Orofacial anomalies, IVH, hemiparesis; dysphagia; hard of hearing, deaf	Deafness, hard of hearing; blindness, visual deficit; syndromes that include developmental delay
6 mo	No response to sudden noise; decrease in sound production; no orientation toward sound; presence of 1 or more high-risk factors	Cooing does not contain a variety of sounds, is limited to 1 to 2 syllables	Does not respond differently to warnings, anger, friendly voice patterns; does not appear to enjoy vocal play
12 mo	No response or localization toward novel sounds; no rhythmic response to music; lack of attention to speech	Little or no babbling; lack of variety of sounds in babbling; jaw fixation during speech	Does not understand familiar "Where is . . . ? questions; expressive vocabulary of less than 3 words; lack of communicative intent
18 mo	Hypernasal or hyponasal speech; lack of response to requests; all items in 12-month group	Less than 4 different consonants in true words; does not babble conversations	Less than 8-word expressive vocabulary; no method of indicating negation (verbal/gestural); lack of successful communication with parent; does not understand common requests
24 mo	Poor speech (for age); poor attention; delayed language; history of multiple episodes of chronic otitis media	Does not name intelligibly at least 10 items; does not use a few 2-word phrases; repetitions effortful	Does not refer to self (name or pronoun); cannot or does not bring objects from another room on request (e.g., diaper or shoe)
30 mo	Uses few consonants; speech very loud or very soft; Says "huh" frequently; does not attend to speech; has speech or language delay; fails hearing examination when ears are not congested	Does not pronounce correctly: /p/, /b/, /m/, /t/, /d/, /n/, /w/, /j/, /y/ in you, /h/ in initial position; does not produce short intelligible phrases; vowel sounds in repetitions incorrect (e.g., "wuh-wuh-what")	Does not repeat 2 numbers correctly; does not use or comprehend verbs; does not communicate in some way
36 mo	Speech or language delay; if parent complains that child is uncooperative or does not follow directions; if child fails hearing examination when ears are not congested	Remains largely unintelligible; parent cannot understand child; child or parent frustrated by difficulty in intelligibility; vowel sounds incorrect, as above; speech effortful (tension or struggle behavior with dysfluency)	Does not use some verb endings (including habitually present be- in Black English); does not understand prepositions: in, on, under, and behind; does not tell what happened when he or she was out (highlights only)
48 mo	Speech or language delay; poor attention; very close observation of speaker's face; fails hearing examination when ears not congested	Does not produce /k/, /g/, and /f/ correctly; /s/, /z/ not produced (may have frontal lisp at this age); amount or severity of dysfluency increasing	Does not describe pictures in detail (unless child is shy); does not name at least 6 animals (without cues) on request; does not answer questions about topics of interest to him or her
60 mo	Omission of /s/, /z/, /(sh)/, /f/, /(th)/ in speech or substitutions between these sounds, except for frontal lisp; speech or language delay; fails hearing examination when ears not congested	Does not produce /s/ initial consonant clusters; makes errors in more than one of following: /s/, /z/, /(sh)/, /ch/, /g in George/, /l/, /r/, /-/, /(th)/; remains dysfluent	Does not describe movie, recent TV program, or other event in a way one can follow; does not give needed information in response to 1 or 2 questions; does not mention more than 10 foods on request

munication between the child and others in his or her environment does not depend entirely on the development of language; it also occurs before language, and language depends, in part, on these early exchanges. Infants and others coo, babble, gesture, and make faces at each other; each responds with attention, with eye contact, and with smiles; infants often attempt to guide these "conversations" by looking at or otherwise indicating objects of interest to them. Games involving verbal imitations of nonsense sounds, imitation of pitch and prosodic patterns, and nonverbal responses to verbal cues develop spontaneously in almost every child's experience. They teach the child that verbal interactions are pleasurable, that responses are related to previous verbal productions, that gestures and verbalizations can relate to the same object or activity, and that people take turns in conversation.

Language acquisition most closely follows a Piagetian model of cognitive development. Before language begins, a child needs to have developed certain concepts that are generally acquired during the first year of life, during the first four stages of Piaget's sensorimotor period. The child needs to develop intention, imitation, representation, and the concept of object permanence. These abilities develop in the normal full-term infant as he or she explores and manipulates the environment.

Infants with various disabilities may not complete these tasks as rapidly as the normal child. The child who is orthopedically disabled is limited in ability to explore his or her environment; the blind child is limited in ability to observe the results of his or her manipulations; the deaf child misses the noise-related results of his or her actions, as well as attention-getting sounds and the speech in his or her environment; the ill child lacks the stamina to explore vigorously and to manipulate his or her environment; the very low birth weight infant must often wait for the addition of ounces or pounds before balance for effective movement can occur. All of these children may require more time to gather sufficient experience to gain these concepts. Therefore, early assessments may show delayed language development.

First uses of words are referential in nature; they refer to the occurrence, nonoccurrence or disappearance, or reappearance of a person or object in the child's environment. The usual first question from a child, a form of What's that? is used as a request for the names of objects or persons occurring in the environment. The child needs a group of words, a lexicon, to ex-

periment with, so that he or she can explore this new method of manipulating the environment. The words and phrases used for this purpose are called referential grammars. Examples of referential grammars are: "milk" (occurrence), "all gone milk" (disappearance), and "more milk" (reappearance).

True language is not used to label the outside world, but to communicate relationships that are salient to the speaker (his or her internal representation of the world). Words and phrases used in this manner are called relational grammars. Full-term normal children reach the stage of developing relational grammars at about 18 months of age.

From the beginning of relational grammars, language becomes increasingly complex as the child's cognitive ability increases. Vocabulary grows to reflect experience, and phrases grow to express more than one relationship in a sentence. As an example, when the child starts using relational grammars he may say, "My ball," "Throw ball," or "Me"; after more experience, he may say, "Throw my ball to me, please." Some questions the pediatrician can ask parents to help elicit information about a young child's vocabulary are found at the end of the chapter.

At first, the child is able to talk only about what is visible in the environment (and may be able to get along with gestures at this stage); this expands through a stage of being able to talk about things that are in some way indexed in the immediate context until he becomes context free and is able to think and talk about his or her experiences without the aid of indexing in the immediate environment of the conversation or thought. The child who is developing normally learns all of this by the end of the fifth year, and language has begun to replace experience as the primary source of new information.

Language clearly augments experience for the developing child. Because of cognitive limits continuing up to early adolescence, all the child's thoughts and language development are firmly rooted in actual experiences. Abstract use of language awaits the cognitive shift that usually occurs at age 11 to 13 years.

P. Gorski

FACTORS AFFECTING LANGUAGE ACQUISITION

Differences in High-Risk Infant Development. The birth of a high-risk infant is followed by a period of anxiety for the parent and includes at least partial separation from the infant. Studies have shown that, after discharge from the hospital, there are differences in interactions between premature infants and their parents and full-term normal infants and their parents. Mothers of preterm infants have less time en face, have less physical contact with their infants, and smile less than mothers of full-term infants. In the first four months, premature infants have been observed to be less attentive in interactions and to look at objects and places more than full-term babies; mothers of premature infants may spend less time in the same room with their infants during their early months, but this difference usually disappears over time. Another characteristic of language development in premature infants has been less frequent vocalization than in full-term infants. The reasons for these differences in style are not clear, and their occurrence should not be considered indicative of negligence or lack of love for the child.

This may reflect the mother's adaptive behavior, perhaps protecting the premature infant's lower sensory thresholds from overload. We must indeed be careful not to mislabel parenting responses as negligent, so long as we ourselves have insufficient understanding of the meaning of particular early parent-infant interactions.

P. Gorski

Obviously, differences in early exchanges between premature infants and their caregivers (as compared to full-term babies) may result in differences in early language development.

Hearing Loss. Even a mild or intermittent hearing loss may adversely affect speech and language development. In children already at risk for speech/language disorders, the effects of even a temporary, mild loss may be magnified. In early language development, hearing loss is often signalled by poor auditory attention on the part of the child, hypernasal or denasal speech, and marked reduction in the production and/or accuracy of consonant production. Children with mild-to-moderate hearing losses, whether conductive or sensorineural in nature, may or may not benefit from amplification. While these children usually do not require the intensive early training of the severely or profoundly hard of hearing, they frequently do need early speech/language therapy to minimize the effects of the hearing deficit on their language development. (Guideline B is a suggested "hand-out" to aid parents of children with hearing loss.)

Blindness. Blindness or severe visual disability places formidable constraints on a child's language learning. Blind children can be expected to follow a different timetable for language acquisition than sighted children; there are also differences in content in their early language. Blind children are often echolalic, particularly children with retrolental fibroplasia; that is, they repeat what is said to them rather than creating their own comments. They frequently store and use "chunks" of language—whole phrases rather than individual words—in their early language period. Programs for blind children aid the child in progressing from echolalia to spontaneous phrase production. Interaction between parent and child and teacher and child is an important part of this process, and the need to talk to the blind child about what he or she is doing should be emphasized with parents. Blind children, like deaf children, need early intervention programs to achieve their maximum potential. Questions about their language functioning should be directed to staff involved in the child's program or to a speech pathologist who is skilled in working with blind children.

Central Nervous System Abnormalities. Low birth weight children and those with birth asphyxia are at risk for CNS compromise; those with evidence of hemiparesis need to be evaluated for orofacial asymmetries and for swallowing or eating disorders. Orofacial weakness increases the difficulty of sound production and places these children at higher risk for speech disorders. High-risk infants with cerebral palsy can be expected to exhibit speech disorders relative to the severity of the involvement. Children with physical disorders of the types described above can be expected to benefit from early intervention.

SPEECH

Speech is a complex motor activity requiring coordination of breathing, laryngeal and pharyngeal function, and orofacial and tongue movement. Children who demonstrate general clumsiness in other areas, even without hard signs of neurologic compromise, can be expected to be slow in developing clear speech. General clumsiness is a common finding in neurologic assessment of preterm infants.

As language skills improve and phrase length increases, respiratory support becomes increasingly important as the real-time requirement for controlled exhalation increases. Many children with chronic lung disease following neonatal respiratory distress syndrome have inadequate air supply. While respiratory distress may improve with age, the very young child devises compensatory strategies that become part of his or her speech production patterns, and children vary in the ease with which they allow changes in these patterns. The result may be atypical prosodic patterns with excessive breaks for inhalation, or sounds may be delayed or disordered as the child continues to have difficulty getting enough breath to support the primary needs of the organism. Speech therapy may be helpful for these children in assuring selection of good compensatory strategies.

Dysphonia. Many very low birth weight children seen in follow-up programs are dysphonic, with high, light voices or hoarse, harsh-sounding speech. Some children speak in a habitual whisper. Almost all of these dysphonic children have had sufficient respiratory distress to require intubation in the nursery; many have had intraventricular hemorrhages. The dysphonia appears to improve over time, but as many as 60 per cent of low birth weight infants continue to be dysphonic at the age of 5 years (ICN Follow-up Clinic, Mount Zion Hospital and Medical Center, San Francisco). Usually the primary caregivers understand most of what these children say, but there may be occasional frustration for both the caregiver and the child when communication is unsuccessful.

Phonologic Delay. Early phonologic development must be considered delayed when it acts as a deterrent to development of a productive vocabulary (Table 12–1). At 18 months of age, normal full-term children are acquiring a rapidly expanding vocabulary. Low birth weight premature infants, at the corrected age of 18 months, have been found to be significantly poorer in phonologic development than normal full-term children. At assessments at 18 to 24 months, phonologic delays sufficient to reduce productive vocabulary potential were found in 63 per cent of tested preterm infants of less than 1500 grams at birth; at subsequent assessments phonologic development was improved relative to age norms in all but 5 per cent (ICN Follow-up Clinic, Mount Zion Hospital and Medical Center).

Developmental Apraxia. Speech deficits that are not so easily understood occur in another group of children. While developmental apraxia is rare, compared to the frequency of phonologic disorder, it is a more serious problem. This is a disorder of motor planning for speech and results in the loss of ability to produce sounds based on the phonologic system. Substitutions are inconsistent; a child may pronounce a word four times, and it will be different each time. Perseveration may also occur, and, after struggling to produce a word, the child may repeat the word (or its approximation) through several attempts at other words. One child in our program, in attempting to say "nurse" in response to a picture, said, "mun," then "luss," then "rum," then "lurse," and finally "nuss." This was followed by responding "nuss" to pictures of a ball, a car, and a bird.

Some children with apraxia are able to repeat words with fair accuracy, but are not able to produce words spontaneously. To determine if apraxia is present it is necessary to use pictures as well as verbal imitation to elicit words. Some children with apraxia also have disordered prosody while others do not. Children suspected of apraxia should be referred to a speech therapist as soon as the suspicion arises.

Dysfluency (Stuttering). Many children go through a period of normal dysfluency at about 3 years of age; in normal full-term children this usually lasts about six months before disappearing spontaneously. This disorder appears to be due to a rapidly expanding language system that exceeds the child's motor ability. In preterm high-risk children this normal dysfluency may cover a longer period and may last for a year or more. If there is no indication of increased muscular tension in the face, neck, and/or shoulders, and no eye blinking, head jerking, or other struggle behavior related to the child's speech, it is appropriate to watch and wait. If tension or struggle behavior exists, the child should be referred to a specialist. This is an area in which patient counseling is often required to assure the parent that the dysfluency should be ignored and that if it is not made an issue of concern for the child, it will most likely disappear spontaneously. Guidelines C, D, and E, at the end of the chapter, may help parents in working with children who have either a speech delay or a problem with fluency.

EVALUATION AND TREATMENT

LANGUAGE DELAY

Table 12–1 and Guideline A, a list of questions to ask parents, will help the pediatrician delineate whether or not there is language delay. Lack of development of speech and language is sometimes the first indication that all is not well with the developing child, and diagnosis of developmental delay may follow a language assessment; the diagnosis of developmental delay should not be based on a speech or language evaluation, however. It is possible for a developmentally delayed child to have an additional language delay. When language is significantly more delayed than overall development, the child is a candidate for speech or language therapy.

> It should be remembered that, when any child visits a pediatrician, he or she will rarely say very much. In addition, the mother may be reluctant to mention her concerns. I recommend active use of the Guidelines at the end of this chapter to obtain the information to assess possible delayed language development.
>
> A. Rosen

Deficit in Contingency. A deficit in contingency is not uncommon in high-risk infants. Although its cause is not known, this type of deficit is one that high-risk, low birth weight children have in common with other at-risk populations, and which occurs much less frequently in full-term, normal children. A conversation with one of these children may go something like this:

Physician: "Hi."
Child: "My mom's here."
Physician: "What's your name?"
Child: "See my hat?"
Physician: "What a nice hat!"
Child: "My dog has spots."

No, the child will not tell you the name of the dog either. Children like this are a great frustration to their parents and to anyone else attempting to converse with them; they are often ostracized by their peers and confused about what is expected of them. This deficit in contingency is a language disorder, and referral to a speech or language specialist is appropriate; however, this is one disorder that usually can be remedied successfully through a program of indirect intervention at home. If the child is 3 years old or younger, a six-month period of watch and wait is indicated if the parent or caregiver is willing to follow these instructions: Set aside a minimum of 15 minutes each day in which to play with your child. During this period, do not attempt to teach your child anything that the child has not requested and do not attempt to make the child talk. Talk about what the child is doing and what you are doing with him or her and respond to any comments the child may make. It should be emphasized that this time should be a play period for the parent's and child's mutual enjoyment. The theory behind the instructions is that if the parent does focus on the child's activities, then the parent will be contingent with the child and will be giving the child a massed experience with contingency; it is the nature of human interaction that most parents will relax their contingency as that of the child improves.

This daily play period is designed to provide focused communication that is pleasurable to both partners. If the child remains noncontingent after six months, he or she should be referred to a specialist. Guideline E gives do's and do not's for parents to use for language development.

Developmental Aphasia. A severe form of language delay, this disorder may occur in any population, including preterm children. Children with this disorder are often labeled autistic, emotionally disturbed, or developmentally delayed. Early diagnosis and treatment of aphasic children affords an improved prognosis.

Autism. Another cause of language delay is, of course, autism. Although many varieties of speech and language disorders have been seen in the children in our high-risk infant follow-up program, autism has not been found. It would appear that preterm and asphyxiated infants are not at higher risk for this disorder than is the full-term population. The development of language in autistic children is a long process when it is successful, and it appears to be crucial if the child is going to avoid institutionalization; so, again, early intervention is recommended.

EDUCATION FOR THE DEAF

There are two schools of thought about the education of the deaf: the oralist tradition and the total communication school. The oralists focus on amplification, speech reading, and speech training. They believe that deaf children should not be exposed to sign language, because they believe that the use of sign language limits the prognosis for oral language.

Those who believe in the total communication approach counter that the deaf cannot learn to hear and that to isolate them from the deaf community and from sign language seriously reduces their acquisition of any language and reduces their ability to function when they become adults.

> By using sign language, the hearing-impaired child avoids constant frustration and, instead, develops a normally increasing interest in effective communication with others.
>
> P. Gorski

This total communication group points to the low success rate for intelligible speech among the deaf-born population (10 per cent) and for successful speech reading (4 per cent) among the deaf population. Their method of teaching, which, as the name implies, makes use of amplification, sign language, finger spelling, speech reading, and speech training, is, at the present time, enjoying increasing acceptance, in part because of recent research that confirms the full linguistic richness of American Sign Language, the sign language of the deaf.[1]

If a child is born deaf or is deafened before he or she has acquired speech, total communication is most apt to succeed. This option requires that other members of the family learn sign language and use it with the deaf child. In some families this has been viewed as an unacceptable hardship. Early stimulation programs for deaf children (if they use total communication) usually provide early training in sign language for the parents as well. Most preschool programs for deaf children that use the total communication approach also provide sign language classes for parents. Parents of deaf children are sometimes bombarded by the competing groups concerning their child's future education. Both groups are strongly committed to their view of what is best for deaf children and attempt to sway the parents to their view. Counseling and support are strongly needed at this time, and the child's pediatrician is often called upon for these.

WHEN TO WORRY

Table 12–1 presents guidelines for identifying anomalies that should trigger enough concern to pursue a referral for hearing, speech, or language evaluation in children between birth and 5 years of age.

WHERE TO FIND HELP

A pediatric audiologist is best located through treatment centers for young deaf and hard-of-hearing children, such as public and private hearing and speech centers and programs associated with medical centers and universities. An audiologist is the best source for a referral for these children.

The ideal speech and language pathologist for the high-risk infant is one with experience with children, a background in linguistics, and experience with neurologic disorders. If the child has motor involvement, a therapist trained to deal with these specific disorders may be needed. It is important that the child, his caregiver, and the therapist be comfortable with one another; without good interaction between the therapist and the child, therapy will be less effective than if there is rapport.

Regional centers are a source for names of therapists, as are nearby medical centers and hearing and speech centers. Speech and language therapists in private practice are often listed in the telephone book. Another way is through word of mouth among colleagues.

Federal Public Law 94-142 guarantees a free and appropriate education for all children. For many years, this was interpreted as all children above the age of 3 years, but recent legislation (PL 99-457)) has extended entitlement from birth to 21 years; but *appropriate* has not been extended to mean the best possible education. The local school district is required to search out, to assess, and to treat appropriately all identified children. The local school district's central assessment team should be notified about the child with special needs before his or her third birthday, to avoid delay in placement in a special needs program. Children may not be assessed or placed in a special program without the parent's consent.

Guidelines

GUIDELINE A: QUESTIONS FOR PARENTS

Questions to ask parents to elicit information about a young child's vocabulary (many conscientious parents, as well as those who are less concerned, usually report a vocabulary significantly smaller than that elicited by this or a similar list of questions).

1. How many words does your child use?
   a. What does he/she call you?
   b. Does he/she call anyone else by name?
   d. What does he/she say when thirsty?
   e. What does he/she say when wanting a toy that is out of reach?
   f. How does he/she say "No"?
   g. Does he/she say "Hi" or "Bye"?
   h. Does he/she say "Go"?
   i. Does he/she say "Up" or "Down"?
   j. What does he/she call a favorite toy, car, ball?
   k. What does he/she call cars, dogs, and cats?
   l. What does he/she say when you ask for or take something he/she has and does not want to give to you?
   m. What does he/she say when you give something to him/her?
   n. What does he/she say when wanting more milk, cookies, play time, and so on?
2. What does he/she do when wanting something that is not within view?

3. Does he/she imitate environmental sounds like cars, dogs, sirens, and the like?
4. Does he/she repeat words overheard in conversations? Swearing?

GUIDELINE B: FOR PARENTS WHOSE CHILD HAS A HEARING LOSS

To help your child understand what you are saying:

DO

1. Get his/her attention. Tap the child on the shoulder, wave your hand, turn the child gently; establish eye contact before speaking.
2. Speak a *little* slower than usual, especially if you are a rapid speaker.
3. Face the child and stand or kneel 3 to 6 feet from him/her while you are speaking.
4. Be sure that the light is at the child's back.
5. Use gestures and facial expressions while you talk.
6. Establish the topic early (example: "About the doll . . .", "Your teacher called . . .," "Where is the truck . . .?")
7. Keep your hands away from your mouth when you are talking.
8. If possible, find a quiet place in which to talk to the child.
9. Be certain the child hears you when you give him/her a compliment.
10. If the child wears hearing aids, check the batteries frequently.

DO NOT

1. Turn your back on the child while you are talking to him/her.
2. Talk to him/her from another room.
3. Yell at the child in an effort to help him/her hear you.

GUIDELINE C: FOR PARENTS WHOSE CHILD HAS SPEECH DELAY

DO

1. Listen for the *meaning,* not for the correctness of sounds.
2. If you are not sure you understood the child, tell him/her what you *think* was said; allow the child to accept or correct your interpretation.
3. Play games with the child that include *sound imitations,* e.g., animal sounds, car sounds, silly sounds.
4. Make *"faces"* with your child; a mirror may be helpful for this.

5. *Sing* with your child.
6. Let the child know that your love and approval are not related to his/her speech. (Avoid giving the message that you love him/her either less or more because of his/her speech.) *Encourage,* but do not force, the child to talk.
7. *Speak as clearly as possible* when you are with your child.
8. *Read* to your child.
9. *Encourage* your child to "read" familiar books to you.

DO NOT

1. *Tease* your child about his/her speech.
2. Attempt to *force* him/her to talk when reluctant to do so.
3. *Withhold* food or toys in an effort to make him/her say a word correctly.
4. *Demand* that he/she say something more clearly.
5. *Punish* the child for his/her speech when you have difficulty in understanding.

GUIDELINE D: FOR PARENTS OF A YOUNG CHILD WITH REDUCED FLUENCY

DO

1. *Listen* when your child talks.
2. *Allow* him/her to say what he/she has to say.
3. *Show an interest* in what he/she is saying.
4. Listen for *meaning,* not for the fluency of speech.
5. *Be as relaxed as possible* when dealing with the child.
6. *Provide a model* of slow, relaxed speech when speaking.
7. *Sing* with your child.
8. When playing with your child, include *noises,* e.g., animal noises, car noises.
9. *Talk* with your child about things of interest to him/her.

DO NOT

1. *Call the child's attention* to his/her dysfluency.
2. Insist that he/she *slow down* or repeat what he/she has been saying.
3. Tell him/her to *think* before speaking.
4. Show by *facial expression* or other reaction that you are upset by his/her speech.
5. *Complete phrases* for him/her.
6. *Demand explanations* for misbehavior. (This causes an unacceptable increase in stress during a period of speech.)

Remember that many children go through a period of dysfluency (stuttering) during the acquisition of language. Almost all of those who remain relaxed about their speech outgrow the dysfluency and develop normal speech and language.

GUIDELINE E: FOR PARENTS WHOSE CHILD HAS LANGUAGE DELAY

To help your child to talk:

DO

1. *Describe* what you are doing in short simple sentences (Example: "I'm washing the dishes," "I'm getting our coats") when you are with your child.
2. Take advantage of every opportunity to *talk* to the child, including social speech. (Example: "Hi," "Thank you," "You're welcome.")
3. *Listen* to your child when he/she does talk and *encourage* the child to do so.
4. *Comment* about the child's topic; continue the conversation. (Example: Child: "Big truck." Caregiver: "I like that truck, too; can you see the driver?")
5. Let the child hear the *names* of people and objects that he/she sees often.
6. When you are playing with your child, include the imitations of cars, animals, fire engines, and the like.
7. Provide some *sound-making toys* for your child.
8. *Accept* as speech any sounds that the child makes.
9. *Make all speech enjoyable.* Give the impression that it is fun to talk and to listen.
10. *Play* with your child with things he/she enjoys for at least 15 minutes a day without trying to teach the child anything directly.
11. Tell him/her you are *sorry* when you do not understand and he/she is becoming frustrated about it.

DO NOT

1. *Urge* the child to talk or make him/her feel you love him/her less because he/she does not speak well.
2. *Criticize* his/her speech to him/her or to others in front of the child.
3. *Laugh* at his/her mistakes or show anger when you do not understand.
4. *Withhold* food or toys in an attempt to force him/her to name them.
5. *Interrupt* the child and ask him/her to repeat something that you did not understand.

Reference

1. Bronowski J, Bellugi U: Language, name and concept. Science 168: 669, 1970.

Recommended Reading

Butler KG: Language processing disorders: Factors in diagnosis and remediation. In Keith R (ed.): Central Auditory Processing Disorders in Children. San Diego, College-Hill Press, 1981.

Ferguson CA: Introduction to Part I: Phonology. In Ferguson C, Slobin D (eds.): Studies in Child Language Development. New York, Holt, Rinehart, and Winston, 1973.

Hatten J, Gorman T, Lent C: Emerging Language 3. Tucson, Communication Skill Builders, 1981.

Hedrik DL, Prather EM, Tobin AR: Sequenced Inventory of Communication Development—Revised. East Aurora, NY, Slossen Educational Publications, 1984.

Kekelis L, Chernus-Mansfield N: Talk To Me. Los Angeles, The Blind Children's Center, Vol 1 and 2, 1986.

Rocisano L, Vatchmink Y: Mother/toddler interaction in preterm dyad and language outcome. Paper presented at the International Conference on Infant Studies, Austin, TX, 1982.

Sachs J: The development of speech. In Carterette EC, Friedman M (eds.): The Handbook of Perception. New York, Academic Press, 1976.

Semel E, Wilig E: Clinical Evaluation of Language Functions. Columbus, Charles Merrill Publishing Company, 1980.

Wilson DK: Voice Problems in Children. Baltimore, Williams & Wilkins Company, 1972.

13

THE EYES OF THE ICN GRADUATE*

SUSAN H. DAY, M.D.

Infants who graduate from the ICN are at risk for many eye problems, including retinopathy of prematurity, ocular consequences of prenatal or neonatal infection, visual loss associated with hydrocephalus, and congenital abnormalities occurring as part of a syndrome.

To assist the pediatrician in the proper care of the eyes of the ICN graduate, this chapter addresses the following issues:

1. Development of the eyes
2. Development of vision
3. Assessment of vision
4. Retinopathy of prematurity

DEVELOPMENT OF THE EYES

The eyes form as an evagination from the brain. In addition to neuroectodermal tissue, components from the surface ectoderm (such as the lens) and the mesoderm (such as blood vessels) also contribute to their development. The most critical time for organogenesis seems to be within the sixth to tenth weeks of gestation, during which any insult may lead to serious congen-

ital abnormalities, such as optic nerve hypoplasia. As the eyes mature, fusion of an embryonic cleft occurs inferiorly. If this fusion is interrupted, then a coloboma of the iris, choroid, retina, and/or optic nerve may result. Further developmental abnormalities may occur as a consequence of persistence of primitive vessels within the eyes (persistent hyperplastic primary vitreous).

In addition to risks related to prenatal formation of the eyes, the premature baby's eyes are at risk for abnormal development *after* birth (see section on retinopathy of prematurity).

DEVELOPMENT OF VISION

In the full-term infant, much of visual development occurs within a "critical" time—the first few months of life. Any factor that limits visual development during this critical period (such as a cataract) may lead to permanent visual loss, i.e., it cannot be corrected at a later date. The specific level of visual functioning has been estimated repeatedly in research settings as approximately 20/400 at birth. By the age of 6 months, some studies have shown that the ability to "see" 20/20 gratings has been reached.

It is not yet clear what effect prematurity has on the development of vision. Although some

* Supported in part by an unrestricted grant to the Department of Ophthalmology, Pacific-Presbyterian Medical Center from Research To Prevent Blindness

studies indicate that gestational age is a key factor in determining the pace of visual development, others indicate that chronologic age is more important, and indeed, some recent research suggests that development of visual acuity is accelerated in the preterm infant.[1]

ASSESSMENT OF VISION

The discharge summary the pediatrician receives from the ICN should include information on the extent to which the eyes have been examined during the hospitalization. Ordinarily a first examination will have been done when the infant was 6 to 8 weeks of age or at 34 weeks corrected age in the tiny premature infant. A baseline examination must be established on initial evaluation. The infant should demonstrate a clear fixing and following response by the age of 6 weeks. Careful follow-through assessments of vision should be done at 3, 6, 9, and 12 months of age.

OFFICE HISTORY AND PROGRESS NOTES

It is critical that the parents' assessment of the infant's vision be obtained when the infant comes to the office for checkups. In situations in which the infant's sight is limited, usually the parents are suspicious of a visual problem long before it is detected by a physician. However, they are often reluctant to mention their concern unless specifically asked, since they hope that their child will "outgrow" any problem. The simple question, "Does your baby see?" should be asked, and specific examples (such as the baby's smiling when the mother smiles, the baby's following a moving object with the eyes) should be noted. Several parental comments warrant careful attention. The parents may report that the child's eyes seem to "wander" without his or her paying attention to any specific object; this, of course, may reflect nystagmus, which can be associated with poor vision. Another worrisome sign is eye poking: An infant who sees poorly may use this behavior or may wave a hand rapidly across the face.

OFFICE EXAMINATION

Three features are important in examination of the eyes of an ICN graduate: the vision, the fundus (red reflex), and the alignment of the eyes.

Vision. How does one examine the developing vision of an infant? Evaluation of the fixation pattern is important. The eyes should remain steady and should be directed toward a specific object of interest. It is important to *assess each eye separately* for this function, since profound visual loss may be present in one eye only. Once central and steady fixation has been ascertained, it is also helpful to determine if the baby seems to follow a moving object. The examiner can simply hold the baby up in front of himself or herself and rock his or her own head from side to side, watching the behavior of the infant's eyes.

If markedly reduced vision is suspected, several tests may help to verify this. The vestibulo-ocular reflex should be elicited by turning in place while holding the infant. Nystagmus will be elicited, but it should be dampened by the fixation reflex if the baby's vision is not impaired. Persistence of nystagmus implies that the infant's vision is poor. The use of a "threat" stimulus to evaluate vision in babies usually is *not* very helpful; however, if a blink reflex is not obtained when a camera flash is triggered just in front of the baby's eyes, then vision is probably reduced.

Red Reflex. In assessing the quality of the *red reflex,* it is best to start at a distance of approximately one foot in front of the baby's eyes, using the direct ophthalmoscope with a $+4.00$ (black number) lens. Note the presence of any media opacities or other irregularity of the red reflex. Then move in toward the eye, gradually diminishing the amount of "plus" lens until a clear image of the retina is obtained.

It is also important to assess the quality of the optic nerve and retina. Often a detailed examination of the fundus is not made if the red reflex appears normal. However, specific abnormalities can be overlooked if the fundus is not examined. I personally recommend the use of dilating drops at least once during the first 6 weeks of life, so that examination of the optic nerve and macula can be more thorough. The use of an agent such as Cyclomydril (combination of cyclopentolate and phenylephrine) is safe and effective.

This procedure will probably not be routine in most offices, however.

Editor

Certain anatomic features can interfere with the quality of the red reflex. If the reflex is absent, then a media opacity (such as a cataract) may be present. Absence of the red reflex warrants immediate referral, since treatment within the critical visual development period can lead to very good vision. The red reflex can be difficult to see if the pupils are very small; sometimes it helps to have the mother or other familiar person talk to the baby from a distance. This stimulus may encourage distance fixation, with subsequent dilatation of the pupil. The presence of heavy pigmentation darkens the red reflex and makes assessment more difficult. The degree of ocular pigmentation roughly parallels that of skin pigmentation. A high refractive error (either myopia or hyperopia) can limit the quality of the red reflex, unless the extreme myopic and hyperopic lenses of the ophthalmoscope are used for viewing.

Finally, if the red reflex is seen extremely easily, this can also be worrisome! In an infant with albinism, the red reflex can even be seen between strands of the iris (so-called transillumination defects). If the iris is hypoplastic (aniridia), then the red reflex is seen as if the child had received dilating drops.

Alignment. The final important aspect of the eye examination is evaluation of alignment. In infants, the position of the corneal light reflex must be assessed. The consistent presence of strabismus warrants further investigation for vision-threatening as well as life-threatening conditions.

CONDITIONS THAT CAN BE TREATED IF RECOGNIZED PROMPTLY

Several conditions found among ICN graduates are treatable if they are recognized and ameliorated within the first 6 weeks of life. Suspicion for one of these conditions should prompt immediate referral, since a delay of even a few days in some conditions can be a critical factor.

CONGENITAL CATARACTS

An abnormality of the red reflex in one or both eyes may lead to the diagnosis of congenital cataracts, which may be partial or total and may involve one or both eyes. They may be detectable on gross inspection, but more often they can be seen only with the use of an ophthalmoscope. Congenital cataracts can be associated with prenatal infections, chromosomal abnormalities, metabolic abnormalities, hereditary conditions, and various syndromes.

CONGENITAL GLAUCOMA

Congenital glaucoma in infants may escape diagnosis for some time. It usually is seen as an enlarged cornea that subsequently becomes cloudy. Prior to the diagnosis, parents may judge the eyes to be beautiful as a consequence of their prominence. However, as the cornea becomes cloudy because of development of intracorneal edema, the child becomes photophobic, and epiphora (chronic tearing) may occur. In fact, congenital glaucoma is often misdiagnosed as a nonpatent lacrimal system. As with congenital cataracts, glaucoma may be associated with prenatal infections and specific syndromes.

HIGH REFRACTIVE ERROR

High refractive errors, especially myopia, occur with greater frequency among premature infants than among term babies. In infants with extreme myopia or hyperopia there will be a poorly focused image on the retina. In extreme cases, amblyopia can develop simply as a consequence of a high refractive error. This error may involve one or both eyes. If one eye is involved, strabismus may provide the presenting clue. If both eyes are involved, sensory nystagmus or abnormal head turning may be the presenting feature. High refractive errors in infants are treatable with either glasses or contact lenses. Special spectacle frames have been available for infants for several years, and special contact lenses have recently been developed.

Contact lenses are prescribed when a refractive error is so high that spectacle lenses would be too thick. (Such is the case in the baby who has had bilateral cataract surgery.) Although hard contact lenses are prescribed occasionally, most infants are given soft contact lenses, which can be worn for longer periods. Contact lenses have associated risks, with infection being the greatest concern, particularly if the child has had previous eye surgery (e.g., for cataract). All parents of a baby with contact lenses should be instructed to remove the lenses immediately if there is any evidence of infection, i.e., redness, discharge, swelling, or irritability).

RETINOPATHY OF PREMATURITY AND OTHER VISUAL PROBLEMS IN ICN GRADUATES

RETINOPATHY OF PREMATURITY

Incidence. A significant percentage of preterm ICN graduates are at risk for retinopathy of prematurity (ROP), although the incidence among children weighing more than 2000 grams at birth is extremely low. The incidence increases significantly in association with birth weights less than 1500 grams and is highest among infants weighing less than 1000 grams at birth, among whom the incidence of cicatricial retrolental fibroplasia is 25 per cent.[2]

Any infant born before 36 weeks of gestation or weighing less than 2000 grams who has received oxygen therapy should be examined by an ophthalmologist. An initial evaluation is usually done prior to discharge from the ICN, but further follow-up is usually recommended at 3 to 6 months of age.

Many studies have been done to assess the various risk factors for retinopathy of prematurity, including arterial oxygen levels, duration of oxygen therapy, and presence or absence of intraventricular hemorrhage. However, numerous cases of ROP have been reported in infants who had *no* neonatal exposure to oxygen therapy.

Is ROP preventable? There has been much discussion of the efficacy of vitamin E administration in the ICN in reducing the severity of ROP. Attempts to reproduce a reduction of severe ROP in multicenter trials have not supported the efficacy of using high doses of vitamin E, and associated side effects have been reported, including retinal hemorrhages, intraventricular hemorrhage, necrotizing enterocolitis, and sepsis.

If ROP occurs, is it treatable? In the early stages of ROP, only observation is indicated, since the vast majority of findings disappear over time. However, certain advanced conditions may warrant treatment of abnormal vessels with freezing techniques, retinal reattachment, and/or vitrectomy procedures. A large collaborative study is presently under way and may provide helpful insight within the near future.

OTHER OCULAR LESIONS

Poor Vision Associated with Neurologic Defects. An infant who has suffered perinatal asphyxia or who has hydrocephalus deserves special attention to visual development. A thorough ophthalmologic examination is indicated to exclude the possibility of optic nerve or retinal disease. For example, cortical blindness is often erroneously diagnosed in association with hydrocephalus when, in fact, optic atrophy has occurred. Dilation of the third ventricle results in stretching of the chiasm that forms its anterior wall, and consequently, optic atrophy may ensue.

In the absence of an ophthalmologic abnormality, the baby's visual performance nonetheless must be followed. Often a child with cerebral palsy *appears* nearly blind within the first two years of life, but suddenly begins to see normally. Thus, great caution must be taken in counseling parents, since the ultimate outcome for such children is so variable.

Epiphora. Chronic tearing occurs in babies as a consequence of nonpatency of the nasal lacrimal system. Usually the distal portion of the nasal lacrimal system is responsible for the symptom. Although the majority of problems resolve spontaneously, there is some risk involved if chronic conjunctivitis or dacryocystitis ensues. Vigorous massage may aid in the opening of the system and should be applied with the index finger, pressing from the inner canthal region downward over the side of the nose. If the problem persists beyond the age of 6 to 8 months, or if chronic infection exists, referral to an ophthalmologist is indicated.

Ptosis. Ptosis can lead to amblyopia if there is partial occlusion of the pupil. One can assess for this finding by looking at the red reflex and judging if the lid interferes with the ability to see the entire pupillary aperture. As an infant with ptosis matures, he or she may attempt to "see around" the ptosis by elevating the chin.

In general, ptosis repair is delayed until the child is several years old, when the tissue planes of the eyelids are more substantial. Exception is made if visual development is jeopardized, when earlier surgery is indicated.

Strabismus. Many pediatricians report a high incidence of transient strabismus in infants. The premature baby is at greater risk for development of strabismus than the term infant. Special "red flags" to watch for are (1) evidence of reduced vision, (2) evidence of poor red reflex, and (3) deviation affecting one eye only.

Infants with any of these findings warrant prompt referral for assessment of reduced vision, determination if it is treatable, and initiation of treatment to reduce the potential for amblyopia during the critical developmental period. Commonly, strabismus is of an intermittent nature. Control of ocular alignment may improve with maturation of the CNS. If intermittent strabismus persists at the age of 6 months, ophthalmologic evaluation is recommended.

If an ophthalmologist has started a child on patching therapy, the mother may direct questions to the pediatrician for clarification of information. Patching is advised when amblyopia has been detected in one eye. Usually this is associated with strabismus (for instance, left esotropia). The goal of patching is to force fixation with the amblyopic eye and thus encourage visual development. Patching therapy is judged effective when the fixation pattern of that eye indicates that vision is as good as in the nonpatched eye. Patching generally does not affect the alignment of the eyes, i.e., strabismus will persist when both eyes are open. An infant being treated with patching should be followed carefully by the ophthalmologist so that occlusion amblyopia of the other eye does not develop.

WHEN TO WORRY

The following are some general areas that should trigger the concern of the pediatrician caring for the ICN graduate.

1. If in the history obtained from the parents they indicate any level of concern that their baby may not see, such as failure of the infant to follow a moving object or "wandering eyes"

2. If the infant has a history of poking at his or her eyes or waving the hands rapidly in front of the face

3. If on examination the nystagmus usually elicited with a vestibulo-ocular reflex is not dampened by the fixation reflex

4. If the infant does not blink to a camera flash just in front of the face

5. If the red reflex is poorly seen or absent

6. If the red reflex is seen too easily (This may be a sign of aniridia, which may be associated with other abnormalities.)

7. If a picture taken of the child looking straight at the camera does not show the red reflex occurring at the same point in both pupils

8. If a clear fixing and following response is not present by a corrected age of 6 weeks

9. If there is any enlargement or cloudiness of the cornea, which might be associated with glaucoma

10. If the child is clearly photophobic or has chronic tearing (also associated with congenital glaucoma)

11. If a child has sensory nystagmus or an abnormal head turn (A high refractive error may be present.)

12. If a child has a history of retinopathy of prematurity of any stage diagnosed in the ICN

13. If a child has chronic tearing associated with nonpatency of the nasal lacrimal system that persists beyond the age of 6 to 8 months, or in such an infant when infection exists

14. In an infant with ptosis in whom the lid interferes with the red reflex

15. In an infant who appears to have strabismus with evidence of reduced vision, a poor red reflex, or deviation affecting only one eye

16. When intermittent strabismus persists at the age of 6 months

SUMMARY

The ICN graduate who has managed the struggle for sheer survival now faces new challenges. Development depends on many systems, and vision is one of the most important. Our goal, then is to ensure the best possible health for the baby's eyes. Awareness of ocular risks associated with neonatal intensive care, careful assessments of the eyes and vision during the critical period (first few months of life in term infants), and knowledge of problems warranting referral are all important to providing a healthy start for the ICN graduate.

References

1. Norcia AM, Tyler CW, Piecuch RE, et al.: A new look at visual acuity in premature infants. Pediatr Res 19:368A, 1985.
2. Phelps DL: Retinopathy of prematurity: An estimate of vision loss in the United States—1979. Pediatrics 67:924, 1980.

Recommended Reading

Dubowitz LMS, Dubowitz V, Morante A, et al.: Visual function in the preterm and fullterm newborn infant. Dev Med Child Neurol 22:465, 1980.

Fletcher MC, Brandon S: Myopia of prematurity. Am J Ophthalmol 40:1912, 1955.

Goren CC, Sarta M, Wand-WU PYK: Visual following and pattern discrimination of facelike stimuli by newborn infants. Pediatrics 56:544, 1975.

Hoyt CS, Nickel BL, Billson FA: Ophthalmological examination of the infant: Development aspects. Surv Ophthalmol 26:177, 1982.

Lucey JF, Dangman B: A reexamination of the role of oxygen in retrolental fibroplasia. Pediatrics 73:73, 1984.

McPherson AR, Hittner HM, Kretzer FL (eds.): Retinopathy of Prematurity. Toronto, B.C. Decker, 1986.

Nelson LB, Rubin SE, Wagner RS, et al: Developmental aspects in the assessment of visual function in young children. Pediatrics 73:375, 1984.

Odom JV, Hoyt CS, Marg E, et al.: Effect of natural deprivation and unilateral eye patching on visual acuity of infants an children: Evoked potential measurements. Arch Ophthalmol 99:559, 1981.

Phelps DL: Vitamin E and retrolental fibroplasia in 1982. Pediatrics 70:420, 1982.

Porat R: Care of the infant with retinopathy of prematurity. Clin Perinatol, February 1984, 123.

Purohit DM, Ellison C, Zierler S, et al.: Risk factors for retrolental fibroplasia. Pediatrics 76:339, 1985.

Shohat M, Reisner SH, Krikler R, et al.: Retinopathy of prematurity: Incidence and risk factors. Pediatrics 72:159, 1983.

Silverman WA, Flynn JT (eds.): Contemporary Issues in Fetal and Neonatal Medicine, 2: Retinopathy of Prematurity. Oxford, Blackwell Scientific Publications, 1985.

Sniderman SH, Riedel PA, Bert MD, et al.: Factors influencing the incidence of retrolental fibroplasia. Retinopathy of Prematurity Conference Syllabus. Columbus, Ross Laboratories, 1981, pp. 406–413.

MANAGEMENT OF PULMONARY SEQUELAE AND SUBSPECIALTY PROBLEMS

14

CHRONIC LUNG DISEASE OF INFANCY

ARNOLD C.G. PLATZKER, M.D.

With recent advances in the care of the neonate with respiratory illness, a new pulmonary sequela has been encountered. Its roots lie in prematurity (i.e., the lack of complete development of the lung at birth), the basic illness or disorder being treated, and the superimposed injury to the lung resulting from oxygen toxicity and assisted ventilation (barotrauma) associated with the treatment of respiratory failure. Because of the nature of the lung injury, it impacts on all of the cellular elements of the lung,[1] affecting both the respiratory and nonrespiratory functions of the lung. While the injury to the lung is diffuse, the development of the lung after birth contributes to a generally good prognosis for the majority of the infants who are afflicted with this disorder (i.e., new terminal units develop, expanding the complement of lung units from 27 million at birth to over 350 million when this phase of lung development is completed at approximately 11 years of age).[2,3]

The original description of bronchopulmonary dysplasia (BPD) by Northway et al.,[4] in 1967, focused on a group of infants with respiratory distress syndrome (RDS) who died after a long course of oxygen therapy and assisted ventilation. Their description of BPD stages was based on the radiologic progression of the pulmonary disease and pathologic findings in the lungs at autopsy. With the passage of time since this original description, it has become increasingly clear that the use of the chest roentgenogram as the sole diagnostic yardstick for this disorder has limitations and, in fact, allows some infants with this disorder to go undetected and thus untreated.

While the majority of infants with BPD are prematurely born and have suffered from RDS,[5-17] they are not alone in contracting this disorder. Premature infants who have never suffered from RDS but who require oxygen therapy, endotracheal intubation, and assisted ventilation for even short periods during the neonatal period are at risk for developing BPD.[18,19] Even preterm or full-term infants who require oxygen therapy or assisted ventilation for treatment of neonatal pneumonia, meconium aspiration syndrome, patent ductus arteriosus, or tracheoesophageal fistula may develop, as a sequela, chronic lung disease that is radiologically and therapeutically indistinguishable from BPD.[20-28] It now appears that infants who have the underlying risk factors of neonatal respiratory illness and, in addition, a family history of asthma or allergy are at a greater risk for this disorder.[29,30] While BPD was originally described in RDS infants alone, it is now clear that it afflicts a broader spectrum of infants who experience neonatal respiratory illness, and thus it is preferable to designate it as chronic lung disease of infancy, rather than bronchopulmonary dysplasia.

Although the most severe cases of chronic lung disease are diagnosed in the nursery, some may initially come to the attention of a pediatrician much later. The infants may fail to grow appropriately, respond inadequately to treatment for upper respiratory tract infection, or require hospitalization for what was initially thought to be a mild respiratory tract infection. They may suffer from recurrent episodes of respiratory illness with some similarity to bronchiolitis, prior to the recognition that the disorder being treated is a distinct form of lung disease. Even in the period between exacerbations, the infant may be noted to have abnormal respiratory function or sometimes only tachypnea. Therefore, this section addresses the wider group of newborn infants who are at risk for this disorder, and it is urged that the entire high-risk group receive close observation, special medical attention, and home care following their discharge from the neonatal unit.

It is clear, then, that the infant who suffers from any respiratory illness in the newborn period and who, for any reason, requires oxygen therapy or assisted ventilation may experience some respiratory sequelae. The diagnosis of BPD is no longer confined to premature infants with RDS, and it can no longer be classified by radiologic stages alone. Therefore, this chapter will address the spectrum of illnesses best described as chronic lung disease of infancy (CLD).

PATHOPHYSIOLOGY

An understanding of the pathophysiology of CLD is useful in understanding the spectrum of disorders that comprise it. In CLD, virtually all of the elements of the lung are injured to some degree.[1,4,31-37] Although the symptoms and clinical findings resulting from involvement of the airway and its mucociliary blanket,[38,39] mucosa, mucous glands,[1] and smooth muscle[30,40] often predominate, the disorder affects the terminal air spaces,[2] interstitium of the lung,[32] and the pulmonary microcirculation[41-43,46,47] as well. Early during the course of oxygen therapy and/or assisted ventilation, defects occur in the mucociliary blanket covering and protecting the airway epithelium.[44,45] The time course of this injury is thought to be quite variable. However, the initial effect of oxygen exposure on the mucus blanket is a reduction in the motility of the cilia, resulting in mucus stasis.[39,48] During the first 4 weeks of oxygen exposure, there is

mucosal injury and inflammatory cell infiltration into the airway mucus membrane, causing exfoliation of the cells lining the airway.[49] The airway mucosa first become edematous; then hypertrophy and hyperplasia of the airway mucus glands and goblet cells follow.[50] This process leads to the secretion of excessive amounts of mucus, associated with reduced development of the mucociliary apparatus needed to remove or clear mucus from the airway. The ciliated cells are replaced by pseudostratified squamous epithelium, which grows in an irregular fashion across the surface of the airway, compromising the cross-sectional area of the lumen. This loss of airway caliber is worsened as some of the smaller airways are occluded by mucus debris and exfoliated airway epithelium. Chronic mechanical obstruction of the airway leads to deformation of airway mucosa, stimulation of cholinergic receptors in the airway mucosa,[49] and further narrowing of the airway from reflex increase in bronchomotor tone. With chronic bronchospasm, the smooth muscle of the bronchi and bronchioles becomes hypertrophied, with the evolution of chronic reduction in airway caliber.

The terminal air spaces, it now appears, sustain more injury from the loss of the type I cell, which covers 80 per cent of the surface of the alveoli, than from injury and loss of the type II cell. This is of interest, since the inadequate secretion of pulmonary surfactant from the type II cell is the major factor in the pathogenesis of RDS.[51] While the immature alveolar type II cell secretes surfactant at a rate inadequate to maintain a complete lining layer, leading to progressive atelectasis and the clinical findings of RDS, the resulting hypoxemia injures the type I cell. The type II cell appears to survive RDS, oxygen toxicity, and barotrauma surprisingly well. In fact, in the repair of the alveolus, the type II cell dedifferentiates and divides, producing type I daughter cells to replace the injured and lost type I cell. With restoration of alveolar lining, the type II cell ceases to divide, and surfactant metabolism again becomes its major role in the lung. In some alveoli, however, the injury to the unit is sufficient to interrupt the integrity of the alveolar wall, with subsequent erosion into the adjacent alveolus. The neighboring alveoli merge into a single giant alveolus. In other areas, alveoli in other stages of repair become atelectatic when their lumina become obstructed by mucus and necrotic cellular debris. Thus the architecture of the lung in CLD is characterized by atelectatic alveoli, as well as normal, large, and even emphysematous alveoli. Because of reduction in the number of alveoli, the alveolar surface area for gas exchange is less than that in infants of comparable age and gestation.

Role of Surfactant Deficiency

The interstitium of the lung sustains injury because of the absence of a confluent layer of surfactant covering the alveolar surface.[52] Pulmonary surfactant normally contributes to the protection of the lung in four principal ways: First, it lowers the surface tension in the alveolus, resisting alveolar collapse during exhalation, while providing more than two thirds of the lung recoil at total lung capacity.[53] A second property of surfactant, resistance to pulmonary edema, derives from the capacity of surfactant to reduce alveolar surface tension.[54-57] A third attribute of a complete surfactant lining layer is its action to contain the underlying, slender, aqueous layer that coats the alveolar epithelium. The presence of the confluent alveolar layer thus acts as a buffer to the direct exposure of the sensitive alveolar epithelial type I cell to the toxic effects of oxygen. An additional role, only recently identified, is the capacity of pulmonary surfactant to act as a major determinant of the pulmonary defense mechanisms.[58] Surfactant has been shown to suppress the early proliferative response of lymphocytes to inhaled antigens without interfering with the effector functions of partially or fully differentiated B and T lymphocytes recruited to the lung.[59] Surfactant also enhances bacterial phagocytosis and intracellular killing by alveolar macrophages.[60] However, during the inflammatory phase of lung repair in CLD, the influx of inflammatory cells, especially phagocytic cells such as alveolar macrophages, may alter alveolar type II cell function as well.

Thus the interruption of the surfactant layer leads to a rise in alveolar surface tension, predisposing to alveolar collapse. The rise in alveolar surface tension also results in a rise in the oncotic gradient across the interface between the pulmonary microcirculation and the alveolar compartment.[61-63] Hypoxia, resulting from atelectasis, elicits constriction of the pulmonary vascular bed and increase in pulmonary vascular resistance. With further increase in the already elevated oncotic gradient, plasma leaks from the microvasculature of the lung into the interstitium.[64,65] This results in thickening of the interstitium and, finally, in the encroachment of edema fluid upon and into the alveolar space. Leukocytes and macrophages enter the interstitium in the inflammatory process, and later, fibroblasts are attracted to the interstitium when the process enters the stage of reconstruction and repair.

Role of the Pulmonary Microvasculature

Inextricably related to the process of injury and repair of the interstitium of the lung is a parallel process that occurs in the pulmonary microvasculature.[36] During the course of RDS and other neonatal respiratory disorders, pulmonary arterial hypoxia results in spasm of the resistance vessels, pulmonary hypoperfusion, increasing pulmonary parenchymal ischemia, and injury to the alveolar epithelium characterized by extensive loss of the delicate alveolar type I cell. With the development of pulmonary hypertension, fluid extravasates across the microvasculature into the alveolar interstitium, forming fluid cuffs around the pulmonary arterioles and capillaries and compressing and narrowing the vessel lumina.[66,67] With sustained hypoxia and pulmonary hypertension, there is continued leakage and, finally, frank extravasation of fluid across the vessel walls that results in ongoing injury to the vessel's endothelium and walls. This process results in perpetuation of the leakage of plasma and, as the defects in the vessel wall enlarge, to leakage of red blood cells and other cellular elements of the blood into the interstitium and alveolus. In most instances, pulmonary hypertension is not a major component of chronic lung disease, and the basis for the pulmonary edema of CLD is posthypoxic injury to the vessel wall; it is a "permeability type" of pulmonary edema.

Pulmonary Edema

With severe CLD, permeability edema is complicated by hypertensive pulmonary edema. With each type of vascular fluid leakage, the distance between gas exchange surface and the pulmonary vascular space is increased, increasing (worsening) the time constant for oxygen and carbon dioxide exchange between the alveolar and vascular compartments and, thus, increasing the magnitude of the disorder of oxygen uptake and carbon dioxide removal from the blood. At present it is unknown whether the vascular injury heals, or — if it heals — whether this occurs by resolution or by a process of fibrosis, which might lead to further reduction in pulmonary capillary blood volume. Indeed, there are as yet no data on the long-term outcome of this injury to the airways, interstitium, and vasculature of the lung. However, during the process of the development of chronic pulmonary edema, described above, the distention of the interstitium with edema fluid encroaches upon and compresses the alveolus, resulting, in some cases, in partial or complete closure of the alveolar duct. With partial closure of the alveolar duct, air enters on inspiration, but becomes trapped during exhalation when rising pleural pressure leads to closure of the alveolar duct. With complete compression of the alveolar duct, the alveoli supplied by the duct remain airless. This mechanism accounts for the finding of both emphysematous and atelectatic areas of the lung in this disorder.

This brief description of the pathologic events resulting from neonatal respiratory illness and treatment with oxygen and assisted ventilation makes it possible to predict the physiologic consequences of the extensive injury to the lung experienced by the CLD infant. Recent findings in infants and children suffering from CLD suggest that the mucosal injury in this disease is diffuse, affecting other mucosal surfaces, such as those lining the middle ear, nasal sinuses, and possibly even the gastrointestinal tract. Further studies are presently under way to clarify the nature and implications of these findings. However, it is already known that CLD is associated with a defect in the structure and motility of the cilia lining the respiratory tract.[39] At present, it is thought that the anatomic and functional abnormalities of the cilia resolve or at least regress as the infant grows and with resolution and repair of the other aspects of lung injury of CLD. However, it remains unclear whether the defect of the cilia is (1) genetic in origin, predisposing the infant to neonatal respiratory illness destined to evolve into CLD; (2) a congenital defect in the cilia, causing only the infant who has neonatal respiratory illness, oxygen exposure, or assisted ventilation to experience CLD; or (3) a response to the lung injury per se.

The impact of the lung injury in CLD on the defense mechanisms and other nonrespiratory functions of the lung, such as clearance from the blood of various endogenous and exogenous substances, including medications, has been poorly studied. While the impact of this injury on mucociliary clearance and chemotaxis, phagocytosis, and bacterial killing have received some study.[39,49] There are no studies of the effects of CLD on the filtration capacity of the pulmonary endothelium.

DIAGNOSIS: EXPECTED FINDINGS

While the classic radiologic staging of this disorder was helpful in initially defining this illness, radiologic staging is no longer possible or desirable. Rather, it is necessary to make the diagnosis of CLD on the basis of the history and assessment of clear-cut physical and laboratory findings.[68] The chest roentgenogram merely documents consistent radiologic features of the illness.[69-71] All premature infants, especially those weighing less than 1500 grams at birth, and full-term infants who had lung disease during the neonatal period that required oxygen therapy or assisted ventilation are at some risk for CLD.[72,73] Infants at greatest risk for significant CLD are those exposed to environmental oxygen tension of 0.30 or greater for at least 30 days and/or to assisted ventilation for more than 7 to 16 days.[22,24,27,40,70-79] A family history of allergy or asthma further increases the risk that neonatal respiratory illness will develop into CLD.[29,30]

CLINICAL FINDINGS

The CLD infant has tachypnea, which is the most sensitive diagnostic index for this illness.[80,81] It is, however, surprisingly difficult to document tachypnea in the small infant, since respiratory patterns change with each change in the infant's activity or state of consciousness. Thus, to observe the infant's respiratory rate under basal conditions, it is necessary to do so during periods of sleep and preferably at the same time each day. In this way, changes in respiratory rate and respiratory effort can be quantified and differences appreciated.

Other associated findings include:

1. Increase in the anteroposterior diameter of the chest. This is the result of airway obstruction from bronchospasm and/or small-airway closure secondary to interstitial pulmonary edema
2. Intercostal retractions—evidence of reduced pulmonary compliance and increased work of breathing
3. Pectus excavatum deformity of the sternum from the molding effect of longstanding retractions and sternal dipping with inspiration
4. Flaring of the alae nasae
5. Coughing, audible wheezing, and coarse and musical rhonchi and moist rales on auscultation of the chest
6. Weak cry
7. Expiratory grunting is an important sign of impending respiratory failure, whether it is con-

tinuous or occurs only during sleep. Many CLD infants will have expiratory grunting during periods of increased ventilation or during stress, as with feeding or crying. The presence of expiratory grunting may indicate impending cor pulmonale and/or pulmonary hypertension. In the latter case, the second pulmonic sound may be prominent or increased, occasionally snapping; an electrocardiogram will confirm the suspicion of right ventricular hypertrophy.[82-84]

8. Possible pulmonary osteoarthropathy in children with longstanding disease

Although the presence of a classic history and typical physical findings make the diagnosis of this illness quite easy, there are infants who, while they are usually asymptomatic, may manifest some or all of the findings of CLD during periods of respiratory illness or when they have had excessively large fluid intake. Thus, obtaining details of a clinical history of neonatal respiratory illness and amount and duration of oxygen therapy and assisted ventilation is an extremely important aspect of making the diagnosis of CLD in infants and in planning for the respiratory care of the infant with recurrent or continuous respiratory illness.

LABORATORY FINDINGS

There are no specific laboratory findings that aid in arriving at the diagnosis of CLD. The laboratory assists in confirming the presence of typical or expected abnormalities of gas exchange. Hematologic findings of increased hematocrit and hemoglobin values are reflections of the impact of chronic hypoxemia, i.e., chronically reduced oxygen saturation of hemoglobin. In cases of severe CLD, hypercapnia may be present. Thus, at each visit of the infant to the physician, blood gases should be assessed.[85,86]

RADIOLOGIC FINDINGS

The radiologic findings in CLD are highly variable and evolve over the first two months after birth or onset of the respiratory illness.[26,70,86-88] The most uniform finding is increased lucency of the peripheral lung fields, associated with a loss of the natural convexity of the diaphragm. The diaphragm appears flattened or, in cases of severe air trapping, concave. However, peribronchial and peribronchiolar thickening, segmental atelectasis, and, occasionally, lobar atelectasis are also noted. Juxtaposed against atelectatic segments of lung are cystic areas. The cystic regions are numerous and best appreciated at the bases of the lungs; in rare instances the cysts achieve large size and lead to compression atelectasis.

Cardiomegaly, although present, is often not appreciated radiographically, because it is hidden by hyperinflation of the lungs. A contrast study of the upper gastrointestinal tract may show gastroesophageal reflux; it is indicated in the CLD infant who has a stormy clinical course in spite of careful medical management of respiratory illness. The newer imaging techniques, especially gastric scintiscan when performed by a skilled pediatric radiologist, increase the sensitivity of detection of gastroesophageal reflux and/or aspiration.[89,90]

PULMONARY FUNCTION FINDINGS

Studies of lung function in CLD have revealed a substantial increase in airway resistances.[40,91] Even infants with a history of RDS, but without CLD, may have a significant increase in airway resistances.[20,30] In the CLD infant, dynamic lung compliance is markedly reduced. As already described, partial airway obstruction and mucous plugging lead to expiratory airway obstruction. This accounts for the increased total lung capacity and enlarged residual volume and functional residual capacity of the CLD infant. This increase in the "trapped" gas volumes is at the expense of the inspiratory capacity and vital capacity. With the patchy nature of the airway obstruction, there is maldistribution of ventilation and thus an increased alveolar-to-arterial (A-a) gradient for oxygen. This, in part, accounts for an increase in the respiratory rate.[80]

In mild and even moderately severe CLD, tachypnea occurs to compensate for the maldistribution of ventilation. Although inadequate to raise the arterial oxygen tension to the expected level, the tachypnea overcorrects the A-a carbon dioxide gradient, which frequently results in reduced arterial carbon dioxide tensions, even in the sleeping child. Oxygen consumption in the CLD infant is increased, resulting in part from the increased work of breathing due to low pulmonary compliance (i.e., reduced lung elasticity).[92,93] This increased oxygen extraction from the blood further worsens oxygenation. In those instances in which the infant has severe mismatching of lung perfusion and alveolar ventilation, the gas transfer defect includes hypercapnia. See Table 14-1 for review of pulmonary function abnormalities and associated clinical findings.

TABLE 14–1. Pulmonary Function Abnormalities in Infants with CLD

Pulmonary Function Finding	Clinical Finding
Increased airway resistance Decreased dynamic lung compliance Partial airway obstruction (mucous plugging)	Expiratory obstruction with wheezing
Results in Increased total lung capacity and Increased residual lung volume—functional residual capacity	
In Addition Decreased vital capacity Maldistribution of ventilation with increased alveolar-arterial (A-a) gradient for oxygen: mild—decreased $PaCO_2$ severe—increased $PaCO_2$ and	Increased respiratory rate
Increased work of breathing Increased oxygen consumption	Poor growth

---

CARDIOVASCULAR FINDINGS

To complete the diagnostic evaluation, studies of the cardiovascular status are necessary. Each CLD infant requires a careful physical examination, with special attention paid to resting heart rate, the location of the precordial impulse, the quality of the cardiac tones, the quality of the pulmonic second sound, and the time between aortic and pulmonic valve closure. Electrocardiography and echocardiography are usually indicated.[84,94] In almost all circumstances a consultation with a qualified pediatric cardiologist is advisable to assure that no subtle clinical finding is missed and that the electrophysical studies are interpreted accurately. Certainly, when clear evidence of cardiac dysfunction or pulmonary hypertension is defined, continued follow-up with the pediatric cardiologist is necessary. In most CLD infants, however, these studies serve primarily as a baseline assessment of cardiac function. Occasionally when an infant does not respond adequately to medical management, repeat cardiac evaluation will disclose that worsening CLD, exacerbation of obstructive lung disease, and chronic

pulmonary edema have led to impairment of right ventricular function. Right ventricular strain and right (or biventricular) hypertrophy, as might be expected, are the most frequently observed abnormalities on electrocardiography or echocardiography. When the CLD infant has pulmonary hypertension as well, two-dimensional echocardiography and, occasionally, cardiac catheterization may be necessary to complete evaluation of the infant—especially to rule out a complicating congenital heart defect or cardiomyopathy.[83,95]

MANAGEMENT OF CHRONIC LUNG DISEASE OF INFANCY: HOME CARE

Care of the CLD infant at home will usually be quite time consuming. Attention to the usual well-baby and pediatric care concerns is necessary, in addition to management of the CLD.[96] (See General Health Issues in Chapter 6.) Immunization of the CLD infant with moderate symptoms with *Hemophilus influenzae* and pneumococcal vaccines should be considered when the infant is old enough to mount an antibody response. Yearly administration of influenza virus vaccine is recommended for all infants over 6 months of age. Attention needs to be focused, as well, on those factors in care that might have an impact on the lung disorder itself. The infant discharged from the ICN with a diagnosis of CLD should be seen regularly by both a skilled pediatrician and an appropriate consultant or multidisciplinary team of specialists from a tertiary care center.[97–100] For the sickest infants, the team should consist of pediatric specialists in lung disorders (i.e., neonatologists, pulmonologists), pediatric subspecialists in otolaryngology, gastroenterology and nutrition, cardiology, neurology, and child development. If the infant was born prematurely a pediatric ophthalmologist and otologist should also be involved in the care.

In addition, critical to the successful home care are the services of pediatric nurses skilled in the care of CLD infants and of pediatric respiratory therapists, medical social workers, nutritionists, and infant developmental assessment specialists. Since the CLD infant is likely to require regular pulmonary function, radiologic, and cardiac assessments, the respective laboratories should be a part of or close to the follow-up clinic, to make it feasible for the consultations and comprehensive clinic assessment to be scheduled on the same day. The CLD infant also requires regular hematologic and serum chemistry studies; if these studies are necessary more frequently than the clinic visits, it may be more convenient for the family to obtain these studies at a laboratory closer to home. In any case, it is advisable to have all of the laboratory studies for an infant performed at the same clinical laboratory, which must have the capability to perform microchemistry determinations.

To present an understandable schema for the management of the CLD infant, it is helpful to examine the continuum of the disorder and to characterize stages that, one must remember, may only exist in theory. These stages are outlined in Tables 14–2 to 14–6. Figure 14–1 portrays the progressive clinical stages of respiratory and, finally, cardiac dysfunction in CLD: (1) tachypnea, (2) airway obstruction, (3) pulmonary edema, (4) hypoxia, and (5) cor pulmonale. CLD infants with a history of tracheal intubation may have sustained a loss of tracheal caliber (i.e., tracheal stenosis). It is necessary to differentiate tracheal from lower airway obstruction seen in CLD prior to developing a treatment plan (for diagnosis and treatment of upper airway obstruction, see chapter 15). The cor pulmonale stage includes infants with alveolar hypoventilation (i.e., hypercapnia), pulmonary hypertension, and hypoventilation sufficiently severe to require assisted ventilation.

In this section, treatment will focus on the care of children with CLD in the home; it will address levels of care necessary to treat the components of lung dysfunction underlying the symptom complex. (See also Appendix A for medications equipment.) Clearly, each CLD infant will have gradations of the various components and will require individualized consideration to determine which aspects of the program should be included in the home care plan. The following discussion includes guidelines for the treatment of the CLD infant that should not, under any circumstances, be taken as a rigid program of care. The CLD infant is in a very dynamic state and will, it is hoped, be experiencing gradual recovery from the illness while achieving substantial growth and development. All of these factors will influence, on a day-to-day basis, the need for various components of the care program. This places particular pressure on the pediatrician and consultants who observe the CLD infant during the transition from hospital to home. Careful instruction of all of the infant's care givers is essential, so that the infant's condition will be monitored accurately and appropriate care administered.

The pediatrician or family doctor plays a central role here in coordinating the activities of the various professionals involved in providing care to these infants; this role is critical to communication between the family and the multitude of other care providers.

Editor

The infant with CLD requires an enormous amount of care. The success of any long-term

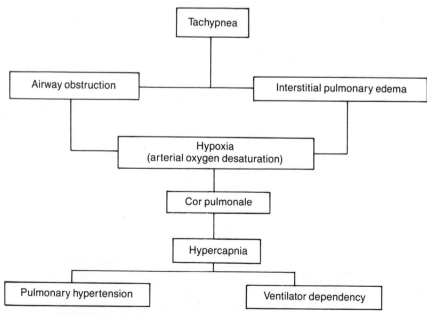

FIGURE 14–1. Chronic lung disease of infancy (CLD) clinical stages.

treatment plan depends on the availability of a good home environment and stable support systems, along with the commitment, competence, and readiness of the patient's parents and others who will participate in the child's care at home. At times, planning for medical foster care will be necessary. Ample time and effort must be directed toward the orientation and training of each patient's home care giver(s). It is important that the care giver(s) understand the pathophysiology of the patient's disease and how each aspect of therapy fits into the overall care plan and also learn to recognize the clinical signs of increased respiratory distress, along with the appropriate intervention to deal with this distress.

Return demonstrations of all of the essential tasks are necessary to ensure that the care giver(s) will be able to function in any urgent situation. Before the infant's discharge from the hospital, the parents should have the opportunity to provide total care responsibilities for the infant under the watchful eye of the neonatal intensive care unit (ICN) staff. These stays should be arranged for periods of 24 to 48 hours; they are particularly helpful if accommodations separate from the ICN environment can be provided for both infant and parents. Depending upon the scope of an infant's home care, the duration of in-hospital training may range from several days to several weeks.

If in-home nursing is to be considered, the nurses who will provide the care should become familiar with the infant in the neonatal unit prior to the baby's discharge. This is essential even if the nurses have a background in pediatrics and have had experience in the care of CLD infants, since each infant is different and will respond differently to various treatments. In addition, the nurses should learn the philosophy of care and become acquainted with the care techniques as practiced by the team caring for the infant in the hospital. A final advantage of a special program of training for the home nurses and parents is that both the family and the nurses assisting them at home will understand and administer the care using the same techniques. This reduces the tensions that naturally occur when persons outside the family must be in the home.

Stage I: Tachypnea

In most instances, once the diagnosis of CLD is established, the infant will require little therapy if his or her symptoms are confined to

tachypnea alone, as characterized in Table 14–2. Tachypnea is defined as a respiratory rate (during sleep) exceeding 45 per minute. The parents and other care givers should be trained to count the infant's respiratory rate during sleep at the same time each day, preferably in the evening. The parents (and other care givers) record the respiratory rate and infant's progress (feeding and activity) daily for the first week the infant is at home. This information should be discussed with the infant's physician in a prearranged telephone call. This recording of sleeping respiratory rate establishes a baseline for comparison if the infant should become ill or manifest other signs of increasing respiratory dysfunction. Retractions, flaring, prolonged expiratory phase of breathing, and wheezing are other physical findings the parents must learn to recognize. With the onset of any of these findings, with anorexia, or with other signs of illness, the infant's pediatrician and the follow-up clinic

TABLE 14–2. Therapy for Chronic Lung Disease of Infancy, Stage I

Clinical Feature	Tachypnea
Clinical Findings	Sleeping respiratory rate >45/min
Evaluation/Monitoring	Sleeping respiratory rate at least twice weekly
	Hemoglobin/hematocrit determination monthly
	Transcutaneous oxygen/carbon dioxide tension or pulse oximetry or arterial blood gas analysis monthly
Pediatric Care	Routine immunization schedule
	Influenza virus immunization each fall
	Consider pneumococcal and *H. influenza* vaccination
	Evaluation by consultant team as indicated for change in symptoms
Home Care	Fluid restriction to 120 to 150 ml/kg/day
	Maintenance of adequate caloric intake to assure weight gain of 10 to 20 gm/day, appropriate growth in length and head circumference
	Avoid exposure to cigarette smoke and air pollutants

When To Worry
1. When sleeping respiratory rate increases by 20% or more
2. When infant develops retractions, flaring, or wheezing
3. When infant's appetite decreases
4. When weight gain is less than 10 to 20 gm/day
5. When infant is exposed to respiratory illness (especially RSV)

need to be informed. The parents' diary provides important, objective, clinical and behavioral information that will aid the physician in responding to the parents' telephone call and in deciding whether the infant should be seen in the office immediately or whether the problem can be handled by telephone. If at any time the sleeping respiratory rate exceeds 20 per cent of the baseline value, the infant requires assessment by the pediatrician.

The infant's fluid intake should be restricted to 150 ml/kg/day to avoid the risk of additional symptoms of worsening interstitial pulmonary edema. The infant should be protected from noxious inhalants, the most prevalent being cigarette smoke. If either parent or any of the care givers smoke, they should abstain from doing so in the home. Infants may even experience increasing symptoms of airway obstruction from exposure to clothing saturated with cigarette smoke.

All of the care givers will require training in cardiopulmonary resuscitation (CPR). The CLD infant, especially if born prematurely, is at a greater than usual risk for experiencing apnea, and therefore CPR training for caregivers is of significant practical importance. Another reason for this training is to reassure the care givers that they have the necessary skills and information to handle temporarily even a dire emergency such as respiratory or cardiopulmonary arrest.

Finally the infant will require monthly assessment of hematocrit and hemoglobin values. The latter provides important evidence of iron sufficiency, as well as whether the infant has been experiencing "occult" hypoxia. With a low hematocrit or hemoglobin value, the infant experiences reduced oxygen-carrying capacity; a rising hematocrit value, particularly when it is elevated or high normal, suggests that hypoxia occurs for a significant portion of the day, producing a rise in red blood cell volume in compensation for chronically reduced hemoglobin oxygen saturation. The presence of hypoxia often goes unrecognized by the parent, particularly if it occurs during sleep when the ambient light is low and when the infant may be unobserved for a period of several hours. Since the small infant spends a large portion of the day asleep, the periods of hypoxemia may, understandably, constitute a majority of the day. Initially it is desirable, therefore, to monitor the transcutaneous and/or arterial oxygen tension regularly in the CLD infant with tachypnea. This information will be especially helpful when it can be obtained after a feeding when the infant may sleep for an hour or more.

Stage II: Airway Obstruction

UPPER AIRWAY OBSTRUCTION

Clinical evidence of airway obstruction is the most common finding in the infant with significant CLD.[72,91,101] Prior to establishment of a treatment plan for the infant with airway obstruction, however, it is essential that the degree of upper (i.e., subglottic) airway obstruction be determined. This is particularly important if the infant required endotracheal intubation, either at birth or in the nursery, for resuscitation or assisted ventilation.[102] Infants who have had endotracheal intubation are at risk for the development of problems ranging from mild narrowing to granulomatous tracheitis, vocal cord paralysis, or cicatricial tracheal stenosis.[103-105] It may, on occasion, be difficult to differentiate between upper and lower airway obstruction, as the symptoms may overlap. The cardinal feature of tracheal stenosis is stridor. The timing of the stridor within the respiratory cycle varies with the location of the tracheal narrowing. However, in tracheal injury following endotracheal intubation, the narrowing of the trachea is most often located in the subglottic space. In this instance, although stridor is present during both inspiration and expiration, the inspiratory component may predominate. A rule of thumb, helpful to the clinician, is that when the stridor is confined to the inspiratory phase of breathing, the tracheal obstruction is above the thoracic inlet, whereas isolated expiratory stridor indicates intrathoracic tracheal obstruction. Stridor in both phases of the respiratory cycle may be associated with tracheal narrowing located in the intrathoracic or extrathoracic trachea. A discussion of the treatment of tracheal stenosis is included in Chapter 15.

LOWER AIRWAY OBSTRUCTION

Symptomatic lower airway obstruction (Table 14–3) is characterized by prolongation of the expiratory phase of breathing. In CLD infants this finding is the earliest, and often the only, indication of lower airway obstruction. Associated clinical findings include the use of accessory muscles of respiration to aid exhalation and expiratory wheezing, occasionally accompanied by coarse and/or musical expiratory

TABLE 14–3. Therapy for Chronic Lung Disease of Infancy, Stage II

Clinical Feature	Airway obstruction
Clinical Findings	Sleeping respiratory rate >45/min
	Prolonged expiratory phase of breathing I:E ≥ 1:2
	Use of accessory muscles of breathing to exhale
	Expiratory wheezing
	Coarse or musical rhonchi
Evaluation/Monitoring	Same as tachypnea (Table 14–2) plus
	1. Weekly office assessment by pediatrician
	2. Blood gas assessment, initially weekly (transcutaneous or arterial)
	3. Serum theophylline (desired range, 15 to 20 μm/ml)
	4. Nutrition assessment
Pediatric Care	Same as tachypnea, Table 14–2
	Consultation at least every 2 to 3 mo during first year
Home Care	Same as tachypnea, Table 14–2, plus
	1. Fluid restriction to 120 ml/kg/day
	2. Bronchodilator medication(s)
	a. Theophylline
	b. Beta-adrenergic aerosols—isoproterenol or isoetharine (see Appendix A, Table A–5, for concentration and method of administration)
	c. Chest percussion and postural drainage
	d. Pharyngeal suctioning

When To Worry
1. As in stage I CLD, plus
2. With increased wheezing
3. With behavioral changes—increased irritability or somnolence

rhonchi. These infants will require regularly scheduled, frequent clinical assessments after discharge from the hospital, with weekly office visits during the first one or two months following discharge from the neonatal unit to assure that the home treatment program is successful in reversing or minimizing the clinical respiratory disability and that adequate respiratory gas exchange is being maintained. These infants should be followed jointly by the pediatrician and, with appropriate consultation from the pulmonary specialist, other members of the follow-up clinic team to permit optimal continuity of care. The CLD infant with obstruction of the lower airway requires transcutaneous and/or arterial blood gas assessment at each clinic visit.[106] In addition, pulse oximetry and transcutaneous and end-tidal carbon dioxide tension measurement are extremely helpful in managing these infants. When the infant is being treated with theophylline, weekly measurement of serum theophylline levels is essential during the initial period after discharge from the hospital; later this assessment is required when the infant manifests any sign of worsening airway obstruction or signs of toxicity. (See Medications, below.)

Frequent nutritional assessment is essential to assure that the infant is receiving an adequate diet and sufficient intake and is achieving adequate weight gain. The nutritional plan for the CLD infant with obstruction of the lower airway includes a more conservative fluid limit of 120 ml/kg/day. The dietary components of the nutritional plan are discussed below in Nutritional Issues in Infants with CLD.

In the CLD infant with findings of lower airway obstruction, bronchodilator therapy is indicated when it is determined that the symptoms are not a sign of excessive fluid intake, i.e., the infant having been fed more than the fluid limit. Not surprisingly this is the most frequent departure of families from the plan of care suggested by the neonatal care team. This is especially true when the infant enjoys or requires a great deal of non-nutritive sucking, is irritable, or cries frequently. The parents usually think that these signs are caused by hunger, and in their desire to provide their infant with the best possible care, they give additional formula feeding, rather than considering other causes of the infant's behavior or consulting with their pediatrician.

Often it is difficult to separate airway obstruction due to damaged airways from pulmonary edema, and a trial of diuretics may help and should be considered.

Editor

Bronchodilator therapy is the mainstay of pharmacologic treatment of lower airway obstruction.[107,108] Theophylline is the bronchodilator of choice for oral administration. The selection and use of a theophylline preparation and aerosol administration of beta-adrenergic agonists is discussed in Medications. Aerosol bronchodilator medications, principally isoproterenol sulfate or isoetharine, are most conveniently administered by bag and mask insufflation of the lungs using a five-breath method. The protocol for administration of these bronchodilators and the instructions for parents are listed in Appendix A, along with a list of the equipment and supplies required. When indicated, it is advisable to have the parents perform chest percussion and postural drainage 15 to 20 minutes after administration of the aerosol, two to four times daily. This short delay following aerosol administration allows sufficient time for the maximal bronchodilator effect to take place and maximizes the effectiveness of the chest therapy in clearing mucus from the airways. There is little to be gained by performing chest percussion and postural drainage more often than every six hours. Rather, there is a decided danger of tiring the infant and interfering with the efficacy of other medications.

Stage III: Interstitial Pulmonary Edema

Interstitial pulmonary edema is a factor in the symptom complex of CLD.[29,36,46,109] However, specific therapy for this aspect of the disorder should be confined to those infants who manifest the clinical findings listed in Table 14–4. These include intercostal retractions, nasal flaring, terminal inspiratory rales, and expiratory grunting, which occurs when the infant is distressed. Infants with these findings of interstitial pulmonary edema are likely also to have tachypnea and signs of expiratory airway obstruction. These CLD infants will require very frequent office visits for evaluation of the adequacy of therapy. Except for the addition of frequent (initially weekly) assessment of serum electrolytes, clinical monitoring is similar to that required by infants with tachypnea and expiratory airway obstruction.

The CLD infant with interstitial pulmonary edema is treated with greater fluid restriction than that recommended for stages I and II. Total fluid intake should not exceed 100 to 110 ml/kg/day. Paradoxically, while the fluid intake for these infants is more severely restricted, their caloric requirements to achieve reasonable growth are increased. Resolution of this dilemma is discussed below in Nutritional Issues in Infants with CLD. The nutritional care of these infants requires frequent consultation with the nutrition experts of the follow-up team. Infants with this disorder appear to have compromised intestinal absorption as well, which is especially severe during periods of increased pulmonary edema. In addition, since they are prone to worsening pulmonary edema, methods other than monitoring only of weight gain must be utilized to detect and confirm "real" weight gain.

TABLE 14–4. Therapy for Chronic Lung Disease of Infancy, Stage III

Clinical Feature	Interstitial pulmonary edema
Clinical Findings	Same as tachypnea and airway obstruction (Tables 14–2 and 14–3) plus 1. Nasal flaring 2. Retractions 3. Moist inspiratory rales 4. Expiratory grunting (when stressed)
Evaluation/Monitoring	Same as tachypnea and airway obstruction (Tables 14–2 and 14–3) plus 1. Serum electrolyte analysis, initially weekly 2. Pulse oximetry (oxyhemoglobin saturation)
Pediatric Care	Same as tachypnea plus 1. Maintain oxygen-carrying capacity of blood (Hgb, Hct in normal range) (see text)

Home Care	Same as airway obstruction, Table 14–3, plus
	1. Fluid restriction to 100 to 110 ml/kg/day
	2. Diuretic therapy (see text)
	  a. Short-term: furosemide 1 to 2 mg/kg/dose, b.i.d., t.i.d., or q.i.d. or
	  b. Long-term: chlorothiazide 10 to 20 mg/kg/dose, b.i.d.
	3. Potassium-sparing diuretic:
	  a. Spironolactone, 1.5 mg/kg, b.i.d. or
	  b. Triamterene, 2.5 to 4.0 mg/kg, b.i.d.

When To Worry

1. As with tachypnea (Table 14–2) or airway obstruction (Table 14–3)
2. When weight gain is too rapid
3. When metabolic alkalosis with low serum chloride develops
4. With gastroenteritis with decreased intake or increased losses of fluid
5. With cyclic improvement and worsening that might be related to aspiration from gastroesophageal reflux

Fluid restriction alone is insufficient treatment for the continuing interstitial fluid loss in these infants. Thus, in addition to the use of medications to treat bronchoconstriction, CLD infants with clinical manifestations of interstitial pulmonary edema should receive diuretic therapy.[110-116] The use of diuretics in CLD and their selection and dosage schedules are discussed in Medications. A distinction is made between the short-term or initial administration of diuretic medications and their long-term use. The impact of long-term use on urinary losses of electrolytes and other minerals is an important consideration in the selection of a diuretic agent. To minimize the loss of potassium and to avoid, if possible, obligatory use of potassium supplementation, the CLD infant requiring long-term diuretic treatment should receive concurrent treatment with a potassium-sparing diuretic[117] (see Table 14–8). The effectiveness of the addition of diuretic medication to the treatment plan is determined by analysis of the parents' diary—the presence of signs of pulmonary edema, i.e., flaring, retractions, expiratory grunting, increased sleeping respiratory rate—as well as the physical examination. Clinical monitoring of blood gases serves to assure the clinician that gas exchange is being maintained and that metabolic alkalosis (rising bicarbonate concentration) secondary to chloride loss has not developed.[118] The latter is particularly important, since metabolic alkalosis depresses the respiratory drive, allowing the arterial carbon dioxide tension to rise, as the respiratory correction of this acid-base abnormality. Measurements of transcutaneous oxygen and carbon dioxide tension, along with pulse oximetry, are essential features of the clinical monitoring of these infants, and pulmonary function studies, i.e., body plethysmography or measurement of respiratory resistance, permit extremely sensitive evaluation of the respiratory status of the CLD infant with pulmonary edema.

Stage IV: Hypoxia and Hemoglobin Desaturation

Hypoxia is a common finding in the CLD infant with airway obstruction and/or interstitial pulmonary edema. However, the magnitude and duration of hypoxia deserve careful investigation and clinical monitoring. A history of "duskiness" of the face or around the eyes or lips or of cyanosis of the tongue, fingertips, or nail beds during sleep, feeding, or crying is alarming and indicates the need for further study. To characterize the magnitude and duration of hypoxia it is necessary to monitor the oxyhemoglobin saturation by pulse oximetry over an extended period, as during a long nap or, preferably, an overnight period that includes feeding and crying. Hypoxia is of particular concern when it is associated with reduction of the hemoglobin oxygen saturation below 90 per cent (measured by pulse oximetry) for even 10 to 15 per cent of the study period. Normal hemoglobin oxygen saturation of 96 per cent in the infant between 1 month and 1 year of age correlates roughly with arterial oxygen tension of 75

to 80 torr, while saturation of 90 per cent is roughly equivalent to arterial oxygen tension of 60 to 65 torr.

The clinician should be aware, however, that the accuracy of pulse oximetry in infants with CLD is yet to be determined.

Editor

The CLD infant with this degree of desaturation is likely to experience worsening pulmonary edema and airway obstruction from hypoxic pulmonary vasoconstriction.[94,119] When transcutaneous oxygen tension (tc PO_2) alone is measured, accurate extrapolation of the tc PO_2 value to hemoglobin oxygen saturation is not possible.[119] For this reason, it is advisable to monitor transcutaneous oxygen tension concurrently with pulse oximetry study.

Many clinicians, however, have noted that tc PO_2 often correlates poorly with actual arterial PaO_2 in CLD infants.

Editor

All infants with a history of cyanosis, who meet the monitoring criteria described above, or who have poor growth will require treatment with oxygen. When the periods during which the CLD infant experiences oxyhemoglobin desaturation are clearly defined by study, it may be possible to limit the use of oxygen therapy to only those periods. This approach is rarely practical or possible, and, therefore, in most cases it is better to use continuous oxygen until the infant's response to this therapy is observed.[120] The latter is always the preferable plan for home oxygen therapy, when the infant's oxygen desaturation has been documented by only a short nap or clinic study.

In the CLD infant with chronic hypoxia, maintaining a normal oxygen-carrying capacity of the blood is essential to providing adequate blood oxygen content. Oxygen therapy alone will not suffice. The infant's hemoglobin should be maintained above 13 grams per dl, and the hematocrit levels should be kept above 39 per cent. In the first three months after birth, blood transfusions may be necessary, but subsequently adequate hemoglobin and hematocrit should be maintained by a sufficient diet and supplemental iron therapy.

Oxygen may be administered by nasal cannula or prongs (see Oxygen Delivery Systems, Appendix A) and should be humidified. It is technically simplest to regulate the amount of oxygen received by adjusting the flow. In this instance, a low-flow (1 to 10 liters/min) oxygen regulator is required. An alternative to regulating oxygen therapy by flow is to use an oxygen concentrator to blend the oxygen to the desired concentration. This alternative is attractive, as it removes the need to have the flow checked carefully each time oxygen therapy is restarted. Oxygen should be humidified and warmed when possible (heated nebulizers are available commercially). Oxygen should be administered at a level sufficient to raise the infant's oxygen saturation above 90 per cent, even during vigorous and prolonged crying. Therefore, oxygen therapy should be adjusted during the pulse oximetry and tc PO_2 study, confirming its need. CLD infants receiving therapy at home will require very close observation. The main goal of implementing oxygen therapy is elimination of continuing or even episodic oxygen desaturation. To monitor the effectiveness of the treatment in the interval between clinic visits, an accurate clinical diary will be needed. In most instances, the amount of care, administration of medication and treatments, and maintenance of the oxygen therapy will necessitate home nursing care for part or all of the day or night (usually, 8 to 16 hours of nursing care during weekdays). Initially the oxygen-dependent CLD infant has weekly follow-up clinic visits.* These infants require the same clinical monitoring as the CLD infant with pulmonary edema (Tables 14–4 and 14–5). A flow sheet that lists the major historical factors from the parents' diary, physical and laboratory findings, clinical monitoring values, medications and their dosages, and oxygen concentration or flow rates should be kept for each CLD infant. In caring for the oxygen-dependent infant, graphing the gas exchange, acid-base values, and clinical findings at each clinic visit is helpful in recognizing even small changes in the infant's condition.

Some pediatric pulmonologists feel that the status of all CLD infants receiving home oxygen supplementation and diuretic therapy is sufficiently unstable to require home monitoring for apnea and bradycardia.[121–124] They recommend that the infant be monitored for apnea at any time he or she is not being directly observed by the parent or other care giver. While this places an additional psychological burden on the parents, some parents will request home apnea monitoring even if they are not familiar with this recommendation. The most reasoned approach is to discuss the apnea-bradycardia monitoring with the family, giving balanced support to the advantages and disadvantages of

_____

* Whenever possible, these assessments should be done in the home, rather than in the clinic. — Ed.

TABLE 14–5. Therapy for Chronic Lung Disease of Infancy, Stage IV

Clinical Feature	Hypoxia — Oxyhemoglobin saturation <90% or PaO_2 < 60 torr
Clinical Findings	Same as interstitial pulmonary edema (Table 14–4) plus 1. Duskiness or frank cyanosis 2. Expiratory grunting at rest 3. Sleeping respiratory rate >45/min
Evaluation/Monitoring	Same as interstitial pulmonary edema (Table 14–4) plus the following at each office visit: 1. Arterial blood gas (acid-base balance) 2. Transcutaneous oxygen and carbon dioxide tension (tc PO_2 and tc PCO_2) 3. Pulse oximetry
Pediatric Care	Same as tachypnea (Table 14–2) Home visits for as much of care and evaluation as possible
Home Care	Same as interstitial pulmonary edema (Table 14–4) plus 1. Nasal oxygen administration 2. Home nursing care when appropriate

When To Worry
1. As in stages I, II, and III (Tables 14–2, 14–3, 14–4)
2. With fever or ambient temperature variations
3. When support systems change or are weak

this form of monitoring. In many metropolitan areas, vendor support for this service is quite adequate, and day-to-day maintenance of the monitors, or even retraining the family in the home on the use of the monitors, is possible. Home monitor use is impractical without the availability of technical support, as described above, on a 24-hour basis.

> Most home monitoring now available is respiratory (impedance pneumography). In infants with CLD, monitoring heart rate or, perhaps, oxygen-saturation monitoring may become more appropriate and effective.
>
> *Editor*

Stage V: Cor Pulmonale and Hypercapnia

Further deterioration in the CLD infant's condition is heralded by alveolar hypoventilation, which will occur as carbon dioxide retention.[124,125] Some of these infants will have associated pulmonary hypertension. Cardiac function may become compromised because of hypoxemia and hypercapnia, but ultimately, cardiac decompensation is caused by the increased right ventricular driving pressure required to propel blood through the constricted pulmonary vascular bed.[126] Cardiac dysfunction may be manifested by right ventricular hypertrophy, but with inadequate response to therapy, biventricular hypertrophy and failure may eventuate. Some indication of cardiac involvement may be seen on the electrocardiogram (e.g., right ventricular strain), and often right ventricular hypertrophy is evident on both the electrocardiogram and echocardiogram.[82, 84,127,128] While these infants may not have clinical findings consistent with pulmonary hypertension, for the reasons already mentioned it is important to eliminate this condition as a factor in the worsening of the respiratory status.[33,129] CLD infants with hypercapnia (i.e., an arterial carbon dioxide tension exceeding 45 torr) or pulmonary hypertension are considered to have functional compromise of right ventricular function — cor pulmonale. For this reason these patients require joint management with a pediatric cardiologist.

PULMONARY HYPERTENSION

When carbon dioxide retention and echocardiographic evidence of cor pulmonale associated with pulmonary hypertension are found, further clinical evaluation is necessary (Table 14–6). Especially in the infant with a history of umbilical artery catheterization during the neonatal period, pulmonary hypertension may be a reflection of systemic hypertension. It is advisable to admit the infant to the hospital for careful studies of the blood pressure during sleep to document whether or not systemic hypertension is a causative factor in the pulmonary hypertension. Then, to rule out hypoxic pulmonary hypertension, a continuous study of oxygen saturation over a 24-hour period is required to determine whether the level of inspired oxygen tension is great enough to raise the arterial oxygen tension to a level sufficient to permit adequate blood oxygen saturation (i.e., greater than 90 per cent) under all levels of activity and states of consciousness. Occasionally it may be necessary to perform cardiac catheterization to rule out cardiomyopathy or "silent" congenital heart disease[83,130] or to determine if the patient's pulmonary vascular resistance can be reduced by oxygen inhalation or pulmonary vasodilators.[82,131,132]

The mainstay of therapy in the CLD infant with isolated pulmonary hypertension is reduction of the hypoxic component. Treatment with an agent to lessen pulmonary vascular resistance may also be indicated. Agents acting to lessen pulmonary vascular resistance include those acting directly on the pulmonary vascular bed (e.g., hydralazine, diazoxide), those acting on adrenergic receptors (e.g., isoproterenol, phentolamine),[133,134] those blocking calcium ion transport (e.g., verapamil, nifedipine),[135-137] and agents inhibiting angiotensin-converting enzyme (e.g., captopril),[137,138] prostaglandins, and cyclo-oxygenase inhibitors (e.g., indomethacin).[139] Unfortunately there is not a great deal of evidence of the efficacy of many of these agents in treating pulmonary hypertension in CLD.[140-143] However, hydralazine is perhaps the most widely used.

The CLD patient with cor pulmonale who is found not to have associated pulmonary hypertension during the work-up described above is suffering from a severe permeability-type of pulmonary edema. The worsening of the clinical findings, if not attributable to excessive fluid intake, may be due to an "occult" infection or aspiration, as discussed below. If results of all of the studies are normal, then it may be advisable to keep the infant in the hospital where all aspects of the program described for the infant with interstitial pulmonary edema can be carried out on a 24-hour basis. A change in diuretic therapy from chlorothiazide to parenteral furosemide is also indicated. Some pediatric cardiologists may advise treatment of the cardiac failure with digoxin, and still others may suggest a trial of afterload reduction with nitro-

---

TABLE 14–6. Therapy for Chronic Lung Disease of Infancy, Stage V

Clinical Feature	Cor pulmonale:
	    Hypercapnia ($PaCO_2 > 45$)
	        +/−
	    Pulmonary hypertension
	        +/−
	    Prolonged ventilator dependence

Clinical Findings	Same as interstitial pulmonary edema (Table 14–4) plus
	    1. Irritability
	    2. Diaphoresis
	    3. Peripheral edema
	    4. Hepatomegaly
	    5. With or without increased or snapping P_2; widening between A_2 and P_2

Management	Admit to hospital for extensive diagnostic evaluation or management
When To Worry	
1. With clinical findings as above
2. With increasing carbon dioxide retention
3. With systemic hypertension

prusside, though neither of these therapeutic approaches has attracted universal support.

Unexplained Worsening of Ventilation in CLD

BACTERIAL INFECTION

When in spite of implemention of appropriate therapy for CLD, the clinical condition of the infant does not improve, careful assessment for other complications must be pursued. First, an *infection* could be a factor in precipitating the exacerbation in the respiratory disease. The most common focus for a bacterial complication of CLD is the middle ear, sinuses, or lung. Bacterial infection of the lower respiratory tract is relatively uncommon and is quite difficult to document, because of the difficulties of identifying new lung involvement in the CLD infant with clinically advanced lung disease and a chest roentgenogram that is diffusely abnormal. Cultures are reliable only if obtained from the lower respiratory tract, which means subjecting the infant to intubation of the trachea or bronchoscopy to obtain uncontaminated culture material. Smearing mucus obtained from pharyngeal suctioning and using Gram stain to search for polymorphonuclear leukocytes and bacteria (especially intracellular bacteria) may provide helpful information. Unfortunately, even with a positive culture, the origin of the infected mucus is in doubt, since both the lung and the nasal sinuses may contribute to mucus collected from the pharynx. If the ears appear infected, tympanocentesis is advised. If the smear and culture of the tympanic aspirate are the same as those from the pharyngeal mucus, the middle ear and/or sinuses are the likely source of the infection and may be contributing to the exacerbation in CLD, either through worsening inflammatory edema of the airway and increasing obstruction or by leading to the development of sinobronchitis (from drainage of infected mucus into the trachea, especially during sleep).

OTHER INFECTIONS

Pulmonary infection caused by microorganisms other than bacteria is another frequent cause of worsening in the condition of a CLD infant. This may be caused by viral agents, such as respiratory syncytial virus or cytomegalovirus (CMV), or by other agents, such as *Mycoplasma pneumoniae*.[69] An infant with CMV infection may have been exposed through blood transfusions in the ICN (although congenital or natural infection with CMV may also occur). In general, CLD infants resist these infections poorly. Since all of these disorders can be identified by cultures and/or serologic tests, attempts to diagnose the specific causative pathogen are important if there is a history suggestive of exposure or if other studies are inconclusive.

GASTROESOPHAGEAL REFLUX

Another cause of worsening lung disease in CLD infants is gastroesophogeal reflux and aspiration.[123,144-148] Infants in whom this occurs experience chronic worsening respiratory disability, with a cyclic course of slight or major improvement followed by inexplicable worsening of symptoms—particularly wheezing. CLD infants are especially prone to this condition when the chest roentgenogram reveals major depression of the diaphragm from pulmonary hyperinflation. The hyperinflation leads to traction on the walls of the esophagus as it passes through the esophageal hiatus; the traction, in turn, disrupts the normal sphincter mechanism of the gastric cardia. Low mean pleural pressure, which is associated with the hyperinflation, encourages reflux of the gastric contents into the esophagus, particularly during transient increases in abdominal pressure that accompany coughing and crying.[146,147]

The treatment is initially medical and entails thickening the formula with rice cereal, encouraging more frequent, smaller feedings, placing the infant in either the prone position with the head of the crib elevated or in an upright sitting position in an infant seat for at least 45 minutes after a feeding. The infant should be treated with metoclopramide (Reglan), in a dose of 0.1 mg/kg three times daily, when gastric scintiscan reveals that the problem is due to or complicated by delayed gastric emptying.[149,150]

> Although gastroesophageal reflux is a common cause of emesis in infants with CLD, we have observed several infants who have developed behavioral responses, including self-induced emesis. This is often difficult to differentiate from gastroesophageal reflux, but should be considered as a possible diagnosis, especially in infants 6 to 12 months of age.
>
> *R. Piecuch*

VENTILATOR DEPENDENCE

The most severe manifestation of CLD is ventilator dependence. The care of infants who require long-term ventilation is discussed in Chapter 16. The major indication for long-term assisted ventilation in CLD infants is hypoventilation with hypercapnia sufficient to lower the arterial pH below 7.25 (in the absence of metabolic acidosis). If the infant's respiratory status is deteriorating rapidly, it is advisable to admit him or her to the hospital for elective initiation of assisted ventilation, to prevent the occurrence of apnea or respiratory arrest. Long-term assisted ventilation at home is possible only if the infant has had a tracheostomy.

MEDICATIONS

Bronchodilator Agents

THEOPHYLLINE

Treatment Plan. To achieve a serum theophylline level of at least 10 μg/ml and less than 20 μg/ml.[101,107]

The initial dose schedule is 10 mg/kg/day with frequency based on the pharmacologic properties of the theophylline preparation used (see Appendix A, Table A–2). Serum theophylline levels should be monitored twice weekly at first to assure that the serum levels remain in the desired range. It is important to remember that some children may excrete theophylline rapidly. Thus the dosage may have to be increased to assure a therapeutic serum level. Usually this can be achieved with a dosage of less than 20 mg/kg/day, although occasionally an infant or child will require a higher dosage so that a serum concentration of greater than 10 μg/ml is maintained.

The clinical response of the pediatric patient to theophylline is also quite variable. While some patients will experience a good therapeutic response with a serum level of 10 μg/ml, others will require levels in the range of 15 to 20 μg/ml. In any case, the therapeutic response must not be achieved at the cost of unfavorable side effects. Tachycardia, anorexia, emesis, sleeplessness, and irritability are some of the side effects of theophylline treatment. When they are observed, the medication should be discontinued temporarily until the theophylline serum level returns to the desired range. Rarely, side effects are observed when the serum level is well below the toxic level. In these cases, theophylline should be discontinued and treatment with another bronchodilator medication begun, or the theophylline dosage should be decreased to a level at which the side effects are no longer observed. If this decrease in dosage is accompanied by reappearance of symptoms, then theophylline should be replaced as the principal bronchodilator by a beta-adrenergic agonist.

Concurrent treatment with other medications may affect the serum theophylline level. For example, treatment with erythromycin usually should be avoided if the patient has had an acceptable clinical response to theophylline. Concurrent treatment with erythromycin retards the excretion of theophylline and may lead to the patient's experiencing toxic serum concentrations of theophylline. *Therefore, each new medication must be evaluated for the potential of interaction with each of the patient's concurrent medications.* (See Appendix A, Table A–2, for preparations and dosage schedules for theophylline.)

BETA-ADRENERGIC AGONISTS

Beta-adrenergic agonist medications have several beneficial pharmacologic properties that may result in improved lung function for infants with chronic lung disease. However, at present only the bronchodilator properties of these medications have actually been documented to be therapeutically beneficial in CLD.[91] The other actions of these medications, e.g., improving ciliary motility, relaxing smooth muscle, inotropic and chronotropic effects on the heart — promoting a shift of potassium from the intravascular space to the intracellular fluid compartment,[151,152] should also be considered when selecting these medications for use in the infant with chronic lung disease. To maximize the potential benefit derived from this class of drugs (i.e., improving bronchomotor tone, increasing ciliary motility, and mucociliary clearance) while reducing the risk of side effects (e.g., excessive increase in heart rate or hypokalemia), it is important to select a route of administration that will deliver the medication to the lung without achieving blood levels that might be accompanied by unwanted side effects.

Administration. In practice, aerosol administration is usually found to be best for beta-adrenergic agonists, and it is most efficacious with respect to freedom from side effects when administered with proper technique. To this end, it is beneficial to time administration of the aerosol with the infant's inspirations. In this manner the aerosol will be directed to the airway, and only minimal amounts of the medication will settle in the buccal mucosa, where it is rapidly absorbed into the circulation. Oral treatment with beta-adrenergic agonists should be reserved for only those instances in which theophylline therapy has not been acceptable and when the beta-adrenergic agonists are not to be used by the aerosol route as well. (See Appendix A, Table A–5, Home Care Instructions: Bronchodilator Aerosol Treatments.)

DIURETICS

The selection of a diuretic medication and its route of administration is based on the acuity of the symptoms of respiratory distress. As previously discussed, diuretic therapy is indicated in the CLD infant only when there is evidence of pulmonary interstitial edema, as characterized by retractions, nasal flaring, and/or auscultatory rales. When these findings have had a rapid onset and have caused serious respiratory distress, then it is prudent to select furosemide as the medication for short-term treatment; furosemide can be administered parenterally by either the intramuscular or intravenous route and has a rapid onset of action (i.e., within 30 minutes).[110-116] For long-term diuretic treatment, especially for a mild form of pulmonary edema, chlorothiazide is a wiser choice of diuretic.[113] Although requiring a longer time to achieve clinical effectiveness, chlorothiazide is nevertheless a very effective agent with a wide therapeutic dosage range. It is calcium sparing, whereas furosemide results in calciuria, and long-term treatment with furosemide eventu-

ally causes bone demineralization and, finally, calcium deposition in the cortex of the kidney. Absorption from the gastrointestinal tract in the small infant is also more predictable with chlorothiazide than with furosemide. However, when either medication is used for a long time, it is essential to monitor closely the concentration of electrolytes in the serum, and electrolyte supplements may be necessary (Table 14–7).

Infants receiving diuretic therapy frequently experience significant loss of sodium and/or potassium from the plasma. Surprisingly the loss of sodium, an extracellular ion, is more easily recognized. The loss of potassium, primarily an intracellular ion, is often masked by an apparently normal or low-normal serum potassium concentration. As the serum potassium concentration falls, potassium is transferred from the intracellular fluid compartment into the plasma, maintaining the serum potassium concentration at nearly normal levels until the total body potassium level becomes dangerously low.[153-154] A low level of total body potassium is often heralded by a falling serum chloride concentration, chloride being a freely diffusable ion that is lost from the body proportionately to both sodium and potassium. Thus when long-term diuretic therapy is contemplated, it is often better therapeutic strategy to couple the initiation of therapy with either furosemide or

TABLE 14–7. Nutritional Management of Chronic Lung Disease of Infancy

STAGE	FLUID RESTRICTION	CALORIC INTAKE NEEDED (KCAL/KG/DAY)	ADDITIVES	SPECIAL CONCERNS
Tachypnea	150 ml/kg of 20 cal/oz formula	100 to 125	1 tsp (5 kcal) Rice cereal/oz of formula (increase to 25 kcal/kg)	Add dietary potassium (banana or avocado)
Airway Obstruction	120 ml/kg of 24 kcal/oz formula or 27 kcal/oz, if needed	115 to 135	Rice cereal, as above, or 2 tsp/oz	Avoid commercial pureed foods (high water content)
Pulmonary Edema	100 ml/kg of 27 kcal/oz cardiac formula	125 to 160	2 tsp/oz Rice cereal or MCT oil Avocado 1.5 kcal/gm	May cause gastrointestinal irritation Potassium supplement Avocado: 8 mEq/gm May require sodium or chloride supplement
TE Fistula				May require continuous tube feeding
GI Mucosal Injury or Short Bowel	Pregestimil 24 kcal/oz formula		Rice cereal	

chlorothiazide with the administration of a potassium-sparing diuretic, i.e., spironolactone or triamterene.[155,156] This approach reduces the losses of potassium from the plasma from the outset of the therapy and may reduce or eventually eliminate the need for potassium supplementation. The latter is highly desirable, since potassium-containing medications are often quite irritating to the gastrointestinal tract.

Since infants receiving diuretic medications have increased loss of fluids and electrolytes in the urine, reduced fluid intake, diarrhea, or vomiting may lead to rapid dehydration and severe electrolyte disturbance. With any of these problems, diuretic medications should be discontinued immediately, and serum electrolyte and BUN determined to assess the electrolyte and hydration status. An elevated BUN value suggests prerenal azotemia, as is seen in dehydration. When there is doubt concerning the status of the infant's hydration following these studies, serum and urine osmolality determinations should resolve this issue. Often, treatment of fluid and electrolyte disturbances entails intravenous rehydration, as the electrolyte concentration of most available oral rehydration solutions is inadequate to compensate for the excessive urinary losses of electrolytes. Finally, with rehydration, the CLD infant may experience rebound pulmonary edema. For these reasons, excessive fluid loss constitutes a medical emergency in diuretic-dependent infants, and it is prudent to care for these infants in the hospital, where the clinical status, hydration, electrolyte balance, and rehydration can be monitored more closely. (See Appendix A, Table A–2, for preparations and dosages of medications.)

ELECTROLYTE SUPPLEMENTS

Following the implementation of diuretic therapy, the diet of the CLD infant should be analyzed carefully, to assure that he or she is receiving a high maintenance intake of potassium chloride and sodium chloride. Even when the potassium intake is adequate prior to the initiation of diuretic therapy, there is no assurance that there will not be excessive urinary potassium loss with long-term diuretic therapy. The infant who has been receiving theophylline therapy may have been experiencing modest diuresis, and, thus, an additional, and perhaps occult, loss of potassium. Most infant formulas contain less than 2 mEq/dl of potassium and provide only sufficient dietary potassium when the infant is fed between 150 and 200 ml/kg/day of the formula. The fluid restriction imposed on all CLD infants is likely to have led to reduced dietary intake of potassium prior to the initiation of diuretic therapy. The concurrent use of a potassium-sparing diuretic with long-term therapy with either chlorothiazide or furosemide may control potassium wasting. If, however, additional potassium supplementation is required, then the initial approach to supplementation should be dietary (Table 14–7). When the infant is already being fed pureed foods, the addition of bananas or avocado should be considered, as they are rich sources of potassium. Avocado, for example, contains approximately 8 mEq/gm of potassium.

A parallel analysis of the infant's dietary intake of sodium chloride is also required. Since sodium is an extracellular ion, its serum losses are generally recognized on the serum electrolyte assay. Unfortunately, infant formulas rarely contain more than 1 to 2 mEq of sodium per deciliter of formula, and breast milk contains only 0.71 mEq/dl.

The preparations recommended for use in electrolyte supplementation are included in the medication section of Appendix A. Their use is indicated when the fluid-restricted infant is not receiving at least 3 mEq of sodium chloride daily or 1 to 2 mEq of potassium chloride daily, and when it is not possible to add a sufficient supplement containing these electrolytes to the infant's diet of pureed or strained food. When the infant is to receive diuretic therapy as well, electrolyte supplementation is indicated.

The recommendation for chloride supplementation is less clear. A reduction in chloride on the serum electrolyte determination usually reflects urinary potassium and sodium losses. When the serum sodium and potassium concentrations are normal in the presence of a low serum chloride level, total body potassium may be reduced, and the low serum chloride level is merely a reflection of the potassium deficiency. The latter is especially likely when analysis of the diet reveals a low or even normal intake of potassium. In this case, potassium chloride supplementation, rather than chloride supplementation, is necessary. If, on the other hand, dietary potassium is adequate, "spot" urinary potassium analysis supports the adequacy of potassium intake, and the serum potassium level is high-normal, then supplementation with a chloride preparation is appropriate. Arginine chloride is the supplement of choice for home administration. It has, however, the disadvantage of being quite insoluble in water, and thus its usual concentration is only 0.5 mEq/ml. Although ammonium chloride is a more potent chloride supplement, it is usually not suitable for administration in the home. Its use requires very frequent laboratory studies to assure that this therapy has not caused an excessive serum chloride level, which can lead to the dissociation of hydrogen from the ammonium ion and result in excessive hydrogen ion accumulation in the serum and metabolic acidosis.

Other Medications

While there has been a great amount of publicity concerning the beneficial effects of glucocorticoid therapy[157-161] and vitamin E therapy,[41,162] there has been no documentation of their effectiveness in the CLD infant. Neither short- nor long-term administration of either of these medications has been confirmed to be of value in the management of CLD. In fact, the potential side effects of glucocorticoids, especially the risk of increased susceptibility to infection, osteopenia, myopathy, cataracts, and fluid retention, as well as a detrimental effect on growth, may outweigh any potential gain from therapy.

OTHER PULMONARY DISORDERS ASSOCIATED WITH CLD

In addition to the sequelae of RDS and other conditions requiring oxygen therapy or mechanical ventilation, there are some neonatal conditions, both pulmonary and extrapulmonary, that may lead to subsequent and sometimes prolonged or chronic respiratory disability. The conditions include (1) infection of the pulmonary parenchyma (e.g., CMV, staphylococcal pneumonia), (2) congenital or acquired airway disease due to congenital anomalies of the airway (see Chapter 16), (3) bulbar or neuromuscular disorders that interfere with deglutition and pharyngeal function and result in pulmonary aspiration, and (4) disorders of the lung, chest wall, diaphragm, or abdominal wall that result in hypoventilation (see Chapter 15). Examples of these include congenital diaphragmatic hernia and eventration of the diaphragm; primary lung hypoplasia; omphalocele-gastroschisis complex; disorders of the muscles of ventilation; disorders of the ribs or vertebrae; and phrenic nerve palsy.

CONGENITAL OR NEONATAL INFECTION

As a consequence of neonatal lung infection, pulmonary function may be abnormal and the lung's airway defense mechanisms also may be impaired. The duration of this disability varies with the extent and type of injury caused by the infective agent. CMV is a multisystem infection and may acutely impair function of the central nervous system, heart, liver, and bone marrow (including the coagulation mechanisms). CMV may also cause interstitial lung disease, of which the major clinical finding is signs of pulmonary edema (unless the infant has some degree of CLD and there are signs of worsening of this condition). If these infants experience long-term interstitial pulmonary edema, they may benefit from diuretic therapy. In some infants, lung disease following CMV infection may be sufficiently severe to cause hypoxia. As in CLD, the hypoxic infant with CMV should be treated with medications that reverse the abnormal pulmonary physical findings and should be monitored in a similar fashion (Tables 14–4 and 14–5).

Staphylococcal pneumonia is an invasive pneumonitis. Pneumothorax and pyopneumothorax are common acute complications of staphylococcal pneumonitis and may lead, over an extended time, to the development of adhesive pleuritis. More often, staphylococcal pneumonia causes destruction of the airway mucosa, with invasion of the pulmonary parenchyma, resulting in residual saccular bronchiectasis. Over the long term, these infants will be very susceptible to recurrent pulmonary infections in the involved segment(s) of the lung, because of the destruction of the airway surface and loss of mucosal mucus–clearance mechanisms. Home care should focus on maintaining optimal respiratory mucus clearance, as described above for the CLD infant with airway obstruction (Table 14–3). During respiratory illness, these infants require monitoring of their hematologic status (complete blood cell count) and bacteriologic examination to exclude bacterial airway infection. Immunizations, similar to those advised for the CLD infant, are indicated to lessen the risk of subsequent bacterial and viral respiratory infections with organisms that might lead to further lung destruction and perhaps the need for surgical resection of the affected lung tissue.

ABNORMALITIES OF THE AIRWAYS

Infants discharged from an ICN often require long-term management of abnormal conditions related to the airways. Continuing airways dysfunction may occur because of congenital malformations of the airways, effects of congenital nonrespiratory disorders, or acquired injuries to the airways. Design of an appropriate plan of care involves anticipation of potential long-term respiratory sequelae of neonatal respiratory tract problems and an appreciation of the fact that the appearance of sequelae may be delayed and modified by postneonatal events.

NUTRITIONAL ISSUES IN INFANTS WITH CLD

Nutrition is the mainstay of the treatment of the infant with CLD. Because of a high work "cost" of breathing from reduced lung elasticity and a higher wasted ventilation, as well as the nutritional cost of "fueling" the process of lung healing, the infant with CLD requires an increased caloric intake in addition to basic nutrition to assure usual growth and development of critical organ systems. The tachypnea and retractions typically seen in infants with CLD attest to the increased work of breathing and explain why these infants, even when their CLD is mild, might not gain weight properly or might not experience adequate growth in length and head circumference when they receive what would ordinarily be a normal caloric intake.[11,12,98] Since fluid restriction is often a part of the care plan for a CLD infant, the challenge of providing adequate nutrition is to supply nutrition of higher caloric density, i.e., sufficient protein but a greater number of total calories in a lower fluid volume.

Many CLD infants are not vigorous feeders, and some may have, in addition, residual gastrointestinal injury from neonatal necrotizing enterocolitis.[79,97] Substantial caution, therefore, must be exercised in prescribing a diet. The basic nutrition philosophy advocates utilizing standard or modified formulas in higher caloric density, i.e., 24 to 27 calories per ounce, or adding usually well tolerated carbohydrate or fatty acid supplements to the standard formulas. While several examples of feeding regimens for the infant with CLD follow, these diets are only examples, not a cookbook (Tables 14–8 to 14–11).

The nutritional plan for each infant must be individualized. Therefore, infants with CLD

TABLE 14–8. Carbohydrate, Fat, and Protein Supplements

	MCT OIL	CONTROLYTE	PROPAC	POLYCOSE LIQUID	AVOCADO
Calories/ml	7.7 kcal/ml 8.25 kcal/gm	40 kcal/15 ml 5 kcal/gm	24 kcal/15 ml 4 kcal/gm	2 kcal/ml	1.5 kcal/gm
Protein (gm)	—	—	0.77 gm/gm powder	—	20 mg/gm
Fat (gm)	93.3	0.24 mg/gm powder	0.08 gm/gm powder	—	153 mg/gm
CHA (gm)	—	0.73 gm/gm	0.05 gm/gm powder	0.5 gm/ml	54 mg/gm
Protein Source	—	—	Whey	—	· · ·
Fat Source	Fractional Coconut oil	Soy oil	Small amount lecithin	—	· · ·
CHO Source	—	Corn starch	Small amount lactose	Glucose polymers	· · ·
Renal Solute Load	—	—	3.33/gm powder	0.062/ml	—
Osmolality (mOsm/kg H_2O)	—	598	?	850	—
Sodium/Potassium (mEq)	1	0.004–0.001/gm powder	0.1–0.13/gm powder	0.025–0.005/ml	0.36 mg/gm (Na) 8.1 mEq/gm (K)
Iron (mg)	—	—	—	—	0.01 mg/gm
Calcium/Potassium (mg)	—	—	6.0–3.1/gm powder	—	0.075 mg/gm (Ca) 0.24 mg/gm (P)
Indications	Patients with fat malabsorption; no EFA	CHO and fat supplement to high cal. 8 gm/tbsp	Protein supplement 6 gm/tbsp	Carbohydrate calorie supplement to be added to liquids	
Comments	Liquid from pharmacy; very expensive	Unflavored powder	Unflavored powder	No flavor	

TABLE 14–9. Nutrition Components in Standard Infant Formulas

	BREAST MILK	WHOLE COW'S MILK	ENFAMIL W/IRON	SIMILAC W/IRON	SMA W/IRON
Calories/100 ml	70	68	68	68	68
Protein (gm/100 ml)	1.2	3.3	1.5	1.55	1.5
Fat (gm/100 ml)	3.6	3.7	3.8	3.6	3.6
CHO (gm/100 ml)	7.2	4.7	6.9	7.2	7.2
Protein Source	Lactalbumin Casein lactoglobulin	Casein	Whey, nonfat milk	Nonfat milk	Nonfat milk, demineralized whey
Fat Source	Human milk fat	Butter fat	Coconut oil, soy oil	Soy oil, coconut oil	Oleo, coconut oil, safflower oil, soy oil
CHO	Lactose	Lactose	Lactose	Lactose	Lactose
Renal solute load (mOsm/100 ml)	8	23	10	11	13
Osmolality	300	288	278	290	300
Na/K (mEq/100 ml)	0.7/1.3	2.2/3.9	0.91/1.74	1.1/2.0	0.65/1.4
Iron (mg/100 ml)	0.05–0.1	0.05	1.25	1.2	1.25
Ca/P (mg/100 ml)	34/14	119/93	46/31	51/39	44/33
Vit A/D (per 100 ml)	190/2.2	138/41.9	208/41.7	250/40	260/41.9
Indications and Comments	Not to be started until 8 mo–1 yr of age	*Without iron* contains 0.1 mg iron/100 ml	*Without iron* contains 0.15 mg iron/100 ml	*Without iron* contains 0.15 mg iron/100 ml	

should be re-evaluated regularly by a nutritionist with specific training and skills in managing the special nutritional problems of small infants, to assure that each infant is prescribed a diet that will permit achievement of the projected rate of growth. Even more important, the addition of a nutritionist to the consulting medical team ensures better continuity in the nutritional management of the CLD infant. Measurements, such as skin-fold thickness, should be obtained to confirm that weight gain is real and not due to edema secondary to "excessive" fluid intake. In many instances, evaluation by a pediatric gastroenterologist is also required. This is particularly true for the infant who has experienced neonatal gastrointestinal difficulties, such as necrotizing enterocolitis or problems associated with gastrointestinal tract deformities such as abdominal wall defects or tracheoesophageal fistula. These infants provide the most difficult challenge and require comprehensive management by a careful, multidisciplinary team. They may require more easily digested formulas and, occasionally, continuous rather than intermittent feedings by gastric tube (i.e., nasogastric or gastrostomy feedings). Patients who have had tracheoesophageal fistula may have very severely reduced distal esophageal peristalsis and/or esophageal stenosis; therefore, solid feedings, when begun, may have to be li-

TABLE 14–10. Nutrition Components in Soy-Based Formulas

	ISOMIL	PROSOBEE
Calories/100 ml	68	68
Protein (gm/100 ml)	2.0	2.0
Fat (gm/100 ml)	3.6	3.6
CHO (gm/100 ml)	6.8	6.9
Protein	Soy protein isolate with added methionine	Soy protein isolate with added methionine
Fat Source	Coconut oil, soy oil	Coconut oil, soy oil
CHO	Corn syrup, sucrose	Corn syrup, solids
Renal solute load (mOsm/100 ml)	13	13

TABLE 14-11.   Nutrition Components in High-Calorie Infant Formulas

	SMA 24	SMA 27	STANDARD CARDIAC FORMULA	HI-CAL CARDIAC FORMULA	PREGESTIMIL	VIVONEX
Calories/ 100 ml	81	90	100	130	68	100
Protein (gm/100 ml)	1.8	2.03	2.72	3.31	1.9	2.2
Fat (gm/ 100 ml)	4.3	4.86	6.18	7.6	2.7	0.1
CHO (gm/ 100 ml)	8.6	9.72	8.43	12.9	9.1	23.1
Protein Source	Nonfat milk, demineralized whey	Nonfat milk, demineralized whey	Same as SMA 24	Same as SMA 27	Casein hydrolysate, W/L-cys, L-tyr, L-try	L-amino acids
Fat Source	Oleo, coconut oil, safflower oil, soy oil	Oleo, coconut oil, safflower oil, soy oil	Same as SMA 24 w/added corn oil (or MCT oil)	Same as SMA 27 w/added corn oil (or MCT oil)	Corn oil, MCT oil	Safflower oil
CHO	Lactose	Lactose	Lactose	Lactose, cornstarch	Corn syrup solids, modified tapioca starch	Glucose oligosaccharides
Renal Solute Load (mOsm/ 100 ml)	10.9	12.3	13.7	22.7	13	
Osmolality	360		364	476	348	550
Na/K (mEq/ 100 ml)	0.8/1.7	0.87/1.9	0.83/2.15	0.96/2.49	1.3/1.9	20/30
Iron (mg/ 100 ml)	1.5	1.7	1.47	1.56	1.3	1
Ca/P (mg/ 100 ml)	53/40	59/43.9	53/39.9	57/44.1	63/42	55.5/55.5
Vit A/D (per 100 ml)	312/50	352/56	303/48.5	320/51.1	209/41.9	278/22
Indications and Comments	SMA 24 and SMA 27: routine feeding when high cal required		Fluid restricted patients or poor feeders, when high-cal intake required; high in protein, low in sodium		For infants with disaccharidase deficiency; galactosemia; cow's milk or soy allergy; expensive	80-gm packet into 300 ml with H_2O needs EFA supplement

quefied to pass through the esophagus. (See Tracheoesophageal Fistula in Chapter 15.)

For all infants with CLD, careful recording of fluid intake is recommended. This should be added to the list of information recorded by the family and other care givers and reviewed by the physician at each office visit. The CLD infant who is not receiving any medications and who is free of symptoms except tachypnea (stage I) should be restricted to a daily fluid intake of 150 ml/kg (Table 14–7). If the infant is fed a standard formula of 20 calories per ounce, he or she will have an intake of 100 kcal/kg/day. If this caloric intake is insufficient and the infant is gaining less than 10 to 20 grams per day, then the formula can be enriched by adding 1 teaspoon of rice cereal to each ounce of formula.

Since each teaspoon of rice cereal contains 5 kcal, the infant will receive an additional 25 kcal/kg/day. Most infants with mild CLD will experience optimal weight gain and, as a side benefit, have less emesis when rice cereal is added to thicken the formula.

When the CLD infant has evidence of airway obstruction (stage II) and also requires treatment with bronchodilator medications, the fluid intake should be restricted to 120 ml/kg/day. To provide an intake of at least 120 kcal/kg/day, a formula of 24 kcal/ounce is utilized. In the infant with a short bowel or otherwise compromised gastrointestinal mucosa, a more "basic" formula usually is required. Pregestimil (20 kcal/ounce) usually is well tolerated by these infants, even when its caloric density is increased to 24 kcal/ounce. Pregestimil is more "digestible" than other formulas because medium-chain triglycerides (MCT) have been substituted for more complex fats, and corn syrup and modified tapioca starch are used for its carbohydrate. An infant prescribed a formula containing 24 kcal per ounce and a fluid limit of 120 ml/kg/day will receive 116 kcal/kg/day if 1 teaspoon of rice cereal is added to each ounce of formula. If the infant still does not experience adequate weight gain, then the caloric density of the formula can be increased to 27 kcal per ounce (with the same fluid limit and addition of 1 teaspoon of rice cereal per ounce of formula, the caloric intake will be 128 kcal/kg/day). An alternative to using a formula of 27 kcal per ounce is to add 2 teaspoons of rice cereal to feedings containing 24 kcal per ounce to provide 136 kcal/kg/day. The only "price" of the latter is thickened formula, which may necessitate much larger holes or crosscuts in the nipple of the bottle, and occasionally some complaints that the infant has become constipated.

The CLD infant with clinical features of both airway obstruction and wet lung (i.e., pulmonary interstitial edema) should be limited to a fluid intake of 100 ml/kg/day. Use of a formula containing 27 kcal per ounce enriched with 2 teaspoons of rice cereal per ounce provides a caloric intake of only 123 kcal/kg/day. Since these infants have the greatest caloric requirements because of the severity of their illness, further alteration of the formula may be needed to provide adequate calories. The first enhancement recommended is to add corn oil (or MCT) to raise the caloric density of the formula to either 30 kcal or 39 kcal per ounce (Table 14–11). Alteration of the formula to 30 kcal per ounce provides 100 kcal/kg/day, and the addition of 2 teaspoons of rice cereal per ounce of formula further increases the caloric intake to 133 kcal/kg/day. Use of a formula of 39 kcal per ounce alone provides 130 kcal/kg/day. Adding 2 teaspoons of cereal to each ounce of formula containing 39 kcal per ounce will provide 163 kcal/kg/day to an infant whose fluid intake is restricted to 100 ml/kg/day.

A word of caution is advisable: the CLD infant with stage III illness may not tolerate formula of such high caloric density. Certainly the infant with coexisting intestinal tract problems is likely to have great difficulty digesting this formula. The early signs of difficulty are likely to be loose stools and emesis. In the tube-fed infant, gastric "residuals" are an even earlier sign of intolerance to this formula. When the infant manifests early signs of intolerance, a formula of lower caloric density must be substituted immediately to avoid more serious side effects. At this point, it is wise to consult the nutrition expert of the consulting team.

Again, remember that emesis can be a behavioral, rather than a physiologic, response in these seriously ill infants.

Editor

Use of special, well-tolerated formulas may be helpful in the treatment of infants with CLD. Vivonex (Table 14–11) contains only minute amounts of fat, in the form of highly absorbable safflower oil, and L-amino acids, rather than protein or a protein hydrolysate. This accounts for its high efficacy in an infant with formula intolerance. However, Vivonex should be used only after consultation with a nutrition expert who should continue to supervise its use. The formula has high osmolality and, without modification, occasionally may be poorly tolerated, especially by the infant with gastrointestinal dysfunction. Other limitations of Vivonex are that its lipid content is inadequate and it does not contain a complement of essential fatty acids (EFA). When Vivonex is used, another source of EFA must be identified, such as regular administration of intravenous lipid or plasma transfusions. Another disadvantage of Vivonex is its high cost. Thus, while it may be a reasonable alternative to the standard formulas for the initial period of nutrition at home for a CLD infant with intolerance to other formulas, the long-range goal should be to substitute a more balanced formula as soon as the infant can tolerate it. Finally, there are other solid foods that can be included in a nutritional plan for the CLD infant. Table 14–8 lists the nutritional contents of avocado, which is 15 per cent lipid by weight (1.5 kcal/gm) and contains approximately 8 mEq/gm of potassium. It is very low in water content, which is also advantageous to planning a diet for the CLD infant. Other solid foods must be introduced with caution, both because they may not be tolerated well and also because the commercially available jars of pureed food are very high in water content, making it difficult to keep track of the infant's fluid intake. Parents should be encouraged to puree food for their CLD infant at home rather than purchasing commercially prepared products.

SUMMARY

Appendix A, Home Care of Infants with Chronic Lung Disease, provides specific information about medications (preparations, dosage schedules, routes of administration) and aerosol treatments (instructions to family and equipment needed), as well as lists of equipment for home care and guidelines for ventilator care.

Care of the infant with CLD is indeed complex and challenging. It requires sophisticated diagnostic and evaluation techniques and must stress nutritional, as well as pulmonary, care. However, with a committed family and care team and a coordinated approach to the management of these infants after discharge from the ICN, their outcome can be excellent. Working with these children and their families can provide a most rewarding experience for the pediatrician.

References

1. Bonikos DS, Bensch KG, Northway WH Jr, et al: Bronchopulmonary dysplasia: The pulmonary pathologic sequel of necrotizing bronchiolitis and pulmonary fibrosis. Hum Pathol 7:643, 1976.
2. Davies G, Reid LM: Growth of the alveoli and pulmonary arteries in childhood. Thorax 25:669, 1970.
3. Hislop A, Reid L: Pulmonary arterial development during childhood: Branching pattern and structure. Thorax 28:129, 1973.
4. Northway WH, Jr, Rosan RC, Porter DY: Pulmonary disease following respirator therapy of hyaline-membrane disease bronchopulmonary dysplasia. N Engl J Med 276:357, 1967.
5. Lewis S: A follow-up study of the respiratory distress syndrome. Proc R Soc Med 61:771, 1968.
6. Shepard FM, Johnston RB Jr, Klatte EC, et al.: Residual pulmonary findings in clinical hyaline membrane disease. N Engl J Med 279:1063, 1968.
7. Bryan MH, Hardie MJ, Reilly BJ, et al.: Pulmonary function studies during the first year of life in infants recovering from respiratory distress syndrome. Pediatrics 52:169, 1973.
8. Harrod JR, L'Heureux P, Wangensteen OD, et al.: Long-term follow-up of severe respiratory distress syndrome treated with intermittent positive-pressure breathing. J Pediatr 84:277, 1974.
9. Watts JL, Ariagno RL, Brady JP: Chronic pulmonary disease in neonates after artificial ventilation: Distribution of ventilation and pulmonary interstitial emphysema. Pediatrics 60:273, 1977.
10. Boros SJ, Orgill AA: Mortality and morbidity associated with pressure and volume-limited infant ventilators. Am J Dis Child 132:865, 1978.
11. Markestad T, Fitzhardinge PM: Growth and development in children recovering from bronchopulmonary dysplasia. J Pediatr 98:597, 1981.
12. Spitzer AR, Fox WW, Delivoria-Papadopoulous M: Maximum diuresis—A factor in predicting recovery from respiratory distress syndrome and the development of bronchopulmonary dysplasia. J Pediatr 98:476, 1981.
13. Morray JP, Fox WW, Kettrick RG, et al.: Improvement in lung mechanics as a function of age in the infant with severe bronchopulmonary dysplasia. Pediatr Res 16:290, 1982.
14. Stahlman M, Hedvall G, Lindstrom D, et al.: Role of hyaline membrane disease in production of later childhood lung abnormalities. Pediatrics 69:572, 1982.
15. Wong YC, Beardsmore CS, Silverman M: Pulmonary sequelae of neonatal respiratory distress in very low birth weight infants: A clinical and physiologic study. Arch Dis Child 57:418, 1982.
16. Shankaran S, Szego E, Eizert D, et al.: Severe bronchopulmonary dysplasia: Predictors of survival and outcome. Chest 86:607, 1984.
17. Truog WE, Jackson JC, Baduara JR: Bronchopulmonary dysplasia and pulmonary insufficiency of prematurity: Lack of correlation of outcome with gas exchange abnormalities at 1 month of age. Am J Dis Child 139:351, 1985.
18. Brown ER: Increased risk of bronchopulmonary dysplasia in infants with patent ductus arteriosus. J Pediatr 85:865, 1979.
19. Stocks J, Godfrey S: The role of artificial ventilation, oxygen, and CPAP in pathogenesis of lung damage in neonates: Assessment by serial measurements of lung function. Pediatrics 57:352, 1976.
20. Coates AL, Desmond K, Willis D, et al.: Oxygen therapy and long-term pulmonary outcome of respiratory distress syndrome in newborns. Am J Dis Child 136:892, 1982.
21. Saigal S, Rosenbaum P, Stoskopf B, et al.: Outcome in infants 501 to 1000 gm birth weight delivered to residents of the McMaster Health Region. J Pediatr 105:969, 1984.
22. Pusey VA, MacPherson RI, Chernick V: Pulmonary fibroplasia following prolonged artificial ventilation of newborn infants. Can Med Assoc J 100:842, 1969.
23. Barnes ND, Hull D, Glover WJ, et al.: Effects of prolonged positive pressure ventilation in infancy. Lancet 2:1096, 1969.
24. Fitzhardinge PM, Pape K, Arstikaitis M, Boyle M, et al.: Mechanical ventilation of infants of less than 1051-gm birth weight: Health, growth, and neurological sequelae. J Pediatr 88:531, 1976.
25. Churg A, Golden J, Fligiel S, et al.: Bronchopulmonary dysplasia in the adult. Am Rev Respir Dis 127:117, 1983.
26. Northway WH Jr: Observations on bronchopulmonary dysplasia. J Pediatr 95:1815, 1979.
27. Rhodes PG, Hall RT, Leonidas JC: Chronic pulmonary disease in neonates with assisted ventilation. Pediatrics 55:788, 1975.
28. Bell FF, Warburton D, Stonestreet B, et al.: Effect of fluid administration on the development of symptomatic patent ductus arteriosus and congestive heart failure in premature infants. N Engl J Med 13:302, 598, 1980.
29. Nickerson BG, Taussig LM: Family history of asthma in infants with bronchopulmonary dysplasia. Pediatrics 65:1140, 1980.
30. Bertrand JM, Riley SP, Popkin J, et al.: The long-term sequelae of prematurity: The role of familial airway hyperreactivity and the respiratory distress syndrome. N Engl J Med 312:742, 1985.
31. Taghizadeh A, Reynolds EO: Pathogenesis of bronchopulmonary dysplasia following hyaline membrane disease. Am J Pathol 82:241, 1976.
32. Rosan RC: Hyaline membrane disease and a related spectrum of neonatal pneumopathies. Pediatr Pathol 2:15, 1975.

33. Reid LM: Bronchopulmonary dysplasia — pathology. J Pediatr 95:836, 1979.

34. Thurlbeck WM: Morphologic aspects of bronchopulmonary dysplasia. J Pediatr 95:842, 1979.

35. Anderson WR, Strickland MB: Pulmonary complications of oxygen therapy in the neonate. Arch Pathol 91:506, 1971.

36. Roberts RJ, Weesner KM, Bucher JR: Oxygen-induced alterations in lung vascular development in the newborn rat. Pediatr Res 17:368, 1983.

37. Sobonya RE, Logvinoff MM, Taussig LM, et al.: Morphometric analysis of the lung in prolonged bronchopulmonary dysplasia. Pediatr Res 16:969, 1982.

38. Rasche RFH, Kuhns LR: Histopathologic changes in airway mucosa of infants after endotrachael intubation. Pediatrics 50:632, 1972.

39. Lee RM, Rossman CM, O'Brodovich H, et al.: Ciliary defects associated with the development of bronchopulmonary dysplasia, ciliary motility and ultrastructure. Am Rev Respir Dis 129:190, 1984.

40. Smyth JA, Tabachnik E, Duncan WJ, et al.: Pulmonary function and bronchial hyperreactivity in long-term survivors of bronchopulmonary dysplasia. Pediatrics 68:336, 1981.

41. Hansen TN, Hazinski TA, Bland RD: Vitamin E does not prevent oxygen-induced lung injury in newborn lambs. Pediatr Res 16:583, 1982.

42. Levin DL, Weinberg AG, Perkin RM: Pulmonary microthrombi syndrome in newborn infants with unresponsive persistent pulmonary hypertension. J Pediatr 102:299, 1983.

43. Stenmark KR, James SL, Voelkel, NF, et al.: Leukotriene C4 and D4 in neonates with hypoxemia and pulmonary hypertension. N Engl J Med 309:77, 1983.

44. Boat TF: Studies of oxygen toxicity in cultured human neonatal respiratory epithelium. J Pediatr 95:916, 1979.

45. John E, McDevitt M, Wilborn W, et al.: Ultrastructure of the lung after ventilation. Br J Exp Pathol 63:401, 1982.

46. Parker JC, Townsley MI, Rippe B, et al.: Increased microvascular permeability in dog lungs due to high peak airway pressures. J Appl Physiol 57:1809, 1984.

47. Dreyfuss D, Basset G, Soler P, et al.: Intermittent positive-pressure hyperventilation with high inflation pressures produces pulmonary microvascular injury in rats. Am Rev Respir Dis 132:880, 1985.

48. Konietzko N, Nakhosteen JA, Mizera W, et al.: Ciliary beat frequency of biopsy samples taken from normal persons and patients with various lung diseases. Chest 80:855, 1981.

49. Johnson DE, Lock JE, Elde RP, et al.: Pulmonary neuroendocrine cells in hyaline membrane disease and bronchopulmonary dysplasia. Pediatr Res 16:446, 1982.

50. Harrison G, Rosan RC, Sloane A: Bronchiolitis induced by experimental acute and chronic oxygen intoxication in young adult rats. J Pathol 102:115, 1970.

51. Young SL, Crapo JD, Kremers SA, et al.: Pulmonary surfactant lipid production in oxygen-exposed rat lungs. Lab Invest 46:570, 1982.

52. Ward JA, Roberts RJ: Effect of hyperoxia on phosphatidylcholine synthesis, secretion, uptake and stability in the newborn rabbit lung. Biochem Biophys Acta 796:42, 1984.

53. Clements JA: Functions of the alveolar lining. Am Rev Respir Dis 115:67, 1977.

54. Jobe A, Ikegami M, Jacobs H, et al.: Permeability of premature lamb lungs to protein and the effect of surfactant on that permeability. J Appl Physiol 55:169, 1983.

55. Guyton AC, Moffatt DS, Adair TH: Role of alveolar surface tension in transepithelial movement of fluid. In Robertson F, van Golde LMG, Batenburg JJ (eds.): Pulmonary Surfactant, 3rd ed. New York, Elsevier, 1984, pp 171–185.

56. Seeger W, Lepper H, Wolf HR, et al.: Alteration of alveolar surfactant function after exposure to oxidative stress and to oxygenated and native arachidonic acid in vitro. Biochem Biophys Acta 835:58, 1985.

57. Seeger W, Stohr G, Wolf HRD, et al.: Alteration of surfactant function due to protein leakage: Special interaction with fibrin monomer. J Appl Physiol 58:326, 1985.

58. Jarstrand E: Role of surfactant in the pulmonary defense system. In Robertson B, van Golde LMG, Batenburg JJ (eds.): Pulmonary Surfactant, 3rd ed. New York, Elsevier, 1984, pp 197–201.

59. Sitrin RG, Ansfield MJ, Kaltreider HB: The effect of pulmonary surface-active material on the generation and expression of murine B- and T-lymphocyte effector functions in vitro. Exp Lung Res 9:85, 1985.

60. O'Neill S, Lesperance E, Klass DJ: Rat lung lavage surfactant enhances bacterial phagocytosis and intracellular killing by alveolar macrophages. Am Rev Respir Dis 130:225, 1984.

61. Matalon S, Cesar MA: Effects of 100% oxygen breathing on the capillary filtration coefficient in rabbit lungs. Microvasc Res 29:70, 1985.

62. Matalon S, Egan EA: Effects of 100% O_2 breathing on permeability of alveolar epithelium to solute. J Appl Physiol 50:859, 1981.

63. Matalon S, Egan EA: Interstitial fluid volumes and albumin spaces in pulmonary oxygen toxicity. J Appl Physiol 57:1767, 1984.

64. Huchon GJ, Hopewell PC, Murray JF: Interaction between permeability and hydrostatic pressure in perfused dogs' lungs. J Appl Physiol 50:905, 1981.

65. Hurley JV: Types of pulmonary microvascular injury. Ann NY Acad Sci 384:269, 1982.

66. Staub NC, Nagano H, Pearce ML: Pulmonary edema in dogs, especially the sequence of fluid accumulation in lungs. J Appl Physiol 22:227, 1967.

67. Staub NC: Pulmonary edema due to increased microvascular permeability to fluid and protein. Circ Res 43:143, 1978.

68. Toce SS, Farrell PM, Leavitt LA, et al.: Clinical and roentgenographic scoring system for assessing bronchopulmonary dysplasia. Am J Dis Child 138:581, 1984.

69. Edwards DK, Dyer WM, Northway WH Jr: Twelve years' experience with bronchopulmonary dysplasia. Pediatrics 59:839, 1977.

70. Edwards DK: Radiographic aspects of bronchopulmonary dysplasia. J Pediatr 95:823, 1979.

71. Edwards DK, Colby TV, Northway WH Jr: Radiographic-pathologic correlation in bronchopulmonary dysplasia. J Pediatr 95:834, 1979.

72. Coates AL, Bergsteinsson H, Desmond K, et al.: Long-term pulmonary sequelae of premature birth with and without idiopathic respiratory distress syndrome in newborns. Am J Dis Child 136:892, 1982.

73. Tooley WH: Epidemiology of bronchopulmonary dysplasia. J Pediatr 95:851, 1979.
74. Anderson WR, Engel RR: Cardiopulmonary sequelae of reparative stages of bronchopulmonary dysplasia. Arch Pathol Lab Med 107:603, 1983.
75. Fisch RO: Long-term consequences of survivors of respiratory distress syndrome. In Nelson G (ed.): Pulmonary Development. New York, Marcel Dekker, 1985, pp 431–466.
76. Johnson JD, Malachowski NC, Grobstein R, et al.: Prognosis of children surviving with the aid of mechanical ventilation in the newborn period. J Pediatr 84:272, 1974.
77. Lamarre A, Linsao L, Reilly BJ, et al.: Residual pulmonary abnormalities in survivors of idiopathic respiratory distress syndrome. Am Rev Respir Dis 108:56, 1973.
78. Outerbridge EW, Nogrady BM, Beaudry PH, et al.: Idiopathic respiratory distress syndrome: Recurrent pulmonary illness in survivors. Am J Dis Child 123:99, 1972.
79. Sauve RS, Singhal N: Long-term morbidity of infants with bronchopulmonary dysplasia. Pediatrics 76:725, 1985.
80. Durand M, Rigatto H: Tidal volume and respiratory frequency in infants with bronchopulmonary dysplasia. Early Hum Dev 5:55, 1981.
81. Gravelyn TR, Weg JG: Respiratory rate as an indicator of acute respiratory dysfunction. JAMA 244:1123, 1980.
82. Melnick G, Pickoff AS, Ferrer PL, et al.: Normal and pulmonary vascular resistance and left ventricular hypertrophy in young infants with bronchopulmonary dysplasia: An echocardiographic and pathologic study. Pediatrics 66:589, 1980.
83. Berman W Jr, Yabek SM, Dillon I, et al.: Evaluation of infants with bronchopulmonary dysplasia using cardiac catheterization. Pediatrics 70:708, 1982.
84. Fouron JC, LeGuennec JC, Villemant D, et al.: Value of echocardiography in assessing the outcome of bronchopulmonary dysplasia of the newborn. Pediatrics 65:529, 1980.
85. Philip AG, Peabody JL, Lucey JF: Transcutaneous pO_2 monitoring in the home management of bronchopulmonary dysplasia. Pediatrics 61:655, 1978.
86. Rome ES, Stork EK, Carlo WA, et al.: Limitations of transcutaneous pO_2 and pCO_2 monitoring in infants with bronchopulmonary dysplasia. Pediatrics 74:217, 1984.
87. Moylan FMB, Shannon DC: Preferential distribution of lobar emphysema and atelectasis in bronchopulmonary dysplasia. Pediatrics 63:130, 1979.
88. Miller KE, Edwards DK, Hilton S, et al.: Acquired lobar emphysema in premature infants with bronchopulmonary dysplasia: An iatrogenic disease. Radiology 108:589, 1981.
89. Reich SF, Earley WC, Ravin TH, et al.: Evaluation of gastropulmonary aspiration by a radioactive technique: Concise communication. J Nucl Med 18:1079, 1977.
90. MacFadyen UM, Hendry GMA, Simpson H: Gastroesophageal reflux in near-miss sudden infant death syndrome or suspected recurrent aspiration. Arch Dis Child 58:87, 1983.
91. Kao LC, Warburton D, Platzker ACG, et al.: Effect of isoproterenol inhalation on airway resistance in chronic bronchopulmonary dysplasia. Pediatrics 73:509, 1984.
92. Weinstein MR, Oh W: Oxygen consumption in infants with bronchopulmonary dysplasia. J Pediatr 99:958, 1981.
93. Field S, Kelly SM, Macklem PT: The oxygen cost of breathing in patients with cardiorespiratory disease. Am Rev Respir Dis 126:9, 1982.
94. Halliday HL, Dumpit FM, Brady JP: Effects of inspired oxygen on echocardiographic assessment of pulmonary vascular resistance and myocardial contractility in bronchopulmonary dysplasia. Pediatrics 65:536, 1980.
95. Abman SH, Wolfe RR, Accurso FJ, et al.: Pulmonary vascular response to oxygen in infants with severe bronchopulmonary dysplasia. Pediatrics 75:80, 1985.
96. Berger LR, Schaefer AR: The premature infant goes home. Am J Dis Child 139:200, 1985.
97. Yu VYH, Orgill AA, Lim SB, et al.: Growth and development of very low birthweight infants recovering from bronchopulmonary dysplasia. Arch Dis Child 58:791, 1983.
98. Vohr BR, Bell EF, Oh W: Infants with bronchopulmonary dysplasia: Growth pattern and neurologic and developmental outcome. Am J Dis Child 136:443, 1982.
99. Koops BO, Abman SH, Accurso FJ: Outpatient management and follow-up of bronchopulmonary dysplasia. Clin Perinatol 11:101, 1984.
100. Sell EJ, Hill S, Poisson SS, et al.: Prediction of growth and development in intensive care nursery graduates at 12 months of age. Am J Dis Child 109:1198, 1985.
101. Rooklin AR, Moomjian AS, Shutack JG, et al.: Theophylline therapy in bronchopulmonary dysplasia. J Pediatr 85:882, 1979.
102. Donnelly WH: Histopathology of endotracheal intubation. An autopsy study of 99 cases. Arch Pathol 88:511, 1969.
103. Papsidero MJ, Pashley NR: Acquired stenosis of the upper airway in neonates—An increasing problem. Ann Otol Rhinol Laryngol 89:512, 1980.
104. Ratner I, Whitfield J: Acquired subglottic stenosis in the very-low-birth-weight infant. Am J Dis Child 137:40, 1983.
105. Gould SJ, Howard S: The histopathology of the larynx in the neonate following endotracheal intubation. J Pathol 146:301, 1985.
106. Mok JYQ, McLaughlin FJ, Pintar M, et al.: Transcutaneous monitoring of oxygenation: What is normal? J Pediatr 108:365, 1986.
107. Nassif EG, Weinberger MM, Shannon D, et al.: Theophylline disposition in infancy. J Pediatr 98:158, 1981.
108. Wanner A: Effects of methylxanthines on airway mucociliary function. Am J Med 79:16, 1985.
109. Spahr RD, Klein AM, Brown DR, et al.: Fluid administration and bronchopulmonary dysplasia: The lack of an association. Am J Dis Child 134:958, 1980.
110. Bland RD, McMillan DD, Bressack MA: Decreased pulmonary transvascular fluid filtration in awake newborn lambs after intravenous furosemide. J Clin Invest 62:601, 1978.
111. Najak ZD, Harris EM, Lazzara A Jr, et al.: Pulmonary effects of furosemide in preterm infants with lung disease. J Pediatr 102:758, 1983.
112. Ali J, Wood LD: Pulmonary vascular effects of furosemide on gas exchange in pulmonary edema. J Appl Physiol 57:160, 1984.

113. Kao LC, Warburton D, Sargent CW, et al.: Furosemide acutely decreases airways resistance in chronic
bronchopulmonary dysplasia. J Pediatr 103:624,
1983.
114. Kao LC, Warburton D, Cheng MH, et al.: Effect of
oral diuretics on pulmonary mechanics in infants
with chronic bronchopulmonary dysplasia: Results
of a double-blind crossover sequential trial. Pediatrics 74:37, 1984.
115. Hazinski TA: Furosemide decreases ventilation in
young rabbits. J Pediatr 106:81, 1985.
116. Patel H, Yeh RF, Jain R, et al.: Pulmonary and renal
responses to furosemide in infants with stage III–IV
bronchopulmonary dysplasia. Am J Dis Child
139:917, 1985.
117. Papademetriou V, Burris J, Kukich S, et al.: Effectiveness of potassium chloride or triamterene in thiazide hypokalemia. Arch Intern Med 145:1986,
1985.
118. Girard P, Polianski J, Brun-Pascaud M, et al.: Ventilatory adaptation to metabolic alkalosis in adult
awake potassium-restricted rats. Respir Physiol
57:23, 1985.
119. Hazinski TA, Hansen TN, Simon JA, et al.: Effect of
oxygen administration during sleep on skin surface
oxygen and carbon dioxide tensions in patients with
chronic lung disease. Pediatrics 67:626, 1981.
120. Campbell AN, Zartin Y, Groenveld M, et al.: Low
flow oxygen therapy in infants. Arch Dis Child
58:795, 1983.
121. Nickerson BG: Bronchopulmonary dysplasia. Chest
87:528, 1985.
122. Werthammer J, Brown ER, Neff RK, et al.: Sudden
infant death syndrome in infants with bronchopulmonary dysplasia. Pediatrics 69:301, 1982.
123. Spitzer AR, Boyse JT, Tuchman DN, et al.: Awake
apnea associated with gastroesophageal reflux: A
specific clinical syndrome. Pediatrics 104:200,
1984.
124. Rich S, Ganz R, Levy PS: Comparative actions of
hydralazine, nifedipine and amrinone in primary
pulmonary hypertension. Am J Cardiol 52:1104,
1983.
125. Milic-Emili J, Ruff F: Effects of pulmonary congestion
and edema on the small airways. Bull Eur Physio-
pathol Respir 7:1181, 1971.
126. DeSa DJ: Myocardial changes in immature infants
requiring prolonged ventilation. Arch Dis Child
52:138, 1977.
127. Riggs T, Hirschfeld S, Borkat G, et al.: Assessment of
the pulmonary vascular bed by echocardiographic
right ventricular systolic time intervals. Circulation
57:939, 1978.
128. Katz AM, Hager WD, Messineo FC, et al.: Cellular
actions and pharmacology of the calcium channel-
blocking drugs. Am J Med 77:2, 1984.
129. Reid LM: Lung growth in health and disease. Br J Dis
Chest 78:113, 1984.
130. Abman SH, Accurso FJ, Bowman CM: Unsuspected
cardiopulmonary abnormalities complicating bronchopulmonary dysplasia. Arch Dis Child 59:966,
1984.
131. Rudolph AM, Paul MH, Sommer LS, et al.: Effects of
tolazoline hydrochloride (Priscoline) on circulatory
dynamics of patients with pulmonary hypertension.
Am Heart J 55:424, 1958.
132. Rich S, Martinez J, Lam W, et al.: Reassessment of the
effects of vasodilator drugs in primary pulmonary
hypertension: Guidelines for determining a pulmo-

nary vasodilator response. Am Heart J 105:119,
1983.
133. Ruskin JN, Hutter AM Jr: Primary pulmonary hypertension treated with oral phentolamine. Ann Intern
Med 90:772, 1979.
134. Klinke WP, Gilbert JAL: Diazoxide in primary pulmonary hypertension. N Engl J Med 302:91, 1980.
135. Melot C, Naeije R, Mols P, et al.: Effects of nifedipine
on ventilation/perfusion matching in primary pulmonary hypertension. Chest 83:203, 1983.
136. Saito D, Haraoka S, Yoshida H, et al.: Primary pulmonary hypertension improved by long-term oral administration of nifedipine. Am Heart J 105:1041,
1983.
137. Rich S, Martinez J, Lam W, et al.: Captopril as treatment for patients with primary pulmonary hypertension: Problem of variability in assessing chronic
drug treatment. Br Heart J 48:272, 1982.
138. Leier CV, Bambach D, Nelson S, et al.: Captopril in
primary pulmonary hypertension. Circulation
67:155, 1983.
139. Rubin LJ, Groves BM, Reeves JT, et al.: Prostacyclin-
induced acute pulmonary vasodilation in primary
pulmonary hypertension. Circulation 66:334, 1982.
140. Perkin RM, Anas NG: Pulmonary hypertension in
pediatric patients. J Pediatr 105:511, 1984.
141. McGoon MD, Vliestra RE: Vasodilator therapy for
primary pulmonary hypertension. Mayo Clin Proc
59:672, 1984.
142. Tifenbrunn LJ, Riemenschneider TA: Persistent pulmonary hypertension of the newborn. Am Heart J
111:564, 1986.
143. Abman SH, Warady Lum BA, et al.: Systemic hypertension in infants with bronchopulmonary dysplasia. J Pediatr 104:928, 1984.
144. Babb RR, Notarangelo J, Smith VM: Wheezing: A
clue to gastroesophageal reflux. Am J Gastroenterol
53:230, 1970.
145. Goyal RK, Rattan S: Mechanism of the lower esophageal sphincter relaxation: Action of prostaglandin
E$_1$ and theophylline. J Clin Invest 52:337, 1973.
146. Christie DL, O'Grady LR, Mack DV: Incompetent
lower esophageal sphincter and gastroesophageal
reflux in recurrent acute pulmonary disease of infancy and childhood. J Pediatr 93:23, 1978.
147. Herbst JJ, Minton SD, Book LS: Gastroesophageal
reflux causing respiratory distress and apnea in newborn infants. J Pediatr 95:763, 1979.
148. Berquist WE, Rachelefsky GS, Rowshan N, et al.:
Quantitative gastroesophageal reflux and pulmonary function in asthmatic children and normal
adults receiving placebo, theophylline, and meta-
proterenol sulfate therapy. J Allergy Clin Immunol
73:253, 1984.
149. Euler AR: Use of bethanechol for the treatment of
gastroesophageal reflux. J Pediatr 96:321, 1980.
150. Strickland AD, Chang JH: Results of treatment of
esophageal reflux with bethanechol. J Pediatr
103:311, 1983.
151. Brown MJ, Brown DC, Murphy MB: Hypokalemia
from beta 2-receptor stimulation by circulating epi-
nephrine. N Engl J Med 309:1414, 1983.
152. Clausen T: Adrenergic control of Na$^+$-K$^+$ homeostasis. Acta Med Scand (Suppl) 672:115, 1983.
153. Gifford RW, Mattox VR, Orvis AL, et al.: Effect of
thiazide diuretics on plasma volume, body electrolytes and excretion of aldosterone in hypertension.
Circulation 24:1197, 1961.
154. Wilkinson PR, Issler H, Hesp R, et al.: Total body and

serum potassium during prolonged thiazide therapy for essential hypertension. Lancet 1:759, 1975.

155. Walker BR, Hoppe RC, Alexander F: Effect of triamterene on the renal clearance of calcium, magnesium, phosphate and uric acid in man. Pharmacol Ther 13:245, 1972.

156. Lawson DH: Adverse reaction to potassium chloride. Q J Med 43:433, 1974.

157. Weichsel JE Jr: The therapeutic use of glucocorticoid hormones in the perinatal period: Potential neurological hazards. Ann Neurol 2:364, 1977.

158. Skubitz KM, Craddock PR, Hammerschmidt DE, et al.: Corticosteroids block binding of chemotactic peptide to its receptor on granulocytes and cause disaggregation of granulocyte aggregates in vitro. J Clin Invest 68:13, 1981.

159. Mammel MC, Johnson DE, Green TP, et al.: Controlled trial of dexamethasone therapy in infants with bronchopulmonary dysplasia. Lancet 1:1356, 1983.

160. Kehrer JP, Klein-Szanto AJP, Sorensen EMB, et al.: Enhanced acute lung damage following corticosteroid treatment. Am Rev Respir Dis 16:256, 1984.

161. Avery GB, Fletcher AV, Kaplan M, et al.: Controlled trial of dexamethasone in respirator-dependent infants with bronchopulmonary dysplasia. Pediatrics 75:106, 1985.

162. Watts JL, Paes BA, Milner RA, et al.: Randomized controlled trial of vitamin E and bronchopulmonary dysplasia. Pediatr Res 15:686, 1981.

Recommended Reading

Abman SH, Wolfe RR, Accurso FJ, et al.: Pulmonary vascular response to oxygen in infants with severe bronchopulmonary dysplasia. Pediatrics 75:80, 1985.

Anderson WF, Strickland MB: Pulmonary complications of oxygen therapy in the neonate. Arch Pathol 91:506, 1985.

Bertrand JM, Riley SP, Popkin J, et al.: The long-term sequelae of prematurity: The role of familial airway hyperreactivity and the respiratory distress syndrome. N Engl J Med 312:742, 1985.

Coates AL, Desmond K, Willis D, et al.: Oxygen therapy and long-term pulmonary outcome of respiratory distress syndrome in newborns. Am J Dis Child 136:892, 1981.

Durand M, Rigatto H: tidal volume and respiratory frequency in infants with bronchopulmonary dysplasia. Early Hum Dev 5:55, 1981.

Fisch RO: Long-term consequences of survivors of respiratory distress syndrome. In Nelson G (ed.): Pulmonary Development. New York, Marcel Dekker, 1985, pp 431–466.

Kao LC, Warburton D, Cheng MH, et al.: Effect of oral diuretics on pulmonary mechanics in infants with chronic bronchopulmonary dysplasia: Results of a double-blind crossover sequential trial. Pediatrics 74:509, 1984.

Koops BL, Abman SH, Accurso FJ: Outpatient management and follow-up of bronchopulmonary dysplasia. Clin Perinatol 11:101, 1984.

Markestad T, Fitzhardinge PM: Growth and development in children recovering from bronchopulmonary dysplasia. J Pediatr 98:597, 1981.

Nickerson BG: Bronchopulmonary dysplasia. Chest 87:528, 1985.

Nickerson BG, Taussig LM: Family history of asthma in infants with bronchopulmonary dysplasia. Pediatrics 65:1140, 1980.

Northway WH Jr: Observations on bronchopulmonary dysplasia. J Pediatr 95:815, 1979.

Reid LM: Brochopulmonary dysplasia—Pathology. J Pediatr 95:836, 1979.

Reid LM: Lung growth in health and disease. Br J Dis Chest 78:113, 1984.

Rome ES, Stork EK, Carlo WA, et al.: Limitations of transcutaneous PO_2 and PCO_2 monitoring in infants with bronchopulmonary dysplasia. Pediatrics 74:217, 1984.

Taghizadeh A, Reynolds EO: Pathogenesis of bronchopulmonary dysplasia following hyaline membrane disease. Am J Pathol 82:241, 1976.

Tooley WH: Epidemiology of bronchopulmonary dysplasia. J Pediatr 95:851, 1979.

Vohr BR, Bell EF, Oh W: Infants with bronchopulmonary dysplasia: Growth pattern and neurologic and developmental outcome. Am J Dis Child 136:443, 1982.

15

MANAGEMENT OF AIRWAYS OBSTRUCTION AND OTHER ABNORMALITIES AFFECTING PULMONARY CARE

CHERYL D. LEW, M.D., SEYMOUR R. COHEN, M.D., JEROME THOMPSON, M.D., and ARNOLD C.G. PLATZKER, M.D.

Major conditions of the upper and lower airways that may require surgical intervention or have an adverse effect on pulmonary outcome will be discussed in this chapter. These include tracheoesophageal fistula and defects of the chest and abdominal walls, which also affect pulmonary function. Specific interventions will obviously depend on the nature, urgency, and severity of the particular anatomic problems.

AIRWAYS OBSTRUCTION

Infants discharged from an ICN often require management of long-term problems relating to the airways. Continuing airways dysfunction may occur because of congenital malformations of the airways, effects of congenital nonrespiratory disorders, or acquired injuries to the airways. Design of an appropriate plan of care involves anticipation of potential long-term respiratory sequelae of neonatal respiratory tract problems and an appreciation of the fact

that the appearance of sequelae may be delayed and modified by postneonatal events.

CONGENITAL MALFORMATIONS

Congenital airways malformations may be divided into extrathoracic and intrathoracic. Extrathoracic airways obstruction occurring in neonates includes choanal atresia, Pierre Robin anomalad, vocal cord paralysis, tracheomalacia, subglottic webs, subglottic hemangiomas, and pharyngeal tumors. Intrathoracic airways obstruction found in neonates includes tracheal stenosis, bronchial stenosis, tracheoesophageal fistula with atresia, and vascular slings and rings.

ACQUIRED AIRWAYS OBSTRUCTION

Acquired airways obstructive problems also may be separated into extrathoracic and intrathoracic. Extrathoracic problems include postintubation injury of the upper airway, such as

157

vocal cord paralysis or subglottic edema and stenosis. Intrathoracic problems include lower tracheal injury due to intubation and secondary to compression of the lower airway due to the dilatation of the great vessels and heart chambers that sometimes is found in complex congenital heart disease.

DISORDERS OF NEUROMUSCULAR CONTROL OF VENTILATION

Infants with congenital disorders affecting innervation of skeletal muscles, congenital myopathy, or birth injury to the spinal cord or peripheral nerves supplying the muscles of respiration are at risk for respiratory insufficiency from birth.

In *phrenic nerve palsy,* usually an injury to the cervical plexus sustained during birth, the pediatrician is alerted to possible diaphragmatic paralysis when the injury is associated with the typical weakness of the hand and forearm on the affected side (i.e., Erb's palsy). However, in some cases the phrenic nerve paralysis may occur alone. In this instance there may be no external clues, except for a history in some infants of a "difficult" vaginal delivery. Usually the injury to the phrenic nerve is temporary, and the infant, while manifesting tachypnea, has little other evidence of respiratory failure. These infants, however, require special surveillance, since they will have reduced ventilatory function and reduced tolerance to respiratory tract infections. Follow-up evaluation should include monthly assessment of blood gases to monitor respiratory function and the use of real-time ultrasound study every two to three months to assess diaphragmatic function. Return of diaphragmatic function, if it occurs, may take three to six months. With long-term paralysis, eventration of the diaphragm may appear, but surgical repair should be postponed, if possible, for at least six months to determine if lung function will improve substantially with return of phrenic nerve function.

Congenital anterior horn cell disease and congenital myopathies present both medical and ethical problems that are beyond the scope of this text.

PATHOPHYSIOLOGIC CONSEQUENCES OF OBSTRUCTION

IMPAIRED VENTILATION

The net physiologic impact of tracheal obstruction is impairment of ventilation. Severe uniform hyperinflation may be the major clinical and radiologic finding. More commonly, however, overdistended lung segments coexist with atelectatic or partially atelectatic segments. Blood gas abnormalities occur whenever the efficiency of gas exchange is diminished. Acute respiratory acidosis is gradually compensated in longstanding upper airway obstruction by renal bicarbonate retention. Less frequently, chronic hypoxemia results from upper airway obstruction.

MUCOUS MEMBRANE INJURY AND BRONCHOSPASM

Mucous membrane injury at the site of upper airway obstruction may complicate and worsen the pre-existing airways obstruction by causing delayed clearance of airways secretions, leading to pooling of mucus and formation of plugs of mucus. Longstanding interruption in the mucociliary blanket and defective mucus clearance may result in increased bronchial reactivity, chronic bronchospasm, and permanent impairment of clearance mechanisms, as well as chronic or recurrent airways infection.

The initial event leading to impaired clearance probably is the alteration of mucociliary blanket function. The mucociliary blanket is a protective barrier of the airways lining, as well as a primary mechanism for movement of mucus from the peripheral to the proximal airways for removal. Mechanical obstruction of the airways interferes with normal mucus flow and the airways cleansing function of the mucociliary blanket. When this flow is interrupted, mucus-producing cells and glands hypertrophy, increasing production of substantially more viscous mucus. Pooling of mucus increases the degree of obstruction. This leads to either aseptic or bacterial inflammation of the airway. Sloughing of the mucociliary blanket also may occur. Submucosal tissues and the associated irritant nerve fibers may be exposed to potentially sensitizing agents in the stagnant mucus, resulting in increased bronchomotor tone and further reduction in airways caliber.

INFECTION

Without relief of airways obstruction, organisms in the mucus may overgrow and cause chronic airways infection, resulting in further mucociliary injury and dysfunction, as well as an abnormal quantity and quality of mucus, which aggravates the pre-existing obstructive process. Bronchial hyperreactivity may worsen with each new episode of infection-injury. Infection and injury at the alveolar level may lead to injury of the interstitium of the lung and eventual pulmonary fibrosis.

MEDICAL METHODS OF TREATMENT

The medical management of an upper airway obstructive disorder is predominantly supportive. While medical management is an important adjunct to the surgical management, in the absence of specific surgical repair it holds the only promise for achieving and maintaining airway patency and thus preserving adequate ventilation.

ADMINISTRATION OF HUMIDIFIED GAS

The first objective of therapy is the prevention or relief of abnormalities in gas exchange. Warmed, humidified air is occasionally administered for inflammatory conditions of the trachea. Oxygen is also administered if the arterial oxygen partial pressure falls below 65 torr. (See discussion of management of airways obstruction and hypoxia in chronic lung disease of infancy, and Tables 14–3 and 14–5.)

POSITIONING

Some young infants benefit from being placed, especially during sleep, in either the Fowler or prone position or occasionally supine with a "roll" under the shoulders. This maximizes airway caliber and promotes efficient air flow. The ideal position is best determined by clinical evaluation and observed improvement in breath sounds. Continuous monitoring of transcutaneous oxygen and carbon dioxide tension, prior to discharge from the hospital, may also be helpful in defining the best positions of each infant. Positioning is a critical form of therapy for the infant with an airway anomaly that cannot be managed surgically. Examples of such conditions include Pierre Robin anomalad and certain congenital heart anomalies in which infants experience airway compression, due to enlargement of the pulmonary artery or left atrium, or vocal cord paralysis.

MEDICATION

To relieve airway obstruction secondary to defective mucociliary function, beta-adrenergic agents (isoetharine, isoproterenol) are administered by aerosol and specifically stimulate mu-

cociliary transport. (See Appendix A.) Furthermore, these agents stimulate goblet cells and mucous glands to produce a thinner, less viscous mucus. Therefore, use of these agents is often indicated even in the absence of overt bronchospasm. The aerosol treatments are particularly efficacious in lowering bronchomotor tone, increasing airway caliber, and removing respiratory secretions if administration is followed by chest percussion and postural drainage three or four times daily.

SURGICAL APPROACHES TO TREATMENT

CHOANAL ATRESIA

Infants with choanal atresia (occurrence one in 8000 births) are at severe risk of respiratory failure if the atresia is bilateral, because of the obligate nasal breathing status of infants less than 3 months of age. In neonates with bilateral atresia, at least one choana must be opened surgically. Patency of the passage is maintained with a polyvinyl tube (usually a portion of an endotracheal tube cut to appropriate length).

The choanal stent may be removed at three months of age, when the infant should be able to breathe by mouth if the choana becomes obstructed. Definitive repair of choanal atresia is performed when the child is 2 to 3 years of age. Infants with unilateral choanal atresia may be managed expectantly, since these children do well unless there is contralateral choanal stenosis or the choana becomes occluded during a respiratory infection. Following the placement of a choanal stent, it is important that the parents receive training and become competent to perform the suctioning required to keep the stent patent and free of secretions. A portable mechanical suction machine will be necessary for home use. (See Appendix A, Home Care of Infants with Chronic Lung Disease.)

PIERRE ROBIN ANOMALAD

The Pierre Robin anomalad is relatively rare (occurrence of one in 30,000 births). Although those infants who experience only mild respiratory distress may be managed medically, infants with the most severe respiratory obstruction may require tracheostomy to guarantee airway patency. Tracheostomy is usually required for 18 to 24 months, when the usual growth of the mandible may result in sufficient airways patency. Results from surgical glossopexy have generally not been satisfactory.

VOCAL CORD PARALYSIS

Vocal cord paralysis may be an isolated consequence of a traumatic delivery, or it may be associated with central nervous system defects such as myelodysplasia and Arnold-Chiari malformation. Post-traumatic vocal cord paralysis may be self-limiting and require only close medical observation until resolution occurs. Unilateral paresis is usually tolerated satisfactorily by the infant and requires no therapy. However, it warrants regular follow-up with endoscopic evaluation. Whenever cord paresis coexists with medical conditions such as Arnold-Chiari malformation, for which medical or surgical intervention is indicated (e.g., relief of hydrocephalus), such therapy should be implemented promptly. Surgical relief of the coexisting problem may lead to adequate resolution of the cord paresis. Bilateral midline cord paresis requires continued use of a tracheostomy to maintain an airway.

SUBGLOTTIC STENOSIS

Subglottic stenosis is an uncommon congenital anomaly. More often it occurs secondary to airways injury following prolonged or traumatic endotracheal intubation. The more severe cases require long-term placement of a tracheostomy tube to guarantee airways patency during a long course of tracheal dilatation procedures and to allow for pulmonary toilet. Periodic endoscopic examinations are necessary to evaluate the injured airway, to assess the healing process, and when appropriate, to remove granulomatous tissue. Laser treatment of granulomatous tissue reduces its mass and allows maintenance of airway caliber following healing of the airway injury. The ultimate goal, with aggressive management and growth of the airway, is removal of the tracheostomy as early in childhood as possible, with restoration of normal laryngeal and bronchial function. (See also Chapter 18, Care of the Infant After Neonatal Surgery.)

SUBGLOTTIC OBSTRUCTION

Subglottic obstruction may also be due to congenital disorders such as hemangioma, hamartoma, or webs of the laryngeal area. Surgical removal is ideal, but the extent of the lesion or other complicating medical problems may dictate that the initial approach be conservative, with long-term placement of a tracheostomy tube to assure airway patency. Once ventilation is established, a definitive medical-surgical plan can be developed.

TRACHEAL AND BRONCHIAL STENOSES

Stenotic lesions of the trachea and bronchi may be diffuse or segmental. They may also result from intrinsic reduction in airway caliber or from external compression from dilated major vessels or aberrant mediastinal structures. Elucidation of the precise nature of the lesion (e.g., vascular rings or slings) through modern imaging techniques allows development of a plan for medical and surgical care. When correction of the underlying cause of airway narrowing is not possible or when it is not sufficient to guarantee patency of the airway, tracheostomy is indicated. However, lesions in the distal portion of the trachea or limited to the bronchial tree are not amenable to tracheostomy placement. In these situations, aggressive and vigorous medical care directed at pulmonary toilet is indicated to promote growth of the child and maintain adequate ventilation.

TRACHEOESOPHAGEAL FISTULA

Surgical correction of esophageal atresia and tracheoesophageal fistula achieves anatomic but not "functional" restoration of the involved passages. Infants with these conditions bear a number of functional disabilities after surgery, which vary in the extent of their clinical expression. Residual upper airway obstruction is experienced by some infants because their tracheas are narrower than normal, even under the best of conditions. In addition, they have a higher incidence of tracheomalacia, which is often associated with congenital defects of the tracheal cartilage, leading to lack of support of the trachea and causing partial or total collapse (even during tidal breathing). The phase in breathing during which tracheal collapse occurs depends on the location of the cartilage anomaly. Inspiratory stridor occurs when the defects are confined to the extrathoracic trachea, whereas expiratory stridor occurs when the defects are confined to the intrathoracic trachea. When the tracheal narrowing is severe and/or the tracheal cartilage defect comprises a large portion of the trachea, severe tracheal obstruction occurs and seriously compromises ventilation. Treatment of life-threatening obstruction includes establishment of a patent airway with placement of an artificial airway (tracheostomy tube) to bypass the tracheal obstruction.

The infant with tracheoesophageal fistula may also suffer respiratory tract obstruction from vocal cord paralysis, which may result from injury to the recurrent laryngeal nerve at the time of corrective surgery. Often this problem is transient, but recovery from vocal cord paralysis may take months, or occasionally it may be permanent. The diagnosis of vocal cord paralysis is made at endoscopy.

Prolonged lower airway obstruction secondary to increased bronchomotor tone is another problem experienced by many infants with tracheoesophageal fistula in the first one to years after birth. As a result of the fistula and gastric spillage into the airway during the period immediately after birth and prior to corrective surgery, these infants experience chronic injury and irritability of the airways. Mild respiratory tract infections may provide the onset of increased bronchomotor tone, manifest clinically by coughing and wheezing. These symptoms also improve with bronchodilator therapy. Further, it is known that these infants have squamous metaplasia of the airway mucosa at the site of the upper airway narrowing, reducing or delaying the clearance of mucus from the airway. Mucous retention alone may trigger bronchospasm in some of these infants; treatment with aerosol bronchodilators, followed by chest percussion, postural drainage, and pharyngeal suctioning, is frequently of great benefit.

The final concern about the infant with tracheoesophageal fistula and chronic respiratory disability is dysmotility of the esophagus, especially of the distal segment. During the process of healing following surgery, the esophagus may become stenotic at the anastomotic site. Gastroesophageal reflux may also occur as a result of the traction that must be applied on the lower esophagus to bring it into apposition with the upper esophageal pouch at operation. The traction may disrupt the integrity of the cardiac sphincter and permit reflux of the stomach contents into the esophagus. This not only raises the likelihood of aspiration, but may also cause esophagitis and worsening of the narrowing at the anastomotic site. Other causes of aspiration in infants with tracheoesophageal fistula are recurrence of the fistula or undetected laryngotracheal cleft. All of the above conditions are very difficult to diagnose.

Recurrent pneumonia in the infant with tracheoesophageal fistula is an indication for a complete study of airway and gastrointestinal function. The requisite studies include contrast radiography, gastric scintiscan, and, finally, esophageal and tracheal endoscopy. When esophageal stenosis is found at esophagoscopy, esophageal dilatation may be performed weekly, as an outpatient procedure, to preserve the caliber of the esophagus and, over time, enlarge the stenotic segment. In very severe cases

of esophageal stenosis, gastrostomy is performed, initial esophageal dilatation is undertaken, and a length of no. 5 surgical silk thread is passed through the nose, pharynx, and esophagus and out the gastrostomy stoma. This establishes a tract for the future dilatations. The thread is secured to the skin at the site of the nose and by the gastrostomy stoma with tape.

Almost half of infants born with tracheoesophageal fistula will have other, nonrespiratory anomalies, e.g., congenital heart disease, obstructive uropathy, radial dysplasia, vertebral defects, anal atresia. The high incidence of this complex of anomalies, the VACTERL complex, as part of the pathology of tracheoesophageal fistula makes multisystem evaluation of these patients essential prior to their discharge home. Follow-up care should include consultation with specialists in the management of each of the infant's problems. Infants with vertebral anomalies, in particular, should be followed closely by a pediatric orthopedist. When vertebral defects are extensive, whether in the thoracic or lumbar region, the early appearance of scoliosis is likely. Such infants may require bracing to avoid a severe scoliotic deformity of the spine—a deformity that will further compromise ventilation. (See also discussion of postoperative care in Chapter 18.)

DEFECTS OF THE ABDOMINAL WALL

An infant born with a congenital defect in the abdominal wall has an excellent prognosis for survival when no other life-threatening birth defects are present. Corrective surgery may be staged, if necessary, by initial closure with skin or interposition of a Silastic patch into the defect in the first few hours after birth. This allows the abdominal cavity to be enlarged to accept the viscera that during fetal life were not enclosed in the abdominal cavity. Definitive correction can then be accomplished electively at some later time.

There are, however, a number of medical consequences of the closure of the abdominal defect in the early hours after birth. The most immediate is the need for oxygen therapy and/or assisted ventilation. This occurs when lung hypoplasia is associated with a congenital abdominal wall defect or when closure of the defect leads to an increase in the intra-abdominal pressure sufficient to cause respiratory failure from restriction of diaphragmatic breathing. With restriction of diaphragm movement following closure of the abdominal wall defect, the infant may require assisted ventilation until the abdominal wall stretches enough to allow a substantial fall in the intra-abdominal wall pressure. If lung expansion is severely curtailed by the tightness of the abdominal closure, oxygen therapy may be required to raise the arterial oxygen tension and oxygen saturation of the blood to appropriate levels.

The preparations for home care should take into account the special medical problems posed by the basic disorder as modified by treatment in the neonatal unit. These infants, as discussed, may have received sufficient long-term oxygen exposure or assisted ventilation to be considered at risk for chronic lung disease. (See Chapter 14, Chronic Lung Disease of Infancy.) However, clinical assessment of these infants is not as easy for the infant with respiratory distress. The infant with an abdominal wall defect may breathe more rapidly during sleep because of the presence of lung hypoplasia, rather than because of chronic lung disease. On the other hand, the infant may have normal lungs but still have tachypnea due to the restriction of diaphragmatic movement caused by the tightness of the abdominal closure. Finally, of course, the infant may have chronic lung disease coexistent with either or both of these alternatives. Predischarge assessment of the infant should therefore include arterial blood gas analysis, as well as transcutaneous monitoring of oxygen and carbon dioxide tension. When technically possible, measurement of lung function by body plethysmography permits more complete assessment of the disability in lung function. When the infant is thought to have chronic lung disease, the guidelines for the treatment plan should be selected from the therapeutic categories listed in Chapter 14. When the infant has lung hypoplasia or restricted lung function, small, frequent feedings should be considered, since large feedings may cause gastric distention and further restriction of diaphragmatic movement, leading to respiratory failure. When lung hypoplasia is severe, pulmonary hypertension may result from the concurrent lack of development of the pulmonary microcirculation. (See Pulmonary Hypertension in Chapter 14.)

The gastrointestinal function of the infant recovering from surgical repair of an abdominal wall defect may also be compromised. This is especially true of the infant with gastroschisis. These infants are born with the viscera outside the abdominal cavity without the normal protective mesenteric covering of the bowel. The bowel often becomes ischemic from cooling and from torsion of the blood supply during delivery. This can lead to severe compromise of bowel function, due to mucosal injury or to necrotizing enterocolitis. Enteric-enteric fistulas may form in the days following closure of the abdominal cavity. Thus, both the abdominal absorptive surface and the flow of feedings through the intestinal tract may be impaired. Occasionally the intestines of these infants are shorter than expected because of intrauterine malrotation, volvulus, bowel ischemia, and resorption of the necrotic portion of the bowel. Thus, before the infant's discharge from the hospital, a careful assessment of gastrointestinal function is required. Selection of an appropriate formula should be based on the extent of the gastrointestinal injury and dysfunction. In addition, some infants may first experience gastrointestinal problems only after discharge from the hospital. This is particularly true of the infant whose neonatal course is very smooth and who is discharged home within the first weeks after birth. Some of these infants may experience late onset of enterocolitis, which occurs only after the infant is taking large feedings. Therefore, the predischarge education of the parents should include the "danger signals" of gastrointestinal dysfunction: emesis, abdominal distention, lack of stools, and melena. In the infant with a history of congenital abdominal wall defect, these symptoms may herald a medical or surgical emergency. The infant will require immediate assessment of the problem by a pediatrician.

DISORDERS OF THE CHEST WALL

Either restriction of chest wall movement by an anatomic deformity or inadequate lung development due to intrauterine failure may result in compromised ventilation after birth. Some of these disorders will eventually prove fatal to the infant. In others, postnatal lung growth may lead to improved lung function. Some of these infants will require home oxygen therapy, and others with more severe restrictive disease may even require assisted ventilation at home. The guidelines listed in Appendix A for oxygen therapy and assisted ventilation of the infant with chronic lung disease apply also to these infants.

DIAPHRAGMATIC HERNIA

Several conditions require special recognition. Mortality is high in infants with congenital left diaphragmatic hernia, even when corrective surgery is performed within the early hours after birth. Fully 50 per cent of those afflicted with this anomaly die in the neonatal period as a result of hypoplasia of the lung and pulmonary vascular bed, which produces profound respiratory insufficiency and persistent pulmonary hypertension (also called persistent fetal circulation). Respiratory sequelae in the survivors vary with the degree of associated hypoplasia of the lung and pulmonary vascular bed and also with the extent of lung injury sustained during the postoperative period, when assisted ventilation is required. These infants should be reassessed prior to discharge from the hospital in a manner similar to that for infants with abdominal wall defects. Treatment should be directed at reversing the abnormal pulmonary clinical findings. (See Chapter 14.)

EVENTRATION OF THE DIAPHRAGM

A second disorder of the chest wall worthy of mention is eventration of the diaphragm. This condition may be congenital, or it may result from diaphragmatic paralysis (see discussion of phrenic nerve palsy earlier). This condition causes respiratory disability due to insufficient ventilation of the affected lung. Diagnosis of this disorder is generally suggested by the anteroposterior and lateral chest roentgenograms. Fluoroscopy aids in defining whether there is associated diaphragmatic paralysis. A decision should be made whether respiration is sufficiently impaired for surgical plication of the diaphragm to be considered. This procedure usually is associated with improvement in lung function and ventilation.

FOLLOW-UP CARE

Infants with a variety of airway, chest wall, or abdominal wall defects may require emergency surgery in the neonatal period. Although there are specific problems particular to many of these defects, the clinical course of these infants is likely to be complicated by some degree of chronic lung disease. The pediatrician will therefore need to evaluate the stage of involvement and follow the guidelines for management of both the chronic lung disease and appropriate nutrition discussed in Chapter 14. The medications and equipment for home care are considered in Appendix A, and ventilatory management at home is covered in Chapter 16. Table 15–1 gives a suggested schedule for follow-up care by the pediatrician (the primary care physician), the pulmonologist, and the otolaryngologist.

WHEN TO WORRY

The most serious complication that may confront the pediatrician in caring for such infants is acute obstruction of the airway. Therefore any clinical evidence of respiratory distress, i.e., wheezing, shortness of breath, or cyanosis, warrants prompt attention and evaluation by a physician on the child's health care team. For children with choanal stents or tracheostomies, the initial measure is lavage and suctioning to remove any secretions that may be causing the obstruction. Accidental dislodgment of the tracheostomy tube should be identified, and the tube replaced if possible. Other emergency measures include administration of oxygen and assisted ventilation by a self-inflatable bag. The patient should then be referred immediately to the otolaryngologist and pulmonologist for further evaluation and therapy, even if the patient appears to improve clinically with the initial measures.

Other less urgent but equally significant clinical findings include bleeding from the tracheostomy site; increased airway secretions, especially purulent or blood-tinged secretions; and severe airway infections, especially those that respond poorly to enteral antibiotic therapy. These findings may appear relatively trivial, but they are often harbingers of more serious underlying problems, such as granulomatous formation within the airway and impending respiratory failure. Children with these findings should always be referred promptly to the pulmonologist and surgeon or otolaryngologist involved in their care.

MANAGEMENT OF COMPLICATIONS

Despite the most vigorous home care, complications are inevitable. These include the development of granulomas within the airway in children who have had a tracheostomy for a long time, tracheobronchial infections, or recurrent parenchymal infections. Table 15–2 considers management of common complications of upper airway disease. (See also Chapter 18.)

When granulomas are suspected or verified by bronchoscopic examination, the usual approach includes antibiotic therapy, increased airway toilet, and surgical resection during bronchoscopic examination.

A patient requiring an indwelling airway appliance, such as a tracheostomy tube, which constitutes a foreign body, has increased susceptibility to infection and to disruption of mucociliary function. Medical management includes a Gram stain and culture of airway secretions, antibiotic therapy, and increased airway toilet.

TABLE 15-1. Management of Airway Obstruction: Routine Follow-up Care

	FREQUENCY*	EVALUATION
Pediatrician	Every week initially, then every 2 weeks to age 6 mo; monthly, age 6 mo to 12 mo	Interval history, growth parameters, nutritional assessment, nutritional counseling, immunizations
Pulmonologist	Biweekly initially, then monthly to age 6 mo; bimonthly, age 6 mo to 12 mo	Interval history, blood gases, transcutaneous oxygen and carbon dioxide monitoring, oxygen therapy, medication adjustments
Otolaryngologist	Every 2 wk to every 3 mo until 12 mo	Interval history, assessment of airway appliances, replacement as necessary, endoscopic examinations

* This schedule is representative of the needs of the typical infant with airway obstructive disease. Precise follow-up intervals must be individualized.

On occasion, bronchoscopic examination may help elucidate the contribution of these factors to concurrent granulomatous growth within the airway.

Recurrent infections are a likely complication, even with optimal airway toilet and home management. To limit the degree of further injury to the airways, a high index of suspicion of interval infections must be maintained. Once infection is suspected or identified (by roentgenography, physical findings, presence of polymorphonuclear leukocytes and bacteria in secretions, or positive cultures of airway secretions), intervention should be aggressive. Most such infections will respond readily to oral antibiotic therapy and the greater frequency of airway toilet than is possible at home. Choice of antibiotics, of course, depends on prevalence of organisms in the community and identification by culture.

Nonbacterial respiratory tract infections are among the most common childhood ailments that have potentially devastating consequences for infants with upper airway obstruction. Aside from the acute impairment of airway function due to inflammation, increased secretions, and airway edema, many respiratory tract viruses induce further severe injury to the airways, which can result in chronic interstitial lung disease. In addition, viral-induced airway injury is frequently complicated by secondary bacterial infections.

Infants with airway obstructive disease may be at particular risk during their first winter for infection with respiratory syncytial virus (RSV). Whenever RSV is a likely cause of an

TABLE 15-2. Management of Common Complications of Upper Airway Disease

COMPLICATION	MANAGEMENT
Infection	
Mild upper respiratory	Symptomatic, supportive, increased attention to toilet of airways
Bacterial infection, otitis media, sinusitis, tracheitis	Culture of accessible secretions, antibiotic therapy, frequent re-evaluation, referral to otolaryngologist and/or pulmonologist for failure to respond to therapy or worsening
Viral bronchiolitis or pneumonia	Immediate supportive care, immediate referral to pulmonologist for assessment and possible hospitalization
Tracheal Granulomas	Antibiotics, increased toilet of airways, immediate referral to otolaryngologist
As indicated by increased secretions, bleeding, stridor, increased obstruction	
Acute Airway Hemorrhage	Supportive care, immediate referral to otolaryngologist
Acute Respiratory Distress	Oxygen, airway suctioning, aerosolized bronchodilator therapy, assisted ventilation with resuscitation bag, immediate referral to pulmonologist for emergency care
As evidenced by severe dyspnea, cyanosis, stridor, air hunger, agitation, depressed sensorium, reduced air movement, apnea	
Accidental Dislodgment of Tracheostomy Tube	Immediate replacement if possible, speak with otolaryngologist regarding follow-up

interval respiratory tract infection, diagnosis should be sought actively by culture and direct antigen-antibody testing, and hospitalization should be considered for close observation for respiratory failure. Recently, aerosolized ribavirin therapy has been reported to reduce the morbidity and duration of acute RSV pneumonia-bronchiolitis in infants with underlying respiratory tract or cardiac disease. Therefore, some consideration should be given to its use in such children. As experience is gained with the technique of continuous aerosol antiviral therapy, more precise identifications for use will undoubtedly be formulated.

PROGNOSIS

Prognosis is dependent on both the specific class of airway obstructive disease and the success of the medical supportive management. The short-term prognosis for most clinical entities remains good for achieving discharge to the home environment.

The long-term prognosis also remains good for most clinical entities, provided adequate somatic growth and reparative airways growth can be accomplished. As airways and parenchymal growth is possible in most children until the age of 8 years or older, we should expect that substantial help for the underlying problem can be achieved if recurrent injury to the airway can be minimized and if nutrition is optimal.

Rarely, surgical reconstructive therapy of parts of the airways may be necessary. In these situations, maximum benefit is derived if the intervention is deferred until growth and optimal medical condition can be achieved.

Recommended Reading

Bland RD: Special considerations in oxygen therapy for infants and children. Am Rev Respir Dis 122:45, 1980.

Cohen SR, Eavey RD, Desmond SM: Endoscopy and tracheostomy in the neonatal period. Ann Otol Rhinol Laryngol 86:577, 1977.

Cotton R, Reilly JS: Stridor and airway obstruction. In Bluestone CD, Stool SE (eds.): Pediatric Otolaryngology. Philadelphia, W.B. Saunders Company, 1983, Vol 2, Ch 64.

Hall CB, McBride JT, et al.: Aerosol ribavirin treatment of infants with respiratory syncytial viral infection. N Engl J Med 308:1443, 1983.

McBride JT: Ribavirin and RSV: A new approach to an old disease. Pediatr Pulmonol 1:294, 1985.

Mok JYQ, McLaughlin JF, Pintar M, et al.: Transcutaneous monitoring of oxygenation: What is normal? J Pediatr 108:365, 1986.

Platzker ACG: Congenital anomalies causing respiratory failure. In Thibeault DW, Gregory GA (eds.): Neonatal Pulmonary Care, 2nd ed. Norwalk, CN, Appleton-Century-Crofts, 1986, pp 657–696.

Reid LM: Lung growth in health and disease. Br J Dis Chest 78:113, 1984.

Richardson MA, Cotton RT: Anatomic abnormalities of the pediatric airway. Pediatr Clin North Am 31:821, 1984.

Todres ID: Respiratory disorders of the newborn. In Bluestone CD, Stool SE (eds.): Pediatric Otolaryngology. Philadelphia, W.B. Saunders Company, 1983, Vol 2, Ch. 65.

16

VENTILATORY MANAGEMENT AT HOME

SALLY L. DAVIDSON WARD, M.D., and THOMAS G. KEENS, M.D.

THE PHYSIOLOGY OF BREATHING

The ability to sustain spontaneous ventilation requires adequate function of neurologic mechanisms that control ventilation, ventilatory muscle function, and lung and airway mechanics. Significant dysfunction of any of these three components of the respiratory system may impair the ability to breathe spontaneously. Respiratory failure occurs when central respiratory drive and/or ventilatory muscle power are inadequate to overcome the respiratory load (Fig. 16–1). These patients will require long-term support of ventilation if the cause of this "imbalance" is not reversible.

CENTRAL CONTROL OF BREATHING

Neurologic control of breathing must ensure adequate ventilation to meet the basal metabolic needs of the body and yet have considerable flexibility so that other complex behavioral and physiologic activities related to breathing may occur.[1,2] This involves integration of automatic and voluntary factors. These systems arise in separate sites in the brain and descend through different neural pathways. The voluntary centers of control, responsible for voluntary ventilation, are located in the motor and pre-

motor cortex and descend in the corticospinal tracts. Automatic control of ventilation, which maintains rhythmic ventilation in response to metabolic needs, originates in the brainstem and descends in the ventral and lateral columns of the spinal cord. The axons from both systems synapse with respiratory motor neurons at segmental levels of the spinal cord where the two control systems are integrated.[3] Since these two systems are functionally and anatomically distinct, lesions of each area result in different clinical syndromes.[3]

Voluntary ventilation and automatic ventilation are modulated differently. The automatic centers receive information regarding the adequacy of ventilation and oxygenation from central and peripheral chemoreceptors. Voluntary ventilation is under cerebrocortical control and, at times, may override automatic control. Automatic control is active during wakefulness and quiet sleep, but during active or rapid eye movement (REM) sleep, voluntary control predominates.[2,3] Thus, ventilation varies with the state of the individual. It becomes less adequate during sleep, and it is nearly unresponsive to modulation by chemoreceptor input during active sleep. It is not surprising that sleep is the most vulnerable period for the development of inadequate ventilation in disorders of respiratory control.[1–3]

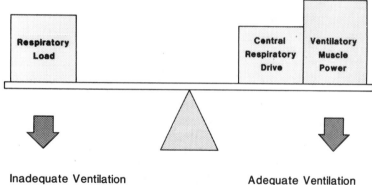

FIGURE 16-1. The respiratory system balance. In order to sustain adequate spontaneous ventilation, ventilatory muscle power and/or central respiratory drive must be sufficient to overcome the respiratory load. Alterations on either side can tip the balance toward respiratory failure.

Inadequate Ventilation   Adequate Ventilation

RESPIRATORY CONTROL OF BREATHING

Immaturity of the respiratory control systems in the infant predisposes to apnea and hypoventilation.[1,4,5] In the older child and adult, hypoxia stimulates ventilation. However, in the preterm and newborn infant, hypoxia depresses central respiratory neurons, resulting in diminished ventilation.[4,5] This depressant effect of hypoxia on ventilation disappears by 1 to 2 months of age. Further, the infant spends 40 to 70 percent of sleep time in active or REM sleep, in contrast to 15 to 20 per cent in the adult.[6] Active sleep is associated with greater variation in respiratory timing and amplitude, resulting in periods of inadequate gas exchange.[7]

NEUROMUSCULAR ROLE IN BREATHING

Ventilation cannot proceed without an intact neuromuscular system to receive the output from neurologic centers of ventilatory control.[8] The diaphragm and intercostal-accessory muscles perform the work of breathing. Respiratory failure can be viewed as inadequate ventilatory muscle power to overcome respiratory loads.[9] For example, ventilatory muscles of normal strength and endurance may fatigue in the face of increased respiratory loads, as in the case of respiratory failure due to increased airways resistance (asthma) or decreased lung compliance (pulmonary edema). On the other hand, weak ventilatory muscles may successfully perform the work of breathing when pulmonary mechanics are optimal, yet fail when pulmonary mechanics change, as during an intercurrent respiratory infection. Ventilatory muscles are striated muscles, and therefore have finite strength and energy requirements, are subject to

fatigue, and have an optimal length from which maximal contractility can be achieved. The factors that predispose to ventilatory muscle fatigue include hypoxia, disuse, malnutrition, hyperinflation, and changes in pulmonary mechanics causing increased work of breathing. The diaphragm of infants has a significantly smaller proportion of fatigue-resistant muscle fibers[10] and is weaker[11] than the diaphragm of older children and adults. Thus the infant is predisposed to ventilatory muscle fatigue.[8-11] Underlying muscle disease will further limit ventilatory muscle endurance.

Infants or children may require prolonged ventilatory support because of failure of neurologic control of ventilation or ventilatory muscle weakness or fatigue. Alteration of pulmonary mechanics and an associated increase in work of breathing are usually an additive factor. Once the decision has been made to institute long-term mechanical ventilation in an infant or child with a stable or progressive disorder, the caretakers should consider the impact of prolonged hospitalization on the life of the child and family. Long-term ventilatory support in the home is for many patients a safe and relatively inexpensive alternative.[12-16] The various conditions that are amenable to long-term ventilatory support in the home, and the steps in discharge planning and follow-up care, will be discussed. (See also Appendix A.)

DISORDERS OF NEUROLOGIC CONTROL OF BREATHING

CONGENITAL CENTRAL HYPOVENTILATION SYNDROME (ONDINE'S CURSE)

Congenital central hypoventilation syndrome (CCHS) or Ondine's curse is defined as the failure of automatic control of breathing.[7,17-21] Since breathing during quiet sleep is neurologically controlled almost entirely by the automatic system, ventilation is most severely affected during quiet sleep in this disorder.[7] However, breathing is also abnormal during active sleep and wakefulness, though usually to a milder degree.[7,17] Disordered ventilatory control may range in severity from relatively mild hypoventilation during quiet sleep with fairly good ventilation during wakefulness to complete apnea during sleep with severe hypoventilation during wakefulness. Other signs of brainstem dysfunction may be present, but are not essential to the diagnosis of CCHS.[17,18] The cause or causes of CCHS are unknown. It is possible that this disorder is due to prenatal damage to areas of the brainstem.

The clinical presentation of CCHS is quite variable, dependent on the severity of the disorder. Some infants will not breathe at birth and will require assisted ventilation in the newborn nursery. Most such infants do not breathe at all during the first few months of life, but will mature to a pattern of adequate breathing during wakefulness. Apnea or hypoventilation persists during sleep. This apparent improvement is due to normal maturation of the respiratory system and does not represent a change in the basic disorder.[1,4,5] In other infants, clinical presentation may be at a later age, with cyanosis, edema, and signs of right-sided heart failure as the first indications of CCHS. These infants have often been thought mistakenly to have cyanotic congenital heart disease. However, cardiac catheterization reveals only pulmonary hypertension. Infants with less severe CCHS may have tachycardia, diaphoresis, and/or cyanosis during sleep. Presumably these infants develop right-sided heart failure if the diagnosis is not made.[22,23] Still others may have unexplained apnea or an apparent life-threatening event.

The diagnosis of CCHS depends on the documentation of hypoventilation during sleep that is not secondary to ventilatory muscle dysfunction or lung disease. Continuous noninvasive monitoring of the adequacy of ventilation during sleep is best accomplished by transcutaneous oxygen and carbon dioxide electrode, oximetry, and expired gas analysis (end-tidal CO_2 monitoring). Intermittent blood gas sampling by arterial puncture or arterialized capillary sampling is not adequate, as it will cause arousal and therefore not represent ventilation during sleep. Although most infants have a decreased ventilatory response to hypercapnia and/or hypoxia, these abnormalities are not seen in all patients.

The treatment of CCHS is to ensure adequate ventilation when the patient is unable to breathe spontaneously.[7,17-21] This requires mechanical assisted ventilation, as no pharmacologic respiratory stimulants have been shown to be effective. CCHS does not resolve spontaneously; therefore, prolonged home ventilatory support is necessary if these patients are to leave the hospital. Positive pressure ventilators via tracheostomy,[24] negative pressure ventilators,[25] or diaphragm pacing[26-28] are options for these patients. Although oxygen administration improves the PaO_2 and relieves cyanosis, this treatment is inadequate, as hypoventilation persists and pulmonary hypertension ensues.[23]

It cannot be overemphasized that CCHS patients may suffer complete respiratory arrest or severe hypoventilation at the onset of sleep. Thus they require continuous observation and/or monitoring so that ventilatory support can be initiated with each sleep episode. In most cases, apnea-bradycardia monitoring alone is not sufficient, as many patients hypoventilate but are not apneic.

As infants grow, ventilatory requirements change rapidly and markedly. Thus the adequacy of ventilation during sleep must be checked every 1 to 3 months on the patient's home ventilator. Progressive pulmonary hypertension and cor pulmonale are not uncommon in these patients and must be assumed to be due to inadequate ventilator settings until proven otherwise.[22,23] Some infants will have progressive pulmonary hypertension even when ventilator settings during sleep are appropriate. This is usually due to hypoventilation during wakefulness. These patients may require some ventilatory support during wakefulness as well, and their prognosis is generally worse than the prognosis of those with a milder disorder.

There is no known cure for CCHS. The disorder appears to be lifelong. There is no documentation of any CCHS patients who have outgrown this disorder. However, with compulsive attention to maintaining the adequacy of ventilation, many patients do well. We currently care for some children with CCHS who attend regular school and have a normal life style while awake.

Acquired central hypoventilation syndrome is caused by conditions resulting in brainstem damage, such as tumors, trauma, neurosurgery, or brainstem hemorrhages.[29] The principles of diagnosis and management are the same as for CCHS.

MENINGOMYELOCELE

Infants with meningomyelocele may have abnormal central ventilatory control most likely due to anatomic disruption of neurons and brainstem nuclei from traction or compression associated with the Arnold-Chiari malformation.[30-34] Some infants are unable to sustain adequate spontaneous ventilation. The decision to consider home ventilation in these infants is clearly a complex one involving ethical and medical decisions. These infants are best managed by a multidisciplinary team.

INFANTS WITH UNEXPLAINED APNEA

Infants with apparent life-threatening events due to unexplained apnea in the absence of chronic hypoventilation are not candidates for long-term ventilatory support. They are usually managed by home apnea–bradycardia monitoring alone.[35] (See Chapter 25.) Some may respond to pharmacologic respiratory stimulants.[36]

VENTILATORY MUSCLE DYSFUNCTION

All causes of ventilatory muscle dysfunction have a similar pattern of respiratory compromise.[8,9,37-40] Weakness of the inspiratory muscles causes inability to fully inflate the lungs, with resulting atelectasis and microatelectasis. Weakness of the expiratory muscles causes ineffective cough, with resulting retention of pulmonary secretions and predisposition to pulmonary infection. Pulmonary infection is the leading cause of morbidity and mortality in patients with neuromuscular disorders and must be aggressively treated.[39,41] If ventilatory muscle weakness is severe enough, hypoventilation may ensue with the need for long-term ventilatory support.[9]

PARALYSIS OF THE DIAPHRAGM

Unilateral or bilateral paralysis of the diaphragm during infancy usually results from phrenic nerve injury; due to birth trauma or following thoracic surgery. Paralysis may be unilateral or bilateral, partial or complete.[42-44]

Eventration of one or both diaphragms may be clinically indistinguishable from diaphragm paralysis, but similar principles of diagnosis and care apply.[37] Cervical spinal cord injury with diaphragm paralysis is a special case in which the intercostal and accessory muscles of respiration are also paralyzed.[45]

Bilateral diaphragm paralysis in infancy results in respiratory failure requiring mechanical assisted ventilation.[44,46] In contrast, in older children and adults, the relative instability of the infant's chest wall prevents the intercostal and accessory muscles from performing the required work of breathing.[8] The diagnosis is suggested by paradoxical inward motion of the abdomen during inspiration. The chest roentgenogram reveals elevation of both hemidiaphragms and, frequently, marked atelectasis. However, these findings may be masked when the infant is treated with assisted ventilation. Transdiaphragmatic pressure measurement, the difference between intra-abdominal and intra-pleural pressure during diaphragm contraction, confirms the diagnosis.[47] Maximal transdiaphragmatic pressure is an indication of diaphragm strength.[11,47] Bilateral diaphragm paralysis usually results in a maximal value of less than 10 to 15 cm H_2O, with normal values exceeding 40 to 50 cm H_2O.[11] Diaphragm motion can be visualized by fluoroscopy or abdominal ultrasound. However, these studies may be misleading because of passive symmetric downward motion of both hemidiaphragms during inspiration. In these instances, phrenic nerve conduction times are used to assess phrenic nerve function.[48]

The initial treatment of respiratory failure due to bilateral diaphragm paralysis is mechanical ventilation. Many infants with phrenic nerve injury will have return of function within weeks to months.[44,46] Some infants do not have sufficient return of function, so that home ventilator care becomes necessary. Bilateral diaphragm plication may result in improved lung volumes.[49,50]

The severity of respiratory compromise from unilateral diaphragm paralysis or eventration varies with the extent of paradoxical upward motion of the paralyzed diaphragm during inspiration. With relatively little paradoxical motion, an infant can be virtually asymptomatic. Marked paradoxical motion may be associated with respiratory failure. Clinical signs of respiratory failure include tachypnea, cyanosis, and poor feeding. Asymmetric chest wall movement with decreased breath sounds on the affected side may be present. The chest roentgenogram reveals an elevated hemidiaphragm. The diagnosis is confirmed by the fluoroscopic or ultrasound finding of upward movement of the paralyzed hemidiaphragm during inspiration.[43,44]

Phrenic nerve function returns in many infants with unilateral diaphragm paralysis; however, this may not occur for up to 6 months after the injury.[44,51] Surgical plication of the paralyzed diaphragm usually improves the respiratory status and should be considered for infants who remain ventilator dependent without clinical improvement.[44,49,50] Following diaphragm plication, many infants can be weaned from mechanical ventilation.[50] Plication does not appear to interfere with the return of phrenic nerve function.

NEUROMUSCULAR DISORDERS

Congenital myopathies are nonprogressive disorders resulting from ultrastructural defects of muscle cells. The diagnosis is made clinically during the first year of life, since the muscle biopsy often reveals nonspecific changes. Patients may have respiratory failure due to ventilatory muscle weakness.[9,38,52,53] Although prolonged ventilatory support may be required, it may be possible to wean some patients from it after several months because of normal maturational changes in chest wall stability.[8] Others will remain completely or partially ventilator dependent.

Spinal muscular atrophy (Werdnig-Hoffmann) is a progressive disorder of anterior horn cells. Patients with spinal muscular atrophy who have respiratory failure in the neonatal period will not survive without ventilatory support. Some families choose long-term ventilatory support for these children in the home. More commonly these patients receive mechanical assisted ventilation for what is thought to be acute respiratory compromise, although they are subsequently unable to be weaned from the ventilator. Because of the progressive nature of this disease, these patients often remain ventilator dependent. Any time mechanical assisted ventilation is instituted for such a patient, for either an acute or chronic problem, the family and caretakers should understand that assisted ventilation may be required for the duration of the patient's life.*

---

*Institution of mechanical ventilation in these infants involves an ethical decision in which the parents should have the opportunity to participate in a fully informed fashion. — Ed.

LUNG DISEASE

Some infants with stable but severe lung disease will require mechanical ventilation for all or part of each day for many months. Bronchopulmonary dysplasia or chronic lung disease of infancy (CLD) is the most common disorder requiring long-term ventilatory support in infancy. Because of the potential for growth of the lung with development of new alveoli, even infants with severe CLD usually improve. (See Chapter 14.) A family, faced with the prospect of many months of hospitalization for their infant during this period of slow improvement, may be willing and able to provide ventilatory support for the infant at home. For successful assisted ventilation in a home setting, an infant's lung disease must be relatively stable, with inspired oxygen concentrations and ventilator settings requiring minimal day-to-day adjustment.[15] Lung disease of this severity may be accompanied by secondary changes in ventilatory muscles resulting in decreased strength and endurance. The resulting ventilatory muscle fatigue contributes to ventilator dependence in these infants.[9]

HOSPITAL MANAGEMENT IN PREPARATION FOR DISCHARGE

The underlying conditions resulting in the need for assisted ventilation are not reversible with specific treatment. However, improvement in pulmonary mechanics will reduce the work of breathing and substantially increase the patient's ability to breathe spontaneously.[9,54] This may allow weaning from assisted ventilation for some portion of the day, significantly improving mobility and quality of life.[15]

Nearly all infants receiving prolonged assisted ventilation develop chronic lung disease with elements of bronchoconstriction, chronic inflammation of the airway and lung parenchyma, and impaired mucociliary clearance. Therapy should be directed toward relief of bronchospasm, clearance of pulmonary secretions, reduction in lung water, treatment of pulmonary infections, and prevention of aspiration.[41] (See Management of Chronic Lung Disease of Infancy in Chapter 14.) Patients with ventilatory muscle weakness, especially, should routinely receive aerosolized bronchodilators administered by positive pressure, followed by intensive pulmonary physiotherapy. Patients should receive the routine immunizations and annual split-virus influenza vaccine.

The goals of long-term ventilatory support are different from those for mechanical ventilation of patients with acute illness[15](Table 16-1).

Weaning children recovering from acute respiratory failure from assisted ventilation is usually done by gradually decreasing the ventilator rate in a uniform fashion throughout the day. However, for the child requiring long-term assisted ventilation, mobility and quality of life are maximized if the child can breathe unassisted for portions of the day.[15] Thus, if possible, the child should be disconnected from the ventilator completely for varying periods during waking hours, even if he or she requires full support during sleep. This allows the ventilatory muscles a rest and recovery period and continues assisted ventilation during the period when the patient is at highest risk for hypoventilation due to the depression of neurologic control of breathing that occurs during sleep.[2] In our experience, the weaning of daytime assisted ventilation is best accomplished by allowing unassisted breathing for short periods, i.e., sprints, increasing the length of each period as tolerated.[55-57] Tolerance for sprinting should be monitored clinically and by measurement of gas exchange, such as continuous end-tidal CO_2 monitoring. Sprinting offers an intense period of ventilatory muscle training. To achieve a maximal training effect, recovery periods with little muscle activity are necessary. Thus the patient's ventilatory needs should be completely or nearly completely met during times of assisted ventilation. Ventilatory muscle fatigue may be masked by assisted ventilation that provides only partial support.

Techniques that have been used for prolonged assisted ventilation in the home include positive pressure ventilation administered through a tracheostomy,[12-16,25] negative pressure ventilator, cuirass,[26] rocking bed,[58] and diaphragm pacing.[27-29,58] However, only positive pressure ventilation through a tracheostomy is adequate for most infants. Electronic portable positive pressure ventilators, which do not require compressed air, provide the greatest flexibility for home care. In infants and small children, air leaks around the tracheostomy are considerable and variable (Fig. 16-2). Thus, using the ventilator in a volume-cycled mode will result in a variable tidal volume delivered to the child at each breath. It is not usually possible to find a tidal volume setting that will consistently achieve adequate alveolar ventilation with this technique. Therefore, we recommend using the ventilator in a pressure-limited mode. This can be accomplished by selecting a high tidal volume, sufficient to compensate for the variable tracheostomy air leak, and adjusting the pressure limit on the ventilator to the desired peak inspiratory pressure. Once the peak inspiratory pressure has been achieved, no further tidal volume is delivered to the patient. This ensures that the lungs are inflated to the same pressure with each breath, regardless of the size of the tracheostomy air leak.

Ventilators used in the home should be equipped with a disconnect or low-pressure alarm, so that inadvertent disconnection of the ventilator from the tracheostomy can be detected and remedied.

Patients tolerate a $PaCO_2$ slightly lower than physiologic, approximately 35 mm Hg, which provides a margin of safety and eliminates any subjective feeling of dyspnea. In the home, ventilator settings cannot be changed frequently to maintain "perfect" blood gas values. Thus, settings should not be changed in response to

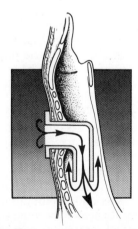

FIGURE 16-2. The relationship of a tracheostomy to the infant trachea is such that a substantial and variable amount of air introduced through the tracheostomy tube from the ventilator leaks out of the respiratory system. These variable leaks can be compensated for by a pressure-limited mode of mechanical assisted ventilation.

TABLE 16-1 Goals of Long-Term Ventilatory Support at Home

1. To optimize child's quality of life: rehabilitation to normal life style and reintegration into family
2. To ensure medical safety of child: normalization of respiratory function and growth
3. To use respiratory equipment safely and properly
4. To prevent or minimize complications

minor variations in blood gas values, but only to correct persistent trends or major abnormalities.

The patient's respiratory status must be stable with use of the home ventilator for at least two weeks prior to discharge. (See Appendix A.) It is difficult to deliver positive end-expiratory pressure (PEEP) using the portable ventilators presently available. Thus, whenever possible, the patient should be successfully weaned from PEEP before changing to the portable ventilator. This may necessitate an increase in other ventilator settings.

Diaphragm pacing is an acceptable method of extended ventilatory support for patients with intact phrenic nerves and diaphragm.[27-29,58] It is most useful for central hypoventilation syndrome and high spinal cord injury. It does not need to be instituted during infancy. It can be substituted for positive pressure ventilation at any time in later life. In our experience, it is better tolerated in children after 2 years of age.

The equipment essential for home care of the ventilator-dependent infant is listed in Appendix A, Table A–7. Service contracts for the maintenance of the ventilator and other respiratory equipment must be arranged. (See Appendix A, Table A–6.) The respiratory equipment vendor should have a troubleshooter who makes weekly home visits and who verifies proper operation of equipment and provides preventive maintenance. Prompt 24-hour availability of the vendor is essential in the event of equipment malfunction. Ideally a back-up ventilator and other essential equipment should be provided to all families, but must be provided when the child lives a long distance from medical or technical assistance. The physical environment of the home should be evaluated, including adequacy of space, grounded electrical outlets, and wiring.[12]

Prior to their child's discharge from the hospital, the family must become familiar with all aspects of his or her care.[12] (See Appendix A.) They must demonstrate competency in equipment operation, tracheostomy care, pulmonary physiotherapy, administration of medications including aerosols, and cardiopulmonary resuscitation. Families need to become adept at recognizing signs of respiratory compromise. Although most families become skilled in these tasks, it is not realistic to expect that they care for their child unassisted in the home. Nurses with pediatric critical care expertise are required to assist the family in the care of their child at home for 16 to 24 hours a day.[12] Before the child's discharge from the hospital, each nurse who will care for him or her at home should receive in-service training in the care of the child, preferably from the child's primary nurse.

Ventilator-assisted children in the home must be closely linked to a medical center capable of providing the subspecialty care required (Fig. 16–3). Prior to home care, arrangements should be made for transportation to the hospital from the home or local emergency room in the event of an emergency. Presently available portable ventilators usually permit the families to transport their ventilator-assisted child for routine visits, although nursing assistance makes this easier. When possible, a local primary pediatrician should be recruited to provide routine pediatric care in the community. The local emergency room or paramedics should be familiar with the child and be able to provide emergency care or transport to the medical center. The local telephone and utility companies must be notified by mail of the patient's location and condition. In the event of a power outage or other interruption of service, the home ventilator patient is then given priority for restoration of service.[12]

HOME MANAGEMENT OF THE VENTILATOR-DEPENDENT CHILD

Ventilator settings should be routinely evaluated every 2 to 3 months so that ventilation meets the changing requirements of the growing child. This usually requires an overnight hospital admission so that continuous noninvasive studies of oxygenation and ventilation may be accomplished during sleep. To minimize elective hospitalizations, other routine procedures can be carried out during these admissions.

Some ventilator-assisted children will also require supplemental oxygen. Supplemental oxygen may be required during spontaneous breathing and/or during mechanical assisted ventilation. Oxygen requirements need to be assessed at regular intervals by means of continuous noninvasive monitoring of oxygenation overnight. Supplemental oxygen is not a replacement for home ventilation in those patients with chronic hypoventilation.

Because mechanical ventilation will not completely meet the ventilatory requirements at all times, even the most successfully managed patients are exposed to periods of alveolar hypoxia and hypoventilation. (See Chapter 14.) Thus, all ventilator-assisted children are at risk for the development of pulmonary hypertension and cor pulmonale.[23,24] The usual clinical findings of right-sided heart failure may not be present until late in the course. Echocardiography may

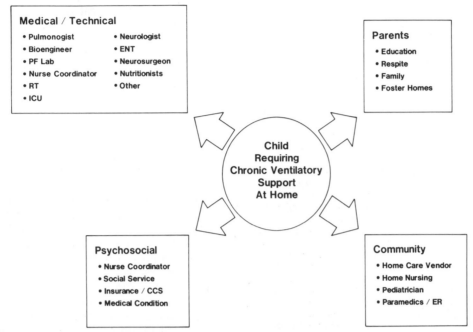

FIGURE 16-3. The complex of medical, psychosocial, and community resources that are required to successfully support the ventilator assisted infant or child in the home.

be a more sensitive method for following function of the right side of the heart. Echocardiography should be used at least every six months to measure right ventricular dimensions, pulmonic valve systolic time intervals, septal morphology, pulmonic valve *"a"* dip, pulmonic valve early systolic closure, and acceleration time of pulmonary artery flow (Doppler). It should be utilized more often if clinically indicated.[59,60] When signs of pulmonary hypertension are discovered, it should be assumed that the level of mechanical ventilation is inadequate until proven otherwise.[22,23] The patient should be hospitalized for continuous noninvasive monitoring of gas exchange and ventilator adjustments. Some patients requiring assisted ventilation only while sleeping may hypoventilate intermittently while breathing unassisted during wakefulness. If this occurs frequently, pulmonary hypertension may result, even if mechanical ventilation at night is adequate.

Common childhood illnesses pose a unique threat to the ventilator-assisted child.[39,41] A number of normal host defenses against disease are either lost or impaired in these patients. For example, breathing via tracheostomy bypasses the normal humidifying and filtering functions of the upper airway, predisposing to inspissated secretions and tracheobronchitis. Ineffective cough leads to impaction and decreased clearance of pulmonary secretions. Inability to increase respiratory rate in response to fever may

lead to dyspnea and hypoxia. Despite preventive and therapeutic measures directed at these problems, even a relatively trivial upper respiratory infection may result in compromise in the ventilator-assisted child. Ventilator adjustments with an increased level of support are usually needed. Patients ordinarily requiring ventilation only during sleep often need support 24 hours a day during illness. Because of these changes in the ventilatory requirements, these patients require hospitalization for blood gas monitoring and frequent ventilator changes.[16] Ventilators with greater flexibility than portable electronic ventilators, e.g., with capability for PEEP, higher rates, higher pressures, higher volumes, are usually required to ensure adequate ventilation during these hospitalizations. After recovery, patients should demonstrate adequate ventilation with use of the home ventilator for several days prior to discharge.

The management of complications of long-term ventilatory support is summarized in Table 16-2.

ROLE OF THE PRIMARY PHYSICIAN

The proper setting for the coordination of care for the home ventilator patient is a medical center capable of providing multidisciplinary support. The physician team should include pe-

TABLE 16–2. Management of Complications of Long-Term Ventilatory Support

MEDICAL PROBLEM	MANAGEMENT
Hypoxia	Evaluate oxygenation by noninvasive monitoring (tcPO$_2$, Sa O$_2$) every 2–3 mo.
Hypoventilation	Evaluate ventilator settings by noninvasive monitoring (P$_{ET}$CO$_2$, tc PCO$_2$) every 2–3 mo.
Chronic Lung Disease	Have a high index of suspicion. The diagnosis of CLD is often missed in ventilator-assisted children. Treatment includes bronchodilators (aerosolized and/or systemic), pulmonary physiotherapy, and diuretics.
Pulmonary Hypertension	Ensure adequate oxygenation and ventilation. Monitor ECG and echocardiogram for signs of pulmonary hypertension every 6 mo.
Pulmonary Infections	Complete immunizations, including influenzae split-virus vaccine. Treat respiratory infections aggressively with antibiotics and pulmonary physiotherapy.
Growth Delay	Give attention to caloric quantity and quality. Assess oxygeneation and ventilation.

diatric pulmonary and rehabilitation specialists. Pediatric surgical and anesthesia services should be available. Consultants from the disciplines of pediatric cardiology, neurology, and gastroenterology are frequently required. Allied health professionals, including the pulmonary nurse coordinator, medical social worker, psychologist, and physical, occupational, and respiratory therapists, provide essential family education and psychosocial support (Fig. 16–3).

Although these infants require specialized care for specific problems, the general pediatrics care for the child as a whole can easily be neglected. Optimal care for the ventilator-assisted infant and child is provided with the active involvement of a primary physician preferably located near the patient's home. The local physician serves a number of important roles that cannot be served by the referral medical center.

The primary pediatrician is in an optimal position to coordinate the community resources for the care of the child (Fig. 16–3). Local emergency medical systems need to be aware of the child and his or her special needs. The primary

pediatrician is the logical resource for emergency care. Coordination of home respiratory equipment vendors, home nursing, and electrical power and telephone service is also greatly facilitated by involved local pediatricians or family physicians. School acceptance of the ventilator-assisted child is often a problem that can be improved if the school knows that a local pediatrician is familiar with the child and willing to serve as a resource for both emergent and nonemergent care.

The primary pediatrician is an expert in the "well-child" needs of children. Immunizations, developmental screening, and attention to the "normal" problems of childhood are often overlooked or inadequately dealt with by subspecialists in the medical center. The primary pediatrician provides continuity to assure that these needs are met.

In the primary care role, the community pediatrician can serve as the link between the family and the referral medical center. When a child is becoming ill, the primary pediatrician is the best person to assess the infant to decide if specialized care is needed or if care can be provided in the community. The role of an emergency care provider cannot be overemphasized, since these children have little pulmonary reserve and can deteriorate quickly.

Finally the primary pediatrician is an excellent resource to provide support for the family. It is often difficult to find community pediatricians who are willing to participate in the care of the infants in these complex situations. However, there can be a great deal of satisfaction for the physician who participates with subspecialists in the care of these infants, and the family often preferentially turns to him or her for advice, support, and the care needs of their child.

SUMMARY

Even with sophisticated management, ventilator-assisted children may succumb to a catastrophe stemming from a simple problem, such as a disconnected ventilator or plugged tracheostomy, emphasizing the need for vigilant care. Other causes of mortality include cor pulmonale and respiratory infections.[16,39,41] However, many home-ventilator–assisted infants do quite well, and home care of these patients can involve safe and relatively inexpensive management techniques. The high motivation of parents for the care of their children in the home often results in high quality of care. After the transition from hospital to home, parent-child relationships and child development are enhanced. Potential for rehabilitation in all aspects of daily living is increased, and many children will experience a near-normal life style.[12]

References

1. Bryan AC, Bryan MH: Control of respiration in the newborn. Clin Perinatol 5:269, 1978.
2. Phillipson EA: Control of breathing during sleep. Am Rev Respir Dis 118:909, 1978.
3. Mitchell RA, Berger AJ: Neural regulation of respiration. Am Rev Respir Dis 111:206, 1975.
4. Rigatto H Control of ventilation in the newborn. Ann Rev Physiol 46:661, 1984.
5. Ready DJC, Henderson-Smart DJ: Regulation of breathing in the newborn during different behavioral states. Ann Rev Physiol 46:675, 1984.
6. Roffwarg HP, Muzio JN, Dement WC: Ontogenetic development of the human sleep-dream cycle. Science 152:604, 1966.
7. Fleming PJ, Cade D, Bryan MH, et al: Congenital central hypoventilation in sleep state. Pediatrics 66:425, 1980.
8. Muller NL, Bryan AC: Chest wall mechanics and respiratory muscles in infants. Pediatr Clin North Am 26:503, 1977.
9. Macklem PT, Roussos CS: Respiratory muscle fatigue: A cause of respiratory failure? Clin Sci 53:419, 1977.
10. Keens TG, Bryan AC, Levison H, Ianuzzo CD: Developmental pattern of muscle fiber types in human ventilatory muscles. J Appl Physiol 44:909, 1978.
11. Scott CB, Nickerson BG, Sargent CW, et al.: Developmental pattern of maximal transdiaphragmatic pressure in infants during crying. Pediatr Res 17:707, 1983.
12. Goldberg AI, Faure EAM, Vaughn CJ, et al.: Home care for life-supported persons: An approach to program development. J Pediatr 104:785, 1984.
13. Goldberg AI, Kettrick R, Buzdygan D, et al.: Home ventilation program for infants and children. Crit Care Med 8:238, 1980.
14. Children with Handicaps and Their Families. Case example: The Ventilator-Dependent Child. Report of the Surgeon General's Workshop. DHHS Publication PHS-83-50194. US Department of Health and Human Services, 1983.
15. Make B, Gilmartin M, Brody JS, Snider GL: Rehabilitation of ventilator-dependent individuals with lung disease: The concept and initial experience. Chest 86:358, 1984.
16. Goldberg AI: The regional approach to home care for life-supported persons. Chest 86:345, 1984.
17. Fishman LS, Samson JH, Sperling DR: Primary aveolar hypoventilation syndrome (Ondine's curse). Am J Dis Child 110:155, 1965.
18. Mellins RB, Balfour HH Jr, Turino GM, Winters RW: Failure of automatic control of ventilation (Ondine's curse). Medicine. 49:487, 1970.
19. Deonna T, Arczynska W, Torrado A: Congenital failure of automatic ventilation (Ondine's curse). J Pediatr 84:710, 1974.
20. Shannon DC, Marsland DW, Gould JB, et al.: Central hypoventilation during quiet sleep in two infants. Pediatrics, 57:342, 1976.
21. Guilleminault C, McQuitty J, Ariagno RL, et al.: Congenital central alveolar hypoventilation syndrome in six infants. Pediatrics, 70:684, 1982.
22. Unger M, Atkins M, Briscoe WA, King TKC: Potentiation of pulmonary vasoconstrictor response with repeated intermittent hypoxia. A Appl Physiol 43:662, 1977.
23. Nattie EE, Bartlett D Jr, Johnson K: Pulmonary hypertension and right ventricular hypertrophy caused by intermittent hypoxia and hypercapnia in the rat. Am Rev Respir Dis 118:653, 1978.
24. Auchincloss JH, Gilbert R: Mechanical aide to ventilation in the home: Use of volume-limited ventilator and leaking connections. Am Rev Respir Dis 108:373, 1973.
25. O'Leary J, King R, LeBlanc M, et al.: Cuirass ventilation in childhood neuromuscular disease. J Pediatr 94:419, 1979.
26. Glenn WWL, Holcomb WG, Gee JBL, Bath R: Central hypoventilation syndrome: Long term ventilatory assistance by radio-frequency electrophrenic respiration. Ann Surg 172:755, 1970.
27. Hunt CE, Matalon SV, Thompson TR, et al.: Central hypoventilation syndrome: Experience with bilateral phrenic nerve pacing in 3 neonates. Am Rev Respir Dis 118:23, 1978.
28. Ilbawi MN, Hunt CE, DeLeon SY, Idriss FS: Diaphragm pacing in infants and children: Report of a simplified technique and review of experience. Ann Thorac Surg 31:61, 1981.
29. Rizvi SS, Ishikawa S, Faling LJ, et al.: Defect in automatic respiration in a case of multiple sclerosis. Am J Med 56:433, 1974.
30. Kirsch WM, Duncan BR, Black FO, Stears JC: Laryngeal palsy in association with myelomeningocele, hydrocephalus, and Arnold-Chiari malformation. J Neurosurg 28:207, 1969.
31. Hoffman HJ, Hendrick EB, Humphreys RP: Manifestations and management of Arnold-Chiari malformation in patients with myelomeningocele. Childs Brain 1:255, 1975.
32. Krieger AJ: Measurement of respiration in Arnold-Chiari malformation. Childs Brain 2:31, 1976.
33. Holinger PC, Holinger LD, Reichert TJ, Holinger PH: Respiratory obstruction and apnea in infants with bilateral abductor vocal cord paralysis, meningomyelocele, hydrocephalus, and Arnold-Chiari malformation. J Pediatr 92:368, 1978.
34. Nickerson BG, van der Hal AL, McQuitty JC, et al.: Central sleep apnea and absent hypoxic and hypercapneic arousal in infants with myelodysplasia. Am Rev Respir Dis (abstract) 125:186, 1982.
35. Kelly DH, Shannon DC, O'Connell K: Care of infants with near miss sudden infant death syndrome. Pediatrics 61:511, 1978.
36. Kelly DH, Shannon DC: Treatment of apnea and excessive periodic breathing in the full-term infant. Pediatrics 68:183, 1981.
37. Shim C: Motor disturbances of the diaphragm. Clin Chest Med 1:125, 1979.
38. Harrison BDW, Collins JV, Brown KGE, Clark TJH: Respiratory failure in neuromuscular diseases. Thorax 26:579, 1971.
39. Vignos PJ Jr: Pulmonary function and pulmonary infection in Duchenne muscular dystrophy. Isr J Med Sci 13:207, 1977.
40. Black LF, Hyatt RE: Maximal static respiratory pressures in generalized neuromuscular disease. Am Rev Respir Dis 103:641, 1971.
41. Johnson EW, Kennedy JH: Comprehensive manage-

ment of Duchenne muscular dystrophy. Arch Phys Med Rehabil 52:110, 1971.

42. Adams FH, Gyepps MT: Diaphragm paralysis in the newborn infant simulating cyanotic heart disease. J Pediatr 78:119, 1971.
43. Smith BT: Isolated phrenic nerve palsy in the newborn. Pediatrics, 49:449, 1972.
44. Green W, L'Heureux P, Hunt CE: Paralysis of the diaphragm. Am J Dis Child 129:1402, 1975.
45. Carter E: Medical management of pulmonary complications of spinal cord injury. Adv Neurol 22:261, 1979.
46. Kreitzer SM, Feldman NT, Saunders NA, Ingram RH Jr: Bilateral diaphragmatic paralysis with hypercapneic respiratory failure: A physiologic assessment. Am J Med 65:89, 1976.
47. Loh L, Goldman M, Newsom Davis J: The assessment of diaphragm function. Medicine 56:165, 1977.
48. Moosa A: Phrenic nerve conduction in children. Dev Med Child Neurol 23:434, 1981.
49. Schwartz MZ, Filler RM: Plication of the diaphragm for symptomatic phrenic nerve paralysis. J Pediatr Surg 13:259, 1978.
50. Schonfeld T, O'Neal MH, Platzker ACG, et al.: Function of the diaphragm before and after plication. Thorax 35:631, 1980.
51. Ahmed S, Gill B: Nonoperative management of postthoracotomy diaphragmatic paralysis in two neonates. Aust Paediatr J 11:81, 1975.
52. Harrison BDW, Collins JV, Brown KGE, Clark TJH: Respiratory failure in neuromuscular diseases. Thorax 26:579, 1971.
53. Keltz H: The effect of respiratory muscle dysfunction on pulmonary function. Am Rev Respir Dis 91:934, 1965.
54. Roussos CS, Macklem PT: Diaphragmatic fatigue in man. J Appl Physiol 43:189, 1977.
55. Leith DE, Bradley M: Ventilatory muscle strength and endurance training. J Appl Physiol 41:508, 1976.
56. Keens TG, Krastins IRB, Wannamaker EM, et al.: Ventilatory muscle endurance training in normal subjects and cystic fibrosis patients. Am Rev Respir Dis 116:853, 1977.
57. Gross D, Riley E, Grassino A, et al.: Influence of resis-

tive training on respiratory muscle strength and endurance in quadriplegia (abstract). Am Rev Respir Dis 117:343, 1978.
58. Hyland RH, Jones NL, Powles ACP, et al.: Primary alveolar hypoventilation treated with nocturnal electrophrenic respiration. Am Rev Respir Dis 117:165, 1978.
59. Gewitz M, Eshaghpour E, Holsclaw DS, et al.: Echocardiography in cystic fibrosis. Am J Dis Child 131:275, 1977.
60. Perkin RM, Anas NG: Pulmonary hypertension in pediatric patients. J Pediatr 105:511, 1984.

Recommended Reading

Bryan AC, Bryan MH: Control of respiration in the newborn. Clin Perinatol 5:269, 1978.

Goldberg AI, Kettrick R, Buzdygan D, et al.: Home ventilation program for infants and children. Crit Care Med 8:238, 1980.

Green W, L'Heureux P, Hunt CE: Paralysis of the diaphragm. Am J Dis Child 129:1402, 1975.

Harrison BDW, Collins JV, Brown KGE, Clark TJH: Respiratory failure in neuromuscular diseases. Thorax 26:579, 1971.

Johnson EW, Kennedy JH: Comprehensive management of Duchenne muscular dystrophy. Arch Phys Med Rehabil 52:110, 1971.

Loh L, Goldman M, Newsom Davis J: The assessment of diaphragm function. Medicine 56:165, 1977.

Macklem PT, Roussos CS: Respiratory muscle fatigue: A cause of respiratory failure? Clin Sci 53:419, 1977.

Mellins RB, Balfour HH Jr, Turino GM, Winters RW: Failure of automatic control of ventilation (Ondine's curse). Medicine. 49:487, 1970.

Muller NL, Bryan AC: Chest wall mechanics and respiratory muscles in infants. Pediatr Clin North Am 26:503, 1977.

Phillipson EA: Control of breathing during sleep. Am Rev Respir Dis 118:909, 1978.

Shim C: Motor disturbances of the diaphragm. Clin Chest Med 1:125, 1979.

17

CYSTIC FIBROSIS

C. MICHAEL BOWMAN, Ph.D., M.D.

GENETICS

The fact that cystic fibrosis (CF) is the most common inherited lethal disease in Caucasians makes it inevitable that cystic fibrosis will ultimately be diagnosed in some ICN graduates. Inherited as an autosomal recessive, CF occurs in approximately 1 in 2000 in the white population.[1] It occurs in 1 in 17,000 among blacks.[2] Because of its pattern of inheritance, any child born to two carriers (carrier rate in whites is approximately 1 in 20) has a 1 in 4 chance of having CF. Thus, a positive family history for CF markedly increases the possibility that an infant with chronic lung disease has CF. Since CF was described as an entity only in the mid to late 1930's, in children dying of CF prior to 1945 or 1950, presumably the diagnosis was pneumonia, failure to thrive, or malnutrition. Thus, a family history that includes early infant deaths prior to 1950 must be considered suspicious for CF.

Recognition

The findings in the high-risk infant that should lead to suspicion of CF are listed in Table 17–1.

Children with meconium ileus are highly likely to have CF.[3] However, children with meconium ileus may be found on later sweat testing not to have CF.[4] It is important to differentiate between the various causes of neonatal gastrointestinal obstruction that can occur in the early newborn period.[5] Whenever a neonate has intestinal obstruction it at least must be considered that meconium ileus or meconium plug syndrome is the cause.

Undernutrition and excessive energy requirements are common problems in premature infants.[6] Again these problems relate to many different diagnoses. However, they are the hallmark of CF as well. The malabsorption in CF results from pancreatic insufficiency.[7–9] This insufficiency leads to fat malabsorption and may even progress to protein calorie malnutrition.[10,11] Children with CF usually demonstrate improved growth and less malabsorption when pancreatic enzymes are supplied along with enteral feedings.[12] However, a neonate who is receiving total parenteral nutrition by central venous catheter would probably not manifest the severe malabsorptive problems typically associated with CF. As a result, a child who grows reasonably well when provided with total parenteral nutrition, but grows poorly when receiving enteral feedings, should be considered a possible candidate for a sweat test. Although a variety of problems, including necrotizing enterocolitis, chronic hypoxia, and chronic heart failure, as well as other diagnoses, are common causes of malabsorption and malnutrition in a premature infant, CF must also be considered. The patient in whom CF is not recognized who develops protein calorie malnutrition may be at in-

TABLE 17–1. Findings in the High-Risk Neonate That May Suggest the Diagnosis of Cystic Fibrosis

1. Meconium ileus
2. Significant malabsorption*
3. Significantly diminished weight gain or the appearance of hypoproteinemia when the feeding route is changed from parenteral to enteral*
4. Chronic pulmonary infection with *Pseudomonas aeruginosa,* especially mucoid strains
5. Progressive pulmonary disease in the absence of recognized continuing insults (consider also chronic aspiration); frequent bouts of "bronchiolitis"
6. Electrolyte imbalance (hypochloremia and/or hyponatremia) out of proportion to the balance between intake and urinary losses (especially in warm environments)
7. Salt crystals on the skin

* In the absence of significant bowel disease

creased risk for respiratory failure and serious infection,[10,13] so early diagnosis of CF and treatment of the malabsorption are essential to the child's well-being when enteral feedings are given.

Most children with CF are recognized by the continued occurrence of respiratory distress.[14-16] This finding is typically diagnosed initially as bronchiolitis or wheezing.[16] The x-ray findings are those of diffuse hyperinflation or linear streaks. In some children with CF, the radiographs may be normal at diagnosis or may be markedly abnormal, occasionally progressing to include lobar atelectasis or pneumothorax.[17] Obviously all of these x-ray changes and respiratory problems are also consistent with the chronic lung disease (CLD) that frequently occurs in premature infants. Thus it may be very difficult to pick out which premature infant with chronic lung disease might have CF. A high index of suspicion must be maintained.

Pulmonary infection is also a chronic problem in patients with CF. Sputum samples or tracheal aspirates frequently grow respiratory pathogens such as *Hemophilus influenzae, Staphylococcus aureus,* or *Pseudomonas aeruginosa.*[18] In addition, these pathogens may also be present in varying amounts, with or without clinical significance, in the respiratory tracts of premature infants with chronic lung disease. As a result, there is again no single finding or pathogen that is diagnostic or strongly suggestive of CF in a given newborn with respiratory problems. One finding that should raise the clinician's suspicion that the baby might have CF is the presence of mucoid strains of *Pseudomonas* or other gram-negative organisms. Such strains are common in patients with CF, but are very uncommon in other respiratory illnesses of in-

fants, children, and adults.[19] Certainly patients with tracheostomy tubes or long-term endotracheal intubation are at risk for harboring *Pseudomonas* species in their airways. However, normal patients with long-term intubation usually have nonmucoid *Pseudomonas* strains. While CF patients may also have nonmucoid strains of *Pseudomonas,* frequently mucoid strains develop later. Such mucoid strains are more resistant to eradication and seem to cause more indolent infection. It has recently been recognized that *Pseudomonas cepacia* can be a particularly devastating pathogen in patients with CF.[20] This organism has not been described as yet in normal newborns or infants.

Many sick neonates have electrolyte imbalance.[21] Such imbalances may be aggravated by multiple organ dysfunction (kidney, gut, heart, lungs) and also by treatments and medications, including diuretics, electrolyte supplements, and restriction of fluid intake. However, patients with CF have increased concentrations of sodium and chloride in their sweat.[22] Thus a patient with persistent hyponatremia and hypochloremia (especially in a warm environment) in whom other factors do not account for such electrolyte imbalances should be considered a candidate for a sweat test. Infants in the ICN are usually monitored too closely to have an opportunity to develop significant hyponatremia. However, many infants who are taking large doses of diuretics do become hypochloremic. Thus it is easy to dismiss a child in the ICN who has hypochloremia as being one who is suffering from the side effects of diuretics. If, in fact, that particular child is not receiving high doses of diuretics, the diagnosis of CF must be considered.

Diagnosis

Currently the diagnosis of CF requires both a history compatible with the disease and the finding of elevated sodium and/or chloride concentrations (positive, 70 mEq/liter; indeterminate, 41-69; negative, 40) in a sample of sweat obtained by the Gibson-Cooke pilocarpine iontophoresis sweat test.[23] Because of significant variation in this test's accuracy from laboratory to laboratory, the consensus is that only findings from a laboratory regularly performing large numbers of sweat tests are acceptable.[24] Laboratories performing sweat tests infrequently may report both false positive and false negative results. For a sweat test to be reliable there must be adequate sample size (in most laboratories, at least 50 mg of sweat).[24,25] Most newborns do not produce large amounts of sweat. As a result, it may be difficult to obtain an adequate sample from a particular neonate. While it is often thought that sweat tests may be inaccurate in newborns, this difficulty reflects primarily the difficulty in getting an adequate sample of sweat. Multiple attempts may be needed to obtain an adequate sample. Once an adequate sample is obtained, however, the electrolyte concentrations can be believed, regardless of the age of the patient (as long as the patient is not severely malnourished, hypochloremic, or hyponatremic). If the result is positive, most CF centers repeat the sweat test to confirm the result. Furthermore, whenever a new family has a child in whom CF is diagnosed, a sweat test must also be obtained in all siblings (whether symptomatic or not) to rule out previously unrecognized disease (risk to siblings is 25 per cent).

Screening of newborns may be useful in the future in the identification of children at risk for CF. Screening techniques proposed in the past have ranged from analysis of meconium to a variety of blood tests and other analyses.[26,27] Currently there are several screening programs of newborns under way utilizing the immunoreactive trypsinogen (IRT) blood test.[28,29] Elevated levels of this protein are not commonly found in the blood of normal newborns and, when found, do not usually persist. Therefore a persistently elevated level of IRT is strongly suggestive of pancreatic difficulties, and, in infants, of CF in particular. In any patient with successive positive IRT tests, a sweat test is necessary. Since routine screening tests (phenylketonuria, thyroid, etc.) are not performed on many neonates in ICN's until several weeks or months of life, an IRT level (which does not require enteral feedings for accuracy and does not require the infant to sweat) may need to be determined separately and relatively early in premature infants who have findings suggestive of CF. In addition, an IRT study may supply very useful supportive data (*not* diagnostic) for an infant who does not sweat sufficiently to allow a useful sweat test. Currently, IRT or other screening tests need further study prior to the establishment of generalized screening programs throughout the country.[30,31]

Patient Care

Table 17–2 presents an overview of the management of an infant with cystic fibrosis.

TABLE 17–2. Sample Home Care Plan for an Infant with CF and CLD*

1. **Diet**
   A. Formulas: standard cow's milk formula, Pregestimil or Portagen, Vivonex (rarely breast milk, *not* soy formula); may need to be increased in caloric density
      1. Amount: 100–180 cc/kg/day
      2. Calories: 120–160 cal/kg/day
      3. Route: oral or by nasogastric tube (if there is a gastrostomy, by gastrostomy tube)
   B. Solids: add as for a similar patient without CF
   C. Supplements: MCT Oil (or safflower oil), Polycose, other commercial supplements (nonfat dry milk powder, instant breakfast drink, etc.)
2. **Medications**
   A. Enzyme replacement: Pancrease or Cotazym-S, $\frac{1}{2}$–2 caps/meal (if needed, Viokase powder, $\frac{1}{8}$–$\frac{1}{2}$ tsp/meal)
   B. Vitamins
      1. Multivitamins: Poly-Vi-Sol or other multivitamins used routinely
      2. A: Aquasol A 5,000–10,000 units/day
      3. D: Vitamin D usually provided by milk and multivitamin
      4. E: Aquasol E 50 IU/day for infants
      5. K: Mephyton 2.5 (infant): 10 mg (older child) orally twice a week, for patients with severe liver disease and/or previous bleeding problems, especially when being treated with antibiotics.
   C. Minerals
      1. Iron: Fer-In-Sol—provide if patient is iron deficient
      2. Zinc: provide if patient is zinc-deficient.
   D. Antibiotics
      1. For pulmonary exacerbations in outpatients: amoxicillin, trimethoprim-sulfa methoxazole, Ceclor, Keflex, cloxacillin, or other antibiotics of similar spectrum, in usual doses recommended for pneumonia
      2. IV antibiotics to cover *Pseudomonas* if patient hospitalized (consider also coverage of *Staphylococcus* and *Hemophilus influenzae*)
      3. Inhalation antibiotics: aminoglycosides – not usually needed for infants
   E. Bronchodilators
      1. Aerosols (with percussion and postural drainage treatments and as needed for wheezing): Bronkosol, Alupent, salbutamol or other, administered with a compressor such as a MediMist or a PulmoAid
      2. Theophylline: in children with frequent wheezing; adjust dose to achieve peak levels of 12–18 μg/ml
      3. Oral beta-agonists: if other bronchodilators are not successful or cannot be tolerated
   F. Others: as indicated (e.g., digoxin, cromolyn, diuretics, steroids, electrolyte supplements)
3. **Percussion and postural drainage**
   1 to 2 times/day when "well," 4–6 times/day when "ill"; often an important reason for hospitalization
4. **Oxygen**
   If needed, sufficient flow (nasal cannula) to maintain $PO_2 \geq 60$ torr at all times (awake, asleep, eating)

* Trade names used are for examples only, not recommendations of one product over another. Consult with the specific CF center providing care when implementing a plan such as this.

Gastrointestinal Problems

ENZYME SUPPLEMENTATION

The mainstay of treatment for malabsorption in infants with CF is pancreatic enzyme supplementation.[12] There has been marked improvement in these preparations over the past 10 to 20 years. Previously, crude extracts of pancreas were used. Such crude enzyme powder is sensitive to inactivation by the acid in the stomach and is, therefore, variable in its effectiveness. More recently, several preparations of microencapsulated enzymes have been released.[12,32] These preparations are relatively resistant to inactivation by stomach acid[33] and appear to provide more uniform and effective control of malabsorption than earlier preparations. One problem is that these newer preparations come in only one size capsule, and it may be excessive for very small infants. It is therefore up to the caregiver to subdivide the capsule into appropriate doses. This can be time consuming and somewhat variable over time. In addition, the microspheres may not pass through a small feeding tube very easily, making these preparations difficult to use in small infants receiving nasogastric feedings.

Since there is no specific dose of enzyme (either the powder or a microencapsulated preparation) for a child of a given weight, treatment is customarily initiated at a relatively low level; stool frequency and consistency are then observed every few days and the dosage adjusted accordingly. Signs of inadequate enzyme supplementation are the continuance of bulky, foul-smelling, or frequent stools, excessive flatulence, poor growth, excessive appetite, abdominal distention, and "colicky" distress. Excessive amounts of enzyme supplements (of either type) may cause severe perirectal rash or skin excoriation as well as constipation. Since it is common to find microspheres in the stool, this finding alone does not indicate that the child is receiving too much supplement or that he or she "can't take" the microencapsulated enzyme supplements. Patients who are receiving non-microencapsulated enzyme preparations may also have oral mucosal damage and oral pain or bleeding. The microencapsulated forms of enzymes can be given in small amounts of such vehicles as cherry syrup, applesauce, or cereal. They can also be adsorbed to the surface of a nipple in karo syrup and then licked off when the patient feeds through the nipple. Conventional powders (such as Viokase) are given in a small amount of formula or food. These powders will cause milk to curdle in a short time and therefore need to be given quickly in a small volume rather than being added to a whole bottle.

DIETARY CONSIDERATIONS

Dietary recommendations vary among CF centers. In general, sick patients with CF require adequate protein and increased calorie intakes.[34,35] Soy-based formula is generally discouraged in patients with CF.[10,13,36] Prolonged use of soy formula can predispose an infant with CF (particularly with unrecognized CF and therefore not receiving enzyme supplements) to protein calorie malnutrition.[10,13] There is controversy about the role of breast milk in the feeding of CF infants. Since early attachment is often challenging during ICN hospitalization, those mothers who are able to continue breast feeding may help themselves emotionally adapt to the diagnosis of CF. Thus, concurrence with the family's desire for feeding preference is probably appropriate, assuming that pancreatic supplementation is adequate and that close office follow-up is possible. One does need to be certain that weight gain is adequate in such infants and that serum protein levels (albumin, total protein, prealbumin) remain in the normal range. There is some justification for administering Pregestimil or other predigested formula for infants with CF.[37] In particular, in cases that are difficult to regulate with enzyme supplements, protein absorption and growth may improve when the child is given a predigested or elemental formula. Unfortunately, such formulas are expensive, and they are not very palatable. As a general rule, therefore, they may not be appropriate, especially for infants who can take all of their feedings by mouth.

Inasmuch as many patients with CF, as well as most ICN graduates, have some catch-up growth to accomplish, caloric intakes of 120 to 150 cal/kg/day may be recommended.[6,38,39] Since there have been no controlled trials comparing growth in paired groups of CF infants with different caloric intakes, it is not possible to define exactly how many calories are needed for growth in these infants. Children with CLD (bronchopulmonary dysplasia or CF) who have increased work of breathing might be expected to need a greater caloric intake than those who have very little lung disease. Furthermore, infants who are hypoxic may need extra calories for sustained growth.[40] In patients with CLD who need fluid restriction[41] (see also Chapter

14) as well as large amounts of calories, calorie-dense formulas (30 to 40 cal/ounce) may be needed. Some CF centers recommend a diet containing less fat. Others utilize a normal diet. In general, while use of fat-restricted diets may minimize the amount of malabsorption and steatorrhea observed, such treatment may also diminish the caloric intake. It is frequently possible, through manipulation of enzyme supplementation, to minimize the amount of steatorrhea even in children receiving regular diets. It is important to avoid essential fatty acid deficiency states. When the weather is hot, in young infants with CF electrolytes should be monitored to assure that the intake of salt and fluid is adequate for the amount of sweating (with its associated loss of sodium and chloride) they do.

VITAMINS AND MINERALS

Vitamin supplementation is recommended in all patients with CF.[42] Most centers suggest routine use of a multivitamin as well as supplementation with fat-soluble vitamins (A and E routinely, plus K in patients with severe liver disease or bleeding tendencies). Average suggested doses include vitamin A (5,000 to 10,000 units/day), vitamin E (50 to 200 IU/day), and vitamin K (depending on size, 2 to 10 mg twice a week).[43] In addition, some infants with CF can be documented to have diminished levels of zinc.[44] Thus, zinc supplementation as well may be beneficial for certain patients. There is some evidence that addition of large doses of other minerals such as selenium may even be harmful in these patients.[45] Maintenance of adequate oxygen-carrying capacity may be difficult in infants who have been chronically ill in the nursery and in those who have significant lung disease. Therefore the addition of iron supplements may benefit some of these infants, in spite of their potential for an inadequate erythroid response to hypoxia.[46]

INTESTINAL OBSTRUCTION

The problem of intestinal obstruction occurs relatively frequently in CF patients. Although excessive use of enzyme supplements may lead to relative constipation, in older patients the appearance of abdominal distention with pain and findings of partial obstruction are more suggestive of a meconium ileus equivalent.[47] This problem stems from the presence of inspissated intestinal secretions in the intestine with partial obstruction or intussusception. Treatment of this problem includes provision of adequate amounts of enzyme supplements orally, as well as enemas, with or without Gastrografin or Mucomyst.[47] The premature infant with necrotizing enterocolitis may have recurrent abdominal distention and partial bowel obstruction.[48] However, the interaction between previous necrotizing enterocolitis and partial small-bowel obstruction in relation to CF is not known. Thus the neonate who has recurrent episodes of abdominal distention may have problems related to either diagnosis or to both.

Pulmonary Problems

COMMON PULMONARY FINDINGS

Pulmonary dysfunction is frequently the finding that leads to recognition of CF.[14-16] This may be in the form of chronic cough, bronchiolitis, recurrent wheezing, or pneumonia. However, the infant who has bronchopulmonary dysplasia (BPD or CLD; see Chapter 14) may routinely demonstrate these findings,[49,50] making it difficult to distinguish them as being related to CF. Children with CF also gradually develop airway colonization with pathogens. These pathogens include *Hemophilus influenzae, Staphylococcus aureus,* and *Pseudomonas aeruginosa.* One might expect the time of colonization to be shortened in a patient with CF who requires use of a ventilator in the ICN compared to children with CF who do not require ventilation. Because of the difficulties encountered in obtaining cultures from the tracheas of small infants who are not intubated, this has not been documented. Furthermore, the problems typical of CLD in neonates are also found in CF patients. In other words, airway reactivity, wheezing, tracheobronchitis, recurrent pneumonia, and hyperinflation are all found in both groups of patients.

Older patients with CF have an increased incidence of airway reactivity (compared to normal individuals) as documented by histamine inhalation challenge tests or reversibility of airway obstruction following inhalation of bronchodilators.[51,52] Patients with BPD also have an increased incidence of airway reactivity and responsiveness to bronchodilators.[53] They also have an increased likelihood of a family history of reactive airway disease.[54] Thus, airway problems could be expected to be magnified even further in the BPD patient who has CF. While most young infants with CF do not require oxygen until they have significant pulmonary deterioration, one would expect that the premature infant with CLD and CF might have a prolonged course of weaning from oxygen. This has not been documented.

CHEST PHYSIOTHERAPY

Physical therapy, with percussion and postural drainage and inhalation of bronchodilators, appears to play an important role in the pulmonary care of most ICN graduates with lung disease, perhaps because of poor mucociliary clearance.[55] Such treatments are rational for CF patients as well. Although it has not been shown that a patient with newly diagnosed CF who does not yet have recognized lung disease will actually benefit from early institution of percussion and postural drainage, the presence of tenacious secretions makes such treatment rational. The ICN graduate with CLD who has impaired mucociliary clearance and increased secretions also requires frequent physical therapy. Administration of bronchodilators by either the oral or inhalation route may improve both airway caliber and mucociliary clearance.[56] The ICN graduate with CF should therefore be sent home with a compressor that allows administration of aerosol bronchodilator medications.

ANTIBIOTICS

The efficacy of routine antibiotic administration to the patient with CF has not been clearly demonstrated. Antibiotics are warranted at some time in the course of all cases of CF.[57] Some centers continually provide antibiotics to all patients with CF on a rotating basis, from the time of diagnosis throughout life. Others provide antibiotics only when there is a pulmonary deterioration (or other obvious indication such as otitis media). Since antibiotic administration is only one part of a complex medical treatment regimen, its efficacy in improving pulmonary function or reducing the rate of pulmonary deterioration in otherwise well infants has not been shown. There appears to be general agreement that antibiotics should be administered relatively freely in CF patients who do have pulmonary deterioration. The impaired mucociliary clearance associated with viral illness puts the patient with CF at increased risk for later bacterial infection of the lung. Furthermore, the prolonged colonization of the airway with the pathogens discussed earlier puts such infants with CF at risk for pneumonia, chronic bronchitis, or bronchiectasis. Antibiotics are probably used more frequently in neonates with CLD than in neonates who do not have CLD. The finding of CF in such a child makes such antibiotic administration even more rational.

IMMUNIZATIONS

Because of the lack of nonimmunized patients with CF, it has not been documented whether administration of vaccines to infants with CF improves the outcome. However, like other children, these infants should be given the routine immunizations of childhood, especially against pertussis, assuming they do not have progressive neurologic disorders or poorly controlled seizures. In addition, young children with CF should probably also receive influenza,[58] pneumococcal, and Hemophilus influenzae vaccines.

Genetic Counseling

Genetic counseling is an important part of the comprehensive care of patients with CF.[59] As noted in the introduction, there are specific recurrence risks for CF in families who have a child with CF. In this way, the diagnosis of CF adds a new dimension to the reproductive planning of families who have a baby in an ICN. In addition to the genetic counseling usually given to an individual set of parents of a child with CF, the parents are usually urged to share the counseling information with their siblings and other family members. In this way the possibility of the carrier state is brought to the attention of appropriate family members. Unfortunately there is no reliable test currently available to detect CF carriers or to diagnose CF in utero. However, major research efforts are under way in both areas.[60]

Recently, it has been possible to use DNA probes to identify restriction fragment length polymorphisms that are tightly linked to the CF gene. These probes have been used successfully for prenatal diagnosis and carrier analysis in cultured amniotic fluid cells or chorionic villi.[61,62,63,64]

Psychosocial Support

Psychosocial support is important for parents of patients with CF and should be initiated at the earliest possible time. The time of diagnosis of CF is a stressful one in all families. However, it has not been shown whether that stress is more easily accepted or more successfully worked through in families in which the patient was seriously ill because of prematurity (or other neonatal problems) or because of CF. Large amounts of literature for parents and well-trained psychosocial personnel are available in virtually every CF center across the country. However, the availability of such personnel at the referral center is not a reason for the primary care giver to retreat from the support his or her patient's family needs. Families of patients with CF must realize that while their children are in need of large amounts of special care, they are not particularly fragile. They may face significant future illness, but they are still children who need to grow and develop as normally as possible within their home environment. This concept may be somewhat easier to convey for the doctor who is accustomed to caring for ICN graduates than for the doctor who normally cares for well infants.

Subspecialist Care

All patients with CF should be referred to the nearest CF center soon after diagnosis (if they did not go there for the sweat test). This referral not only improves the record keeping and statistics of the National Cystic Fibrosis Foundation, but more importantly, it provides the family contact with subspecialists (including pulmonologists, gastroenterologists, nutritionists, physical therapists, nurses, and social workers) who are able to provide the multiple types of care and counseling that families of CF patients require. It also allows the patient and family to have contact with other families and children with CF. When families are first presented with the diagnosis of CF, they frequently have many questions about the disease, the diagnosis, and what the future holds. These can initially be answered with most assurance and accuracy by personnel who have cared for a large number of such patients. However, the family's primary care giver can and should provide essential support and reassurance.

The young patient with CF also has need for routine medical care. Pediatric care needs are compounded in the child with CF who was also a premature infant and who has the problems associated with an extended stay in an ICN. In such a setting, patient management should be shared by the primary physician, the neonatal follow-up clinic, and the CF center. It is important to have easy communication between all

members of the health care team, regardless of their particular contribution to the patient's care. Specific guidelines should be given to the family recommending whom they should contact for what kinds of problems. Unfortunately, because of the wide spectrum of clinical problems in infants with CF, no general rule can be given about when a patient should see which type of physician. The single most important aspect of this "shared care" is the maintenance of open communication between the primary physician and the CF center. In that way, danger signs can be listed that are particularly relevant to the specific patient, and the family can be counseled appropriately. Most patients with CF require only intermittent contact at the CF center as long as they are getting routine medical follow-up from their primary physician. However, not all hospitals are able to provide the inpatient care necessary to give optimal pulmonary toilet and administer medication to young infants with CF. As a result, most CF centers have particular preferences about which hospitals in their referral areas are appropriate for the admission of a young infant with CF when there is deterioration of his or her status. The problems of prematurity, CLD, and other sequelae of ICN care only make that difficulty worse. As a result, ICN graduates who have CF should probably be hospitalized almost exclusively at tertiary centers.

Pulmonary Function

The quantitation of pulmonary function in young infants (whether they have CLD or CF) is difficult. Oxygenation measurements are helpful in defining the course of lung disease.[65] Chest radiographs are also useful, and scoring systems have been proposed for quantitation of roentgenographic findings.[66] Unfortunately, conventional pulmonary function testing is not readily available for children below the age of 5 or 6 years. However, great progress is being made in the development of pulmonary function tests to assess pulmonary pathophysiology in infants who are below the ages at which they can cooperate.[67,68]

RESOURCES

Both local and national offices of the Cystic Fibrosis Foundation are available as sources of information both to members of the medical team and to parents. It is generally recommended that both families and medical personnel with general questions about CF contact their closest CF clinical center first. Depending on the information requested, personnel at that center may answer the question or refer the questioner to either the local CF chapter (often listed in the phone book) or the national CF group. Questions about fund raising, donations, volunteer work, or other nonmedical concerns should probably be initially directed to the local CF chapter. The address of the National Cystic Fibrosis Foundation is 6000 Executive Boulevard, Suite 510, Rockville, Maryland, 20852; phone (301) 881-9130.

Overall, patients with CF present many challenges to the personnel who provide their care. That care is complex, prolonged, and expensive. It requires the dedication of all concerned (patient, family, health care team) for it to be provided effectively. Both medical and psychosocial problems will be magnified in a patient with CF who also is an ICN graduate. However, neither CF nor neonatal problems necessarily condemn an infant to a short, painful, and tragic life. The course of CF, ranging from mild to severe disease manifestations, is impossible to predict for any given patient at the outset. Thus the care of these children requires both hope and reality. It is in this context that the practice of medicine, for the patient, the family, and the health care provider, can be its most challenging and its most rewarding.

References

1. Steinberg AG, Brown DC: On the incidence of cystic fibrosis of the pancreas. Am J Hum Genet 12:416, 1960.
2. Kulczycki LL, Schauf V: Cystic fibrosis in blacks in Washington, D.C. Am J Dis Child 127:64, 1974.
3. Donnison AB, Schwachman H, Gross RE: A review of 164 children with meconium ileus seen at the Children's Hospital Medical Center, Boston. Pediatrics 37:833, 1966.
4. Shigemoto H, Endo S, Isomoto T, et al.: Neonatal meconium obstruction in the ileum without mucoviscidosis. J Pediatr Surg 13:475, 1978.
5. Jones TW, Schutt RP: Alimentary tract obstruction in the newborn infant; A review and analysis of 132 cases. Pediatrics 20:881, 1957.
6. Reichman BL, Chessex P, Putet G, et al.: Partition of energy metabolism and energy cost of growth in the very low-birth weight infant. Pediatrics 69:446, 1982.
7. Oppenheimer EH, Esterly JR: Pathology of cystic fibrosis. Review of literature and comparison with 146 autopsied cases. Perspect Pediatr Pathol 2:241, 1975.
8. Imrie JR, Fagan DG, Sturgess JM: Quantitative evaluation of the development of the exocrine pancreas in cystic fibrosis and control infants. Am J Pathol 95:697, 1979.
9. Lapey A, Kattwinkel J, di Sant'Agnese PA, et al.: Steatorrhea and azotorrhea and their relation to growth and nutrition in adolescents and young adults with cystic fibrosis. J Pediatr 84:328, 1974.
10. Fleischer DS, DiGeorge AM, Barness LA, Cornfield D: Hypoproteinemia and edema in infants with cystic fibrosis of the pancreas. J Pediatr 64:341, 1964.
11. Nielson OH, Larsen BF: Incidence of anemia, hypoproteinemia, and edema in infants as presenting signs of cystic fibrosis. J Pediatr Gastr Nutr 2:545, 1982.
12. Cho Y, Aviado D: Clinical pharmacology for pediatricians. Pancreatic enzyme preparations with special reference to enterically coated microspheres of pancrelipase. J Clin Pharmacol 21:224, 1981.
13. Abman SH, Accurso FJ, Bowman CM: Persistent morbidity and mortality of protein calorie malnutrition in young infants with CF. J Pediatr Gastr Nutr 5:393, 1986.
14. di Sant'Agnese PA: Pulmonary manifestations of fibrocystic disease of the pancreas. Dis Chest 27:654, 1955.
15. Lamarre A, Reilly BJ, Bryan AC, et al.: Early detection of pulmonary function abnormalities in cystic fibrosis. Pediatrics 50:291, 1972.
16. Lloyd-Still JD, Khaw KT, Schwachman H: Severe respiratory disease in infants with cystic fibrosis. Pediatrics 53:678, 1974.
17. Schwachman H, Holsclaw DS: Pulmonary complications of cystic fibrosis. Minn Med 52:1521, 1969.
18. Huang NN, Van Loon EL, Sheng KT: The flora of the respiratory tract of patients with cystic fibrosis of the pancreas. J Pediatr 59:512, 1961.
19. Reynolds HY, di Sant'Agnese PA, Zierdt CH: Mucoid *Pseudomonas aeruginosa:* A sign of cystic fibrosis in young adults with chronic pulmonary disease? JAMA 236:2190, 1976.
20. Isles A, Maclusky I, Corey M, et al.: *Pseudomonas cepacia* infection in cystic fibrosis: An emerging problem. J Pediatr 104:206, 1984.
21. Usher RH. The special problems of the premature infant. In Avery GB (ed.): Neonatology: Pathophysiology and Management of the Newborn, 2nd ed. Philadelphia, J.B. Lippincott Company, 1981, pp 247–250.
22. di Sant'Agnese PA, Darling R, Perera G, et al.: Abnormal electrolyte composition of sweat in cystic fibrosis of the pancreas. Pediatrics 12:549, 1953.
23. Gibson LE, Cooke RE: A test for concentration of electrolytes in sweat in cystic fibrosis of the pancreas utilizing pilocarpine by iontophoresis. Pediatrics 23:545, 1959.
24. Report of the Committee for a Study for Evaluation of Testing for Cystic Fibrosis. J Pediatr 88:711, 1976.
25. Denning CR, Huang NN, Cuasay LR, et al.: Cooperative study comparing three methods of performing sweat tests to diagnose cystic fibrosis. 66:752, 1980.
26. Stephan U, Busch EW, Kollberg H, et al.: Cystic fibrosis detection by means of a test strip. Pediatrics 55:35, 1975.
27. Robinson PG, Elliott RB: Cystic fibrosis screening in the newborn. Arch Dis Child 51:301, 1976.
28. Wilcken B, Towns SJ, Mellis CM: Diagnostic delay in cystic fibrosis: Lessons from newborn screening. Arch Dis Child 58:863, 1983.
29. Reardon MC, Hammond KB, Accurso FJ, et al.: Nutritional deficits exist before 2 months of age in some infants with cystic fibrosis identified by screening test. J Pediatr 105:271, 1984.
30. Ad Hoc Committee Task Force on Neonatal Screening. CF Foundation: Neonatal screening for CF: Position Paper. Pediatrics 72:741, 1983.

31. Farrell PM: Early diagnosis of cystic fibrosis: To screen or not to screen — An important question. Pediatrics 73:115, 1984.

32. Nassif EG, Younoszai MK, Weinberger MM, et al.: Comparative effects of antacids, enteric coating, and bile salts on the efficacy of oral pancreatic enzyme therapy in cystic fibrosis. J Pediatr 98:320, 1981.

33. Gow R, Bradbear R, Francis P, et al.: Comparative study of varying regimens to improve steatorrhea and creatorrhea in cystic fibrosis: Effectiveness of an enteric-coated preparation with and without antacids and cimetidine. Lancet 2:1071, 1981.

34. Huang NN, Holsclaw D, Hilman BC, et al.: Dietary care. In Huang NN (ed.): Guide to Drug Therapy in Patients with Cystic Fibrosis. Atlanta, The National Cystic Fibrosis Research Foundation, 1972.

35. Shepherd R, Cooksley WGE, Cooke WDD: Improved growth and clinical, nutritional and respiratory changes in response to nutritional therapy in cystic fibrosis. J Pediatr 97:351, 1980.

36. Fleischer DS, DiGeorge AM, Auerbach VH, et al.: Protein metabolism in cystic fibrosis of the pancreas. J Pediatr 64:349, 1964.

37. West CD, Wilson JL, Eyles R: Blood amino nitrogen levels: Changes in blood amino nitrogen levels following ingestion of proteins and a protein hydrolysate in infants with normal and with deficient pancreatic function. Am J Dis Child 72:251, 1946.

38. Berry HK, Kellogg FW, Hunt MM, et al.: Dietary supplement and nutrition in children with cystic fibrosis. Am J Dis Child 129:165, 1975.

39. Hubbard VS, Mangrum PJ: Energy intake and nutritional counseling in cystic fibrosis. J Am Diet Assoc 80:127, 1982.

40. Huse DM, Feldt RH, Nelson RA, Novak LP: Infants with congenital heart disease: Food intake, body weight and energy metabolism. Am J Dis Child 129:65, 1975.

41. Kao LC, Warburton D, Sargent CW, et al.: Furosemide acutely decreases airways resistance in chronic bronchopulmonary dysplasia. J Pediatr 103:624, 1983.

42. Chase HP, Long MA, Lavin MH: Cystic fibrosis and malnutrition. J Pediatr 95:337, 1979.

43. Farrell PM, Hubbard VS: Nutrition in cystic fibrosis: Vitamins, fatty acids, and minerals. In Lloyd-Still JD (ed.): Textbook of Cystic Fibrosis. Littleton, MA. John Wright–PSG Inc., Publishers, 1983, pp 263–292.

44. Jacob RA, Sandstead HH, Solomons NW, et al.: Zinc status and vitamin A transport in cystic fibrosis. Am J Clin Nutr 31:638, 1978.

45. Snodgrass W, Rumack B, Sullivan J, et al.: Selenium: Childhood poisoning and cystic fibrosis. Clin Toxicol 18:211, 1981.

46. Vichinsky EP, Pennathur-Das R, Nickerson B, et al.: Inadequate erythroid response to hypoxia in cystic fibrosis. J Pediatr 105:15, 1984.

47. Jaffe BF, Graham WP III, Goldman L: Postinfancy intestinal obstruction in children with cystic fibrosis. Arch Surg 92:337, 1966.

48. Avery GB, Fletcher AB: Nutrition. In Avery GB (ed.): Neonatology: Pathophysiology and Management of the Newborn, 2nd ed. Philadelphia, J.B. Lippincott Company, 1981, pp 1049–1051.

49. Bancalari E, Abdenour GF, Feller R, Gannon J: Bronchopulmonary dysplasia: Clinical presentation. J Pediatr 95:819, 1979.

50. Smyth JA, Tabachnik E, Duncan WJ, et al.: Pulmonary function and bronchial hyperreactivity in long-term survivors of bronchopulmonary dysplasia. Pediatrics 68:336, 1981.

51. Mitchell I, Corey M, Woenne R, et al.: Bronchial hyperreactivity in cystic fibrosis and asthma. J Pediatr 93:744, 1978.

52. Larsen GL, Barron RJ, Landay RA, et al.: Intravenous aminophylline in patients with cystic fibrosis. Am J Dis Child 134:1143, 1980.

53. Kao LC, Warburton D, Platzker ACG, Keens TG: Effect of isoproterenol inhalation on airway resistance in chronic bronchopulmonary dysplasia. Pediatrics 73:509, 1984.

54. Nickerson BG, Taussig LM: Family history of asthma in infants with bronchopulmonary dysplasia. Pediatrics 65:1140, 1980.

55. Lee RMKW, Rossman CM, O'Brodovich H, et al.: Ciliary defects associated with the development of bronchopulmonary dysplasia: Ciliary motility and ultrastructure. Am Rev Respir Dis 129:190, 1984.

56. Wood RE, Wanner A, Hirsch J, Farrell PM: Tracheal mucociliary transport in patients with cystic fibrosis and its stimulation by terbutaline. Am Rev Respir Dis 111:733, 1975.

57. Hyatt AC, Chipps BE, Kumor KM, et al.: A double-blind controlled trial of anti-*Pseudomonas* chemotherapy of acute respiratory exacerbations in patients with cystic fibrosis. J Pediatr 99:307, 1981.

58. Cate TR, Miller GB, Mostow SR, Ruben FL: Influenza vaccines 1982–1983. ATS News p 6, 1982.

59. Valentine GH: The reproductive counseling process. Comments based on experience. Clin Pediatr 16:233, 1977.

60. Branchini BR, Salituro GM, Rosenstein BJ: Identification of the major 4-methylumbelliferyl p-guanidino-benzoate-hydrolyzing plasma protein in cystic fibrosis: Implication for intrauterine and heterozygote detection. Pediatr Res 17:850, 1983.

61. Dean M, O'Connell P, Leppert M, et al.: Three additional DNA polymorphisms in the **met** gene and D7S8 locus: Use in prenatal diagnosis of cystic fibrosis. J Pediatr 111:490, 1987.

62. Tsui L-C, Buchwald M, Barker D, et al.: Cystic fibrosis locus defined by a genetically linked polymorphic DNA marker. Science 230:1054, 1985.

63. White R, Woodward S, Leppert M, et al.: A closely linked genetic marker for cystic fibrosis. Nature 318:382, 1985.

64. Farrall M, Rodeck CH, Stanier P, et al.: First-trimester prenatal diagnosis of cystic fibrosis with linked DNA probes. Lancet 1:1402, 1986.

65. Phillips AGS, Peabody JL, Lucey JF: Transcutaneous PO$_2$ monitoring in the home management of bronchopulmonary dysplasia. Pediatrics 61:655, 1978.

66. Brasfield D, Hicks G, Soong SJ, et al.: The chest roentgenogram in cystic fibrosis: A new scoring system. Pediatrics 63:24, 1979.

67. Godfrey S, Mearns M, Howlett G: Serial lung function studies in cystic fibrosis in the first five years of life. Arch Dis Child 53:83, 1978.

68. Godfrey S, Bar-Yishay E, Arad I, et al.: Flow-volume curves in infants with lung disease. Pediatrics 72:517, 1983.

Recommended Reading

Cho Y, Aviado D: Clinical pharmacology for pediatricians. Pancreatic enzyme preparations with special reference to enterically coated microspheres of pancrelipase. J Clin Pharmacol 21:224, 1981.

Donnison AB, Schwachman H, Gross RE: A review of 164

children with meconium ileus seen at the Children's Hospital Medical Center, Boston. Pediatrics 37:833, 1966.

Gurwitz D, Corey M, Francis PWJ, et al.: Perspectives in Cystic Fibrosis. Pediatr Clin North Am 26:603, 1979.

Lloyd-Still J (ed.): Textbook of Cystic Fibrosis. Littleton, MA, John Wright–PSG, Inc., Publishers, 1983.

Lloyd-Still JD, Khaw KT, Schwachman H: Severe respiratory disease in infants with cystic fibrosis. Pediatrics 53:678, 1974.

Matthews LW, Drotar D: Cystic fibrosis — A challenging long-term chronic disease. Pediatr Clin North Am 31:133, 1984.

Nassif EG, Younoszai MK, Weinberger MM, et al.: Comparative effects of antacids, enteric coating, and bile salts on the efficacy of oral pancreatic enzyme therapy in cystic fibrosis. J Pediatr 92:320, 1981.

Shepherd R, Cooksley WGE, Cooke WDD: Improved growth and clinical, nutritional and respiratory changes in response to nutritional therapy in cystic fibrosis. J Pediatr 97:351, 1980.

Waring WW: Current management of cystic fibrosis. Adv Pediatr 23:401, 1976.

Wood RE, Boat TF, Doershuk CF: State of the art. Cystic Fibrosis. Am Rev Respir Dis 113:833, 1976.

18

CARE OF ICN GRADUATES AFTER NEONATAL SURGERY

ALFRED A. DE LORIMIER, M.D.

This chapter focuses on special problems of infants who are born with either congenital anomalies or tumors that require surgery in the newborn period or those who require operation for complications of other problems during their neonatal course. It is not meant to be a complete discussion of the surgical problems found in either newborns or infants and will not deal with issues related to care in the immediate neonatal period. Rather, it will focus on issues that will be brought to the physician caring for these infants after discharge from the nursery.

SURGICAL PROBLEMS INVOLVING THE NECK

The most significant postsurgical problems in this area are lesions that make up the cystic hygroma–lymphangioma spectrum.

Congenital Problems

CYSTIC HYGROMA

A true cystic hygroma is a congenital abnormality that is well circumscribed and can be completely resected. Since this problem is resolved after operation, it is possible to reassure the parents that their infant should ordinarily not be expected to have any further problems. Occasionally, however, small satellite lesions may be present, which may enlarge later and may require a second, or even a third, surgical extirpation. The ultimate outcome should still be complete recovery. The problems that may occur later are related to the necessarily very aggressive resection of the tumor from the brachial plexus. Occasionally this produces lymphedema of the face or extremity until collateral drainage develops. Because this may take up to a year, parents may require reassurance. Another problem may result from occlusion of the subclavian vein, leading to the development of collateral venous plexuses that are visible at the shoulder and neck and may be unsightly and long lasting.

LYMPHANGIOMA

Lymphangiomas are extremely radioresistant tumors that may be very large and occasionally are fatal. These tumors, as opposed to cystic hygromas, infiltrate adjacent structures; therefore, complete resection is uncommon. Recurrence of tumor is likely, and repeated surgical debulking will be required. The goal of these procedures is to approximate symmetry of the face, neck, and extremities. The major problems encountered in these infants include lesions that develop in the scars of previous surgical resections and form blisters that are subject to secondary infection and lymphangitis. Long-term antibiotic administration may be required in such situations. The usual course of a lymphangioma in children requires repeated surgical procedures, with an ultimate goal of symmetry and stability of the lesion by approximately 4 or 5 years of age.

HEMANGIOMA

Although ICN graduates are not particularly prone to hemangiomas, compared with other infants, their course may be complicated by these lesions. In particular, there may be concern when a hemangioma involves the airway in infants who already have some respiratory difficulty secondary to their neonatal course. The possibility of airway involvement by hemangioma must be considered in an infant with visible hemangiomas who experiences worsening respiratory symptoms. In this situation, consultation with a surgeon is recommended. The glottic or subglottic areas of the larynx are most commonly affected. The child may need a tracheostomy for 1 to 3 years while awaiting spontaneous regression of the hemangioma.

PIERRE ROBIN SYNDROME

In general, surgical procedures that have been suggested for infants with Pierre Robin syndrome are not helpful. Symptomatic airway obstruction will require tracheostomy, and gastrostomy may be indicated in some instances to facilitate feeding if swallowing is impaired. (See Chapters 14 and 24.)

COMPLICATIONS OF NEONATAL COURSE

TRACHEOSTOMY

The issues for the parents and physician of an infant discharged from the ICN with a tracheostomy chiefly have to do with tracheostomy care and the timing for removal of the tube.

Tracheostomy Care (See Also Chapter 15 and Appendix C.). The major issue in tracheostomy care is careful suctioning of the tube with an end-hole catheter. The catheter should not be passed beyond the end of the tube, since doing so may result in further trauma to the mucosal lining of the airway. Another very important aspect of tracheostomy care is to pay strict attention to humidification, particularly in very dry climates. A common problem is the development of granulation tissue around the tracheostomy site, leading to bleeding and mucopurulent discharge. The purulent discharge will usually contain *Staphylococcus aureus* or *pseudomonas* organisms; However, antibiotics are not automatically indicated, usless there is cellulitis of the surrounding skin of the neck. By the trimming away or cauterizing of granulomatous tissue, the purulent drainage can usually be controlled. Small areas can be cauterized with silver nitrate sticks. Parents may be supplied with these for use at home, but if granulation tissue protrudes very prominently, surgical resection may be required. In general, management of this problem should be directed by the surgeon who performed the tracheostomy.

Removal of the Tracheostomy Tube. Whether or not a tracheostomy tube can be removed, of course, depends upon the indications for its placement initially. In infants with bilateral laryngeal nerve palsy, tracheostomy is permanent. Airway involvement with hemangioma will require tracheostomy for several years, until the tumor has regressed. Residual tumor encroaching on the airway may be resected with laser or direct excision. When the indication for tracheostomy was subglottic stenosis, careful periodic assessment is needed to determine the child's readiness for a surgical procedure that will enlarge and stabilize the airway.

A major group of ICN graduates with tracheostomies are those who have required long-term assisted ventilation. (See Chapter 16.) In these children, plugging the tracheostomy opening for a time will identify whether the airway is sufficiently patent for removal of the tube. However, evidence of persistent obstruction of the airway may indicate growth of granulation tissue into the trachea compromising the lumen. Removal of the granulation tissue may establish a satisfactory airway. In addition, various degrees of tracheomalacia develop in the area of the tracheostomy, with resulting collapse and obstruction with exhalation. In infants or children, if a tracheostomy is to be removed, the associated exuberant granulation tissue and tracheomalacia can be treated by excision of the tracheostomy tract and primary closure of the wound. The importance of education and support cannot be overemphasized in the home care of an infant with a tracheostomy. (See Appendix C for guidelines for tracheostomy care.)

Speech Development. Some children who

have long-term tracheostomies experience some degree of difficulty in their speech development, despite their ability to close off the tracheostomy site with their chins and thereby vocalize. It is useful to teach some of these children (and their parents) sign language, to reduce frustration and encourage communication. It is advisable to refer any child with a tracheostomy for speech evaluation at the age when speech would be expected.

SURGICAL PROBLEMS OF THE CHEST

TRACHEOESOPHAGEAL FISTULA

The physician caring for children who have undergone an operation to repair esophageal atresia or a tracheoesophageal fistula (TEF) must be aware that many ongoing problems are likely to be encountered. Parents are commonly so relieved and overjoyed at taking their infant home that they often appear not to have understood the long-term implications of his or her condition. Primarily they fail to understand that the surgical procedure did not correct all of the infant's difficulties. Common problems that may persist after repair of TEF or esophageal atresia include tracheomalacia, esophageal dysmotility, gastroesophageal reflux, stricture of the lower esophagus, and recurrent or previously undiscovered fistula. (See also Chapter 15.)

Tracheomalacia. Virtually all TEF infants have some degree of tracheomalacia. The collapse of the trachea may be confined to the area of the fistula, or the entire intrathoracic and cervical trachea may be affected. As a result, these infants have a chronic barking cough, usually until 4 or 5 years of age. The family can be reassured that this is an expected finding that will ultimately resolve. Infants with tracheomalacia who have both inspiratory and expiratory problems may experience increased difficulties during viral infections, and tracheostomy may become necessary if their breathing is seriously impaired.

Esophageal Dysmotility. All infants with TEF also have esophageal dysmotility, which necessitates careful, slow feeding. The esophagus in these patients does not have normal peristalsis; at best it is a passive conduit. However, periods of focal or massive spasm will develop in varying degrees and cause obstruction. Solid foods must often be "chased" with liquids to facilitate their progress through the esophagus.

Choking episodes may occur during the periods of spasm. Eventually the children learn to identify the sensation of the spasms and thus learn to avoid feeding during these episodes. For some time, however, it can be very frustrating for the infant and parents, because the crying from hunger is replaced by the panic of choking. Much patience is required until unimpeded swallowing is assured.

Gastroesophageal Reflux. At least 20 per cent of infants with TEF have problematic gastroesophageal (GE) reflux. Infants with GE reflux may have episodes of vomiting and choking (apparent life-threatening events), persistent vomiting with poor growth, episodes of aspiration tracheobronchitis and pneumonia, or anemia from esophagitis. In some, gastroesophageal reflux may cause fibrosis at the anastomosis site and subsequent development of a stricture. The definitive test to identify GE reflux is overnight placement of an esophageal pH probe. Any of the complications of GE reflux warrants an antireflux fundoplication.

Stricture of the Lower Esophagus. Approximately 2 per cent of children with TEF have an associated stricture of the lower esophagus not specificically related to reflux. Esophageal dilatation is usually effective in relieving the stricture, but occasionally direct surgical excision is necessary. Infants with stricture of the esophagus have choking episodes that occur with every feeding, in contrast to children with GE reflux in whom vomiting occurs intermittently and inconsistently.

Recurrent or Separate Fistula. Some infants with TEF may suffer recurrence of their fistula or may have an undiagnosed, second, H-type fistula at a level higher than the primary lesion. This latter possibility must be considered in infants with persistent coughing with virtually every swallow. Referral to the child's surgeon without undue delay is recommended.

WHEN TO WORRY

1. When a child fails to fall within the normal growth curve or at least to maintain consistent parallel growth. (Some TEF infants appear to be naturally small.)

2. When a child coughs with every swallow —Consider recurrent or secondary fistula.

3. When a child chokes and/or vomits with every feeding—Consider the possiblity of an anastomotic or lower esophageal stricture.

4. When a child has persistent vomiting with poor growth—Consider gastroesophageal reflux that may require surgical correction.

5. When a child has significant, severe choking episodes, recurrent tracheobronchitis, or pneumonia indicating aspiration—Consider the need for surgical intervention for TEF or reflux.

ROUTINE FOLLOW-UP

A child who has had TEF should be followed up by his or her surgeon, as well as the primary physician. The primary physician should pay careful attention to how much the child eats at each feeding, how long it takes, and what problems are associated with or following feedings. Parental reassurance and education concerning when to call the primary physician are essential for the child's and family's well-being.

DIAPHRAGMATIC HERNIA (SEE ALSO CHAPTER 15)

The problems after discharge home experienced by infants born with diaphragmatic hernia are related primarily to the amount of lung hypoplasia that has occurred. For those who have very little hypoplasia, a completely normal outcome can be expected. Children with more severe degrees of hypoplasia will have increased pulmonary problems, including bronchospastic disease, increased susceptibility to infection, and impaired exercise tolerance. Many children have some GE reflux after repair of a diaphragmatic hernia, and aspiration is a serious risk, given their impaired pulmonary function.

SURGICAL PROBLEMS IN THE ABDOMEN

It is beyond the scope of this chapter to deal with all the specific tumors and lesions that may occur in the newborn. For the physician providing pediatric surveillance of an infant after neonatal surgery, the main issues of care center on complications subsequent to abdominal surgery.

OBSTRUCTION

Regardless of the original reason for the operation, anyone who has had a laparotomy is at risk for developing bowel obstruction, because of adhesions. At least 5 per cent of patients who have abdominal surgery will have intestinal obstruction at some later time. The incidence is probably higher among infants who have had a complex operation during the neonatal period.

Parents should be advised to call their physician promptly if their child becomes irritable and appears to have abdominal cramps, particularly if there is bilious vomiting. The symptoms of obstruction are directly related to the site of the lesion. If the lesion is high in the intestine, obstruction may be associated with intense cramping, vomiting soon after the onset, and only minimal distention. With a lower lesion, cramping pain and abdominal distention occur early, while vomiting develops relatively late. An absence of stooling may be also noted. In assessing children with possible obstruction, listening to bowel sounds is virtually no help. Abdominal radiography, supine and upright or lateral decubitus position, will identify abnormal bowel distention with air-fluid levels. Occasionally, a small-bowel study with barium contrast will be needed.

WHEN TO WORRY

When a child with an abdominal scar:

1. Does not feel well, is irritable, and has abdominal cramps
2. Has bilious vomiting
3. When parents report pain and abdominal distention, vomiting, and absence of stooling

The physician should:

1. Obtain a plain film of the abdomen in supine and lateral decubitus or upright position to detect dilated loops of bowel and air-fluid levels
2. Establish gastric decompression with a *large* (at least 10 F) nasogastric tube with multiple side holes (preferably a sump catheter) connected to constant vacuum
3. Begin an intravenous infusion of Ringer's lactate solution with 20 mEq KC1 added
4. Send the child to the surgeon for further management

It is important to remember that a child with cramping abdominal pain and an abdominal scar has a bowel obstruction until proven otherwise. Even if the plain film of the abdomen is normal, obstruction may be present, and surgical exploration may be necessary, because there is no means to distinguish accurately between a simple and a gangrenous obstruction.

ABDOMINAL WALL DEFECTS

GASTROSCHISIS (SEE ALSO CHAPTER 15)

Although gastroschisis usually is not associated with other congenital abnormalities, infants born with this condition do have problems after discharge home. In utero, the bowel floats in the amniotic fluid for a time and becomes enveloped by fibrous inflammatory membrane. The blood supply to the bowel may also be impaired, resulting in compromised integrity of the mucosa, with areas of defective absorption or even ulceration. Infants with this condition, therefore, tend to develop malabsorption or sepsis. When an infant born with gastroschisis becomes ill, antibiotic administration should be initiated earlier than in other infants, because of their propensity for sepsis. In addition, because of malabsorption, they may have diarrhea and difficulty maintaining normal growth. Special dietary measures may be needed, and parents may need both education and reassurance with respect to their infant's nutritional care. Occasionally, parenteral nutrition may be required for several months to supplement enteral nutrition.

OMPHALOCELE (SEE ALSO CHAPTER 15)

Infants with a small omphalocele in the newborn period are not likely to have other abnormalities. However, a large omphalocele is frequently associated with other anomalies. It is therefore important to look for abnormalities of the kidneys and heart. Infants with a large omphalocele positioned cephalad toward the costal margins tend to have hypoplastic lungs. These infants usually require assisted ventilation in the nursery, and later the child may have a small chest and reduced pulmonary function. Persistence of a communication between the peritoneum and pericardium may result in herniation of bowel later on. Repair of a very large omphalocele usually requires insertion of prosthetic mesh material, and bulging or herniation of this material may occur. In addition, the mesh may ulcerate through the skin. Therefore, most surgeons will remove all of the graft, which often requires several staged procedures. Obviously, infants born with omphalocele (or gastroschisis) are at risk for bowel obstruction from adhesions as a result of their abdominal surgical procedures, and the physician must be alert to this

possibility (see When to Worry, later). These infants often have very poor growth, although no specific malabsorption syndrome associated with this anomaly has been documented. Therefore, nutritional care plays an important role in their management.

SHORT-BOWEL SYNDROME

The major reasons for extensive resection of bowel in the ICN are necrotizing enterocolitis, intestinal atresia, or volvulus. Depending upon the amount and location of the bowel resected, this surgery may result in malabsorption and malnutrition. Clark[1] has reviewed the management of short-bowel syndrome in high-risk neonates. The pediatrician supervising the care of infants with short bowel needs some understanding of the pathophysiology of the various problems, as well as knowledge of how much bowel was removed from the specific infant under his or her care. In addition, the physician needs to be aware of special formulas and nutritive additives that may be important for the patient. Intestinal adaptation can be expected to require as long as two years to develop, before a normal diet will be tolerated.

Some infants with difficult-to-manage growth failure may require parenteral nutrition at home. A discussion of this management is beyond the scope of this book, but it is reviewed by Kerner.[2]

NUTRITION

Many of the infants who are finally discharged from the ICN with short bowel have had an extremely stormy course during their hospitalization. By the time of discharge they should be tolerating enteral feedings and gaining weight.

Special Formulas. Most infants with short-bowel syndrome will require some type of special formula for the first few months at home. This will generally be recommended by the surgeon or gastroenterologist who has supervised the infant's care in the hospital and may include elemental feedings with formulas such as Vivonex, Pregestimil, or CHO-Free mixed with Polycose and triglycerides. Other formulas available include Osmolite, which is an isosmolar elemental formula capable of delivering 1 cal/ml. (See Tables 14–10 and 14–11 for a list of contents of special formulas and their osmolarity.)

Special Supplements. All infants with short bowel should receive multivitamins, as well as calcium and vitamin D supplements to prevent metabolic bone disease. Some of the infants with proximal resections will also require parenteral magnesium and supplementation with iron and folate (which also may need to be given parenterally if the infant does not tolerate them when given orally). Infants who have had a distal resection involving the ileum require parenteral vitamin B_{12} supplements as well.

Method of Feeding. Feedings and medication will be tolerated better by many of these infants if they can be administered by continuous drip. For this reason it may be useful if gastrostomy is performed and a constant perfusion pump used to administer the formula best tolerated by the infant.

PROBLEMS RELATED TO EXTENT AND TYPE OF BOWEL RESECTION

Although it is important for the pediatrician to be aware of the extent of the resection, it must be remembered that it is not possible to quantitate exactly the amount of remaining bowel. It is generally considered that more than 50 per cent of the small bowel must be removed before significant malabsorption occurs. However, survival has been documented in infants with as little as 15 cm of small bowel remaining after surgery. The site of resection is also obviously very important. Resection of the jejunum is usually tolerated relatively well. Although most nutrients are completely absorbed in the jejunum, when the jejunum is resected the ileum has a phenomenal capacity to adapt and compensate for the loss of jejunal function. However, when ileum is resected, rapid bowel transit time frequently results. The ileocecal valve is ordinarily a physiologic barrier that prolongs intestinal transit time and also prevents colonic bacteria from migrating into the small bowel. Hence the presence or absence of the ileocecal valve may influence the clinical course. The colon is important for absorption of water and excretion of potassium. The severity of diarrhea following ileal resection is to some extent dependent upon the amount of contiguous colon that was also removed.

The remainder of the gastrointestinal tract also undergoes some changes after small-bowel resection. Gastric hypersecretion may contribute to malabsorption, as the pH of the chyme is below the optimal pH for digestive enzymes. Decreased levels of cholecystokinin and secretin may also interfere with ideal enzyme produc-

tion. With malabsorption, unabsorbed bile salts enter the colon where they are deconjugated to free bile acids by the colonic microflora, producing a watery diarrhea. The enterohepatic absorption of bile salts is also affected, producing a depleted pool of bile acid, impaired fat micelle formation, and steatorrhea.

Medications. There is some evidence that cimetidine may be effective in the treatment of gastric hypersecretion in the early course of some cases of short-bowel syndrome. It has therefore proved useful to measure stool pH or to perform gastric analysis to detect gastric hypersecretion. However, this treatment should be required only in the early months after resection, since it is a transient phenomenon. Some clinicians have also used cholestyramine and colestipol (ion exchange resins) to combine with unabsorbed bile acids to help prevent the watery diarrhea that occurs in these infants. Recent evidence suggests that the benefit of cholestyramine is actually due more to a direct effect in reducing bowel motility than to its effect on absorption of bile acids. Others have attempted to use antiperistaltic agents to help reduce stool frequency. Pancreatic enzymes should not be necessary, unless pancreatic insufficiency, such as cystic fibrosis, is present.

OSTOMY CARE AND CLOSURE

A high percentage of infants with short-bowel syndrome will have some type of ostomy for the first several months to 1 year of age. Guidelines for ostomy care are given in Appendix C.

Timing for closure of an ostomy will depend upon the initial reason for the ostomy, the well-being of the infant, and whether the infant will benefit nutritionally by early closure. Generally, ostomy closure is delayed until the child is about 1 year of age, if at all possible. The reason for this is that adhesion formation appears to be greater when the surgical closure is done sooner. However, when a child who has a high ileostomy is having difficulty with absorption and nutrition, the benefits of closure of the ileostomy and restoration of the terminal ileum and colon to the intestinal tract might outweigh the concern about adhesion formation. If the infant has had necrotizing enterocolitis, it is important to consider a contrast enema to ensure that stricture of the bowel has not occurred beyond the ostomy.

WHEN TO WORRY

1. When a consistent (albeit somewhat slow at first) growth in weight, length, and head cir-

cumference is not sustained following the infant's discharge from the hospital

2. When there is severe growth retardation at 5 to 6 months (corrected age) and head circumference has not entered onto the normal growth curve. In such an infant, serious consideration should be given to the need for parenteral nutrition, since this period is a critical one for brain growth and development.

3. If there is no evidence of improved adaptations of the intestine to tolerating a more normal type of diet by 2 years of age, a complicating problem may be present, or this child may have a chronic malabsorption problem.

GASTROSTOMY

Infants who are discharged home from the ICN with gastrostomies in place are subject to three problems. First, irritation occurs around the gastrostomy site, occasionally resulting in low-grade, spreading cellulitis. This will require antibiotics for staphylococcus aureus. Second, exuberant growth of granulation tissue around the tube produces purulent discharge and bleeding, which are readily treated by excising and/or cauterizing the granulation with silver nitrate sticks. The third problem, which is not uncommon, is dislodgment of the gastrostomy tube. It is very important for the physician to instruct the parents that if the tube comes out, it must be replaced promptly. They should understand that if reinsertion is delayed more than a few hours, a surgical procedure may be necessary to replace the tube. This is a problem that merits their calling the doctor immediately, and the physician should have a plan ready to manage the problem promptly and calmly. Usually the parents are supplied with extra Foley catheters, or their equivalent, and before the infant's discharge from the nursery have been instructed how to insert these. (See Gastrostomy Care in Appendix C).

HIRSCHSPRUNG'S DISEASE

Hirschsprung's disease in the newborn is treated by colostomy or ileostomy. The definitive pull-through operation probably will not be done until the child is 9 to 12 months of age, when the pelvis is large enough for a good surgical outcome to be obtained. Until that time, care of these infants is concerned largely with management of the problems associated with ostomy care and supportive care for the child and family.

After the definitive pull-through surgery, both the physician and the parents should be aware of two significant problems common in these children. The first is that, because the anal sphincter is also affected and very likely to be spastic, some of the internal anal muscle is removed at the time of surgery. However, in perhaps 20 per cent of cases, the remaining sphincter is still too spastic, and a second surgical procedure is needed to prevent obstructive symptoms. Abdominal distention plus diarrhea characterize the tight anal sphincter of Hirschsprung's disease. A further internal anal sphincterotomy might be necessary in these patients.

In addition, infants and children with a tight internal sphincter have acute evidence of dilated bowel loops and air-fluid levels on abdominal radiographs, which appear exactly like a small-bowel obstruction. If this occurs the pediatrician should immediately pass a large rectal tube into the rectum, which will release a large amount of gas and liquid stool and relieve the obstruction. The emergence of this picture is another indication for anal sphincterotomy.

WHEN TO WORRY

1. When a child who has had pull-through operation for Hirschsprung's disease develops abdominal distention and vomiting. Radiographs of the abdomen should be obtained, and a large rectal tube should be passed to rule out anal sphincter constriction as the cause of the obstruction.

SMALL LEFT-COLON SYNDROME

An infant discharged from the nursery with a diagnosis of neonatal small left colon syndrome may indeed have Hirschsprung's disease or some other bowel malfunction. The physician should be alert for any signs of colonic obstruction and advise the parents to notify him if the child has irritability associated with abdominal cramps or vomiting. He should also observe the child's nutrition and growth closely, and any suggestion of bowel dysfunction warrants contrast enema study.

IMPERFORATE ANUS

In providing care for a child born with imperforate anus, as in the management of other intestinal problems, the physician must know the level of the original lesion, i.e., whether it is above or below the level of the levator ani muscle. If it is below the levator ani, then some normal, internal sphincter smooth muscle should be present, and the infant can be expected to develop good sphincter control. If the original lesion was above the level of the levator ani, no internal sphincter muscle is present, and bowel control will be an ongoing problem for the child, because only smooth muscle contracts continuously without fatiguing. Toilet training involves learning the conscious control of the puborectal, external sphincter, and skeletal muscles. Many of these infants may lack even the sensory mechanism to enable them to identify colon distention and need for evacuation, and therefore they cannot know when to consciously contract the skeletal muscle sphincter.

A second major concern is bowel dysmotility, which is part of the anomaly, and all children born with imperforate anus, regardless of the size of the original lesion, have some degree of constipation. It is therefore important to establish daily colon evacuation to gain anal control and to prevent constant staining.

INGUINAL HERNIA

The incidence of hernias goes up with increasing prematurity, and so does the possibility of incarceration (see also Chapter 6). Therefore in a preterm infant with a hernia, surgical repair should be accomplished as soon as possible (usually the surgery is done prior to the infant's discharge from the ICN). It should be stressed that hernia repair in the preterm infant is not a simple procedure and should be done by a pediatric surgeon or a surgeon who frequently does the procedure *in infants*. Once the repair has been accomplished, follow-up care is the same as for any child with abdominal surgery.

HYDROCELE

Hydroceles rarely require surgical intervention. Almost all of them should resolve by 2 years of age. The only circumstances in which surgical intervention should be considered are excessive size that is unacceptable cosmetically and failure to resolve after the child reaches two years of age.

UNDESCENDED TESTES

Undescended testes are a common occurrence in preterm infants. Usually the testes will descend in a matter of months after term, and repair should be not considered until the child is one year of age. Operative repair for undescended testes prior to one year of age is technically difficult, because the tissues are fragile, and there is risk of damage to the vas deferens and blood supply. It is probably safe to tell the parents that if the testes have not descended by the age of 1 year (age corrected for prematurity), they are unlikely to descend spontaneously. Nevertheless, operation can be delayed until some time between 1 and 2 years of age. Hormonal therapy, such as administration of human chorionic gonadotropin or nasal instillation of luteinizing hormone releasing hormone, has been used, but its efficacy remains questionable. There remains uncertainty as to whether a testis is normal if it has not descended by the time a child is 1 year of age.

URINARY TRACT ANOMALIES

For the most part, children with complex urinary tract anomalies are observed closely by their surgeon or urologist. Important concerns that may come to the pediatrician's attention relate to urinary tract infection or hematuria. Discussion of the child's specific problems with the surgeon or urologist soon after discharge from the hospital is desirable, so that the joint management and communication with parents are coordinated appropriately.

When a child is discharged home with a nephrostomy tube in place, it is important that the parents be instructed that if the tube comes out it must be replaced immediately.

SUMMARY

The most frequent neonatal surgical problems affecting the neck, chest, abdomen, and genitourinary tract that will present ongoing management issues for the pediatrician have been discussed in this chapter. Graduates of an ICN who have required surgical treatment may be discharged home with a tracheostomy, gastrostomy, or intestinal ostomy, which may be closed later when the child has achieved sufficient growth. Guidelines to assist the pediatrician in managing these situations are provided in Appendix A and Appendix C.

References

1. Clark JH: Management of short bowel syndrome in the high-risk infant. Clin Perinatol 11:189, 1984.

2. Kerner JA Jr (ed.): Manual of Pediatric Parenteral Nutrition. New York, John Wiley & Sons, 1983.

Recommended Reading

Aaronson IA, Bowie MD, Cywes S, et al.: Massive small bowel resection in a neonate: Four-year follow up. Arch Surg 110:1485, 1975.

Adzick NS, Harrison MR, Glick PL, et al.: Fetal cystic adenomatoid malformation: Prenatal diagnosis and natural history. J Pediatr Surg 20:483, 1985.

Bohane TD, Hada-Ikse K, Biggar WD, et al.: A clinical study of young infants after small intestinal resection. J Pediatr 94:552, 1979.

Cannon RA, Byrne WJ, Ament ME, et al.: Home parenteral nutrition in infants. J Pediatr 96:1098, 1980.

Filston HC, Izant R (eds.): The Surgical Neonate: Evaluation and Care. New York, Appleton-Century-Crofts, 1978.

Grand RJ, Watkins JB, Torti FM: Progress in gastroenterology. Development of the human gastrointestinal tract. A review. Gastroenterology 70:790, 1976.

Hoffman AF, Poley JR: Role of bile acid malabsorption in pathogenesis of diarrhea and steatorrhea in patients with ileal resection: I. Response to cholestyramine or replacement of dietary long chain triglyceride by medium chain triglyceride. Gastroenterology 62:918, 1972.

Koldovsky O: Digestion and absorption. In Stave U (ed.): Perinatal Physiology. New York, Plenum Publishing Corp., 1978, p 317.

Murphy JP Jr, King DR, Dubois A: Treatment of gastrohypersecretion with cimetidine in the short-bowel syndrome. N Engl J Med 300:80, 1979.

Peevy KJ, Speed FA, Hoff CH: Epidemiology of inguinal hernia in preterm neonates. Pediatrics 77:246, 1986.

Tilson MD: Pathophysiology and treatment of short bowel syndrome. Surg Clin North Am 69:1273, 1980.

19

NEUROSURGICAL PROBLEMS IN THE INFANT

MICHAEL S.B. EDWARDS, M.D., and
MARJORIE E. DERECHIN, R.N., M.S.

The majority of pediatric neurosurgical problems recognized in the neonate that require management are related to spina bifida and hydrocephalus. Other problems, such as craniosynostosis, rarely require immediate surgical intervention, but must be followed and evaluated as the infant grows.

SPINA BIFIDA

Spina bifida is a general term used to describe a continuum of congenital anomalies of the spine that range from asymptomatic spina bifida occulta (failure of fusion of the posterior vertebral arch or arches) to open spinal defects (spina bifida aperta) that are associated with neurologic involvement.

SPINA BIFIDA OCCULTA

The most benign form of spina bifida is a defect in the lamina of the lumbar or sacral spine that has no associated nervous tissue involvement. This anomaly is observed on plain spine radiographs in 30 per cent of the general population. In an undertermined proportion of these patients, however, there may be underlying nervous tissue involvement that produces

tethering of the spinal cord. The presence of a tuft of hair, hemangioma, dermal sinus tract, or subcutaneous lipoma is the signature of potential underlying nervous system involvement and in conjunction with spina bifida (bony involvement) should alert the pediatrician to this possibility. Neurologic involvement may be present despite a normal neurologic examination. Involvement of the lowest sacral roots or cord segments may produce bowel or bladder dysfunction that is very difficult to diagnose in the neonate. Obviously, if there is neurologic dysfunction, which is often manifest by a foot deformity, loss of leg-foot sensation, or reflex asymmetry, the likelihood of tethering of the cord is very high. Plain spine radiographs in neonates are difficult to evaluate, because the posterior neural arch is cartilaginous and poorly ossified. Computed tomography (CT) and, more recently, magnetic resonance imaging (MRI) may help confirm the presence of a bony defect and/or underlying nervous system involvement. Metrizamide myelography in conjunction with CT is the definitive neurodiagnostic test for evaluation of intraspinal anatomy and the presence or absence of a tethered cord that may be caused by dermal sinus with or without a dermoid tumor, lipomyelomeningocele, thickened filum terminale, diastematomyelia, or meningocele. The presence of a tethered cord caused by one of these conditions, with or without neurologic dysfunction, is an indication for surgical intervention within the first three months of life. If the tethered cord is left untreated, it is probable that progressive neurologic and/or urologic dysfunction will result.

SPINA BIFIDA WITH MENINGOMYELOCELE

The most severe form of this anomaly is open spina bifida with meningomyelocele, which results from an abnormality in neurulation at 26 to 28 days of gestation. When the neural tube does not close, neither the posterior aspect (lamina) of the vertebral arches nor the posteriorly situated muscle, skin, and soft tissues will develop normally. The lumbar and sacral regions are most frequently involved, although spina bifida may occur at any level of the spine. Typically, defects occur on or near the midline; they may vary in size and may involve one or many spinal segments, and different amounts of skin may be missing. The level of the spine that is affected determines the severity of the neurologic dysfunction. Low sacral lesions may produce only bowel and bladder dysfunction and spare lumbar nerve roots that subserve ambulation. Lesions producing loss of neurologic function cephalad to the L-4 nerve root cause such severe paralysis that independent ambulation, even with braces, is unlikely. The L-4 nerve root is critical because it supplies the quadriceps muscle, which causes the knee joint to lock and thereby allow ambulation. The controversy concerning selection of infants in whom surgical management is appropriate is beyond the scope of this chapter.

Neonatal Management. If an open defect is to be repaired, in most instances surgery is performed within 24 hours of birth to reduce the chance of meningitis, which appears to be a negative prognostic factor for long-term intellectual development. Approximately 75 to 80 per cent of infants will develop hydrocephalus following closure of the meningomyelocele sac. In some infants, progressive ventricular enlargement will be detected on cranial sonograms before external signs of increased intracranial pressure, such as a full fontanelle, increasing head circumference, or irritability, are apparent. Therefore, cranial sonograms are obtained every two days, and a shunt is implanted at the first signs of progressive hydrocephalus.

Urinary Tract Management. Because of the involvement of the lower sacral nerve roots (S-2 to S-4), bladder function is always impaired. Careful urologic studies, including ultrasound and intravenous pyelography, should be performed after the spinal defect is closed, and appropriate management to assure adequate bladder drainage becomes a part of long-term care for the infant. Rarely the presence of posterior urethral valves may be associated with meningomyelocele and produce severe upper urinary tract (kidney) disease. If the infant does not void soon after birth, this possibility must be considered.

Previously, upper urinary tract disease secondary to a neurogenic bladder was the major cause of long-term morbidity and mortality in children with myelodysplasia. With the use of clean intermittent catheterization in conjunction with pharmacologic management, this is no longer the case; in fact, by employing this regimen, continence may be established in up to 80 per cent of children.

Orthopedic Management. Orthopedic evaluation and management can usually be delayed until the child's condition is stable after closure of the defect and/or shunt procedure. The most common problems noted are foot and leg deformities secondary to lack of innervation and/or hip dislocation.

Management of Chiari Malformation. All children born with meningomyelocele have an associated Chiari type II hindbrain malformation that consists of elongation of the cerebellar tonsils, fourth ventricle, and brainstem through the foramen magnum into the cervical spinal canal (Fig. 19–1A and 1B). Extension through the foramen magnum causes obstructive hydrocephalus. In addition, the microscopic anatomy of the brainstem is abnormal.

The Chiari II malformation may be associated with brainstem dysfunction. Symptoms may occur immediately after repair of the meningomyelocele, or onset may be delayed by months. Symptoms consist of stridor, difficulty feeding and swallowing, regurgitation, and aspiration. Some or all of these symptoms may develop. The overall incidence of symptomatic Chiari II malformation is unknown, but is estimated to be 18 per cent. In the majority of symptomatic patients, symptoms occur before 3 months of age.

Treatment remains controversial. First and foremost, hydrocephalus and/or a shunt malformation must be excluded, because this is the most correctable cause of Chiari II symptoms. An occipital cervical laminectomy has been advocated by some authors, but others feel that the

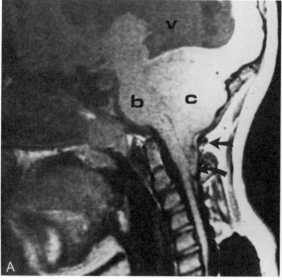

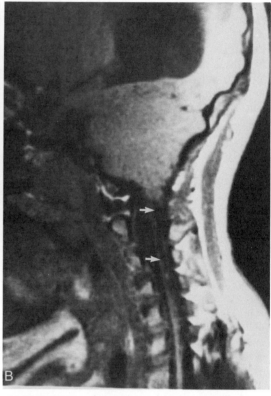

FIGURE 19–1. *A,* Parasagittal MRI of a 14-year-old with myelodysplasia and Arnold-Chiari malformation, type II. Straight arrow: foramen magnum with cerebellar tonsils extending into the cervical canal; curved arrow: tip of the cerebellar tonsils at C3; v: enlarged lateral ventricles; b: abnormal shape of the brain stem (pons); c: cerebellum. No fourth ventricle is seen. *B,* Parasagittal MRI of the same patient. White arrows point to mild hydromyelia of the cervical cord.

procedure is of little benefit. While infants with minor symptoms usually survive, the prognosis for survival in infants with severe symptoms remains poor. The morbidity in surviving infants is high, and because of bilateral vocal cord paralysis, gastrostomy and tracheostomy are often required to avoid aspiration. It is important to recognize the earliest symptoms of Chiari malformation because, once initiated, they may progress rapidly; early surgical intervention has the best chance of preventing deterioration.

Neurologic Management. Finally, the pediatrician must be aware that the neurologic dysfunction associated with spina bifida should remain static. Any evidence of progression of neurologic dysfunction, such as increased spasticity, weakness, or sensory loss should lead to early re-evaluation. Progression may result from an occult shunt malformation that produces hydrocephalus or hydromyelia, hydromyelia secondary to the Chiari II malformation, or late tethered cord—all of which can be repaired surgically.

Team Management. After being discharged from the ICN, these infants should be seen frequently in a multidisciplinary spinal defects clinic during the first year of life. Close follow-up is usually necessary to avoid neurologic and/or urologic deterioration and to provide the appropriate orthopedic management (corrective surgery and bracing) to allow early ambulation when possible. With aggressive management in a multidisciplinary clinic setting, unselected infants have a 70 per cent chance of having a normal IQ (greater than 80), 70 per cent will be able to ambulate independently, and 80 per cent will achieve urinary continence.

When To Worry

SPINA BIFIDA OCCULTA

1. In the presence of a tuft of hair, hemangioma, sinus tract, lipoma, or other sign of possible underlying neurologic involvement
2. With evidence of bladder dysfunction
3. With foot deformity, loss of distal leg-foot sensation, or reflex asymmetry

MENINGOMYELOCELE

1. In infants (usually less than 3 months of age) who develop symptoms of stridor, difficulty feeding and swallowing, regurgitation, and aspiration. (These may be indicative of symptomatic Chiari II malformation with brainstem dysfunction.)

2. In infants with increasing head circumference or ventricular enlargement on cranial sonogram

HYDROCEPHALUS

Hydrocephalus is an abnormal accumulation of cerebral spinal fluid (CSF) within the cerebral ventricles that results from an abnormality of some aspect of the process of absorption of CSF. Overproduction of CSF occurs only in the rare instance of a choroid plexus papilloma. The old classification of hydrocephalus as communicating or noncommunicating is of little use, because almost all hydrocephalus is the result of obstruction at some site in the CSF pathways. Therefore, hydrocephalus is best described by noting the sites at which flow is obstructed, such as the aqueduct, basal cisterns, and sagittal sinus. The cause can vary from congenital anatomic obstruction to infection or hemorrhagic neoplastic causes.

Diagnosis

In infants, once hydrocephalus is suspected, ultrasonography is the best technique for evaluating ventricular size and the effectiveness of medical or surgical management. Ultrasonography is advantageous because it can be performed at the bedside, does not require sedation, and does not use ionizing radiation (Fig. 19–2A and 2B). It is limited by the need for an acoustic window such as a fontanelle, by the inherent difficulty of imaging the posterior fossa, and by difficulties inherent in evaluating the subarachnoid spaces overlying the cerebral hemispheres. CT and MRI can also give excellent anatomic information. When ventricles are enlarged, MRI can often show abnormal CSF flow into the brain parenchyma surrounding the ventricles (Fig. 19–3A to 3C). After the infant is discharged, the circumference of the head should be measured weekly for three months, and sonograms should be obtained monthly to evaluate the size of the ventricles. In neonates, especially premature infants, brain compliance is slight, and the ventricles may dilate while head circumference remains stable and the fontanelle is soft; therefore, sonography is essential for the evaluation of intracranial dynamics.

Management

CONGENITAL HYDROCEPHALUS

Infants born with congenital overt hydrocephalus are best managed by ventriculoperitoneal shunting performed after neurodiagnostic and etiologic evaluation. Complete neurodiagnostic testing can help in the choice of the correct shunting system. In most instances, a shunt placed from the right lateral ventricle to

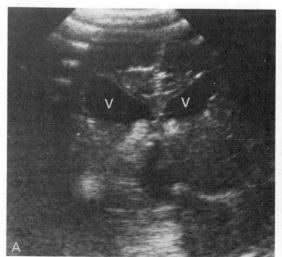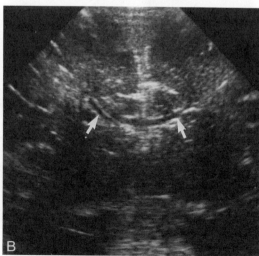

FIGURE 19–2. *A,* Coronal sonograph of a four-day-old infant with myelodysplasia and hydrocephalus. Both ventricles (V) are dilated. *B,* Sonograph of the same patient 24 hours after placement of a ventriculoperitoneal shunt. The ventricles are barely visible (arrows) and are now of normal size.

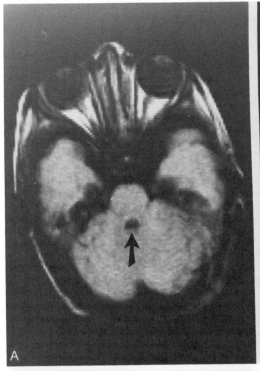

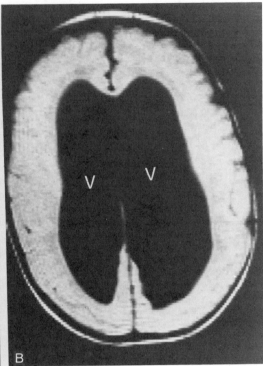

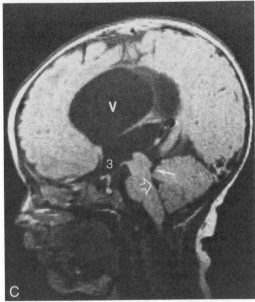

FIGURE 19–3. *A,* Axial MRI of a two-month-old child with aqueductal stenosis and hydrocephalus. Arrow: normal size for the fourth ventricle. *B,* MRI of the same patient at a lower level, showing dilated lateral ventricles (V). *C,* Midsagittal MRI of the same patient, showing the dilated lateral ventricles (V) and third ventricle (3). The aqueduct of Sylvius is occluded (straight closed arrow) just cephalad to the fourth ventricle (open arrow).

the peritoneum is adequate. However, in some instances a suprasellar arachnoid cyst can obstruct flow between the lateral ventricles, and it may be necessary to place 2 ventricular catheters: a single catheter extending through the lateral ventricle into the cyst and a direct fenestration of the cyst followed by placement of a shunt. In infants with the Dandy-Walker malformation, it is frequently necessary to place a catheter in the lateral ventricle as well as the posterior fossa cyst to control hydrocephalus.

HYDROCEPHALUS AFTER INTRAVENTRICULAR HEMORRHAGE

Hydrocephalus that develops secondary to prematurity and hemorrhage into the germinal matrix represents a more complex management problem. With improved ICN management, the incidence of severe intraventricular hemorrhage (IVH) has decreased, and the majority of infants with IVH do not require neurosurgical intervention. Complicated IVH with parenchymal cerebral hemorrhage or associated with ventricular dilatation, however, may require ventricular shunting. When IVH and ventricular enlargement are present, aggressive medical management is usually the initial therapeutic approach of choice. If, however, ventricular dilatation continues and appears to be impinging on the cortical mantle, then some form of ventricular drainage, either permanent or temporary, may be necessary.

In very small neonates, especially those in whom ventricular protein or red blood cell count is high, a subcutaneous ventricular catheter reservoir can be used to aspirate CSF and control hydrocephalus. This technique carries less risk of infection than external ventricular drainage and can be used in some infants for up to one month before conversion to a ventriculoperitoneal shunt, or until hydrocephalus is reversed.

Ventriculoperitoneal shunting remains the primary surgical technique for controlling hydrocephalus when medical management fails. Infection and obstruction, however, are more likely in premature infants. Obstruction may occur because high protein content secondary to the original hemorrhage makes CSF extremely viscous; the content of fibrinogen and fibrin products is more critical than the absolute protein value, however. Serial lumbar punctures and/or aspiration of CSF from a subcutaneous reservoir can reduce CSF protein content to a level less than 300 to 400 mg/dl, which reduces the likelihood of obstruction. Systemic administration of antibiotics with antistaphylococcal activity is begun preoperatively and continued for 48 to 72 hours postoperatively; vancomycin is our drug of choice. Preoperative use of antibiotics and meticulous surgical technique have allowed us to keep our overall infection rate below 5 per cent.

INFECTION

When infection occurs, it is usually associated with placement or revision of a shunt. In rare instances, an existing systemic infection may cause a secondary shunt infection in infants with severe sepsis or in those with ventriculoatrial shunts. However, the appearance of signs and symptoms of shunt infection may be delayed by weeks or months after surgical intervention. The primary symptoms are usually irritability and fever, but in some children infection may manifest itself as multiple shunt malfunctions.

> **In infants with ventriculoatrial shunts, infection may occur insidiously as prolonged direct-fraction hyperbilirubinemia or with a picture similar to that of subacute bacterial endocarditis, with petechiae and hematosplenomegaly. These infants may also have nephritis secondary to their shunt.**
>
> *Editor*

The organism found most frequently is *Staphylococcus epidermidis,* but attempts should be made to culture low-virulence anerobic organisms, especially when multiple shunt malformations occur. Aspiration of fluid from the shunt reservoir most often produces positive results. If the shunt is functioning but infected, treatment includes administration of appropriate systemic antibiotics as indicated by Gram stain and CSF culture results. After CSF has remained sterile for 72 hours, the shunt can be removed and a new one placed in a different site. Antibiotics are continued for seven to ten days after the shunt is replaced. If the CSF does not become sterile within three to five days, or if symptoms and signs worsen despite systemic antibiotics, intrashunt administration of antibiotics is used until the CSF is sterile for 72 hours and continued after the shunt has been replaced.

If the shunt is obstructed at the peritoneal end, it should be externalized until CSF becomes sterile and then replaced with a new shunt. A shunt that is obstructed at the ventricular end in the face of infection must be removed; an external ventricular drainage system is placed, and antibiotics are administered until the CSF is sterile for 72 hours, after which a new shunt can be placed. We have had no recurrence of infection after replacement of shunts using the above management approaches.

FOLLOW-UP OF INFANTS WITH SHUNTS

After a shunt has been placed, infants are followed-up serially at least every three months during the first year of life with neurologic and developmental testing, sonography, and measurement of head circumference. Sonography is the most critical diagnostic test for evaluating shunt function while the fontanelle remains open. In most infants the size of the ventricles decreases toward normal by three to five days after placement of the shunt; a lack of improvement may indicate either shunt malfunction or cerebral atrophy. In such instances a radionuclide shunt study with quantitative analysis can be used to determine active flow rates within a shunt. Static pictures may show a site of obstruction or abdominal cyst formation. After the fontanelle has closed, CT or MRI should be carried out at six-month intervals until age 3 years and at yearly intervals thereafter. If clinical symptoms or signs (Table 19–1) suggest that the shunt is malfunctioning, an emergency scan should be obtained. Plots of head circumference over time may help define subtle changes in shunt function. Even if the child appears to be healthy, sequential scans should be obtained to determine slowly progressive shunt failure that causes enlargement of the ventricles. Prompt diagnosis and management of even the most subtle shunt malfunction are critical to prevent additional brain injury.

Shunt Function. Evaluation of shunt function by palpation of the shunt reservoir can lead to erroneous conclusions. Neither refilling nor lack of refilling of the reservoir is an accurate indication of shunt function. Failure of the res-

ervoir to refill may be associated with small ventricles and decreased CSF volume in a functioning shunt, whereas rapid refilling may be associated with a patent ventricular catheter that is obstructed at the peritoneal end. If clinical symptoms and/or signs suggest shunt failure, sonography, CT, or MRI should be performed immediately.

The relation of the duration of shunt failure to clinical symptoms and signs is particular to each child. In infants, especially those with widely open cranial sutures, the duration may be long (days). In older children with adqueductal stenosis who are shunt dependent, however, progression to lethargy and coma may occur within hours of shunt failure. Rapid evaluation is mandatory if the diagnosis suggests shunt obstruction.

Outcome. The prognosis for neonatal hydrocephalus depends strongly on etiology, severity of the hydrocephalus at birth, and the presence or absence of infection. However, one half to two thirds of infants born with overt hydrocephalus, if treated appropriately, are likely to have an IQ of 80 or greater. Children with communicating hydrocephalus or myelodysplasia do better than children with Dandy-Walker malformations and adqueductal stenosis.

In one study of long-term follow-up of infants who received shunts for progressive ventricular dilatation from IVH, only 18 per cent had normal neurologic development, and most were severely handicapped. This suggests that the poor outcome in infants with IVH is caused by many factors, since ventricular dilatation due to ventricular obstruction caused by aqueductal stenosis does not result in such a poor outcome. It is probable that these infants have experienced hypoxia, ischemia, and subsequent cerebral atrophy, which contribute to a poor outcome. Others have not found the outcome after IVH to be quite so grim (see Appendix D).

TABLE 19–1. Symptoms Of Shunt Malfunction

Infants
Enlargement of baby's head
Fontanelle full and tense (when infant's head is upright and quiet)
Prominent scalp veins
Swelling or redness along shunt tract
Downward deviation of eyes (sunset eyes)
Fever
Vomiting
Irritability
Sleepiness
Seizures

Toddlers
Head enlargement
Fever
Vomiting (abdominal pain)
Headache
Irritability and/or sleepiness
Seizures
Loss of previous abilities (sensory or motor)

Children and Adults
Fever
Vomiting (abdominal pain)
Headache
Vision problems
Irritability and/or tiredness
Personality change
Loss of coordination or balance
Swelling or redness along shunt tract
Seizures
Difficulty in waking or staying awake

When To Worry

1. When head growth is more rapid than expected from growth curves, or with fullness of the fontanelle

2. In an infant with a ventriculoatrial shunt: when prolonged hyperbilirubinemia or signs associated with subacute bacterial endocarditis or nephritis are present

3. In infants with any shunt: when fever, irritability, vomiting, or change in general neurologic status occur

MUSCLE DISEASE

Hypotonia, which occurs as a result of various insults that affect the brain or motor unit, may be seen in neonates. Hypotonia must be differentiated from weakness per se (secondary to early gestation or severe illness), even though weakness is usually a feature of hypotonia in the neonate or young infant.

When suspended with the abdomen held on the examiner's hand, the term infant assumes a straight posture. The truly hypotonic infant will be limp and drape himself over the examiner's hand. Shoulder girdle tone may be assessed by holding the infant vertically with the examiner's hands under the infant's axillae. Full-term infants will adduct their arms, but hypotonic infants will slip through the hand. At term, the normal infant has flexor tone in all limbs. (See Chapter 9.)

In general, hypotonia affects the axial musculature more than it affects the extremities. A variety of metabolic, traumatic, and genetic causes may produce hypotonia. The diagnosis of benign congenital hypotonia can be made only after all other possibilities have been excluded. All other aspects of the neurologic examination are normal. Results of additional tests, such as serum enzymes (creatine phosphokinase) electrophysiologic tests, and muscle/nerve biopsies, are normal. The prognosis for infants with benign congenital hypotonia is excellent. (For more detailed information on hypotonia, see Recommended Reading.)

CRANIOSYNOSTOSIS

Craniosynostosis is a developmental disorder characterized by premature closure of one or more of the cranial sutures and/or sutures of the skull base. Cranial sutures allow the normal, rapid growth of the brain during infancy and early childhood. The human brain grows more rapidly during the first six months of life than it does during the remainder of infancy and childhood. Eighty per cent of brain growth has occurred by two years of age. Normally sutures remain open (fibrous union) into young adulthood.

Etiology

Possible factors in craniosynostosis include infection, metabolic bone disorders, abnormali-

ties of the cranial base suture, and local trauma such as cephalohematoma. A majority of simple synostoses may be caused by deformation of the skull either in utero (fetal head constraint) or extra utero (hypotonia) that causes occipital flattening and subsequent suture closure. Sagittal synostosis is most common in males (80 per cent). A single suture or several sutures may be involved. If the facial skeleton is also involved, as in Crouzon's disease or Apert's syndrome, the term *craniofacial dysmorphism* is used. Carpenter's syndrome (acrocephalopolysyndactyly), Chotzen's syndrome (acrocephalosyndactyly, type III), and many other rare conditions are also associated with craniosynostosis.

Diagnosis

In most infants, the diagnosis can be made from clinical findings (Table 19–2). Plain skull radiographs may show the involved suture and confirm the shape of the cranial vault. CT can be used to evaluate suture anatomy and potential intracranial malformations and/or hydrocephalus. CT is particularly helpful for the evaluation of lambdoid synostosis, a condition for which plain skull radiographs are frequently inconclusive. Familial cases are rare.

TABLE 19–2. Simple Synostosis

HEAD SHAPE	SUTURE	CHARACTERISTICS
Scaphocephaly	Sagittal	Frontal bossing Narrow biparietal diameter Elongated AP diameter Increased head circumference
Brachycephaly	Bilateral coronal	Increased biparietal diameter Decreased AP diameter Hypoplastic supraorbital rims
Plagiocephaly	Unilateral coronal Unilateral lambdoid	Asymmetric head shape Ear displaced anteriorly Flat forehead (coronal) Flat occiput (lambdoid)
Trigonocephaly	Metopic	Triangular forehead Ridge middle forehead Hypotelorism

Treatment

Surgical correction is the mainstay of treatment. A wide-strip craniectomy that includes the suture extending from the coronal to lambdoidal sutures will correct the abnormal head shape rapidly if performed in an infant less than six months of age. Lambdoid synostosis is also treated by simple craniectomy. Unilateral and bilateral synostoses that affect facial features require a craniofacial team approach. These infants frequently have multiple medical and neurologic conditions, such as hydrocephalus, that require aggressive management. A good correction can be obtained by more extensive surgery that includes advancement of the supraorbital rim(s) and opening of the basal sutures.

Apert's syndrome (acrocephalosyndactyly) occurs in 1 per 160,000 live births and is characterized by bilateral coronal synostosis, midface and mandibular hypoplasia, fusion of phalanges, and a significant incidence of hydrocephalus. Developmental delay is very common. Aggressive management of hydrocephalus, when present, and correction of coronal suture synostosis has improved the outlook for these infants.

Crouzon's disease (craniofacial dysostosis) is characterized by hypoplasia, premature closure of the coronal sutures, and midfacial and maxillary hypoplasia; the phalanges are not fused. Crouzon's disease is caused by an autosomal dominant genetic pattern. The incidence of hydrocephalus and mental retardation is less than in Apert's syndrome, but early intervention is critical to prevent of loss of vision and to maximize outcome.

With modern techniques of craniofacial surgery, a wide variety of disorders of the skull base can be corrected with minimum morbidity and mortality. The ability to recognize these abnormalities in infancy and perform corrective surgery early has significantly improved the intellectual and social outcome for these children.

When To Worry

1. When an infant's skull growth appears asymmetric with no other apparent reason
2. When facial or ear asymmetry develops
3. If skull growth is less than normal

Recommended Reading

Spina Bifida, Meningomyelocele

Hoffman HJ, Taecholarn C, Hendrick EB, et al.: Management of lipomyelomeningoceles. Experience at the Hospital for Sick Children, Toronto. J Neurosurg 62:1, 1985.

McLone DG, Dias L, Kaplan WE, et al.: Concepts in the management of spina bifida. Concept Pediatr Neurosurg 5:97, 1985.

Naidich TP, McLone DG, Fulling KH: The Chiari II malformation: IV. The hindbrain deformity. Neuroradiology 25:179, 1983.

Park TS, Hoffman HJ, Hendrick EB, et al.: Experience with surgical decompression of the Arnold-Chiari malformation in young infants with myelomeningocele. Neurosurgery 13:147, 1983.

Hydrocephalus

Allan WC, Dransfield DA, Tito AM: Ventricular dilation following periventricular-intraventricular hemorrhage: Outcome at one year. Pediatrics 73:158, 1984.

Allan WC, Holt PJ, Sawyer LR, et al.: Ventricular dilatation after neonatal periventricular intraventricular hemorrhage. Am J Dis Child 136:589, 1982.

Amacher AL, Wellington J: Infantile hydrocephalus: Long-term results of surgical therapy. Childs Brain 11:217, 1984.

Chaplin ER, Goldstein GW, Myerberg DZ, et al.: Posthemorrhagic hydrocephalus in the preterm infant. Pediatrics 65:901, 1980.

Cooke RWI: Early prognosis of low birthweight infants treated for progressive posthaemorrhagic hydrocephalus. Arch Dis Child 58:420, 1983.

Hagberg B, Naglo A-S: The conservative management of infantile hydrocephalus. Acta Paediatr Scand 61:165, 1977.

Kreusser KL, Tarby TJ, Kovnar E, et al.: Serial lumbar punctures for at least temporary amelioration of neonatal posthemorrhagic hydrocephalus. Pediatrics 75:719, 1985.

Krishnamoorthy KS, Shannon DC, DeLong GR, et al.: Neurologic sequelae in the survivors of neonatal intraventricular hemorrhage. Pediatrics 64:233, 1979.

Levene MI, Starte DR: A longitudinal study of post-haemorrhagic ventricular dilatation in the newborn. Arch Dis Child 56:905, 1981.

Liethy EA, Gilmour RL, Bryson CQ, et al.: Outcome of high-risk neonates with ventriculomegaly. Dev Med Child Neurol 15:162, 1983.

Lorber J: The results of early treatment of extreme hydrocephalus. Dev Med Child Neurol 16:21, 1968.

McComb JG: Recent research into the nature of cerebrospinal fluid formation and absorption. J Neurosurg 59:369, 1983.

McComb JG, Ramos AD, Platzleer AC, et al.: Management of hydrocephalus secondary to intraventricular hemorrhage in the preterm infant with a subcutaneous ventricular catheter reservoir. Neurosurgery 13:295, 1983.

McCullough DC, Bakar-Martin LA: Current prognosis in overt neonatal hydrocephalus. J Neurosurg 57:378, 1982.

Ment LR, Duncan CC, Scott DT, et al.: Post-hemorrhagic hydrocephalus: Low incidence in very low birth weight neonates with intraventricular hemorrhage. J Neurosurg 60:343, 1984.

Palmer P, Dubowitz LMS, Levene MI, et al.: Developmental and neurological progress of perterm infants with intraventricular hemorrhage. Am J Dis Child 56:905, 1981.

Muscle Disease

Berg BO: Child Neurology. A Clinical Manual. Greenbrae, CA, Jones Medical Publishers, 1984, pp 250–256.

Swaiman ST, Wright FS: The practice of Pediatric Neurology, 2nd ed. St. Louis, C.V. Mosby Company, 1982.

Craniosynostosis

Furuya Y, Edwards MSB, Alpers CE, et al.: Computerized tomography of cranial sutures: I. Comparison of suture anatomy in children and adults. J Neurosurg 61:53, 1984.

Furuya U, Edwards MSB, Alpers CE, et al.: Computerized tomography of cranial sutures: II. Abnormalities of sutures and skull deformity in craniosynostosis. J Neurosurg 61:59, 1984.

Swaiman ST, Wright FS: The Practice of Pediatric Neurology, 2nd ed. St. Louis, C.V. Mosby Company, 1982.

20

THE NEWBORN AND HOST DEFENSE

PEGGY S. WEINTRUB, M.D., and DIANE W. WARA, M.D.

The host defenses of the newborn have been studied extensively in an attempt to explain the increased frequency and severity of infections during infancy. Several detailed reviews have been written on the subject and are listed in Recommended Reading at the end of this chapter. Multiple components of the immune system must mature and interact to assure optimal protection from the foreign microbial agents that cause disease in the newborn and infant. Table 20–1 summarizes the components of the immune system and compares quantities and function in normal term infants and preterm infants to levels in adults. This chapter will summarize briefly what is known about host defenses in the newborn, with particular emphasis on the high-risk newborn.

GENERAL PRINCIPLES

Antibody, produced by mature B lymphocytes, coats or opsonizes bacteria and prepares them for phagocytosis. Decreased production of specific antibody results in increased frequency and severity of bacterial infections, especially from bacteria with primarily polysaccharide surface antigens *(Streptococcus pneumoniae, Hemophilus influenzae, Escherichia coli,* meningococcus). Normal cellular immunity (T cell)

is essential for the production of antibody by B lymphocytes. T lymphocytes include subpopulations: T-helper cells, which promote antibody production, and T-suppressor cells, which restrict the production of antibody. In addition, T lymphocytes are primarily responsible for cytotoxicity, which may result directly in the destruction of virus-infected cells. T cells produce numerous soluble factors (lymphokines), which modulate interactions among different cell types. Thus, abnormal cellular immunity may result in increased infection from bacteria, virus, or protozoa. Nonspecific host defenses enhance the effects of the antibody and cell-mediated immune systems. A series of low molecular weight serum proteins, complement components, when activated sequentially, result in opsonization of bacteria. Following opsonization, bacteria are removed from the circulation by cells and organs of the reticuloendothelial system. Following uptake or phagocytosis, bacteria are destroyed.

B CELL (ANTIBODY-MEDIATED) IMMUNITY

B cell development begins early in fetal life. The lymphoid stem cell matures into a pre-B cell, recognized by staining for intracytoplasmic

IgM, and later IgG and IgA. It progresses next to an immature B cell, with membrane-associated IgM, and then to a B cell committed to the production and secretion of a specific immunoglobulin (Ig) isotype and antibody. Although normal numbers of B cells with membrane-associated immunoglobulin can be detected by eight weeks of gestation, Ig synthesis and secretion are minimal. At delivery, IgM production precedes that of other immunoglobulins and predominates for several months. The secretion of isotypes (IgM, IgG, and IgA) is decreased in newborn infants when cord blood lymphocytes are compared with adult peripheral blood mononuclear cells. Deficient newborn Ig synthesis is probably related to inadequate T-helper cell promotion or antibody production. Increased T-suppressor cells, immature B cells, or immature antigen-presenting cells may contribute to decreased Ig production by newborn B cells.

At birth, Ig levels are determined both by intrauterine production and by antibody transported across the placenta. Immunoglobulin levels have been studied in the newborn period in both healthy and high-risk infants. Normally little or no immunoglobulin is made in utero. IgG is actively transported across the placenta at approximately 34 weeks of gestation, and levels of IgG at birth are greater than or equal to maternal levels in term newborns. All IgG subclasses appear to be transported well, and the proportion of each subclass in the infant mirrors that in the mother. Thus the IgG antibody repertoire of the term infant directly reflects the mother's and her prior exposure to specific organisms.

Serum levels of IgA and IgM are insignificant in the healthy term infant, as these isotypes are unable to cross the placenta. The fetus responds to intrauterine infection by production of IgM antibody, and thus the presence of significant amounts of IgM in cord blood may reflect congenital infection.

In premature infants, Hobbs[1] has shown a linear correlation between gestational age and the logarithm of IgG levels. Infants less than 32 weeks of gestation frequently have levels less than 400 mg/dl (compared to approximately 1100 mg/dl at 40 weeks). IgG levels in infants who are small for gestational age (SGA) are decreased when compared to those of normal-sized infants of similar gestational age. IgG may also be decreased in postmature infants following birth. In a single study of 64 infants born at less than 36 weeks of gestation, IgG levels decreased with increasing age; in many infants IgG

dropped to very low levels (less than 200 mg/dl) by age three to four months. IgM levels did increase with age, indicating early synthesis of IgM but not IgG. By five to eight months of age, there was a wide range of IgG levels (100 to 646 mg/dl). One ICN follow-up clinic has shown an increased risk of infection in infants with low IgG levels.

The ability to produce unique antibody in response to a specific antigen (not only absolute Ig levels) is an additional important consideration in evaluation of B cell immunity. The sequential development of the ability to produce antibody to discrete antigens with different characteristics has been shown experimentally in fetal life in several species. In the human neonate and infant, there also is evidence to support the sequential development of the ability to respond to specific antigens. For example, infants less than two years of age form poor antibody in response to polysaccharide antigens. In addition, the infant's antibody response to some antigens may be decreased in the presence of passively acquired maternal antibody. Infants produce suboptimal antibody following measles immunization until one year of age. The infant's decreased antibody response is presumably secondary to residual maternal antibody. Both premature and term infants produce adequate specific antibody to protein antigens. Following immunization with DPT vaccine at two, four, and six months postnatally, seroconversion occurred in more than 80 per cent of preterm infants after the second month immunization and in 100 per cent after the fourth month immunization. Eighty per cent seroconversion to pertussis was achieved after the fourth month dose of vaccine. Seroconversion to all three polio serotypes was shown in 89 per cent of 37 premature infants by six months postnatal age; this is comparable to responses found in term infants.

Although IgG and IgM are synthesized by the newborn within the first year of life, significant production of IgA antibody is delayed until after age 1 year. Breast milk and colostrum may provide IgA antibody to eliminate gut pathogens in the newborn, to coat the intestinal mucosa and thus decrease the entrance of foreign antigens into the circulation, and to provide minimum amounts of serum IgA. Studies suggest that breast-fed newborns have decreased frequency and severity of infection from intestinal pathogens. In addition, evidence supports a decreased incidence of allergy in breast-fed infants born to atopic families.

Overall, many ICN graduates may have low

TABLE 20–1.   Components of the Immune System: Quantity and Function in Newborns When Compared to Healthy Adults

	NORMAL INFANT	PRE-TERM INFANT
B-cell Immunity		
Quantitative IgG	Increased	Decreased
Quantitative IgM	Decreased	Decreased
Quantitative IgA	Decreased	Decreased
Antibody response to protein antigen	Normal	Normal
Antibody response to encapsulated organisms	Decreased	Decreased
T-cell Immunity		
Absolute lymphocyte count	Increased (4000/dl)	Decreased
Per cent T-cells	Decreased (50%)	Normal
Absolute no. T-cells	Normal	Normal
Per cent T-helper cells	Normal	Increased
Per cent T-suppressor cells	Normal	Decreased
Functional T helper	Decreased	Decreased
Functional T suppressor	Increased	Decreased
Sensitization to dinitrochlorobenzine (DNCB)	Decreased	Decreased
Proliferative response to phytohemagglutinin	Normal	Normal
Proliferative response to allogeneic cells	Normal	Normal
Cytotoxic reactions (natural killer, antibody dependent)	Decreased	Decreased
Cytokine production		
Interferon gamma	Decreased	Unknown
Interleukin 2	Decreased	Unknown
Interleukin 1	Normal	Unknown
Nonspecific Mediators		
Complement activation		
Alternative pathway	Decreased	Decreased
Classic pathway	Normal	Decreased
Phagocytic cells		
Neutrophils		
Cell numbers	Normal	Normal
Chemotaxis	Decreased	Decreased
Neutrophil adherence	Decreased	Decreased
Phagocytosis	Normal	Normal
Intracellular killing	Normal	Normal
Monocytes		
Phagocytosis	Decreased rate	Unknown
Intracellular killing	Normal	Normal
Splenic Function	Abnormal	Abnormal

levels of IgG at delivery, prolonged periods of hypogammaglobulinemia before endogenous Ig production begins, and increased susceptibility to infection. Few investigators have evaluated the role of gamma globulin (IgG) administration in high-risk infants. Some studies have suggested therapeutic benefit, while others do not find this therapy valuable. Controlled trials are now under way in high-risk infants (or during the follow-up period) with the newer intravenous preparations of gamma globulin. It should be noted that commercially available intravenous gamma globulin is prepared at a pH of 6.4 to 6.8 to decrease particle aggregation. Its rapid administration to a small premature, therefore, may result in metabolic acidosis.

Although antibody response to some antigens may be delayed, responses to antigens such as DPT are close to normal. Therefore the recommendations of the American Academy of Pediatrics (see Chapter 6) should be followed closely for infants with relatively normal immunity. As live viral vaccines may result in disseminated disease in infants with primary immunodeficiency, these immunizations should be deferred if one suspects primary immunodeficiency or infection with HIV.

T CELL (CELL-MEDIATED) IMMUNITY

In the normal term infant, the mean number of circulating lymphocytes is approximately 4200 per deciliter (range 2000 to 7300 per deciliter). Between 50 and 60 per cent of these lymphocytes are T cells (as measured by rosetting techniques). Although the percentage is slightly decreased when compared to adult normals, the absolute numbers of T cells are normal because of the relative lymphocytosis in the newborn. The percentage of T-helper cells is slightly decreased at birth, while the percentage of T-suppressor cells is increased.

The functional capacity of T cells has been measured in a variety of ways, including blastogenic responses to nonspecific mitogens, such as phytohemagglutinin (PHA) or to alloantigens in a mixed lymphocyte culture, and sensitization of skin with dinitrochlorobenzene (DNCB). The lymphocyte response to PHA is seen early in gestation in the peripheral blood lymphocytes (approximately 14 weeks gestation) and is normal to increased at the time of delivery. The response to alloantigens reaches the level of term infants by 20 weeks of gestation. Mature lymphocytes may reach the developing fetus either from the maternal circulation or from nonirradiated intrauterine transfusions, yet graft-versus-host disease (GVHD) usually is not seen in the newborn (unless the infant has a primary T cell immunodeficiency). The absence of GVHD in normal newborns who have received viable histoincompatible T lymphocytes from their mothers suggests that the newborn's cellular immunity is relatively intact.

Other measures of T cell function are diminished in the newborn. Newborns are less easily sensitized to DNCB than are adults. Cord blood lymphocytes produce lower levels of lymphokines, such as gamma interferon, important in the regulation of T cell function and/or in the destruction of virus. It is clear that additional information is necessary to define the nature and significance of T cell abnormalities beyond the newborn period, particularly in high-risk infants.

In the high-risk nursery population and in ICN graduates, other factors may influence cell-mediated immunity. Various levels of immunocompetence have been noted in these populations, depending upon inclusion criteria and methods of evaluation. Premature infants, like term neonates, have decreased sensitization to DNCB. SGA infants have reduced numbers of T cells when compared with controls who are average for gestational age. The percentage of T lymphocytes remains decreased (44 per cent in SGA compared with 72 per cent in healthy newborns) at three months post partum. These SGA infants also showed decreased response to PHA at term; no data are available at the three-month follow-up. In contrast, another study indicates that noninfected infants with intrauterine growth retardation (IUGR) have T cell proliferative responses equal to age-matched controls. Factors other than IUGR and prematurity may also affect T cell function in ICN graduates. Congenital infections, the use of steroids to lessen pulmonary disease, or multiple transfusions may decrease T cell function. (See section, Special Problems.)

NONSPECIFIC HOST DEFENSE

HUMORAL FACTORS, PHAGOCYTIC CELLS, RETICULOENDOTHELIAL SYSTEM

Humoral Factors. In the newborn infant, nonspecific aspects of host defense, such as humoral mediators (other than antibody, phagocytic cells, and the reticuloendothelial system), are extremely important. Of the humoral factors, complement components have been studied most extensively. Most of these proteins are synthesized at low levels early in gestation, with a rapid increase during the third trimester. Although classic pathway complement activity of cord blood may be decreased compared to maternal activity, term infants have 60 to 100 per cent of the activity of controls when compared to normal adults. More commonly, abnormalities of the alternative pathway have been described in term infants. Preterm neonates have diminished classic and alternative complement pathway activity when compared to term infants. Although adult levels of complement activity are normally attained at approximately three to six months postnatal age in term infants, the maturation of the pathway in high-risk infants has not been studied.

Phagocytic Cells. The role of phagocytic cells in newborn host defense is widely appreciated. Normal numbers of these cells usually are present (except during overwhelming infection-sepsis) in the normal newborn, the high-risk newborn, and the ICN graduate; however, a wide range of functional abnormalities have been reported. Chemotaxis is approximately 20 per cent of adult values in both term and preterm infants and is decreased even further in preterm infants with proven sepsis. This decreased locomotion to the site of infection may be related to the abnormalities of neutrophil adherence also seen in this population. Abnormal migration of neutrophils may also be related to deformability of the cells; this, too, is diminished in newborns. Numerous studies of phagocytosis in neonates have been performed and have been reviewed recently. Briefly, neutrophil phagocytosis and intracellular killing are probably normal in term and preterm infants, though bactericidal activity is less effective in "stressed" neonates at any gestational age. Neonatal monocytes have slowed rates of phagocytosis; however, their bactericidal capacity is comparable to that of adults.

Reticuloendothelial System. Splenic function assumes increased importance in the newborn as well, because of the decreased ability in the infant to form specific antibody. The spleen normally removes deformed or "pocked" red blood cells from the circulation; therefore, increased numbers of pocked erythrocytes reflect decreased splenic function. Splenic function is probably abnormal in both premature and term newborns. Term newborns have increased numbers of pocked erythrocytes, and the more premature the infant the greater the number. No information is available concerning the maturation of splenic function in nursery graduates.

SPECIAL PROBLEMS

It is clear from the preceding sections that host defenses are immature in the newborn period and that these alterations may be even more pronounced in premature, SGA, and postmature infants. A number of problems, in addition to immaturity, may arise during the initial hospitalization or the follow-up period and contribute to relative immunodeficiency in these infants.

Syndromes with Immunodeficiencies. Primary immunodeficiency is frequently part of a more complex congenital syndrome. The related disorders, rather than the immunologic problem, may be responsible for the ICN admission. The following are typical examples: Infants with DiGeorge syndrome and dysembryogenesis of the third through fifth branchial pouches initially are noted to have congenital heart disease and hypocalcemia. They may or may not have the characteristic abnormal facies. Associated thymic hypoplasia results in abnormal cell-mediated immunity and recurrent infections. As these infants are susceptible to GVHD, all donor blood products should be irradiated. Therefore, early diagnosis is essential. Infants with Wiskott-Aldrich syndrome may require intensive-care support for bleeding episodes secondary to thrombocytopenia, while the eczema and immunologic abnormalities may be noted later during follow-up. The purpose of this chapter is not to provide a complete list of congenital immunodeficiency disorders, but it should be remembered that many of these syndromes are likely to be noted in the nursery or within several months of discharge from the hospital.

> Parents with one child who suffers from immune deficiency disorder may desire prenatal diagnosis in subsequent pregnancies. The immune deficiency disorders than can be diagnosed in utero at the present time include severe combined immune deficiency with enzyme deficiency, immunodeficiency with biotin deficiency, ataxia-telangiectasia, Wiskott-Aldrich syndrome, and chronic granulomatous disease.
>
> *M. Abbott*

Secondary Immunodeficiencies. Secondary immunodeficiencies may also manifest themselves after the infant's discharge from the ICN; those related to prematurity or IUGR have already been discussed. Additional etiologic factors in secondary immune dysfunction in such infants include (1) treatment with steroids, (2) malnutrition, (3) congenital infections, and (4) pediatric acquired immunodeficiency syndrome (PAIDS) (see below).

Steroid therapy has been used for brief periods in nursery patients, both to prevent and to treat pulmonary disease. Although such short courses of therapy are benign in the immunologically mature host, there is some evidence that they may contribute to long-term effects in newborns. For a variety of reasons, some degree of *malnutrition* is common in ICN patients and ICN graduates. Abnormalities in all areas of host defense have been described in children with malnutrition. These deficiences do have clinical significance; they predispose to increased morbidity and mortality from infection.

Immunologic consequences of *congenital infections* have been reviewed by Starr.[2] Of the "TORCH" complex infections, only congenital rubella has been associated with clinically significant defects (usually B cell) in immunity. Infants with congenital cytomegalovirus infection, syphilis, or toxoplasmosis may have increased immunoglobulins, but are generally felt to have normal immune responses. No specific immune dysfunction has been described in survivors of neonatal herpes simplex.

PEDIATRIC ACQUIRED IMMUNODEFICIENCY SYNDROME

In 1981, acquired immunodeficiency syndrome (AIDS) was described in homosexual men with abnormal cell-mediated immunity, opportunistic infections such as *Pneumocystis*

TABLE 20-2. Pediatric Aids: Risk Factors by Age Group

	<5 YEARS	5-12 YEARS	13-18 YEARS
Perinatal exposure	79%	17%	—
Transfusion	15%	9%	2%
Hemophilia	1%	42%	1%
IV drug use	—	10%	5%
Sexual contact	—	17%	75%
Unknown	5%	5%	17%

TABLE 20-3. Perinatal Risk Factors for AIDS

IV drug-using mother	61%
IV drug-using father	11%
Mother of Haitian descent	22%
Bisexual partner	4%
Maternal blood transfusion	1%

carinii pneumonia, or malignancies such as Kaposi's sarcoma. Subsequently, AIDS was observed in intravenous drug users and recipients of blood products, including hemophiliacs. In 1983, pediatric AIDS was independently described in three geographically distinct areas associated with three major risk factors: (1) intravenous drug-using mothers, (2) Haitian ancestry, and (3) blood transfusions. Subsequently, vertical transmission of an infectious agent was suggested by the discovery of three affected female siblings born to an intravenous drug-using, prostitute mother. Histocompatibility typing of the siblings and mother documented that each child had a different father, excluding a genetic etiology for the observed immunodeficiency.

As of September 1, 1987, over 500 children and over 35,000 adults with AIDS had been reported to the Centers for Disease Control. These numbers reflected a doubling of incidence in both adults and children since January 1, 1986. Today, with the possible exception of protein-calorie malnutrition, infection with HIV is the major cause of severe cellular immunodeficiency in children.

Transmission and Epidemiology. The most frequent means by which children are infected with HIV is from an infected mother, as the majority of children less than 13 years of age diagnosed with AIDS are infected during the perinatal period (Table 20-2). Other routes include sexual contact (abuse), infected needles, and infected blood products. The most common means of transmission of HIV in infants in utero is through an infected mother. In the majority of these instances, the mother's risk factor is intravenous drug abuse, although other perinatal risk factors exist (Table 20-3). Perinatal transmission through cervical secretions and possibly through breast milk has been suggested.

The second most frequent risk factor for pediatric AIDS in children under age five years has been receipt of contaminated blood products. In 1982, a child with AIDS who had received a platelet transfusion from an infected donor was reported. The other blood products most commonly associated with HIV infection are Factors VIII and IX concentrates for patients with hemophilia. At present, techniques for processing concentrates inactivate HIV. These techniques, as well as antibody testing of all blood donors, have significantly reduced the incidence of new HIV infection in recipients of blood products.

Although the virus has been detected in saliva, tears, and urine, only two possible cases of HIV transmission through casual, nonsexual contact with excretions or secretions have been reported. In both cases the infants received contaminated blood products after birth, developed AIDS, and were cared for at home by mothers skilled in nursing. Neither mother used gloves or other precautions while handling her infant's secretions and excretions. Both mothers developed antibody to HIV. Recently, three health care workers, each of whom came into contact with HIV-infected blood while they had open skin lesions, converted from seronegative to seropositive for HIV. The above examples are meant to illustrate the rare occurrence of infection with HIV by routes other than sexual contact or intravenous infection with contaminated blood or blood products.

Clinical Manifestations. HIV infection in pediatric patients has a clinical course that is similar but not identical to that of adult patients. The incubation period for pediatric AIDS (exposure to onset of clinical AIDS) ranges from weeks to years (eight months median). Many observations remain unexplained, including the variable progression of the syndrome and the fact that some, but not all, infants born to HIV-positive mothers are infected. It is currently estimated that children born to infected mothers have a 50 to 60 per cent risk of HIV infection. In a single, limited study of mothers who had had one previously infected child, two thirds of 20 subsequent children were also infected. The infection of the neonates did not correlate with the

TABLE 20–4. Clinical Presentation in 62
Infants with Symptomatic HIV Infection

	NUMBER	PERCENTAGE
Failure to thrive	55	89
Chronic pneumonia (interstitial)	42	68
Recurrent febrile episodes	60	97
Recurrent bacterial sepsis	28	45
Diarrhea	54	87
Encephalopathy	40	65
Skin rash (eczema-like)	13	20
Chronic parotid swelling	8	13
Cardiomyopathy	3	5
Nephropathy/nephritis	3	3

clinical status of the mother; some healthy, antibody-positive women had infected infants whereas some women with AIDS had uninfected offspring. It has been suggested that the variability of transmission from mother to fetus may reflect the presence or absence of other infections (such as cytomegalovirus or Epstein-Barr virus), differences in pathogenicity of "strains" of HIV, or time during gestation of maternal "viremia."

The incubation period from HIV infection to the development of initial symptoms is approximately eight weeks. Because many children with AIDS acquire the infection in utero, clinical manifestations may begin during the neonatal period. Approximately 60 per cent of children with AIDS are diagnosed before their first birthday.

Many of the clinical manifestations seen in adults affected with HIV are also observed in children. These include fevers, weight loss (failure to thrive), malaise, chronic or recurrent diarrhea, lymphadenopathy, hepatosplenomegaly, and recurrent or persistent thrush (Tables 20–3 and 20–4). Increased susceptibility to bacterial infections in children with HIV often is manifested by draining otitis media and/or recurrent episodes of septicemia and meningitis. The most common pathogens are Streptococcus pneumoniae, Staphylococcus aureus, and Escherichia coli. These signs and symptoms may persist for weeks to months before the development of clinical symptoms indicative of AIDS and may include opportunistic infection, diffuse interstitial pneumonitis, and malignancy. Children appear susceptible to all of the opportunistic infections seen in adults with AIDS. Pneumocystis carinii pneumonia (PCP) occurs in 70 per cent of children with AIDS. Other opportunistic infections that have been identi-

fied in children include invasive Candida esophagitis, invasive herpes simplex, disseminated varicella, cryptosporidium, and atypical mycobacterium. Lymphoid interstitial pneumonitis (LIP) is common in children with AIDS (30 to 60 per cent). Isolated case reports of children with LIP suggest that the long-term prognosis is better in children with AIDS and LIP than in others.

Two clinical aspects of HIV in children deserve specific attention. The first is central nervous system manifestations, which occur in 15 to 50 per cent of children infected with HIV and are characterized by an acquired microcephaly and a progressive loss of developmental milestones. Seizures, although uncommon, do occur. Pyramidal tract signs, such as truncal ataxia, may be seen. Computed tomography of the brain either is normal or shows cortical atrophy and/or basal ganglia calcification. In most cases, results of cerebrospinal fluid examination are normal except for the recovery of HIV. It was initially believed that most neurological involvement in AIDS was secondary to opportunistic infections. It is now clear that HIV is a neurotropic virus.

The second aspect deserving specific mention is the observation of dysmorphic features in children with AIDS. Recently, a group of children who were infected perinatally were noted to have severely dysmorphic features, including microcephaly, prominent box-like forehead, flattened nasal bridge, wide palpebral fissures, hypertelorism, blue sclerae, and shortened philtrum. These features are not specific to all children with HIV infection.

Diagnosis. Children with suspected exposure to HIV, such as a potentially infected mother or a history of blood transfusion, who demonstrate the clinical manifestations described above should be evaluated for pediatric AIDS. To confirm the diagnosis of pediatric AIDS, infection with a retrovirus must be documented. In an infant it is often difficult to interpret a positive antibody test to HIV, because the IgG antibody measured may reflect maternal antibody rather than the infant's own production. At present, no reliable method for detecting IgM antibody to HIV is available. If it is necessary to document HIV infection in an infant under one year of age, cultures for HIV or detection of HIV antigen should be performed. However, success in culturing virus from patients varies considerably.

Laboratory abnormalities found in children with pediatric AIDS are numerous. The earliest findings include polyclonal hypergammaglobulinemia and T-cell immunodeficiency, as evidenced by elevated quantitative immunoglobulins and diminished proliferative response of peripheral blood mononuclear cells to antigen or mitogen. Lymphopenia and abnormal helper/suppressor T-cell ratios, while frequently present in adults with AIDS, may not be found in children with AIDS, and these studies should not be used to diagnose pediatric AIDS.

Recognizing that larger numbers of HIV-infected women will be found in areas with a high prevalence of HIV, the San Francisco Health Department developed perinatal AIDS guidelines. The current recommendations are to assess pregnant women for seropositivity if intravenous drug use has occurred since 1979 or if the mother has had more than five sexual partners since that same year. If the woman is seropositive for HIV antibody during the first trimester, the fetus is considered at risk and appropriate counseling is carried out. If the test for HIV antibody is negative during the first trimester and the mother continues at risk, then antibody testing is repeated during the third trimester. In all deliveries of infants of high-risk mothers, health care professionals should gown, glove, and mask. The placenta should be considered to be highly infectious and handled appropriately. Suctioning of the newborn should utilize wall suction devices. Until the infant is proven to be HIV-antibody negative, all excretions and blood should be regarded as infectious and caregivers should glove to obtain blood, start intravenous infusions, and handle excretions.

In San Francisco, it is recommended that newborns be evaluated for seropositivity to HIV if a mother is seropositive or is at risk for HIV but was not tested for antibody during pregnancy. Recommendations for follow-up of infants born to high-risk mothers include the following: (1) Cord blood should be tested for antibody to HIV; if cord blood is antibody positive, the infant should be re-evaluated at age 12 months when maternal antibody has been catabolized. (2) If the infant is clinically ill, peripheral blood mononuclear cells should be cultured for virus in an effort to document active infection. (3) Immunological function should be followed as indicated. (4) An infant is considered at high risk for clinical AIDS if virus is detected in peripheral blood mononuclear cells or antibody persists beyond 12 months.

A PRACTICAL APPROACH

We have briefly reviewed the information on host defenses at term and in the postnatal period, including, when possible, data on infants cared for in ICN's. Physicians caring for these patients after discharge may see infants who seem to have an increase in the number or the severity of infections. The following is meant to provide some guidelines for evaluation of the status of these children. The evaluation begins with a careful history and physical examination. Special attention should be directed to the types of infections, the response to therapy, growth parameters, and family history. Physical examination should include careful note of the amount of lymphoid tissue present, as well as other stigmas associated with congenital immunodeficiencies (i.e., eczema, petechiae, telangiectasia, albinism, and the like). Live viral vaccines should not be given until the results of an immunologic work-up are available and normal immunity is documented.

Recurrent bacterial infections, particularly with encapsulated organisms, suggest a defect in antibody production, or (less commonly) in the complement pathway. Screening tests of B cell function include quantitative immunoglobulins: IgG, IgM, and IgA. Care must be taken to compare the values obtained with age-matched controls. Both decreased and elevated values may indicate a need for further evaluation. In children with a decrease in all Ig classes (total less than 250 mg/dl) the total number of B cells with surface immunoglobulin should be quantitated. B cells are absent or markedly decreased in patients with congenital hypogammaglobulinemia. Infants with low IgG but detectable IgA and IgM are more likely to have transient hypogammaglobulinemia; they typically have normal numbers of B cells. Gamma globulin therapy is indicated for patients with the congenital form and for those with the transient form who have significant morbidity from infections. As previously mentioned, patients with elevated immunoglobulin values may also need further evaluation; increased levels can be seen in several immune deficiencies, as well as in congenital and perinatal infections—including PAIDS. Therefore the direction of the evaluation will depend on the clinical circumstances.

Complement-deficient patients can also be susceptible to increased bacterial infections. A total hemolytic complement, measured as CH_{50}, is a sensitive and inexpensive screening test; no further evaluation is needed if it is normal. If the CH_{50} is decreased the patient should be referred to an immunologist for further testing. It is important to make the diagnosis of complement deficiencies, because, although the components themselves cannot be replaced, therapy is available (i.e., vaccination with appropriate vaccines and prophylactic use of anti-biotics).

Severe fungal, protozoan, or viral infections, particularly in conjunction with failure to thrive, are suggestive of T cell or combined T cell and B cell defects. The total lymphocyte count is usually a good reflection of the number of circulating T cells (see Table 20–1). Skin testing can be a helpful screening test of function if it is positive, but its usefulness is limited in children under age two years. If T cell deficiency is suspected because of clinical symptoms, an absence of lymphoid tissue, or persistent lymphopenia, then T cell numbers and T cell functional assays (such as mitogen stimulation) should be performed. Treatment for these disorders can include administration of trimethoprim-sulfamethoxazole for prevention of *Pneumocystis carinii* pneumonia, gamma globulin, thymic factors, and lymphokines and bone marrow transplantation. These patients should be referred to a pediatric immunologist.

Phagocytic defects should be considered in patients with recurrent *Staphylococcus aureus* or gram-negative infections, especially those with osteomyelitis, bacterial lymphadenitis, cutaneous abscesses, and/or pneumonia. The initial procedure in detection of these problems is a complete blood count to determine both the absolute neutrophil count and the neutrophil morphology. Intracellular metabolism and killing to diagnose chronic granulomatous disease are evaluated with a nitroblue tetrazolium dye test and then a killing curve. Tests are not clinically available to measure the chemotaxis, deformability, and adherence of phagocyte cells.

It is difficult to recommend precise guidelines of when to investigate the ICN graduate for an immune defect. If the possibility seems likely, a significant portion of the laboratory evaluation (such as the absolute neutrophil and lymphocyte counts and quantitative immunoglobulins) is easily obtained by the primary physician. Infants with worrisome recurrent infection but normal screening tests should be referred to an immunologist for more definitive testing.

Much remains that is not known about immunologic problems of the ICN graduate, and the primary physician should never feel that seeking help is inappropriate.

References

1. Hobbs JR, Davis JA: Serum γ-gobulin levels and gestational age in premature babies. Lancet 1:757, 1967.
2. Starr SE: Immunologic aspects of congenital infections. Clin Perinatol 8:509, 1981.

Recommended Reading

Bernbaum J, Anolik R, Polin RA, et al.: Development of the premature infant's host defense system and its relationship to routine immunizations. Clin Perinatol 11:73, 1984.

Cates KL, Rowe JC, Ballow M: Curr Probl Pediatr 13(8):1, 1983.

Conley ME, Beckwith JB, Mancer JFG, et al.: The spectrum of the DiGeorge syndrome. J Pediatr 94:883, 1979.

Ferguson AC, Cheung SC: Modulation of immunoglobin M and G synthesis by monocytes and T lymphocytes in the newborn infant. J Pediatr 98:385, 1982.

Goldman AS, Garza C, Nichols B, et al.: Effects of prematurity on the immunologic system in human milk. J Pediatr 101:901, 1982.

Host Defense in the Fetus and Neonate (Conference Proceedings). Pediatrics (Suppl) 63:705, 1979.

Miller ME: Host Defenses in the Human Neonate. Monographs in Neonatology. New York, Grune & Stratton, 1978.

Miyagawa Y, Sugita K, Komiyama A, et al.: Delayed in vitro immunoglobulin production by cord lymphocytes. Pediatrics 65:497, 1980.

Notarangelo LD, Chirico G, Chiara A, et al.: Activity of classical and other native pathways of complement in preterm and small for gestational age infants. Pediatr Res 18:281, 1984.

O'Duffy JF, Isles AF: Transfusion induced AIDS in four premature babies. Lancet 2:1346, 1984.

Oleske J, Minnefur A, Cooper R, et al.: Immune deficiency syndrome in children. JAMA 249:2345, 1983.

Pabst HF, Kreth HW: Ontogeny of the immune response as a basis of childhood disease. J Pediatr 97:517, 1980.

Scott GB, Buck BE, Leterman JG, et al.: Acquired immunodeficiency syndrome in infants. N Engl J Med 310:76, 1984.

Stites DP, Carr MC, Fudenberg HH: Ontogeny of cellular immunity in the human fetus. Development of responses to phytohemagglutinin and to allogenic cells. Cell Immunol 11:257, 1984.

Wara DW, Brunner WC, Ammann AJ: Graft versus host disease: Pathogenesis, recognition, prevention and treatment. Curr Prob Pediatr 8:1, 1978.

Welsh JK, May JT: Anti-infective properties of breast milk. J Pediatr 94:1, 1979.

Pediatric AIDS

Amman AJ, Cowan MJ, Wara DW, et al.: Acquired immunodeficiency syndrome in an infant; possible transmission by means of blood product administration. Lancet 1:956, 1983.

Barnes DM: Brain function decline in children with AIDS. Science 232:1196, 1986.

Cowan MJ, Hellmann D, Chudwin D, et al.: Maternal transmission of acquired immune deficiency syndrome. Pediatrics 73:382, 1984.

Marion RW, Wiznia AA, Hutcheon G, et al.: Human T cell lymphotropic virus III (HTLV-3) embryopathy. A new dysmorphic syndrome associated with intrauterine HTLV-3 infection. Am Dis Child 140:638, 1986.

Minkoff H, Nanda D, Menez R, et al.: Pregnancies resulting in infants with AIDS and ARC: Clinical and long-term follow-up of mothers. Pediatr Res 20:297A, 1986.

Oleske J, Minnefor A, Cooper R, et al.: Immune deficiency syndrome in children. JAMA 249:2345, 1983.

Rubenstein A, Bernstein L: The epidemiology of pediatric acquired immunodeficiency syndrome. Clin Immunol Immunopathol 40:115, 1986.

Rubenstein A, Sicklick M, Gupta A, et al.: Acquired immunodeficiency with reversed T4/T8 ratios in infants born to promiscuous and drug addicted mothers. JAMA 249:2350, 1983.

Scott GB, Buck BE, Leterman JG, et al.: Acquired immunodeficiency syndrome in infants. N Engl J Med 310:76, 1984.

Scott GB, Fischl M, Klimas N: Mothers of infants with AIDS: Evidence for both symptomatic and asymptomatic carriers. JAMA 253:63, 1985.

Shaw, GM, Harper ME, Hahn BE, et al.: HTLV-3 infections in brains of children and adults with AIDS encephalopathy. Science 227:177, 1985.

Ziegler JB, Cooper DA, Johnson RT, et al.: Postnatal transmission of AIDS-associated retrovirus from mother to infant. Lancet 1:896, 1986.

21

INFECTIOUS DISEASE ISSUES IN THE CARE OF THE ICN GRADUATE

ANN M. ARVIN, M.D.

Infection is a well-recognized complication of the clinical course of the high-risk newborn in the intensive care nursery (ICN). Infectious diseases pose a continuing problem for many of these infants in the first few years of life. Their care during the months following discharge requires attention to three major categories of problems related to infection. These include (1) proper follow-up of infectious diseases or exposures to pathogens that were identified while the infant was still in the ICN; (2) early identification of infections that become symptomatic or are acquired following discharge from the ICN and the proper management of these infections; and (3) efforts to avoid the exposure of the high-risk infant to certain important pathogens after discharge and the proper management of such exposures if they do occur.

FOLLOW-UP OF INFECTIONS DURING THE IMMEDIATE NEONATAL PERIOD

There are several infectious diseases that may be identified in the immediate newborn period that require careful follow-up during the first few years of life to provide appropriate care and to ensure accurate diagnosis. Follow-up of focal infections caused by bacteria or *Candida* in the newborn period is usually straightforward and is dictated by the site of the initial infection. For example, the infant who has had bacterial meningitis will require periodic re-evaluation by the primary pediatrician, for common sequelae, including hearing deficits, abnormalities of motor function, and delays in language and intellectual development. The monitoring for sequelae is the same regardless of the pathogen that caused the meningitis, e.g., group B streptococcus, *Escherichia coli, Candida,* although the risk of sequelae is probably greater for gram-negative pathogens. The early detection of deficiencies allows appropriate intervention, such as hearing aids or infant stimulation programs, which will be of major value to the child. Infants who have had bone or joint infections with bacteria or with *Candida* are at high risk for altered bone growth or joint deformities that may need orthopedic management. Lobar bacterial pneumonia may leave the infant at greater risk for repeated bacterial respiratory infections. If a documented urinary tract infection occurs in the newborn period, it is especially important to rule out an anatomic defect. Even if such an anomaly has been ruled out, urinalysis and urine culture are advisable several times in the first year of life to be certain that the infant is not having recurrent asymptomatic infection of the urinary tract.

Congenital Infections

A more complex problem concerns the follow-up of infants suspected of having had congenital infection. The evaluation of these infections, which include toxoplasmosis, syphilis, rubella, and cytomegalovirus, is often incomplete or inconclusive at the time of the infant's discharge from the ICN. The symptoms of congenital infection are typically nonspecific, e.g., intrauterine growth retardation, and may not evolve or appear until the infant is several weeks old. The primary pediatrician must identify new findings in the evolving syndrome, determine whether the appropriate diagnostic evaluation has been carried out, and interpret the laboratory results. The concept that intrauterine infections can be diagnosed by a single serum sent for "TORCH" titers is incorrect, with the possible exception of some cases of toxoplasmosis. Often follow-up clinical samples are required to confirm or exclude a suspected intrauterine infection. The primary pediatrician must be aware of the need to continue the work-up for several of these infections and must be aware of the clinical problems that may arise long after discharge. The following paragraphs summarize some details related to infectious diseases that fall into this category.

TOXOPLASMOSIS

Prospective studies have documented that the majority of cases of congenital toxoplasmosis are asymptomatic in the newborn period. In many cases the only manifestation may be intrauterine growth retardation. In some nurseries it is the practice to obtain a serologic test for toxoplasmosis from all high-risk infants. The common clinical findings that suggest the need to rule out congenital toxoplasmosis include intrauterine growth retardation, chorioretinitis or other ocular abnormalities, hepatosplenomegaly, and microcephaly or hydrocephalus. Any of these findings may be obvious at the time of follow-up examination without having been appreciated in the ICN. Congenital toxoplasmosis is relatively rare in the United States, with an estimated frequency of 3300 cases per year. However, it is important to screen infants with nonspecific but compatible symptoms because toxoplasmosis is an intrauterine infection that

should be treated.[1] Even among asymptomatic infants who are identified by routine screening as having congenital toxoplasmosis, there is a very high incidence of later onset of chorioretinitis due to the pathogen. The goal of the early diagnosis and treatment of these infants is to prevent retinitis and other potential neurologic sequelae.

As has been carefully described by Remington,[1] the first clue to the diagnosis of congenital toxoplasmosis is often the detection of an elevated Sabin-Feldman dye titer in serum from the mother or the infant. If a borderline or high titer is detected, it is important to measure the titer of IgM antibody to toxoplasmosis in serum from the mother and the infant. If the Sabin-Feldman titer is significantly elevated or if IgM antibody is detected, most infants should be treated presumptively until the diagnosis can be confirmed. It is seldom possible to make a conclusive diagnosis based upon a cord blood toxoplasmosis titer or on a single serum sample from the infant. The confirmation of the diagnosis is made by following the Sabin-Feldman dye titer in the infant's serum and by repeated testing of the infant for IgM antibody to toxoplasmosis. If the infant's dye titer declines and there is no evidence that the infant's body has begun to make its own antibody to toxoplasmosis by four to six months of age, or if the infant does not develop an IgM response to the agent, then it is unlikely that the infant has congenital toxoplasmosis. However, the diagnosis of congenital toxoplasmosis may require a series of titers in the first few months of life because of the variability in the rate of disappearance of IgG antibody to toxoplasmosis which has been acquired transplacentally from the mother and the variability of the onset of production of IgG antibodies to the pathogen by the infant. In addition, IgM antibodies cannot be detected in all infants who are subsequently proved to have had congenital toxoplasmosis.

Details concerning the treatment of congenitally infected infants should be sought from an infectious disease consultant when the diagnosis of congenital toxoplasmosis is made, because the recommendations change as new information is acquired. At present, the treatment regimen consists of pyrimethamine and sulfadiazine. Treatment with these drugs also requires the administration of folinic acid. Spiramycin is the second drug that is used for treatment of congenital toxoplasmosis, alternating with the pyrimethamine and sulfa regimen. This drug must be obtained through the FDA. Follow-up care of patients being treated for this infection is complicated by the need for hematologic monitoring, by the difficulty of getting the drugs, and by unavailability of the drugs in pediatric formulation.

SYPHILIS

The diagnosis of congenital syphilis usually has been made by the time of discharge of the high-risk neonate, since the clue to the diagnosis of this infection is usually the cord blood VDRL or the VDRL in serum obtained from the mother during pregnancy. The only specific clinical findings of intrauterine syphilis are the cutaneous lesions that contain the spirochete or "pseudoparalysis" with classic bone changes on radiographs. Otherwise the infant may have the typical nonspecific findings suggesting intrauterine infection, especially intrauterine growth retardation and hepatosplenomegaly. If the possibility of intrauterine exposure to syphilis is not noted until the infant is a few months of age, the problem of management may be solved quickly by determining whether the infant was treated in the ICN with ampicillin or penicillin in doses sufficient for the treatment of congenital syphilis. If any question remains it is important to pursue the diagnosis in the infant, because even treatment initiated at several months of age may prevent some of the sequelae of the infection. The diagnosis is made by testing the infant's serum, by means of the VDRL test (or an equivalent nonspecific test), followed by a confirmatory determination of FTA-ABS titer if the VDRL is positive. Antibodies may still be detected by either test in infants who have been adequately treated. If the infant was not treated in the newborn period, it is necessary to determine whether the mother received treatment for syphilis during pregnancy. Most infants of untreated mothers should be given a course of aqueous penicillin, 50,000 U/kg/day in two doses for 10 days. It is generally recommended that CSF be obtained prior to the treatment of these infants to try to document the existence of CNS infection, but a more conservative approach is to treat all infants for the possibility of CNS infection regardless of the CSF findings. If the mother was treated appropriately, the infant can be followed for the disappearance of the antibody from the serum in the first few months of life as evidence that the antibody was only transplacentally acquired and was not a marker for active infection in the infant.

CYTOMEGALOVIRUS

Infection with cytomegalovirus (CMV) may occur in utero or as a consequence of perinatal exposure to the virus. The current evidence suggests that symptomatic infection of the fetus is the result of primary CMV infection of the mother during pregnancy.[2] Most of the 1 per 100 infants who excrete the virus in their urine at the time of birth have acquired transplacental infection from a mother who had experienced primary CMV infection prior to conception. The risks for the latter group of infants in terms of subtle sequelae are not well defined, but are probably minimal in most healthy term infants. CMV infection can also be acquired perinatally by infants of seropositive mothers from exposure to cervical virus at the time of delivery or to breast milk. The infant of a seronegative mother may be infected with CMV through transfusions required during the immediate newborn period or possibly by exposure to fresh breast milk from a seropositive woman. The majority of infants with congenital CMV infection are asymptomatic at birth.

When to Worry. Findings that suggest the initiation of a work-up for congenital CMV include intrauterine growth retardation, microcephaly, hepatosplenomegaly, chorioretinitis, prolonged and unexplained jaundice, and neutropenia or thrombocytopenia. Some manifestations of intrauterine infection may not occur until the infant is a few weeks old and may therefore present a diagnostic problem for the primary pediatrician, e.g., hepatosplenomegaly, jaundice, and petechiae.

The diagnosis of congenital CMV infection is made by isolation of the virus from urine obtained within the first three or four weeks of life. Perinatally acquired infection is diagnosed by detection of the virus in urine obtained after four weeks of life from an infant whose urine culture in the immediate newborn period was negative for the virus. Serologic diagnosis usually is not helpful for the diagnosis of congenital CMV infection, because of the confusion caused by transplacentally acquired IgG antibody to CMV and because the assays for IgM antibody to CMV are difficult to standardize and have a high frequency of false positive and false negative results. In many cases, no urine sample may have been obtained in the first months of life, so that it is difficult to distinguish between congenital and perinatally acquired infection. Until more information is available concerning the consequences of CMV infection for the high-risk premature infant, it is appropriate to observe all infants who are excreting CMV for the less obvious sequelae of this infection.

Careful evaluation of hearing and of developmental milestones is important, whether the infection is likely to have been intrauterine or acquired perinatally. These children should be observed for subtle developmental problems related to speech and language, in particular.

Finally, infants who acquire CMV in the perinatal period may at several weeks of age have a syndrome of protracted pneumonia.[3] These infants develop a diffuse pneumonia that could cause serious illness in a high-risk infant whose pulmonary status remains compromised. This syndrome is clinically very similar to the diffuse pneumonia in infants which is caused by *Chlamydia*.

It is also important to advise the parents of infants who are shedding CMV that there is a risk for transmission of the virus to CMV-susceptible individuals who are in continued close contact with the infant. The virus is shed in the urine for the first few years of life and also is present in the saliva of these infants. The virus is shed in the same quantity and for the same period whether the infection was acquired in utero or postnatally. The major risk is exposure of CMV-susceptible pregnant women, which might cause primary CMV infection during pregnancy and result in damage to the fetus. Since the CMV immunity status of most individuals is not known, it is best to advise limited contact of pregnant women with CMV-infected infants. This recommendation should be handled with great care to avoid the social problems that occur if it is applied in an extreme fashion. The focus should be upon avoiding direct contact with urine and saliva. It should also be pointed out that CMV is *not* a highly contagious virus, and careful hygiene is likely to reduce the risk of transmission significantly. In cases in which the infant of a seronegative mother has acquired CMV while in the ICN, it is important to advise the mother that careful technique should be used during subsequent pregnancies. These women should also be observed for seroconversion, so that if pregnancy occurs it will be known whether the acquisition of antibody to CMV preceded the conception. Women who are known to be CMV seropositive need not be considered at significant risk from exposure during pregnancy to an infant with CMV.

RUBELLA

Congenital rubella, like toxoplasmosis and CMV, may be asymptomatic in the newborn period. Clinical findings that lead to the suspicion of this infection include intrauterine growth retardation, cataracts, chorioretinitis, hepatosplenomegaly, petechiae and thrombocytopenia, "blueberry muffin" rash (dermal erythropoiesis), and patent ductus arteriosus or peripheral pulmonic stenosis. Most infants undergo inadequate work-up for this infection during the newborn period because the serologic approach to diagnosis is limited by the presence of transplacentally acquired antibody to rubella. The diagnosis can be excluded if the mother is proved to be seronegative. If congenital rubella is strongly suspected, the definitive diagnosis requires obtaining viral cultures for rubella from the infant. This virus can be reliably recovered from the infant's pharynx for several years; it is also often present in the urine. Therefore the diagnosis of congenital rubella can be confirmed even if the possibility is not considered until the infant is several months old, when some manifestations such as deafness, cataracts, or hypotonic motor function are noted. Rubella is highly contagious, and children with congenital rubella are a potential source for infection of susceptible pregnant women.

HEPATITIS B

Hepatitis B infection is rarely symptomatic in the newborn period, even among high-risk premature infants. At present, hepatitis B is not transmitted to infants by transfusion of blood products, which are adequately screened, but the virus is transmitted perinatally from a chronically infected mother. There is a small risk of intrauterine infection, which accounts for less than 5 per cent of cases.[4] Hepatitis B is a particular problem among populations with a high frequency of endemic hepatitis B infection.

When to Worry. Asian-Americans, as well as recent immigrants from Asian countries, immigrants from certain areas of Africa, intravenous drug abusers, or mothers with occupational or household contact with chronic carriers of hepatitis B are among the groups in which this infection has a high incidence. The optimal prenatal management of pregnant women with these risk factors includes screening the mother for hepatitis B surface antigen. If a mother is found to be a chronic carrier, or if a mother is known to have had acute hepatitis B infection during pregnancy, it is necessary to begin prophylaxis in the infant by administration of hepatitis B immune globulin within 12 hours after birth. Screening newborns for hepatitis B surface antigen usually is not helpful, because the virus is rarely transmitted prior to delivery and the presence of surface antigen in cord blood does not mean that the infant is already infected. The infant should then receive three doses of hepatitis B vaccine, the first of which should be given within the first week of life, with subsequent doses at one and six months.

In some cases surface antigen positivity in the mother may not be recognized until the infant has been discharged from the ICN. Such infants should be tested for hepatitis B surface antigen. If the infant's serum is already positive, it will not be helpful to give hepatitis B immune globulin or vaccine. However, if the serum is still negative, hepatitis B vaccine should be given to the infant. The infant is not always infected as a result of perinatal exposure, but the risk of exposure persists if the mother remains a chronic carrier. If the infant's serum is already positive for hepatitis B surface-antigen, it is important to repeat the assay to determine whether the infection resolves or whether the infant also has become a chronic carrier. Persistence of the antigen for more than the first year of life would suggest chronic infection of the infant. Chronic hepatitis B infection has implications for the health of the child, i.e., risk of chronic active hepatitis or hepatocellular carcinoma. Intimate contact is required for the transmission of hepatitis B. Hepatitis B vaccine is not recommended except for individuals who have household contact with a known carrier. There should be no restriction on school placement for the infant with hepatitis B.

The chief responsibility of the primary physician is to make certain that follow-up doses of the hepatitis B vaccine are given at the appropriate time to infants who were exposed to hepatitis B in the perinatal period.

Hepatitis vaccine is very expensive, and often these high-risk families cannot easily afford the cost. If the first dose of vaccine (0.5 cc) is given in the nursery, and the hospital pharmacy charges the entire 3-cc vial to the patient's hospital bill, the vial can be given to the parent or physician to be kept in the physician's office for the subsequent doses of vaccine.

A. Rosen

INFECTIONS THAT BECOME SYMPTOMATIC OR ARE ACQUIRED AFTER DISCHARGE

As mentioned in the previous discussion, many infants with congenital toxoplasmosis, syphilis, cytomegalovirus infection, and rubella are asymptomatic in the immediate newborn period and may be evaluated for these infections only because of new findings noted after discharge from the ICN. Perinatally acquired CMV and hepatitis B infections often are also asymptomatic. While the specific diagnosis of these infections is important for appropriate care of the infant, these pathogens rarely cause life-threatening illness. However, there is a group of viral and bacterial pathogens to which infants may be exposed in the perinatal period that can cause rapidly progressive illness in an infant who was considered to be doing well. The inoculation of the infant with these agents is usually unsuspected. Herpes simplex is an example, as is "late-onset" group B streptococcal infection.

HERPES SIMPLEX

Infections with herpes simplex virus (HSV) are usually the result of perinatal exposure. There are a few reported cases of probable intrauterine infections, but these infants usually are identified in the immediate newborn period by the presence of cutaneous lesions and other stigmas, such as microcephaly and chorioretinitis. In infants who are exposed to HSV in the perinatal period the incubation period is variable. The range may be from two to three days of age to as long as six weeks. It is not unusual for mothers of infants with HSV to lack any history of recurrent genital HSV.[5] This may be the result of asymptomatic genital infection in the mother, or it may be a consequence of the infant's having acquired herpes simplex from another source. Because the attack rate for HSV infection is clearly related to prematurity, it is important to be aware of this possible diagnosis in the high-risk premature infant who returns with the development of mucocutaneous lesions compatible with HSV. This infection can now be diagnosed within a few hours by making a smear of the lesion and obtaining a direct immunofluorescence stain for HSV. A Tzanck smear of lesions may also be prepared, but this method is less reliable.

The cutaneous lesions may appear at any location and often are not associated with mucous membrane lesions at the time of onset. Infection of the mucous membranes of the eye is more common than oral infection in the newborn. The early diagnosis of mucocutaneous lesions of HSV is important, because antiviral therapy is available and is much more effective if initiated before the onset of invasive infection. It is also important to recognize that many infants with HSV infection do not have mucocutaneous lesions.[6] Symptoms in infants with disseminated HSV include lethargy, poor feeding, and transient low-grade fever. In other infants there are sudden onset of lethargy, poor feeding, and focal or generalized seizures, i.e., symptoms of HSV encephalitis. Infants with HSV encephalitis are typically older than those with disseminated infection. Most cases occur from the second to the fourth week of life. The work-up for HSV encephalitis requires electroencephalography, computed tomography, and brain biopsy for definitive diagnosis. Serologic studies do not eliminate the possibility of HSV infection, since these infections may occur in seronegative cases; also, the production of antibody in the infected infant may require two weeks or longer. There is no assay for HSV IgM antibody that will aid the diagnosis. The specific diagnosis of neonatal HSV requires viral cultures of lesions or of brain tissue. Culture of the oropharynx may be positive for HSV, even if lesions are not visible. It is also worthwhile to review the mother's history and to re-examine her for evidence of genital infection and obtain cultures from the cervix.

Infants with HSV in the newborn period typically develop recurrent skin lesions. This is the case even among infants who did not have skin lesions as part of the initial presentation of the infection. These recurrent lesions need to be considered from two points of view. The first concerns the risk to the infant. It is clear that in treated infants relapse may occur, and dissemination of encephalitis may develop as a consequence. The second problem is the risk of transmission of the virus to close contacts, but this problem can be managed by careful hand washing. The transmission of HSV 1 or HSV 2 to older children and adults is not associated with a significant risk of life-threatening infection. Caregivers or others in close contact with the infant need be advised only to take usual precautions by washing their hands with soap and water after handling the infant when a recurrent skin lesion is present and to avoid touching their own mouths or eyes before washing.

> The fear of contagion throughout communities and schools must be combated with the sensible approach outlined above. The developmental consequences of hysteria far exceed the risks from protected exposure to a child with herpes lesions.
>
> *P. Gorski*

To prevent the acquisition of HSV by high-risk infants, it is necessary to advise parents to avoid exposing the infant to individuals with fever blisters or cold sores. It is clear that HSV 1 infection can be acquired by infants and that these infections are as devastating as HSV 2 infections. This can be communicated prior to discharge of the infant, but it is worthwhile to emphasize the point in follow-up visits as well.

BACTERIAL PATHOGENS

In evaluating illness in the ICN graduate, it is important to keep in mind the "late-onset" presentations of neonatal bacterial infections. Organisms that have colonized the infant during the hospitalization can become invasive and cause serious infections after discharge. Among bacterial pathogens, group B streptococcus, *Staphylococcus aureus,* and *Escherichia coli* and other gram-negative enteric organisms are important. Although group B streptococcus and *E. coli* infections usually occur in the first few weeks of life, these organisms may be pathogenic to high-risk infants up to several months of age. Other, less common, organisms such as *Listeria monocytogenes* and *Hemophilus* species can occasionally cause sepsis or focal infections in infants who are a few weeks of age.

When to Worry. The late-onset manifestations of these bacterial infections tend to be localized. The major sites for focal infections include the central nervous system and the bones and joints. Bacterial pneumonia also may occur. *Candida albicans* is a fungal pathogen that resembles these bacterial agents in its ability to cause late-onset infections. This pathogen is a particular problem for very low birth weight infants who have had central vascular lines and hyperalimentation. The primary pediatrician should remember that in infants who have been treated in the newborn period for group B streptococcus, *E. coli, Candida,* or other infections, relapse may occur with reinfection by the same pathogen in the same or a new site, e.g., *E. coli* meningitis followed by *E. coli* septic arthritis.

In addition to the "neonatal" bacterial pathogens, bacterial infections secondary to the organisms that commonly cause bacteremia in young children may be a special risk to the ICN graduate. These include *Streptococcus pneumoniae* (pneumococcus) and *Hemophilus influenzae* type B. These organisms are the most frequent agents in meningitis, bacterial pneumonia, and joint infections in the first few years of life. *Neisseria meningitidis* (meningococcus) is the third major bacterial pathogen that causes sepsis and meningitis. There is no definite evidence that high-risk infants are any more likely to develop systemic infections with these bacteria than other young infants, but the ability to localize the infection may be limited in the high-risk infant. Pneumococcus and *H. influenzae* type B are recognized as causing "outpatient bacteremia"; i.e., the infection may occur as fever without localizing findings. It is important to consider obtaining blood cultures in a high-risk infant with unexplained fever, in addition to providing close clinical follow-up. If a culture is positive prior to the onset of focal infection, it may be possible to treat early and thus prevent these complications. Similarly, a positive culture may lead to the earlier identification of a focal infection, such as meningitis.

An additional bacterial agent acquired by vertical transmission is *Chlamydia trachomatis*. The diseases caused by this agent are both preventable and treatable. The clinical expression of *Chlamydia trachomatis* in children takes two forms, conjunctivitis and pneumonia. The incidence of both forms varies with the socioeconomic status of the mother (conjunctivitis: 10 to 70 cases per 1000 live births; pneumonia: 5 to 40 cases per 1000 live births). The pneumonia caused by *Chlamydia trachomatis* has a classic presentation: an afebrile tachypneic infant, one to three months of age, with a staccato cough and interstitial infiltrates on a chest x-ray. Additional laboratory testing usually reveals an elevated eosinophil count (greater than or equal to 300/cu mm) and elevated IgG and IgM. Oral erythromycin shortens the duration of the pneumonia.

M. Abbott

VIRAL RESPIRATORY INFECTIONS

The respiratory viruses that can cause significant morbidity for the ICN graduate include respiratory syncytial virus; parainfluenza viruses I, II, and III; influenza A and B; and, less commonly, adenovirus. There is a high likelihood that primary infection with any of these viruses will cause lower respiratory tract disease in any infant. When such infections occur in an infant who has pre-existing pulmonary disease, the risk of respiratory compromise is significant.

Respiratory Syncytial Virus. Respiratory syncytial virus (RSV) is the most common viral pathogen that is likely to cause lower respiratory infection.[7] Epidemics of RSV infection occur every year in the winter and spring months, so that most cases in high-risk infants occur during these months. Older children and adults have immunity to RSV, which protects them from lower respiratory disease in most cases but does not prevent transient upper respiratory infection. The virus is shed in respiratory secretions and is readily spread by large-particle aerosol if there is close contact between the infected individual and the infant. The virus is also spread by hand contact.

The clinical symptoms of RSV infection in the infant may be the expected ones of pneumonia or bronchiolitis; however, in a small preterm infant, the symptoms may be nonspecific. A prominent finding in these infants is apnea. It is important to be aware of this symptom of RSV infection because it can result in an apparent life-threatening event (ALTE) that is not recognized as related to infection, or it can be considered the recurrence of symptoms of apnea the infant may have had prior to discharge. In general, if the apneic episodes are related to RSV

infection, the symptoms are transient and resolve within a few days.[8] RSV infection can also compromise the high-risk infant directly by copious, thick nasal secretions. The diagnosis of RSV infection can now be made within a few hours by direct immunofluorescence staining of a smear of respiratory secretions.

Bronchiolitis due to RSV infection is a relatively uncommon clinical presentation in the first few months of life. However, it can be a source of serious disease in high-risk infants who are six months to two years of age. The pathologic findings are characterized by obstruction of the small airways with necrotic debris sloughed from the respiratory mucosa. Occlusion of the small airways can further compromise an infant with residual lung disease. Lower respiratory tract disease caused by RSV not infrequently results in the need for assisted ventilation in infants with persistent chronic lung disease. These infants should be evaluated early and frequently during the clinical course of viral respiratory illness. Hypoxemia and hypercarbia may be significant but underestimated clinically in the early phases of the infection. In addition, the appearance of new findings on a chest radiograph may lag behind the clinical illness. Tachypnea, decreased activity, and poor feeding may be the prominent clinical findings. At this time, the management of these infections is supportive in most cases, but a further reason for specific diagnosis of RSV infections is the availability of ribavirin, an antiviral drug that may benefit infants with RSV pneumonia or bronchiolitis.

Parainfluenza Viruses. Parainfluenza I, II, and III are possible causes of viral pneumonia in infancy. Parainfluenza epidemics are less predictable than RSV epidemics and may be the cause of sporadic cases of viral respiratory illness at any time during the year. Parainfluenza infections are recognized most commonly as the cause of laryngotracheobronchitis and croup. The consequences of viral pneumonia with these pathogens resemble those of RSV infection. The edema and mucosal inflammation associated with croup can be a serious cause of morbidity in small, premature infants, particularly those with sequelae of prolonged intubation, e.g., subglottic stenosis. The additional airway compromise caused by the infection can lead to the need for reintubation in these infants.

Influenza Viruses. Influenza A and B are relatively unusual pathogens in viral pneumonia of infancy. The epidemics of these viral infections are also less predictable from year to year, so that infants may not be exposed to these viruses as consistently as they are to RSV. However, if a high-risk infant develops influenza A or B infection, the consequence can be a very severe pneumonia requiring major respiratory support. Consideration should be given to influenza vaccination of the adult caregivers of these children.

Adenovirus. Adenovirus differs from the other respiratory viruses in that it is a DNA virus that has the propensity to cause a more systemic illness than the respiratory viruses, e.g., it may cause hepatosplenomegaly as well as pneumonia. Adenoviral infection is an uncommon cause of pneumonia in infants, but when it occurs, it can cause a severe, necrotizing process that may have long-term sequelae.

PATHOGENIC AGENTS JEOPARDOUS TO HIGH-RISK INFANTS

There are several pathogens that can cause serious infections in the high-risk infant and that should be considered in evaluation of an infant's home environment. The following list is not exhaustive, but is intended to focus upon the more common problems that may arise.

RESPIRATORY VIRUSES

Viral respiratory pathogens are a major cause of morbidity for the graduate of the ICN. Although it is impossible to eliminate exposure of high-risk infants to all of these pathogens, there are strategies for minimizing exposure. This is an important consideration, because the risk of lower respiratory disease from these pathogens, in addition to being associated with primary infection, is also related to the age at acquisition of primary infection. If a child acquires his or her first infection with RSV at two or three years of age, instead of during the first year, the risk of lower respiratory illness and possible sequelae is reduced. Respiratory viral pathogens are usually brought into the home by older siblings and adults, a circumstance that is unavoidable during an epidemic period. However, direct contact with the infant can be minimized when symptoms are present. Clinical studies of RSV transmission have shown that a distance greater than 6 feet is sufficient to prevent airborne transmission of the virus and that careful hand washing or avoidance of hand contact by infected persons also reduces transmission. Thus it is not necessary to isolate the infant from other family members to reduce the risk of acquisition of respiratory viral infections.

The problem of respiratory viral infection also has implications for the kind of child care provided for the high-risk infant. Attendance at a group child care center is likely to result in a high rate of acquisition of respiratory viral infections by a high-risk infant. The risks of these exposures should be weighed carefully against the benefits of the child care provided. Whenever possible, infants who have chronic pulmonary disease should probably be cared for individually or in a "family" day care center with only one or two other children.

> This risk of exposure to viruses complements the neurological interest in protecting recent ICN graduates from the sensory overloading common to the environments of most large day care centers.
>
> *P. Gorski*

PERTUSSIS

Pertussis in the high-risk premature infant can be a very serious clinical problem. In addition to the respiratory compromise caused by this infection, pertussis can interfere seriously with the ability to maintain the infant's nutrition, because of vomiting induced by the paroxysmal cough. The central nervous system complications of pertussis can also be an important cause of morbidity. Pertussis is most often transmitted from school-age children to infants in the home. The high-risk infant should be protected from exposure to pertussis by vaccination of the other children in the household. In many ICN graduates there will be no contraindication to the administration of pertussis vaccine; however, the degree of protection acquired depends upon the number of vaccine doses the infant has received. Therefore the immunization status of the infant's contacts is an important issue. (See Chapter 6.)

MEASLES

As measles vaccination programs have improved, infants are less likely to be exposed to the disease. At present the population groups most likely to be susceptible to measles and that might be sources of exposure to high-risk infants are adolescents and young adults. If a high-risk infant is exposed to measles, it is particularly important that the recommendations for exposed infants be followed.[9] Depending upon the interval between the occurrence of the exposure and its identification, the infant should receive either immune globulin or measles vaccine. If the infant receives vaccine, it is important to provide a follow-up dose if the initial dose was given during the first 12 months of life.

VARICELLA-ZOSTER VIRUS

Primary infection with varicella-zoster virus causes varicella (chickenpox). The virus can be transmitted from individuals who have chickenpox or herpes zoster. The yearly epidemics of varicella are associated with high attack rates among preschool and younger school-age children. Thus, high-risk infants with older siblings may have household exposure to varicella. Most infants born to women who grew up in the United States have transplacentally acquired antibody to varicella-zoster virus. These antibodies usually protect infants from serious infection during the first six to nine months of life. Most preterm infants also probably have sufficient antibody.[10] However, early gestation, very low birth weight infants may lack equivalent titers at birth and theoretically could lose the protection of passive antibody sooner. Severe varicella has not been described in such infants, but the cohort of very low birth weight survivors is small enough that the circumstances may not have occurred yet. If one of these infants, or an infant whose mother has not had varicella, is exposed to varicella, the optimal management would consist of checking the varicella-zoster antibody titers of the infant and, within 72 to 96 hours after exposure, administering varicella-zoster immune globulin to infants with no detectable antibody. If a high-risk infant develops varicella, the infant should be observed carefully for progressive or disseminating infection. Antiviral therapy may be a consideration if the clinical illness is severe.

TUBERCULOSIS

While tuberculosis control has been very successful in most of the population in the United States, there are subpopulations at high risk for this disease. The risk factors relate primarily to socioeconomic variables, the same variables that may also be involved in the birth of a high-risk infant. It is important, when one is evaluating the home environment prior to an infant's discharge from the ICN, to ask whether any adults in the household have a history of tuberculosis or chronic cough. Grandparents as well as parents should be screened, since grandparents may be primary caregivers for the infant. If there is any question, adults can be tested for skin test reactivity. If the infant is exposed to an adult with active tuberculosis, an initial chest radiograph should be obtained and repeated skin testing carried out. Because an infant may show no response to the skin test, and because the attack rate is high among infants with direct exposure to tuberculosis, consideration should be given to beginning INH prophylaxis during the period of skin test follow-up, even if the skin test and chest radiograph are normal. "Empiric" prophylaxis is an issue because the period from the occurrence of primary tuberculosis in infants to dissemination of the infection is very short, i.e., as little as four to six weeks.

VIRAL DIARRHEA PATHOGENS

Rotavirus is the most common cause of diarrhea in the first two years of life. The infection can be diagnosed by means of an enzyme-linked immunoabsorbent assay. Methods to reduce the risk of exposure of infants to this and related viral diarrheal pathogens have not been identified. Management of the high-risk infant, as of any infant, requires supportive care to prevent dehydration. Refeeding can be a problem after viral diarrhea, due to relapses caused by secondary malabsorption.

BACTERIAL DIARRHEA PATHOGENS

Salmonella, Shigella, and *Campylobacter* are the common bacterial pathogens of diarrhea in the United States. These pathogens may result in significant diarrheal disease, which may be dangerous to the high-risk infant. Bacterial enteritis can cause damage to the mucosa of the gastrointestinal tract, which may interfere with nutrition for a prolonged period. *Salmonella* is of particular importance as a pathogen in this context, because of its propensity to cause bacteremia and focal infections in infants.[11] Salmonella may also cause meningitis in infants. Since these infections are introduced into the home by older children and adults, it is important for the family's primary physician to carry out a very careful work-up of clinical syndromes that suggest enteric bacterial infections in other family members. The theoretical issue of the development of chronic carrier status should not lead to the deferral of antibiotic treatment of salmonella infection in infants. A blood culture also is indicated when this pathogen is identified in the stool of a high-risk infant.

Shigella can cause significant morbidity as a gastrointestinal tract pathogen, but it does not carry the same risk of systemic infection, even among high-risk infants. Shigella infection should be treated with oral antibiotics, according to the sensitivity of the organism.

Campylobacter infections are a prominent cause of bacterial diarrhea, but they also have limited potential for causing systemic infection. The clinical course of campylobacter diarrhea appears to be altered by early treatment with antibiotics, so that an attempt to diagnose it is worthwhile. Because campylobacter infection must be treated with erythromycin, rather than ampicillin or trimethoprim-sulfa, laboratory identification of the pathogen is needed.

Infectious disease problems are of primary importance to the practitioner. When working with premature infants, especially those with chronic health or developmental problems, the diagnosis and management of infectious disease create a great deal of anxiety.

B. Bernsten

References

1. Remington J: Toxoplasmosis. In Remington J, Klein J (eds.): Infectious Diseases of the Fetus and Newborn Infant. Philadelphia, W.B. Saunders Company, 1983, p 144.
2. Stagno S, Pass RF, Dworsky M, et al.: Congenital cytomegalovirus infection: The relative importance of primary and recurrent maternal infection. N Engl J Med 306:945, 1982
3. Stagno S, Brasfield DM, Brown MD, et al.: Infant pneumonitis associated with cytomegalovirus, chlamydia, pneumocystis and ureaplasma: A prospective study. Pediatrics 68:322, 1981.
4. Wong VCW, Ip HMH, Reesink HW, et al.: Prevention of the HBsAg carrier state in newborn infants of mothers who are chronic carriers of HBsAg and HBeAg by administration of hepatitis B vaccine and hepatitis B immune globulin. Lancet 2:921, 1984.
5. Yeager AS, Arvin AM: Reasons for the absence of a history of recurrent genital infections in mothers of neonates infected with herpes simplex virus. Pediatrics 73:188, 1984.
6. Arvin AM, Yeager AS, Bruhn FW, Grossman M.: Neonatal herpes simplex infection in the absence of mucocutaneous lesions. J Pediatr 100:715, 1982.
7. Hall CB, Douglas RG: Modes of transmission of respiratory syncytial virus. J Pediatr 99:100, 1981.
8. Anas N, Boettrich C, Hall CB, et al.: The association of apnea and respiratory syncytial virus infection. J Pediatr 101:65, 1982.
9. Measles. In Klein JO (ed.): Report of the Committee on Infectious Diseases (Redbook), 19th ed. Evanston, IL, American Academy of Pediatrics, 1982, p 135.
10. Wang EL, Prober CG, Arvin AM: Varicella-zoster virus antibody titers before and after administration of zoster immune globulin to neonates in an intensive care nursery. J Pediatr 103:113, 1983.
11. Davies PA, Gothefors LA: Bacterial Infections of the Fetus and Newborn Infant. Philadelphia, W.B. Saunders Company, 1984, p 128.

22

CARE OF THE INFANT WITH HEART DISEASE

DAVID TEITEL, M.D.

Infants with congenital heart disease in the newborn period comprise a substantial proportion of the population of the ICN. Of the 1 per cent of infants with congenital heart disease, approximately one half develop significant symptoms in the first week of life, necessitating medical intervention. Not included are those infants, predominantly prematurely born, who develop symptoms of congestive heart failure as a result of a persistently patent ductus arteriosus or infants with persistent pulmonary hypertension of the newborn, who have severe cyanosis, usually after asphyxia or aspiration. Congenital heart disease in infants may occur in several different ways. A large proportion of infants will be asymptomatic, with or without clinical findings suggestive of heart disease. Of those infants who are symptomatic, half have cyanosis, either with or without respiratory distress, and half have congestive heart failure with no significant cyanosis. Those infants with congestive heart failure will have either good peripheral perfusion with evidence of a high-output state or poor perfusion with evidence of a low-output state. Tables 22–1 and 22–2 summarize the various ways heart disease occurs in the newborn, with lesions grouped into hemodynamic categories. There is considerable overlap in these, and multiple lesions may coexist, so that these tables are presented only as a general guide.

This review will address each hemodynamic group in turn. I shall discuss the presentation of each group and important specific findings for particular lesions within the group, review the neonatal care, and then focus on management after discharge from the nursery. Management will be determined by the particular problems that may arise, possible medical or surgical interventions to alleviate such problems, and the relative risk of intervention vs the risk of significant morbidity if the illness is untreated. Although great strides have been made to increase the likelihood of healthy survival of infants with critical heart disease, neonatal management is often palliative, and significant problems may arise in the first several months of life.

CYANOTIC HEART DISEASE

Transposition of the Great Vessels

Infants with transposition of the great vessels are cyanotic because the systemic and pulmonary circulations are functionally separate. Poorly oxygenated systemic venous blood returns to the systemic arteries via the aorta, which is transposed over the right ventricle. Pulmonary blood flow is normal or increased in the presence of a systemic-pulmonary communica-

TABLE 22–1. Congenital Heart Disease Associated with Cyanosis in the Newborn and Infant, Grouped According to Hemodynamic Category

Transposition Group
  D-Transposition of the great vessels
  Double-outlet right ventricle with D-position (type 2)
  Taussig-Bing malformation
  Isolated ventricular inversion
  Complex syndromes with malposed great vessels (e.g., asplenia syndrome)
Decreased Pulmonary Blood Flow
  Tricuspid insufficiency
  Tricuspid stenosis-atresia
  Ebstein's malformation
  Hypoplastic right ventricle
  Tetralogy of Fallot
  Severe pulmonary stenosis-atresia with intact ventricular septum, VSD, or single ventricle, with normal or malposed vessels

TABLE 22–2. Congenital Heart Disease Associated with Congestive Heart Failure in the Newborn and Infant, Grouped According to Hemodynamic Category

High-Output Congestive Heart Failure
  1. Normal systemic arterial oxygen saturation
    Ventricular septal defect
    Endocardial cushion defect
    Patent ductus arteriosus
    Aortopulmonary window
    Arteriovenous malformation
  2. Decreased systemic arterial oxygen saturation
    Total anomalous pulmonary venous connection without obstruction
    Tricuspid atresia with large VSD
    Single ventricle equivalents without pulmonary stenosis
    Truncus arteriosus communis
Low-Output Congestive Heart Failure
  1. Left-ventricular inflow or outflow tract obstruction
    Total anomalous pulmonary venous connection with obstruction
    Cor triatriatum
    Supravalvular or valvular mitral stenosis
    Hypoplastic left-heart syndrome
    Subvalvar or valvar aortic stenosis
    Interrupted aortic arch
    Coarctation of aorta
  2. Intrinsic myocardial dysfunction
    Primary cardiomyopathies
    Coronary artery abnormalities
    Glycogen storage diseases
    Myocarditis
    Infiltrative diseases (e.g., congenital leukemia)
  3. Extrinsic myocardial dysfunction
    Dysrhythmias (supraventricular tachycardia, congenital heart block)
    Endocrine or metabolic causes (e.g., hypoglycemia, hypocalcemia, adrenal insufficiency)
    Sepsis
    Perinatal asphyxia
    Anemia-polycythemia
    Hypovolemia

tion, such as a ventricular septal defect or patent ductus arteriosus. The infants have cyanosis and various degrees of respiratory distress in the first days of life. After stabilization of the infant's condition, cardiac catheterization and balloon atrial septostomy are performed. The septostomy permits highly oxygenated pulmonary venous blood to cross to the left atrium and ventricle and pass to the aorta and permits poorly oxygenated systemic venous blood to cross to the left atrium and ventricle and pass to the lungs for reoxygenation. The infants remain somewhat cyanotic, but as long as systemic arterial oxygen saturation is greater than about 75 per cent at rest, oxygen delivery is adequate and acute decompensation attributable to tissue hypoxia is unlikely. In a few centers, corrective surgery (an atrial baffle or arterial switch procedure) is performed in the first week of life on selected infants. Most infants, however, are discharged from the hospital after septostomy alone, and surgery is performed when the infant is between 2 and 18 months of age.

The greatest problems that may arise in these infants, once home, are consequences of cyanosis, which may cause acute or chronic morbidity by several different mechanisms. Acutely, severe cyanosis may cause tissue hypoxia, which results in anaerobic metabolism, lactic acidosis, and possibly death. Cyanosis may be severe if the atrial septostomy is inadequate, or it may become severe if the communication closes. To ensure that the atrial communication is adequate prior to discharge from the nursery, arterial blood gases should be measured, and oxygen

tension should be at least 30 torr. After discharge, any evidence of increasing cyanosis, either by inspection or by a history of increasing irritability or poor feeding, should alert the physician to repeat arterial blood gas measurements. Some physicians measure transcutaneous oxygen tension during regular office visits as another indicator of the adequacy of systemic oxygen delivery. It is important to realize that oxygen delivery is determined not only by systemic arterial hemoglobin oxygen saturation but also by systemic blood flow and hemoglobin concentration. Systemic blood flow is usually normal in these infants and cannot be increased significantly by drugs. Hemoglobin concentration, however, is critically important to monitor. It normally falls over the first 4 to 10 weeks of life, causing a decrease in systemic oxygen delivery. Cyanosis, however, will stimulate erythropoietin production and maintain or increase hemoglobin concentration. This erythropoietic response will occur only if iron stores are adequate. These infants must be given oral iron supplementation, and hemoglobin concentration and red cell indices must be monitored frequently.

It's nice to know that a single test like a hematocrit, which almost any pediatrician's office can do, can be so valuable in the management of such a complex problem. Most private pediatricians cannot do transcutaneous oxygen measurements in their offices; but this usually can be done at the local hospital.

A. Rosen

Even if systemic oxygen delivery is adequate to prevent acute tissue hypoxia, cyanosis may still cause serious morbidity. When oxygen delivery is chronically subnormal, there is a persistent stimulus to red blood cell production, and polycythemia may occur. A hematocrit level above 65 per cent increases blood viscosity and may cause cerebral, pulmonary, gastrointestinal, or cardiac ischemic events. As well, the hypoxemic infant is more susceptible to serious bacterial infections, and the presence of a systemic-venous-to-systemic-arterial communication increases the likelihood of cerebral abscess and other infections caused by bacteremia. Ischemic events are far more likely in infancy than either cerebral abscess or endocarditis, however. Moreover, ischemic events are more likely with iron deficiency anemia than with polycythemia, probably because of the greater rigidity of iron-deficient red cells. Thus, cyanosis without progressive polycythemia must not be considered benign unless iron deficiency has been excluded. Cyanosis also appears to increase blood coagulability, which would increase the likelihood or severity of ischemic events. Aspirin or other antiplatelet agents may be useful if surgery must be postponed. I would also emphasize that, although endocarditis is rare in infancy, prophylaxis should be given to those infants at risk for bacteremia, and the presence of fever or other signs of infection should be vigorously investigated and treated.

In addition to polycythemia, inadequate systemic oxygen delivery causes metabolism to shift toward activities vital to survival. Growth requires up to 30 per cent of total body oxygen consumption in the normal newborn lamb and probably about 15 per cent in the human. Inadequate oxygen delivery suppresses the metabolic

activity related to growth, and thus failure to thrive commonly occurs in hypoxemic infants. Several mechanisms of growth suppression may come into play, including decreased caloric intake, suppression of DNA replication by intracellular hypoxia, and redistribution of blood flow away from anabolically active tissues. Growth patterns of cyanotic infants must be monitored closely; growth retardation should be considered an indication of inadequate oxygen and substrate delivery that requires intervention. Because severe growth retardation cannot be fully reversed, even after its cause has been eliminated, it must be anticipated and treated early.

Even in the absence of polycythemia and growth retardation, cyanosis may be deleterious to the developing infant. Studies of children with transposition of the great vessels have shown developmental abnormalities in those undergoing late repair in the absence of obvious ischemic events. Developmental delay may be caused by repeated minor ischemic events or by subnormal oxygen delivery during rapid brain development, emphasizing the importance of both maintaining maximal oxygen delivery prior to surgical correction and performing surgery as early as is feasible.

In those infants with large systemic-to-pulmonary communications, arterial oxygen saturation is adequate, but congestive heart failure may occur. Excessive pulmonary blood flow increases interstitial fluid and decreases lung compliance, thereby increasing the work of breathing. In addition, increased cardiac work associated with increased cardiac output may result in inadequate delivery of oxygen because of increased demand rather than decreased supply. The symptoms and signs of congestive heart failure and its treatment are discussed in the next section. Pulmonary vascular disease may progress much more rapidly in infants with large ventricular septal defects when associated with transposition of the great vessels. If surgery is delayed, cardiac catheterization should be repeated within the first six months to evaluate the pulmonary vascular bed. The absence of significant symptoms in this group of patients should not lull the physician into a false sense of security.

Cyanotic heart disease is thus associated with significant morbidity and mortality in infancy. Ischemic events, growth retardation, serious infections, and developmental delay all may occur. Congestive heart failure and pulmonary vascular disease may occur in the presence of large shunts. The physician should closely monitor severity of cyanosis, hematologic status, and growth and development. The patient should be referred for surgical correction or palliation immediately if any abnormalities are detected that are not remediable by medical intervention. Even in the absence of problems, surgical correction should be attempted as early as is feasible (i.e., when patient age or size does not significantly increase morbidity of surgery). In simple transposition of the great vessels, many centers perform elective surgery by two months of age. The presence of a large ventricular septal defect markedly increases surgical morbidity, because ventriculotomy must be performed, usually in the systemic (right) ventricle. In these patients, surgery may be delayed for several months, but concern for the development of pulmonary vascular disease must be extremely high. The presence of more complex lesions (e.g., single ventricle) may exclude corrective surgery, and palliation should be performed only when necessary.

DECREASED PULMONARY BLOOD FLOW

Approximately one half of infants with cyanotic heart disease have normally related great vessels, but pulmonary blood flow is decreased. Inflow obstruction of the right ventricle may occur at the tricuspid valve alone (tricuspid atresia or stenosis) or as part of the hypoplastic right heart syndrome. Outflow obstruction may be complete (pulmonary atresia) or partial (pulmonary stenosis), but severe enough to cause a right-to-left shunt. Any of these lesions may be associated with ventricular septal defect (e.g., tetralogy of Fallot).

These infants have cyanosis and hyperventilation in the newborn period but without true respiratory distress. Cyanosis may not be immediately apparent because the ductus arteriosus is patent at birth and may be of adequate size to allow normal pulmonary blood flow. When the ductus arteriosus begins to close, cyanosis will become apparent during feeding or crying. The immediate care of these infants includes decreasing oxygen requirements (ensuring a neutral thermal environment), correcting any metabolic derangements (hypoglycemia, hypocalcemia, or hemoglobin or electrolyte abnormalities) and infusing prostaglandin E_1 to maintain patency of the ductus arteriosus. After stabilization, the infants undergo definitive investigation (echocardiography and usually cardiac catheterization), so that long-term therapy can be determined. In many infants with tetral-

ogy of Fallot, pulmonary blood flow across the narrowed outflow tract is adequate, so that early surgical intervention is not necessary. In other lesions, immediate definitive surgical correction is possible. For example, severe pulmonary stenosis or atresia with an intact ventricular septum and a normal right ventricle may be corrected by a simple pulmonary valvotomy or pulmonary outflow patch. Unfortunately, many newborns do not have surgically correctable lesions but require palliative surgery. This may be achieved by a variety of approaches. Usually some form of aortopulmonary shunt is carried out to connect a systemic and pulmonary artery, either directly (e.g., Blalock-Taussig anastomosis between a subclavian artery and branch pulmonary artery) or via an artificial tube (e.g., a Goretex shunt between the ascending aorta and main pulmonary artery). Other techniques to increase pulmonary blood flow include enlarging the right ventricular outflow tract with an artificial patch (in severe tetralogy of Fallot or pulmonary atresia) or increasing the size of a ventricular septal defect when the right ventricle and pulmonary outflow tract are normal (in tricuspid atresia with ventricular septal defect). Right ventricular outflow enlargement is becoming more popular because it does not distort the branch pulmonary arteries and allows the right ventricle and main pulmonary artery to develop normally, making later definitive surgery more feasible. The infant is discharged from the nursery when arterial oxygen saturation is adequate and the infant is feeding well.

Once home, these infants should be cared for in a fashion similar to those with transposition of the great vessels. The most common and serious morbidity results from cyanosis. Palliative procedures such as shunts allow only a fixed amount of blood to enter the pulmonary arteries. As the infant grows, pulmonary blood flow becomes inadequate. There is also a fairly high incidence of shunt obstruction that results in reduced pulmonary blood flow. In tetralogy of Fallot, infundibular narrowing tends to progress over the first few months of life, and thus pulmonary blood flow may become inadequate rapidly. The physician must carefully monitor the color and hematologic status of the infant to ensure that iron intake is adequate. The parent should be alert to any changes in the infant, particularly increasing cyanosis or irritability or decreasing feeding or activity.

Hypercyanotic Episodes. These infants may also develop hypercyanotic episodes. These episodes tend to occur in the early hours of the morning, but can occur at any time of day. They begin with fussiness and increasing cyanosis. The infants then become inconsolable, crying persistently and becoming more cyanotic. The episodes may end spontaneously, or they may be terminated by fainting or a generalized seizure. The mechanisms for hypercyanotic episodes are uncertain. Some investigators have described infundibular spasm that causes increased right ventricular outflow tract obstruction in infants with tetralogy of Fallot. However, true muscle spasm is probably uncommon. Similar episodes also occur in infants with pulmonary atresia and aortopulmonary shunts who do not have a right ventricular outflow tract. A variety of changes in the loading conditions of the heart probably occur, directing blood away from the lungs. For example, in tetralogy of Fallot, a decrease in the preload of the right ventricle will decrease its end-diastolic volume, accentuate the narrowing of the outflow tract in systole, and thus increase the right-to-left ventricular shunt. A decrease in systemic vascular resistance will increase blood flow to the systemic arteries and away from the pulmonary arteries. This occurs even in pulmonary atresia, in which the shunt flow is proportional not only to the size of the shunt but also to the relative resistances of the pulmonary and systemic vascular beds. A decrease in both preload and systemic vascular resistance occurs during sleep, when there is venous pooling and systemic vasodilation. The increased incidence of hypercyanotic episodes during cardiac catheterization can also be explained on this basis: sedation causes systemic vasodilation, and venous pooling occurs when the infant is placed in a supine position and muscle movement is limited. Once a hypercyanotic episode begins, the infant becomes irritable and cries vigorously. This increases intrathoracic pressure, which is transmitted to the pulmonary vascular bed. An increase in pulmonary resistance further directs blood away from the lungs, increasing cyanosis. Progressive systemic arterial hypoxemia causes pulmonary vasoconstriction, which also increases pulmonary resistance. Moreover, crying and irritability increase oxygen consumption so that, while oxygen delivery is rapidly decreasing, demand is increasing.

The vicious circle of progressive cyanosis leading to further decreases in pulmonary blood flow and arterial oxygen tension is difficult to terminate. If the infant is at home, the parent should place the baby in the knee-chest position to increase systemic vascular resistance and direct blood flow back to the lungs. Efforts should be made to placate the infant to decrease oxygen consumption and pulmonary resistance. If the infant is in the hospital, further interventions may be undertaken if necessary. Oxygen administration increases oxygen delivery by that amount of oxygen that can be dissolved in blood. This is not a large amount, but, in the presence of severe hypoxemia, oxygen may be doubled. Oxygen administration also causes pulmonary vasodilation, which increases blood flow. Drug administration is rarely necessary, but morphine or propranolol may be given. Morphine decreases oxygen consumption, relaxes the infant, and may relieve infundibular spasm (if it is present). Propranolol decreases oxygen consumption and may also relieve infundibular spasm. In addition, propranolol decreases heart rate and thus increases the end-diastolic volume of the right ventricle. In tetralogy of Fallot this would decrease the degree of right ventricular outflow tract obstruction in early systole and thus markedly increase pulmonary blood flow. Finally, propranolol increases systemic vascular resistance, which also redirects blood to the lungs.

> In anticipation of possible hypercyanotic episodes, one might consider having oxygen and/or medication available at home for some families. In any case, they should have printed instructions which could be used by the technicians who staff the 911 emergency medical service in many communities.
>
> *A. Rosen*

The long-term management of infants who have had hypercyanotic episodes is controversial. These episodes do occur more frequently in anemic infants, probably because the diminished oxygen delivery at rest creates a smaller reserve. Transfusion may thus abolish hypercyanotic episodes; we give a transfusion to any infant who has had one episode and whose hematocrit is under 40 per cent. Many physicians begin oral propranolol, which has been shown to decrease the incidence of hypercyanotic episodes. In our institution, infants with tetralogy of Fallot in whom anemia is not the cause of hypercyanotic episodes undergo surgery after their first episode. We feel that the risk of surgery, even in the young infant, is less than the risk of morbidity from future episodes. If the pulmonary arteries are of insufficient size to attempt closure of the ventricular septal defect, an outflow patch alone is performed. In infants with more complex cyanotic heart disease, a decision between medical and surgical management may be more difficult, but we are still inclined to perform surgery to improve pulmonary blood flow if possible. Other complications, including polycythemia, retardation of growth and development, and brain abscess, occur with frequency similar to that seen in transposition of the great vessels and require no further discussion here.

Congestive Heart Failure. Infants with this group of lesions may also have congestive heart failure. Pulmonary blood flow may be excessive because of a left-to-right ventricular (mild tetralogy of Fallot or tricuspid atresia with ventricular septal defect) or aortopulmonary shunt. These infants should be treated as described in the section on congestive heart failure. Congestive heart failure usually resolves as the infant grows. In these infants, pulmonary vascular resistance should be assessed within the first year of life.

In asymptomatic infants without excessive cyanosis, hypercyanotic episodes, or congestive heart failure, we still follow the dictum that surgical correction should be performed as early as possible, to improve oxygen delivery and separate the two circulations. In infants with tetralogy of Fallot this can usually be accomplished late in the first year of life. In infants in whom the right ventricle is inadequate a Fontan operation or some modification of it (connecting the right atrium to the pulmonary arteries with or without an artificial tube) can be performed when the arteries are of adequate size. We prefer to wait until after the age of two years, since the morbidity of surgery is high in younger children. There are still a significant number of children in whom "correction" (i.e., separation of the two circulations to achieve normal arterial oxygen tension) cannot be accomplished, usually because the pulmonary arteries are too small. These infants should be treated conservatively; when there are signs of inadequate oxygen delivery (polycythemia with hematocrit greater than 65 per cent, hypercyanotic episodes, or growth retardation), a further palliative shunt should be performed.

Summary

In summary, infants with cyanosis attributable to decreased pulmonary blood flow are a heterogenous group who often require palliation at birth and may have more definitive surgery within the first few years of life. The major problems are caused by cyanosis, hypercyanotic episodes, polycythemia, anemia, infection, and, rarely, congestive heart failure. These infants should be cared for carefully, and urgent cardiology consultation should be requested if there is any evidence of a change in clinical status that may be attributable to cyanosis.

CONGESTIVE HEART FAILURE

Increased Pulmonary Blood Flow (High-Output Failure)

Infants with acyanotic heart disease and increased pulmonary blood flow may have congestive heart failure in the newborn period. These infants can be divided into two groups: those with a left-to-right shunt and normal systemic arterial oxygen tension, and those in whom systemic venous and pulmonary venous blood mix at some level in the heart or blood vessels, thus mildly decreasing systemic arterial oxygen tension. In the absence of obstruction to pulmonary blood flow, however, the presentation of these two groups of infants is similar, and is attributable to excessive blood flow to the lungs (Table 22–2).

Unlike infants with cyanotic heart disease, these infants usually do not have symptoms in the first few days of life. Pulmonary vascular resistance is high at birth and does not permit a large amount of blood to enter the lungs. There is a rapid fall in resistance over the next few weeks of life, which then permits a large proportion of the systemic output to be redirected into the pulmonary circulation. Congestive heart failure is rarely evident until pulmonary blood flow exceeds systemic by two and a half to three times (except in the premature infant). This increase in pulmonary blood flow will occur earliest when there is a large runoff to the pulmonary circulation throughout systole and diastole. Thus, infants with truncus arteriosus and aortopulmonary window have congestive heart failure often within the first two weeks of life. Infants with ventricular septal defects and endocardial cushion defects will have heart failure in the first two months of life if the communications are large enough, because these shunts are primarily systolic. Lastly, shunts at the atrial level may be associated with heart failure only after several months of life (if at all), since right ventricular compliance for accepting blood decreases very slowly, and thus, left-to-right atrial shunting occurs only intermittently during ventricular diastole. Therefore, infants who are admitted to the ICN with congestive heart failure generally have truncus arteriosus or multiple-level shunts permitting shunting throughout much of the cardiac cycle or are prematurely born infants with either ductal or ventricular

---

TABLE 22 – 3. Therapy for Congestive Heart Failure

Decrease Oxygen and Substrate Demand
 Maintain neutral thermal environment
 Treat infection, especially associated fever
 Elevate head of bed
 Diuresis
  Agents include furosemide, spironolactone, hydroclo-
   rothiazide, metolazone
 Systemic arterial and venous vasodilation
  Agents include prazosin, captopril, hydralazine, ni-
   troglycerine, nitroprusside
Increase Oxygen and Substrate Delivery
 Maintain hemoglobin concentration normal (or high)
 Maintain adequate caloric intake (150 to 200 kcal/kg/
  day)
 Inotropic support
  Oral agent, digoxin (amrinone, milrinone, prenalterol
   may become available)
 Systemic arterial vasodilation
  See above

---

level shunts (these infants can develop heart failure with much less pulmonary blood flow).

Congestive heart failure in the newborn results in tachypnea with respiratory distress, tachycardia, diaphoresis, and poor feeding and growth. The symptoms are caused by several mechanisms. Pulmonary blood flow is excessive and causes increased interstitial fluid, which in turn increases the work of breathing. To maintain adequate systemic blood flow in the face of large redirection of left ventricular output to the lungs, sympathetic activity is extremely high. This increases cardiac output, heart rate, and basal metabolism, particularly of brown fat. Oxygen consumption thus rises because of the increased cardiorespiratory work and metabolic rate. This increased oxygen and substrate demand directs consumption away from anabolic processes, suppressing growth. Growth is further suppressed because respiratory distress limits the infant's ability to feed. Regurgitation is a frequent complicating factor in young infants with congestive heart failure, further limiting substrate availability.

OPTIMAL OXYGEN DELIVERY

Therapy may be oriented in many directions (Table 22 – 3). However, each therapeutic method must be focused toward increasing oxygen or substrate delivery or toward decreasing demand. To minimize oxygen demand, work of breathing should be reduced and normal metabolic processes should be controlled. Diuretics are the mainstay in decreasing the work of breathing, because they decrease interstitial edema. Furosemide, spironolactone, thiazides, ethacrynic acid, and metolazone may be used individually or in various combinations to maximize diuresis while adequate circulating volume is maintained. Electrolyte and blood urea concentrations should be monitored frequently during aggressive diuresis. To decrease further the work of breathing, elevating the head of the infant's bed is helpful and has the added benefit of decreasing regurgitation. Oxygen may be used if pulmonary edema causes alveolar hypoxia, but this is rare. Moreover, increasing arterial oxygen tension decreases pulmonary vascular resistance, which may significantly increase the magnitude of the left-to-right shunt and aggravate the heart failure. Afterload reduction is a relatively new but promising therapy in high-output failure. Reducing systemic vascular resistance increases the proportion of left ventricular output that goes to the body. Systemic blood flow, which is usually normal prior to therapy, does not actually increase; rather, left ventricular output and pulmonary blood flow decrease. Prazosin, hydralazine, and captopril have all been used with equivocal results. Unfortunately, systemic vascular resistance is usually low in high-output failure and cannot decrease greatly without an unacceptable decrease in systemic blood pressure. In addition, pulmonary vascular resistance may decrease to a similar degree during therapy, limiting the effectiveness of these agents.

ANEMIA

At this juncture it is important to discuss the critical role that the normal fall in hemoglobin concentration plays in the decline of pulmonary vascular resistance over the first few weeks of life. If hematocrit were maintained at levels greater than 45 per cent in these infants, pulmonary vascular resistance would fall much less, causing a smaller increase in pulmonary blood flow. These infants must therefore be monitored for adequate iron stores and hemoglobin concentration. If heart failure cannot be controlled by the usual techniques, blood transfusions should be considered in the anemic infant.

Oxygen demand may be decreased by ensuring that the infant is in a neutral thermal environment and is normothermic. Exposure to heat and, particularly, to cold markedly increase metabolic rate and thus oxygen consumption. Substrate delivery must also be monitored. To grow normally, infants with congestive heart failure may require up to 150 to 200 kcal/kg/day. If this is not possible by normal feeding, supplementation with calorically dense substances (e.g., medium-chain triglycerides, Polycose) or nasogastric feeding may be necessary. Fluid restriction has no role in the long-term management of infants with heart failure. Caloric intake must not be sacrificed, and excessive fluid retention should be controlled by diuresis.

INOTROPIC AGENTS

The use of inotropic agents is controversial. Digoxin has been a mainstay in the treatment of young infants with high-output failure. The rationale is to improve oxygen delivery by increasing cardiac output. However, sympathetic activity increases markedly in infants with high-output failure, and the myocardium is probably maximally stimulated. In fact, the left ventricle often ejects four to six times more than its normal output. Moreover, the vast majority of any increase in output that could be achieved by inotropic agents would be delivered to the lungs, further increasing the work of breathing. The therapeutic-toxic ratio of digoxin is also very small, and vigorous diuresis often causes hypokalemia, increasing the likelihood of digoxin toxicity. Thus, many cardiologists do not recommend the early use of digoxin in neonates with congestive heart failure associated with increased pulmonary blood flow. They begin with digoxin only if all other methods fail and surgery is being considered.

PROBLEMS AFTER DISCHARGE

Once the infant is discharged from the hospital, care should be monitored closely. Problems that may arise include recurrence or exacerbation of heart failure, bacterial endocarditis, recurrent respiratory tract infections, and development of pulmonary vascular disease. Congestive heart failure may be manifested by tachycardia, tachypnea, diaphoresis, poor feeding, or failure to thrive. Heart failure occurs when the heart is not supplying the body with adequate oxygen and substrate to maintain normal metabolic function, which, in the child, includes growth. The only finding of heart failure may be failure to thrive, and it is critically important to monitor the infant's weight gain on discharge from hospital. To confirm that failure to thrive results from heart failure rather than inadequate caloric intake, we measure resting oxygen consumption and calculate caloric intake. The normal infant's oxygen consumption is approximately 150 ml/kg/min. In heart failure, oxygen consumption of over 200 ml/kg/min is common. If heart failure is considered to be the cause of failure to thrive, the physician should treat the infant along the lines just described. If failure to thrive cannot be controlled medically, surgery should be considered. Failure to thrive is the primary indication for closure of a ventricular septal defect in the first few months of life; pulmonary vascular changes do not occur that early, and spontaneous closure is likely, so that surgery is deferred unless growth retardation supervenes.

> When following a baby with congenital heart disease, we often focus on proper weight gain as a recordable indicator of well-being. Many times we nervously look at weight gain to make sure that a rapid increase is truly weight gain and not evidence of heart failure. This is especially true for the baby who is always a little symptomatic. Diaphoresis as an indicator of heart failure must be viewed with the understanding that many babies perspire profusely shortly after falling asleep and that that is nothing for the parents to be concerned about.
>
> *A. Rosen*

PULMONARY VASCULAR DISEASE

Pulmonary vascular disease is the most critical problem facing the infant with high pulmonary blood flow. Development of irreversible vascular changes in the pulmonary bed is caused by shear forces on the endothelial surfaces of the small arterioles. These forces are determined by the velocity and volume of blood passing through the vessels and the systolic and diastolic pressures that impinge upon the vessel walls. Alveolar or systemic arterial oxygen tension may affect shear forces. Hypoxemia constricts pulmonary arterioles, and the resultant decrease in luminal size increases the pressure and velocity of blood passing through them. The rapidity of development of pulmonary vascular disease can be predicted by the pathophysiology of the cardiac lesion in question. Truncus arteriosus, with extremely high pulmonary blood flow and systolic and diastolic pulmonary hypertension, may be associated with irreversible changes within the first six months of life. Endocardial cushion defects and large ventricular septal defects, in which pulmonary blood flow and systolic pressure are high, often show irreversibility within 18 months, whereas atrial septal defects, in which only pulmonary blood flow is high, do not show irreversibility until the third decade of life or later. As mentioned earlier, cyanotic infants with increased pulmonary blood flow can develop pulmonary vascular disease at an extremely early age, based on the added effects of hypoxemia on the pulmonary vascular bed. There is also a group of infants in whom irreversible pulmonary vascular disease develops early because the normal postnatal drop in resistance does not occur. These infants appear to maintain much of the fetal musculature around their pulmonary arterioles after birth. Pulmonary blood flow does not increase greatly, and congestive heart failure does not occur. However, the small luminal size and the subsequent high-velocity and high-pressure blood flow lead to early development of endothelial damage. These infants often have endocardial cushion defects in association with trisomy 21, and appear cyanotic, especially when crying, at a very early age.

Pulmonary vascular disease can be prevented only if the physician recognizes the potential for its development and advises surgery when the risk appears too high. Currently the only method of accurately determining pulmonary arterial pressures and resistance is by direct measurement during cardiac catheterization. During catheterization, pulmonary vasodilators may be given to assess the reactivity of the pulmonary bed. When reactivity begins to decrease, irreversible changes are likely to occur, and thus surgery must be considered. Prior to catheterization, noninvasive studies, such as physical examination, electrocardiography, and echocardiography, can demonstrate the progression of right ventricular hypertension and alert the cardiologist to perform catheterization. Awareness of the likelihood of development of pulmonary vascular disease for each lesion permits catheterization and surgery to be planned logically. Generally, infants with truncus arteriosus are catheterized within the first two months of life, and surgery is performed by two months of age. In complete endocardial cushion defects, catheterization is usually performed by six to eight months of age, with surgical correction performed soon thereafter. Ventricular septal defects have a great tendency to close spontaneously, so we try to delay intervention as long as possible. If the infant grows normally but shows evidence of right ventricular hypertension on examination and noninvasive studies, catheterization is usually performed by nine months of age. Depending on the pulmonary vascular resistance and the reactivity of the pulmonary bed, surgery is either recommended or delayed. If surgery is delayed, the infant should be reassessed by catheterization no less than every six months if pulmonary hypertension exists, since a decrease in reactivity signaling irreversible changes may occur quickly.

SUMMARY

In summary, those infants with high-output congestive heart failure in early infancy usually have nonrestrictive ventricular or arterial communications. Congestive heart failure causing failure to thrive is the most common problem in the first few months of life. Heart rate, respiratory rate and effort, diaphoresis, and especially feeding and weight gain should be monitored closely on an outpatient basis. Heart failure often worsens between four and eight weeks of age as a result of the normal decrease in hemoglobin concentration, which decreases oxygen delivery and also causes a fall in pulmonary vascular resistance, further increasing the left-to-right shunt. Therapy should be aimed at decreasing oxygen demand, ensuring caloric intake, and perhaps redirecting blood away from the lung (by red blood cell transfusions) and toward the body (by vasodilators). Respiratory tract infections should be anticipated and treated aggressively. Surgery should be considered when heart failure cannot be controlled medically or when the risk of pulmonary vascular disease becomes greater than that of surgery. All of these children should be followed in close collaboration with a pediatric cardiologist.

Low-Output Failure

Congestive heart failure in the newborn may also occur with low cardiac output; i.e., the left ventricle is unable to eject enough blood to maintain adequate oxygen delivery and perfusion pressure (see Table 22–2). The infants appear pale, cool, tachypneic, and in respiratory distress, with poor pulses and perfusion. They usually develop significant metabolic acidosis and have significant organ dysfunction. Low-output heart failure on a cardiac basis is caused either by obstruction of inflow to or outflow from the left ventricle or by intrinsic or extrinsic dysfunction of the myocardium. Obstruction to left ventricular outflow of blood is the most common cause of low-output failure, and coarctation of the aorta and hypoplastic left-ventricle syndrome are the most common causes of obstruction. Myocardial dysfunction may be caused by a wide variety of processes (Table 22–2), but is usually caused by metabolic derangements, such as hypoglycemia, polycythemia, or perinatal asphyxia.

SUPPORTIVE THERAPY

When an infant has low-output failure, it is important to correct the metabolic derangements rapidly, support the circulation, and define the cause of the failure so that specific therapy may be instituted. Metabolic derangements, such as metabolic acidosis, hypoglycemia, hypocalcemia, and hypoxia, should be evaluated and treated. Oxygen, with or without ventilatory support, is indicated if the infant is hypoxemic or hypercarbic. The circulation should be supported by volume infusion if there is no evidence of volume overload, by diuresis if there is, and inotropic agents, such as dopamine or isoproterenol, to improve myocardial function. Isoproterenol is particularly useful in the infant without significant tachycardia (140 beats/min), since increasing heart rate alone can greatly increase output. Rapid anatomic diagnosis should be made by echocardiography and other noninvasive tests. If outflow of blood from the left ventricle appears obstructed, prostaglandin E_1 should be infused to open the ductus arteriosus and allow the right ventricle to supply blood to the body, until surgery can be performed. If echocardiography is not available and obstruction cannot be excluded, prostaglandin E_1 should be infused until the infant is admitted to an institution where the diagnosis can be made. All infants with either inflow or outflow obstruction to the left ventricle should undergo surgery, if possible, since deterioration is the rule in untreated lesions. Those infants with intrinsic myocardial dysfunction should be treated supportively, and specific therapy may be instituted for specific problems (e.g., treatment of the dysrhythmia in supraventricular tachycardia).

HOME CARE ISSUES

The infant is discharged from the ICN once the hemodynamic status is stable and he or she can feed normally. The residual hemodynamic difficulties are extremely variable, depending upon the underlying lesion and the success of any specific intervention. However, the problems that may develop in these infants are similar, as are the signs of impending problems. The treatment will again vary, depending on the lesion. Major complications depend on the ability of the left ventricle to perform and the residual

stresses on the ventricle that oppose its performance. If the function of the left ventricle is inadequate, its filling pressure increases, which also causes right ventricular filling pressure to increase. Both pulmonary venous and systemic venous pressures will be elevated, leading to respiratory distress, poor feeding, hepatomegaly, and failure to thrive. As in high-output heart failure, hemoglobin concentration should be maximal. The major problem in obstructive heart disease is serious, and potentially irreversible, myocardial damage that may occur prior to clinical evidence of heart failure; the physician must therefore consider other indices of cardiovascular compromise.

The infant should be monitored frequently over the first few months of life. Feeding and weight gain are most critical. A careful history of respiratory distress and diaphoresis, particularly during feeding, may uncover problems. Historical evidence of myocardial ischemia should be sought and would be suggested by increasing irritability and episodes of uncontrollable crying. Physical examination should be directed toward assessing perfusion and pulses, blood pressure, liver size, and respiratory status. Heart failure in infants with nonobstructive disease should stimulate the physician to institute or increase medical therapy. Diuretics are still the mainstay of treatment. They not only decrease interstitial pulmonary fluid, but also decrease preload to more normal levels and improve myocardial performance. Inotropic agents are far more useful in low-output than in high-output heart failure. Myocardial function may be impaired because of intrinsic abnormalities of the myocardium or by inadequate myocardial perfusion. Afterload reduction may also improve these infants. Unlike high-output failure, low-output failure is associated with decreased renal blood flow and thus with increased renin secretion. The subsequent production of angiotensin II and aldosterone raises systemic vascular resistance to supranormal levels. This increase in afterload further obstructs the left ventricle and decreases its output. Vasodilators, particularly angiotensin-converting enzyme inhibitors (e.g., captopril), cause a marked decrease in resistance and an increase in cardiac output. As in high-output failure, caloric intake should be maximized, and supplementation with high-density substances is often beneficial. (See also Chapter 14, Section on Nutrition in CLD.)

Obstructive heart disease requires intensive follow-up. Since progressive myocardial damage can occur in the absence of symptoms, these infants should be under the care of a cardiologist who can perform periodic echocardiography and other noninvasive tests to assess myocardial hypertrophy and fibrosis. Symptoms are usually a sign of severe impairment, and unless unfeasible, surgery is warranted. In coarctation of the aorta the physician should measure upper and lower limb pressures, even after repair. The presence of hypertension or a differential between blood pressures of 20 torr or more demands full cardiovascular assessment. Hypertension in the absence of coarctation of the aorta is not caused by congenital heart disease, so that a noncardiac cause must be sought.

SUMMARY

Low-output failure secondary to obstructive heart disease is a serious problem that usually requires urgent surgery. In those infants with nonobstructive low-output failure, symptoms can generally be controlled by a combination of diuretic, inotropic, and afterload-reducing agents, in association with good caloric intake and maximal hemoglobin concentration. Follow-up should be frequent, directed toward assessing growth and signs of congestive heart failure. In addition, infants with obstructive heart disease should be evaluated regularly by a pediatric cardiologist.

BACTERIAL ENDOCARDITIS

Bacterial endocarditis is rare in infancy. However, if persistent fever is found in any infant with congenital heart disease, blood cultures should be obtained to exclude endocarditis as the source. Although embolic phenomena and other, cutaneous, manifestations of endocarditis are rare, hematuria and splenomegaly are more common and should be sought. Endocarditis will most likely occur when a high-velocity jet of blood crosses a narrow orifice, generating low-flow eddies downstream in which the bacteria multiply. Thus, patent ductus arteriosus, ventricular septal defect, and aortic stenosis are most commonly associated with endocarditis. More commonly, however, bacterial endocarditis is seen in infants after surgery in which artificial material may be present along with a high-velocity jet of blood. Endocarditis occurs most frequently in the pulmonary artery distal to an aortopulmonary shunt, but it can also

TABLE 22-4. Recommendations for Prevention of Bacterial Endocarditis

1. **Cardiac Conditions***
   Endocarditis prophylaxis *recommended*
   > Prosthetic cardiac valves (including biosynthetic valves)
   > Most congenital cardiac malformations
   > Surgically constructed systemic-pulmonary shunts
   > Rheumatic and other acquired valvular dysfunction
   > Idiopathic hypertrophic subaortic stenosis
   > Previous history of bacterial endocarditis
   > Mitral valve prolapse with insufficiency†
   Endocarditis prophylaxis *not recommended*
   > Isolated secundum atrial septal defect
   > Secundum atrial septal defect repaired without patch 6 or more months earlier
   > Patent ductus arteriosus ligated and divided 6 or more months earlier
   > Postoperative coronary artery bypass graft surgery
2. **Procedures for Which Endocarditis Prophylaxis is Indicated**
   All dental procedures likely to induce gingival bleeding (not simple adjustment of orthodontic appliances or shedding of deciduous teeth)
   Tonsillectomy and/or adenoidectomy
   Surgical procedures or biopsy involving respiratory mucosa
   Bronchoscopy, especially with a rigid bronchoscope‡
   Incision and drainage of infected tissue
   Genitourinary and gastrointestinal procedures§

---

*Common conditions, list not all-inclusive.
†Definitive data to provide guidance in management of patients with mitral valve prolapse are particularly limited. It is clear that, in general, such patients are at low risk of developing endocarditis, but risk-benefit ratio of prophylaxis in mitral valve prolapse is uncertain.
‡The risk with flexible bronchoscopy is low, but the necessity for prophylaxis is not yet defined.
§See Pediatrics 75:607, 1985.

occur in conduits or next to ventricular defect patches prior to endothelialization.

Persistent fever, however, is more likely to be caused by pulmonary infections or heart failure itself than by endocarditis. Pulmonary infections decrease the infant's ability to feed and increase oxygen consumption by increasing respiratory work and body temperature. Any suspected infection must therefore be treated aggressively, and recurrent infections must be considered an indication for surgery. General recommendations for prevention of bacterial endocarditis are given in Table 22-4.

ASYMPTOMATIC HEART DISEASE

Many newborns have clinical findings suggestive of heart disease but are without symptoms. Although these infants may not be gradu-

TABLE 22-5. When to Worry: Natural Morbidity of Congenital Heart Disease

PATHOPHYSIOLOGIC PROCESS	FINDING	POTENTIAL MORBIDITY/PRESENTATION
Cyanosis	Hematocrit 65%	Hyperviscosity may cause ischemic events.
	Iron deficiency	Predisposes to ischemia (particularly cerebral) in cyanotic heart disease
	Chronic hypoxemia	May lead to delay in growth and development
	Episodic "spells"	Hypercyanotic episodes may cause irreversible ischemic events.
	Irritability	May indicate increasing hypoxemia
Congestive heart failure	Decreased intake	Will lead to growth retardation
	Sweating, grunting	Signs of increased failure
	Regurgitation	Often sign of failure; leads to inadequate intake
	Improvement	Be sure improvement in failure is *not* due to progressive pulmonary vascular disease
Obstruction	Poor pulses	Inadequate systemic blood flow, with rapid deterioration possible
	Hypertension	In coarctation, leads to arteriolar (cerebral and coronary) damage
	Hypertrophy	As noted on ECG or echocardiogram, may lead to fibrosis with irreversible myocardial damage
Infection	Endocarditis	Persistent fever, embolic phenomena, hematuria, particularly with high-velocity (VSD, aortic stenosis) jets
	Cerebral abscess	Fever, vomiting, altered neurologic status, in cyanotic heart disease
	Pneumonia	Increased respiratory distress and fever in high pulmonary blood flow lesions

ates of the ICN, I would like to address two issues about them. A large number of newborns have heart murmurs that are heard in the first several days of life. The etiology of these murmurs is varied. The ductus arteriosus may remain patent for several days, and, as it constricts, a murmur may be heard. This murmur is rarely the usual continuous murmur of patent ductus arteriosus found in the older infant, but is usually systolic and nonspecific in nature. Transient tricuspid insufficiency occurs frequently in asphyxiated infants and is often indistinguishable from a ventricular septal defect. Innocent intracardiac flow murmurs are common, because of the large increase in cardiac output that occurs at birth. Probably the most common cause of a murmur in the newborn is (physiologic) peripheral pulmonary artery stenosis. In the fetus, very little blood passes through the right and left pulmonary arteries, because right ventricular output is diverted through the ductus arteriosus to the descending aorta and placenta. At birth, blood flow through these arteries increases more than 10-fold. Not surprisingly, turbulence occurs in the relatively small fetal vessels when flow increases dramatically. The murmur is systolic and generally best heard in the axillae; it usually disappears in the first few months of life, because of rapid growth in the pulmonary arteries. Because there are so many "normal" murmurs in the newborn, a murmur without symptoms is usually not caused by structural heart disease. These infants should be evaluated by the pediatrician alone during the first month of life.

> The general pediatrician's evaluation during the first month of life usually includes an EKG, chest x-ray and serial physical examinations.
>
> *M. Abbott*

If the infant remains asymptomatic, evaluation by a pediatric cardiologist can be deferred for six to eight weeks. By this time, many of the asymptomatic murmurs will have disappeared, and evaluation of the infant will be greatly facilitated when the common newborn murmurs can be excluded.

Conversely, the infant without symptoms who has evidence of abnormal pulses or blood pressures should be evaluated immediately by a pediatric cardiologist. As I have already discussed, left ventricular outflow obstruction is a serious problem that may rapidly cause an irreversible low-output state. We have seen several infants with coarctation of the aorta who were healthy on discharge from hospital, but who, two or three weeks later, arrived seriously ill in the emergency room. This deterioration is probably caused by slow closure of the ductus arteriosus. If all pulses appear diminished, severe aortic stenosis must be excluded. If only lower-limb pulses are diminished, coarctation of the

TABLE 22–6. Morbidity Associated with Common Surgical Procedures

PROCEDURE	MORBIDITY	PRESENTATION/MECHANISM
Atrial baffle (TGV)	Atrial dysrhythmias	Episodic discomfort, possible heart failure
	Venous obstruction	Systemic: may cause increasing head size, hepatomegaly, pleural effusions
		Pulmonary: may lead to respiratory distress, recurrent pneumonia, failure to thrive
	Right ventricular dysfunction	May lead to tricuspid insufficiency and congestive heart failure
VSD closure (VSD, ToF, truncus, ECD)	Residual shunt	Possible congestive heart failure
	Ventricular scar	Ventricular dysrhythmias
	Hemolysis	Particularly if small residual shunt persists
	Endocarditis	From patch and residual shunt
Right ventricle to pulmonary artery conduit (truncus, PA)	Ventricular scar	Ventricular dysrhythmias
	Endocarditis	From conduit
	Obstruction	Conduit narrowing may lead to right ventricular hypertension and failure
Right atrium to pulmonary artery conduit (TA)	Atrial dysrhythmias	Episodic discomfort, possible heart failure
	Systemic venous hypertension	Ascites, peripheral edema, low-output heart failure
	Endocarditis	From conduit
Aortopulmonary shunt	Endocarditis	*Common*, because of high-velocity shunt flow
(ToF, PA, TA)	Heart failure	Excessive pulmonary blood flow
	Cyanosis	Either shunt narrowing or pulmonary vascular disease

TGV = D-Transposition of great vessels; VSD = ventricular septal defect; ToF = tetralogy of Fallot; ECD = endocardial cushion defect; PA = Pulmonary atresia, TA = tricuspid atresia

aorta is likely. The pediatrician should check the pulses in both the upper and lower extremities in all infants prior to discharge from the hospital and after two weeks of age. If there is any doubt about the adequacy of the pulses, blood pressures in the upper and lower extremities should be measured; if doubt persists, evaluation by a cardiologist should be obtained immediately.

SUMMARY

The infant in the ICN with heart disease may have one of a variety of cardiac lesions, but the lesions can be grouped into only a very few hemodynamic categories. Postdischarge care can be simplified if the lesion is placed into one of these categories. Potential problems may thus be defined, and care tailored to address the specific problems that may be encountered (Table 22–5 lists when to worry.) Close monitoring of growth is critical in all forms of heart disease. The timing of surgical intervention varies among lesions and cardiac care centers, depending on the relative risks of natural morbidity vs surgical morbidity (Table 22–6) and the

likelihood of spontaneous resolution of the lesion. The pediatrician can direct the full care of the infant during this critical period of development, but only if he or she is aware of all the issues that may arise.

Recommended Reading

General

Adams FH, Emmanouilides GC: Moss' Heart Disease in Infants, Children and Adolescents, 3rd ed. Baltimore, Williams & Wilkins Company.

Goor DA, Lillehei CW: Congenital Malformations of the Heart. New York, Grune & Stratton.

Rowe RD, Freedom RM, Mehrizi A, Bloom KR: The Neonate with Congenital Heart Disease. Philadelphia, W.B. Saunders Company, 1981.

Rudolph AM: Congenital Diseases of the Heart. Chicago, Year Book Medical Publishers, 1974.

Therapy

Arnold WC: Efficacy of metolazone and furosemide in children with furosemide-resistant edema. Pediatrics 74:872, 1984.

Artman M, Parrish MD, Boerth RD, et al.: Short-term hemodynamic effects of hydralazine in infants with complete atrioventricular canal defects. Circulation 69:949, 1984.

Boucek MM, Chang R, Synhorst DP: Vasodilators and ventricular septal defect: Comparison of prazosin, minoxidil, and hydralazine in a chronic lamb model. Pediatr Res 18:859, 1984.

Koch-Weser J: Captopril. N Engl J Med 306:214, 1982.

Levine TB, Franciosa JA, Cohn JN: Acute and long-term response to an oral converting-enzyme inhibitor, captopril, in congestive heart failure. Circulation 62:35, 1980.

Loggie JMH, Kleinman LI, VanMaanen EF: Renal function and diuretic therapy in infants and children: i.e. I, II, III. J Pediatr 86:408,657,825, 1975.

Prevention of bacterial endocarditis: Statement for health professionals. Committee on Rheumatic Fever and Bacterial Endocarditis, Council on Cardiovascular Diseases in the Young. Pediatrics 75:603, 1985.

Soyka LF: Pediatric clinical pharmacology of digoxin. Pediatr Clin North Am 28:203, 1981.

Wettrell G, Anderson KE: Clinical pharmacokinetics of digoxin in infants. Clin Pharmacokinet 2:17, 1977.

Surgery

Engle MA, Diaz S: Long-term results of surgery for congenital heart disease (reference list). Circulation 65 (Pt 1 and 2):415, 1982.

Engle MA, Perloff JK: Congenital Heart Disease after Surgery: Benefits, Residua, Sequelae. New York, Yorke Medical Books, 1983.

Gersony WM, Krongrad E: Evaluation and management of patients after surgical repair of congenital heart diseases. Prog Cardiovasc Dis 18:39, 1975.

Graham TP: Assessing the results of surgery for congenital heart disease: A continuing process. Circulation 65:1049, 1982.

Morriss JH, McNamara DG: Residua, sequelae and complications of surgery for congenital heart disease. Prog Cardiovasc Dis 18:1, 1975.

23

ENDOCRINE PROBLEMS IN THE HIGH-RISK INFANT

MARTIN A. GOLDSMITH, M.D.

In the following section six topics in pediatric endocrinology are addressed that the practitioner may encounter when caring for the ICN graduate. This material is presented in an abbreviated fashion for quick reference in keeping with the scope of this book; however, the reader is directed to Recommended Reading for more detailed discussion of these topics and to the list of standard references on endocrinology at the end of the chapter.

HYPOTHYROIDISM

Congenital hypothyroidism resulting from thyroid dysgenesis occurs in approximately 1 in 4000 live births. This includes absence of detectable thyroid tissue as well as ectopic glands. Most of these cases will be detected in newborn thyroid screening programs that measure thyroid-stimulating hormone (TSH) in infants with low T_4 values. A small percentage of infants with ectopic glands, however, will have compensated hypothyroidism (normal T_4 and elevated TSH), and the condition will therefore not be detected by screening programs. Infants with thyroid dysgenesis have a permanent disorder and require lifetime replacement therapy with levothyroxine.

There are a number of transient disorders, on the other hand, that do not require lifetime therapy. One such disorder, transient hypothyroxinemia, occurs in 25 to 50 per cent of premature infants. It is postulated that incomplete hypothalamic maturation results in serum T_4 levels lower than those in full-term infants. Since TSH levels are not elevated, as they would be in a term infant with thyroid dysgenesis, it appears that in some premature infants the hypothalamus is less sensitive to low serum T_4 levels. In these infants the thyroid gland is anatomically normal, T_4 levels are usually normal by six weeks of life, and the infants develop normally. Chowdhry et al.,[1] in a double-blind study, assessed the effect of thyroid replacement on 23 very low birth weight infants (less than 1250 grams, 25 to 28 weeks' gestation). They found no difference in growth or intellectual and motor development at one-year follow-up and therefore do not recommend therapy for these infants. Thyroid function is often depressed even further in the sick premature infant whose biochemical profile may resemble the ill adult's with the "euthyroid-sick" syndrome. Here, the serum T_4 level is normal or low, the TSH level is normal, and the free T_3 is low. It is unlikely that further studies are necessary, or that levothyroxine therapy is warranted in this situation.

Other transient disorders that occur in infants with a normal thyroid gland include transient hyperthyrotropinemia (TSH level is high and T_4 is normal) and transient hypothyroidism (TSH level is high and T_4 is low). The cause of transient hypothyroidism is often not apparent. It is a rare condition in term infants, but appears to be more common in prematures. It may also be seen in infants cleaned with iodine-containing antiseptics, in infants born to mothers with iodine deficiency, and in infants born to mothers treated with thionamides for hyperthyroidism.

Any preterm infant with a low T_4 level and an elevated TSH level has hypothyroidism and requires the same evaluation as a term newborn. The T_4 and TSH measurements should be repeated to document the abnormality, a technetium scan of the thyroid should be obtained, and appropriate thyroid medication should be prescribed. Most newborns require 25 to 50 μg/day of levothyroxine. The serum T_4 should be kept in the normal range for age, and growth and development should be monitored at regular intervals. If the clinical picture is in any way confusing to the physician, consultation with a pediatric endocrinologist is appropriate.

INFANT OF THE MOTHER WITH GRAVES' DISEASE

The pediatrician is challenged with several questions when faced with the infant born to a woman with Graves' disease. First, since thionamide medication given to the mother can cross the placenta, the newborn can develop transient hypothyroidism. Fortunately this is usually mild and corrects within a few days. (See previous section, Hypothyroidism.)

The potentially more threatening problem is neonatal thyrotoxicosis, which may not be evident until several days after delivery. Feeding difficulties, diarrhea, jitteriness, poor weight gain, and tachycardia suggest the diagnosis. An elevated T_4, resin T_3 uptake, and free T_3 values confirm it. When sustained tachycardia is a part of the clinical presentation, aggressive therapy is essential to prevent congestive heart failure. Initially, propranolol (2 mg/kg/day orally every eight hours) can be lifesaving. Propylthiouracil (5 to 10 mg/kg/day orally every eight hours) and iodide (Lugol's solution, one drop every eight hours, started two hours after the propylthiouracil) can control the hyperthyroidism. The etiology of this condition is not fully understood, and a varying natural course has been observed by different investigators. In some infants the disorder has lasted a few weeks, while others have been affected for months or years.

In the infant who does not develop either transient hypothyroidism or thyrotoxicosis, the question of the appropriateness of breast-feeding arises, since thionamides are present in breast milk. Since, theoretically, hypothyroidism could develop in the nursing infant, assessment of the serum T_4 on a regular basis would be required. Alternatively, it might be simpler to provide the usual replacement dose of levothyroxine to the infant while nursing. Although these two choices sound intrusive, we do not feel that maternal thionamide use should be considered a routine contraindication to breast-feeding. Kampmann et al.[2] studied the concentration of propylthiouracil in serum and breast milk in nine lactating mothers and demonstrated that only small amounts are actually present in milk, i.e., a dose unlikely to cause hypothyroidism in the infant.

PREMATURE THELARCHE

Thelarche has only recently been described in premature infants. It is not known if the incidence is higher than in term infants, but the pathophysiology and clinical significance are similar. The normal term infant may be born with breast tissue, which often regresses after several weeks or months. If it reappears at toddler age, without other signs of true sexual precocity, then this is benign premature thelarche. It may wax and wane and requires no specific management outside of clinical observation. The cause appears to be intermittent estradiol secretion by ovarian follicles that mature transiently before undergoing involution. If there are no signs or symptoms of sexual precocity, such as linear growth acceleration, pubic or axillary hair, vaginal discharge or menses, then the case can be followed clinically. At times, a radiograph of the wrist to determine bone age and measurement of serum estradiol and serum gonadotropins appropriately complement the history and physical examination. If development of breast tissue appears to be rapid, or if other signs are present, consultation with a pediatric endocrinologist is warranted.

HYPERGLYCEMIA

Hyperglycemia is not uncommon in low birth weight infants and is thought to result from insulin resistance in some infants and pancreatic beta cell immaturity in others. In such infants, hyperglycemia is exacerbated by asphyxia, intracranial hemorrhage, and infection. The onset is usually within the first few days of life, and the usual course is one of a gradual return to euglycemia over seven to ten days. Although insulin therapy is unnecessary in most cases, the course in some infants may be prolonged, and insulin is required to correct severe hyperosmolarity, polyuria, and weight loss.

In contrast, insulinopenic diabetes mellitus may not become evident until days to months after birth. These infants require insulin and continual monitoring of glucose, and many eventually outgrow their insulin needs. However, two of the patients reported by Traisman[3] required insulin therapy into adulthood.

HYPOGLYCEMIA

Hypoglycemia is a common complication among high-risk infants in the ICN, particularly among prematures, infants with intrauterine growth retardation, and infants born to mothers with poorly controlled diabetes. These infants ordinarily do not require complex evaluation, and their problem will have resolved prior to discharge. There are, however, a number of circumstances in which it is appropriate to evaluate further, vigorously pursue precise diagnosis, and institute treatment. These include hypoglycemia that persists for more than several days and severe hypoglycemia requiring an infusion of more than 10 per cent glucose over a period of days to correct the hypoglycemia. In addition, the cause of the hypoglycemia should be investigated when it is associated with:

1. Term, uncomplicated birth
2. Metabolic acidosis in the absence of hypoxia
3. A midline defect of the skull or face
4. Prolonged hyperbilirubinemia or increased liver enzymes
5. Microphallus

The evaluation of these infants is complex and should involve consultation with a pediatric subspecialist in endocrinology or metabolism.

SHORT STATURE

A child can be characterized as short when his or her stature is more than 2.5 standard deviations below the mean for the population. The need to investigate its cause depends on the growth velocity, the parents' heights, and the presence of any symptoms or signs suggesting

underlying disease. Readily available, standardized growth curves for full-term healthy infants provide useful and time-tested tools for the clinician who must decide if further evaluation, beyond a thorough history and physical examination, is necessary. That decision is not always simple and can be more difficult with the ICN graduate. Several investigators have analyzed the growth patterns in preterm and small for gestational age infants and compared these patterns to those in healthy term infants. (See Chapter 5.) There is great heterogeneity in the growth patterns of these infants, and particularly among those who have been very ill.

In evaluating growth in ICN graduates, the pediatrician might consider the following questions:

1. Does the child have any dysmorphic features suggesting one of the many syndromes often associated with short stature?
2. Is there a history of abnormal eating behavior or poor child-parent interactions, suggesting a psychosocial basis for the poor growth?
3. Does the history point toward a particular system that should be investigated?

If the history and physical examination do not indicate any of the above, routine screening tests (CBC, blood chemistry profile, thyroid studies) should be performed. If these are also normal, the physician may entertain the diagnosis of growth hormone deficiency, and an exercise-induced serum growth hormone level should be determined. This study is a good screening tool in a cooperative child who is old enough to exert himself or herself on request; however, most children require provocative stimulation studies (see Recommended Reading). If the growth hormone levels are consistently below 7 ng/ml, a bone age and a lateral skull radiograph should be obtained, and the child referred to a pediatric endocrinologist.

INDICATIONS FOR FURTHER EVALUATION AND REFERRAL

The following general guidelines are suggested as indications for more complex evaluation and referral to a pediatric endocrinologist.

1. For initial evaluation of any infant with hypothyroidism
2. If the clinical picture in an infant being treated for hypothyroidism is in any way confusing
3. In premature thelarche, if the breast tissue appears to develop rapidly or if other signs of sexual precocity are present

4. In an infant born to a mother with Graves' disease who manifests tachycardia, diarrhea, or jitteriness

5. When hypoglycemia is either persistent or severe, or follows the circumstances outlined on page 242.

6. In any child whose growth is more than 2.5 standard deviations below the mean for the population and who is growing poorly

SUMMARY

In-depth discussion of the endocrine conditions that may affect ICN graduates is beyond the scope of this book; however, Recommended Reading should be helpful to the pediatrician who is beginning to evaluate a possible endocrine problem.

References

1. Chowdhry P, Scanlon JW, Auerbach R, et al.: Results of controlled double-blind study of thyroid replacement in very low-birth-weight premature infants with hypothyroxinemia. Pediatrics 73:301, 1984.
2. Kampmann JP, Hansen JM, Johansen K, et al.: Propylthiouracil in human milk: Revision of a dogma. Lancet 1:736, 1980
3. Traisman HS: Diabetes mellitus in infancy. In Traisman HS (ed.): Management of Juvenile Diabetes Mellitus. St Louis, C.V. Mosby Company, 1980, pp 208–211.

RECOMMENDED READING

Hypothyroidism
Cheron RG, Kaplan MM, Larsen PR, et al.: Neonatal thyroid function after propylthiouracil therapy for maternal Graves' disease. N Engl J Med 304:525, 1981.
Cuestas RA: Thyroid function in healthy premature infants. J Pediatr 92:963, 1978.
Delange F, Dalhem A, Bourdous P, et al.: Increased risk of primary hypothyroidism in preterm infants. J Pediatr 105:462, 1984.
Fisher DA, Klein AN: Thyroid development and disorders of thyroid function in the newborn. N Engl J Med 304:702, 1981.
Hadeed AJ, Asay LD, Klein AH, et al.: Significance of transient postnatal hypothyroxinemia in premature infants with and without respiratory distress syndrome. Pediatrics 68:494, 1981.
Klein AH, Stinson D, Foley B, et al.: Thyroid function studies in preterm infants recovering from respiratory distress syndrome. J Pediatr 91:261, 1977.
LaFranchi S: Hypothyroidism, congenital and acquired. In Kaplan SA (ed.): Clinical Pediatric and Adolescent Endocrinology. Philadelphia, W.B. Saunders Company, 1982, pp 82–95.
l'Allemand D, Gruters A, Heidemann P, et al.: Iodine-induced alterations of thyroid function in newborn infants after prenatal and perinatal exposure to povidone-iodine. J Pediatr 102:935, 1983.

Morissette J, Dussault JH: Commentary: The cut-off point for TSH measurement or recalls in a screening program for congenital hypothyroidism using primary T$_4$ screening. J Pediatr 95:404, 1979.
New England Congenital Hypothyroidism Collaborative: Characteristics of infantile hypothyroidism discovered on neonatal screening. J Pediatr 104:539, 1984.
Refetoff S, Ochi Y, Selenkow HA, et al.: Neonatal hypothyroidism and goiter in one infant of each of two sets of twins due to maternal therapy with antithyroid drugs. J Pediatr 85:240, 1974.
Uhrmann S, Marks KH, Maisels MJ, et al.: Thyroid function in the preterm infant: A longitudinal assessment. J Pediatr 92:968, 1978.

Neonatal Graves' Disease
Burrow GN: Hyperthyroidism during pregnancy. N Engl J Med 298:150, 1978.
Fisher DA: Pathogenesis and therapy of neonatal Graves' disease. Am J Dis Child 130:133, 1976.
Hollingsworth DR, Mabry CC: Congenital Graves' Disease. Four familial cases with long-term follow-up and perspective. Am J Dis Child 130:148, 1976.

Premature Thelarche
Collett-Solberg PR, Grumbach MM: A simplified procedure for evaluating estrogenic effects and the sex chromatin pattern in exfoliated cells in urine: Studies in premature thelarche and gynecomastia of adolescence. J Pediatr 66:883, 1965.
Kenny FM, Midgley AR Jr, Jaffe RB, et al.: Radioimmunoassayable serum LH and FSH in girls with sexual precocity, premature thelarche and adrenarche. J Clin Endocrinol Metab 29:1272, 1969.
McKiernan J: Premature thelarche in preterm infants. J Pediatr 105:171, 1984.
McKiernan JF, Hull D: Breast development in the newborn. Arch Dis Child 56:525, 1981.
Mills JL, Stolley PD, Davies J, et al.: Premature thelarche: Natural history and etiologic investigation. Am J Dis Child 135:743, 1981.
Nelson KG: Premature thelarche in children born prematurely. J Pediatr 103:756, 1983.
Styne DM, Kaplan SL: Normal and abnormal puberty in the female. Pediatr Clin North Am 26:123, 1979.

Hyperglycemia In Infancy
Cowett RM: Pathophysiology, diagnosis and management of glucose homeostasis in the neonate. Curr Prob Pediatr 15:30, 1985.
Dweck HS, Cassady G: Glucose intolerance in infants of very low birth weight: I. Incidence of hyperglycemia in infants of birth weights 1,100 grams or less. Pediatrics 53:189, 1974.
Goldman SL, Hirata T: Attenuated response to insulin in very low birthweight infants. Pediatr Res 14:50, 1980.
Pagliara AS, Karl IE, Kipnis DB: Transient neonatal diabetes: Delayed maturation of the pancreatic beta cell. J Pediatr 82:97, 1973.
Pollak A, Cowett RM, Schwartz R, et al.: Glucose disposal in low-birth-weight infants during steady-state hyperglycemia: Effects of exogenous insulin administration. Pediatrics 61:546, 1978.
Rudolph N, Minsky AA: Transient neonatal diabetes— Possible therapeutic use of glucagon. J Pediatr 86:475, 1975.
Schiff D, Colle E, Stern L: Metabolic and growth patterns in transient neonatal diabetes. N Engl J Med 287:119, 1972.
Schwartz R: Should exogenous insulin be given to very low

birth weight infants? J Pediatr Gastroenterol Nutr 1:287, 1982.

Vaucher YE, Walson PD, Morrow G: Continuous insulin infusion in hyperglycemic, very low birth weight infants. J Pediatr Gastroenterol Nutr 1:211, 1982.

Zarif M, Pildes RS, Vidyasagar D: Insulin and growth-hormone responses in neonatal hyperglycemia. Diabetes 25:428, 1976.

Hypoglycemia

Cornblath M, Poth M: Hypoglycemia. In Kaplan SA (ed.): Clinical Pediatric and Adolescent Endocrinology. Philadelphia, W.B. Saunders Company, 1982, pp 479–518.

Drash AL: Causes of hypoglycemia. In Lifshitz F (ed.): Pediatric Endocrinology: A Clinical Guide. New York, Marcel Dekker, 1985, pp 479–518.

Lovinger RD, Kaplan SL, Grumbach MM: Congenital hypopituitarism associated with neonatal hypoglycemia and microphallus: Four cases secondary to hypothalamic hormone deficiencies. J Pediatr 87:1171, 1975.

Pagliara AS, Karl IE, Haymond M, et al.: Hypoglycemia in infancy and childhood: I. J Pediatr 82:365, 1973.

Pagliara AS, Karl IE, Haymond M, et al.: Hypoglycemia in infancy and childhood: II. J Pediatr 82:558, 1973.

Stanley CA, Baker L: Hyperinsulinism in infants and children: Diagnosis and therapy. Adv Pediatr 23:315, 1976.

Short Stature

Babson SG: Growth of low-birth-weight infants. J Pediatr 77:11, 1970.

Kaplan SL: Growth. In Rudolph AM (ed.): Pediatrics, 17th ed. Norwalk, Appleton-Century-Crofts, 1982, pp 83–105.

Martell M, Falkner F, Bertolini LB, et al.: Early postnatal growth evaluation in full-term, preterm and small for dates infants. Early Hum Dev 1: 313, 1978.

Sann L, Darre, Lasne Y et al.: Effects of prematurity and dysmaturity on growth at age 5 years. J Pediatr 109:681, 1986.

Schaff-Blass E, Burstein S, Rosenfield RL: Advances in diagnosis and treatment of short stature, with special reference to the role of growth hormone. J Pediatr 103:801, 1984.

Tanner JM, Whitehouse RH: Clinical longitudinal standards for height, weight, height velocity, weight velocity, and stages of puberty. Arch Dis Child 51:170, 1976.

Villar J, Smeriglio V, Martorell R, et al.: Heterogeneous growth and mental development of intrauterine growth-retarded infants during the first 3 years of life. Pediatrics 74:783, 1984.

Standard Endocrinology References

Bacon GE, Spencer ML, Hopwood NY, et al. (eds.): Practical Approach to Pediatric Endocrinology, 2nd ed. Chicago, Year Book Medical Publishers, 1982.

Collu R, Dacharone JR, Guyda H (eds.): Pediatric Endocrinology. New York, Raven Press, 1981.

DeGroot LJ (ed.): Endocrinology. New York, Grune & Stratton, 1979, (3 vol).

Frasier SD (ed.): Pediatric Endocrinology. New York, Grune & Stratton, 1980.

Hung W, August GP, Glasgow AM (eds.): Pediatric Endocrinology. New Hyde Park, NY, Medical Examination Publishing Company, 1983.

Job J-C, Pierson M (eds.): Pediatric Endocrinology. New York, John Wiley & Sons, 1981.

Kaplan SA (ed.): Clinical Pediatric and Adolescent Endocrinology. Philadelphia, W.B. Saunders Company, 1982.

Kaplan SA (ed.): Symposium on Pediatric Endocrinology. Pediatr Clin North Am vol 26, no. 1, 1979.

LaCauza C, Root AW (eds.): Problems in Pediatric Endocrinology. Proceedings of Serono Symposia, vol 32. New York, Academic Press, 1980.

Lifshitz F (ed.): Pediatric Endocrinology: A Clinical Guide. New York, Marcel Dekker, 1985.

Smith DW: Growth and Its Disorders. Major Problems in Clinical Pediatrics, Vol 15. Philadelphia, W.B. Saunders Company, 1977.

Williams RH (ed.): Textbook of Endocrinology, 7th ed. Philadelphia, W. B. Saunders Company, 1985.

24

HEALTH SUPERVISION AND ANTICIPATORY GUIDANCE FOR INFANTS WITH CONGENITAL DEFECTS

JOHN C. CAREY, M.D.

About 2 per cent of infants have a congenital defect or malformation syndrome that is of medical, surgical, or developmental significance and is recognized in the newborn period.[1,2] Down syndrome, meningomyelocele, and craniofacial malformations comprise the most commonly occurring of the congenital disorders that demand multidisciplinary involvement. The purpose of this chapter is to review the natural history of selected congenital malformations and multiple anomaly syndromes and to present guidelines for the routine health supervision and primary care of these infants.

Caring for children with medically complicated malformations is challenging for the primary care practitioner: It requires a commitment of responsibility that is both similar to the care of any child with a chronic illness and different, because of the genetic and psychosocial meaning of congenital defects. As outlined by Stein,[3] the pediatric practitioner has three alternatives when confronted with the issue of long-

term care of a child with a chronic illness: (1) The child can be referred to a subspecialist or multidisciplinary team for total management. (2) The pediatrician can manage the case entirely on his or her own. (3) The practitioner can elect for joint management of the case with the appropriate subspecialist or team.[3] Because the pediatrician is both a primary care giver and a specialist in the health aspects of children, he or she is the ideal practitioner to coordinate the necessary continuous and comprehensive care. Given knowledge of the natural history of the individual disorder and the willingness to assume responsibility for supportive care, the pediatrician, working with consultants, is able to engineer effectively the care of infants with complicated defects. Besides the complex process of referral and coordination with specialists, the pediatrician can provide the direct services for normal health care maintenance, intercurrent illnesses, long-term support, and help with the special requirements of health supervision. Four general issues regarding the initiation and provision of health supervision for children with medically complicated defects will be discussed in more detail in the ensuing paragraphs.

ISSUES IN MANAGEMENT

CORRECT DIAGNOSIS

The most crucial issue in the initial planning of health care management for a child with multiple congenital anomalies is correct diagnosis. Of all children recognized to have a multiple malformation syndrome in the newborn period about one third will have the Down syndrome, one third will have another recognizable syndrome, and about one third will not fit a known syndrome.[4] The actual diagnostic process of a child with multiple congenital anomalies may seem overwhelming, because of the large number of relatively uncommon disorders and the continual description of "new syndromes." It is difficult for the primary care practitioner to keep up with the literature on such a specialized topic. However, the approach to the diagnosis of a child with multiple malformations is as much in the domain of primary pediatrics as is the evaluation of anemia or developmental delay. Texts on the more common disorders are available in most libraries. Reviews of the principles of approach and catalogues of the more common disorders are included in Recommended Reading.

The importance of accurate diagnosis cannot be overemphasized. Although the labeling process may seem to be stigmatizing and merely an academic exercise, correct diagnosis of a syndrome provides prediction, as it does in any clinical problem. Precision in diagnosis is of benefit to the family and in the care of the child. An accurate syndrome diagnosis helps in the following clinical settings:

1. Recurrence risk in genetic counseling. The recognition of a known syndrome will usually provide information on etiology and genetic aspects of the disorder.

2. Relative prediction of prognosis. Each syndrome has its own particular natural history and its own individual risk for developmental disorders. Although exact diagnosis will not provide a "crystal ball" for the future of an individual child, the clinician is able to discuss these concerns with some guidelines.

3. Appropriate laboratory testing. In the evaluation of a child with multiple congenital anomalies, many expensive and invasive diagnostic procedures are considered. Accurate diagnosis will eliminate the need for unnecessary testing and will focus the evaluation.

4. Treatment or management issues. Exact diagnosis, coupled with knowledge of natural history, will lead to establishment of priority of management and treatment plans for the future. Necessary referrals can be outlined, and particular complications can be screened for. Although many of the syndromes that are associated with developmental disabilities do not have "treatment" in the usual medical sense, many are associated with specific areas of disability, and, thus, available knowledge may be helpful in future educational planning. In addition to the aforementioned clinical themes, correct diagnosis is important for a family, because it may take them from a place of confusion, uncertainty, and mystery to a place that has, at least, some concrete order and a framework of expectations.

INFORMATION ON THE NATURAL HISTORY

The second issue regarding health supervision for infants with congenital anomalies pertains to the gathering of current and accurate information on *natural history*. Each condition has its own set of problems for which the child is at risk as part of the syndrome. Families will desire knowledge about the implications of the individual condition. However, accurate prediction of risk for certain complications depends on the quality of the published studies that examine the frequency of occurrence of the particular complication. Investigations concerning the clinical course and prognosis of a particular condition are often limited, because of the rarity of a disorder and because of selection and ascertainment biases.[5] These factors need to be taken into consideration when one is predicting the chance that a child will develop an adverse complication associated with a condition. Despite the methodologic limitations of most investigations of the natural history of malformation syndromes, the studies do give the clinician some feeling for the specific at-risk problems and the range of frequency of the complications. Much of this chapter will be an attempt to outline guidelines for observing the child for the specific medical complications of the selected conditions. In this way, as in the guidelines for health supervision in regular well-child care, problems can be anticipated and the course ideally altered.

PROVIDING PSYCHOSOCIAL SUPPORT

The third issue in planning long-term care of the child with multiple congenital defects involves the professional's commitment to provide the necessary psychosocial support. Besides the complex task of coordinating the care of the child with the subspecialist and/or multidisciplinary team, the pediatric practitioner is in the ideal position to help the family cope with the emotional and social issues of rearing a child with a chronic illness or disability. This commitment requires time and energy and special knowledge of the impact of a chronic condition on a family. Listening to individual parental concerns, acknowledging uncertainty, and validating that most feelings are natural responses to the situation are only a few of the objectives that one can include in routine well-child visits. Distribution of reading material and referral to appropriate parent support groups can also occur in the primary care setting.

> The ultimate developmental task for children with chronic illness or disability is to integrate into their self-concept their sameness, *as well as their difference,* with other children. Toward supporting this goal, pediatricians should ask and talk with the child about the full range of universal childhood experience, not limiting his or her regard for the child to the problematic medical condition.
>
> P. Gorski

PROVIDING GENETIC COUNSELING

The last general issue regarding care of the infant with multiple congenital anomalies is consideration of referral for genetic counseling. The genetic aspects of isolated malformations and multiple anomaly syndromes are extremely complex and have helped precipitate the emergence of the subspecialty of clinical genetics. The practitioner needs to decide whether he or she feels comfortable with the biologic and genetic aspects of the individual condition. If so, then the informational aspects of the genetic counseling process can be carried out in the primary care domain. However, the sharing of up-to-date information on the natural history and genetics of a condition is only one aspect of the genetic counseling process.[6] Other issues, such as options for reproductive decision making, current developments in the prenatal diagnosis of genetic disorders, and the meaning of genetic disease in society, make the biomedical and psychosocial issues complex. Thus, referral for genetic counseling is always an appropriate option in any family who has questions about any of these issues.

Long-Term Care of Children with Common Congenital Disorders

The remainder of this chapter will deal with the long-term care of children with the more common congenital disorders that require multidisciplinary consultation. Although the importance of the developmental and psychosocial issues in the care of children with these disorders cannot be overemphasized, they are beyond the scope of this book, and the following discussion will emphasize the medical aspects of the individual conditions.

CHROMOSOMAL DISORDERS

Down Syndrome

Down syndrome is the most common multiple congenital anomaly syndrome in man. About 1 of 800 to 1000 infants have the condition. Although J. Langdon Down recognized this pattern of malformation in the nineteenth century, the fact that the syndrome was due to trisomy of chromosome 21 was not discovered until 1959. The syndrome includes a consistent pattern of phenotypic variations and structural malformations that, taken together as a cluster, lend themselves to making the diagnosis even prior to determination of the chromosome result. Furthermore, infants with Down syndrome are at risk for a number of specific abnormalities, in addition to developmental disability. All children who have the Down syndrome have a developmental disorder that, as they get older, will result in enough limitation of performance to cause them to fall into the retarded range. It is this aspect of the natural history of the condition, along with the risk for congenital heart disease, that provides most of the impact of the disorder on the family in the childhood period. These implications, as well as other common medical manifestations, will be discussed in detail below.

DIAGNOSIS

Diagnosis and counseling of the family of a newborn with Down syndrome is both a challenge and an opportunity. The challenge consists of synthesizing the complex information in a meaningful fashion and providing support at the time of diagnosis. Since families remember the experience of the informing interviews, the opportunity to be a helper is a unique one. Some of the practical issues of the informing interview are discussed in the reviews by Irvin et al.[7] and Myers.[8] The initial days after the diagnosis will usually focus on the actual diagnostic process itself. The assumptions by the clinician in making a phenotypic diagnosis of the Down syndrome are not easy to understand for many parents, especially since most of the physical characteristics are subtle and not clearly abnormal. The frequency of individual characteristics useful in the diagnosis of the syndrome are available in many sources[9,10] and will not be reviewed here.

A karotype is always indicated, even in a child in whom the clinical diagnosis seems certain, because of the different genetic implications of the various chromosome findings. All children who have the classic phenotype will have trisomy of the long arm of chromosome 21. About 90 to 95 per cent of affected children will have complete trisomy 21, i.e., 47 chromosomes, with an extra freestanding chromosome 21. Less than 10 per cent will have mosaicism or a partial trisomy due to a robertsonian translocation or other rearrangement. The cytogenetic aspects of the Down syndrome have been reviewed in depth by Thuline and Pueschel.[11] In addition, the complex information surrounding the epidemiology of trisomy 21 has been summarized by Hook.[12]

For the practitioner to develop a health supervision plan for children with Down syndrome, it is important to summarize the associated complications and natural history. Table 24–1 outlines the more common medical problems of children with Down syndrome and recommendations for management, diagnostic testing, and referral. The significant medical manifestations and prognostic issues will be discussed in more detail below.

Infant-Childhood Mortality. Most recent studies on mortality in children with Down syndrome show an improvement in survival, compared to earlier investigations.[14,15] Congenital heart disease is the most significant factor in determining survival in children with the Down syndrome. In the absence of congenital heart disease, more than 90 per cent of children with Down syndrome are alive at age 10 years. However, even after excluding children with heart defects, there is some increase in infant and early childhood mortality in children with this syndrome. Most of this increased risk is in the first two years of life and is usually accounted for

by infectious disorders. The overwhelming number of infants without heart disease will live to adulthood.

Congenital Heart Disease. About 30 to 40 per cent of infants with the Down syndrome will have an associated congenital heart malformation as part of the syndrome.[16] An endocardial cushion defect accounts for about half of all cases, with isolated ventricular septal defect, atrial septal defect, and tetralogy of Fallot comprising the other defects most commonly occurring in these children. Some malformations that usually are noted in the newborn period, such as coarctation of the aorta and transposition of the great vessels, are rare in the syndrome and thus emphasize the nonrandom occurrence of the types of heart defects associated with the syndrome.

In addition to the structural defects, there is some controversy whether an infant with Down syndrome and cardiac disease has a propensity for early development of pulmonary hypertension.[17] Although the issue remains unclear, the controversy strengthens the argument for early cardiac evaluation of children with a heart defect. Sondheimer and colleagues[18] recommend that all children with Down syndrome, even those without an audible heart murmur, be referred for cardiac evaluation sometime in the first nine months of life. The minimal evaluation by the primary care practitioner in the newborn period should include an electrocardiogram and chest radiograph, along with clinical examination. Since children with an endocardial cushion defect may not have an obvious murmur, the apparent absence of a murmur should not eliminate one's suspicion.

Hearing Loss. Significant hearing loss of both a conductive and sensorineural nature occurs in about 40 to 60 per cent of children with Down syndrome.[19] At least half of the children with hearing loss will have binaural loss. The hearing loss is usually of a degree that can potentially affect language acquisition and educational achievement. Although the pathogenesis of the conductive hearing loss is not usually delineated in the studies, it can be presumed that some of it is related to chronic serous otitis media. Thus, children with Down syndrome who have chronic otitis media or middle ear infusions should be referred for otologic evaluation as early as possible. Routine audiologic evaluation, including impedance testing, of all infants with Down syndrome before the age of 9 months is recommended. Yearly follow-up into the school-age years should be routine for health maintenance of the child.

TABLE 24-1. Anticipatory Guidance and Health Maintenance in Children with Down Syndrome

AGE GROUP (YR.)	DEVELOPMENTAL THEMES/ STRATEGIES	AT-RISK MEDICAL COMPLICATION		
		Specific Complications	Frequency (%)	Referrals/Suggested Diagnostic Tests
Infancy (0-1)	Diagnosis, cause Supportive care Degree of disability Uncertainty/supportive	Congenital heart disease	30-40	Cardiac evaluation (newborn) Cardiology referral by 8 mo
	Recurrence risk/ genetic counseling	Serous otitis media/hearing loss	40-60	Audiologic evaluation with typanogram by 8 mo
	Coping with implications Parents groups/infant preschool programs* Reading material	Congenital hypothyroidism	1	T_4, TSH in neonatal period
		Ocular abnormalities	20-60	Ophthalmologic consult. if strabismus, nystagmus, etc.
Early Childhood (1-4)	Coping with child rearing/supportive care Routine developmental testing in office Discussion of plastic surgery Dental hygiene	Serous otitis media/hearing loss	40-60	Audiologic evaluation yearly
		Speech problems	common	Speech evaluation*
		Atlantoaxial subluxation	20	Lateral neck films once, 3-4 yr
		Refractive errors	30-50	Yearly visual testing in office Ophthalmology consult. at 4 yr
Late Childhood (4-12)	Educational planning Psychometric evaluation Advocacy issues Obesity/nutritional guidance; activities Special Olympics	Keratoconus	1-8	Ophthalmology consult. yearly after 10 yr
		Thyroid disorders	3-5	T_4, TSH yearly after 10 yr

* Many of the developmental, psychological, and educational aspects of care will occur routinely through preschool and school programs. These suggestions are included here as a guideline.

Thyroid Disorders. These children are at risk for various forms of thyroid disease throughout childhood, beginning with an increased risk for congenital hypothyroidism[20]; therefore, all infants should be tested in the newborn period. After the newborn period, most of the thyroid disorders reported in individuals with Down syndrome have occurred in adolescents and adults. However, thyroid dysfunction can occasionally occur early in childhood in Down syndrome.[21,22] Because of this, annual thyroid studies are suggested in these children. Evaluation of thyroid function is especially recommended in any infant or school-age child with macroglossia, hoarseness of voice, change in growth velocity, or school problems, all common findings in Down syndrome.

Atlantoaxial Subluxation. Children with Down syndrome are at increased risk to develop atlantoaxial subluxation and its neurologic complications. This issue has recently come to surface because of the involvement of these children in the Special Olympics. The atlantoaxial instability of C1-C2 is probably a consequence of the hypotonia and joint laxity seen in the syndrome. Pueschel et al.[23] observed that 17 per cent of an unselected population with Down syndrome had atlantoaxial instability, as defined by lateral radiographs of the upper cervical spine. Of this group, 15 per cent had neurologic symptoms due to spinal cord compression related to the C1-C2 subluxation. Because of this finding, it is recommended that routine radiographic examination of the cervical spine be done for all patients with Down syndrome aged two years and older. The examination should include lateral views of the neck in both flexion and extension. Individuals with atlantoaxial subluxation need close follow-up for neurologic status, and those with neurologic signs or symptoms should be restricted in strenuous activities and referred for neurosurgical evaluation. The Committee on Sports Medicine of the American Academy of Pediatrics also recommends that lateral cervical radiographs be obtained for all children with Down syndrome who wish to participate in sports.[24]

Ophthalmologic Abnormalities. These children are at increased risk for a number of ocular complications.[9] The most common problems are strabismus and nystagmus, and thus the routine child-care examinations in the first three years of life should include a high index of suspicion for these signs. Because of the increased frequency of refractive errors and retinal abnormalities, yearly ophthalmologic evaluations should probably start in infancy. Certainly, referral to an ophthalmologist should occur in infancy if nystagmus, strabismus, or cataracts are present. Because of the frequency of refractive errors, routine referral to an ophthalmologist for evaluation at age 4 years is warranted, and children over 10 years need annual eye examinations, because of the increased occurrence of keratoconus.

Growth and Development. A thorough review of the developmental disability that occurs in children with Down syndrome is beyond the scope of this chapter. There will always be some degree of psychomotor retardation, ordinarily manifesting itself in the first year of life. Helping a family cope with developmental and behavioral issues is clearly a part of the daily practice of the primary care provider. The range of developmental limitation in Down syndrome is wide, and ultimate prediction of performance is impossible during infancy. When tested, the majority of school-age children will fall into the moderate range of retardation, but approximately 20 per cent will have a milder degree of performance limitation.

Growth of young children with Down syndrome can be followed during the early years of life by using the curves that have been developed from infants with the syndrome.[25] Such standards can be placed in the medical chart as would any growth curve. In this way, if linear growth or weight gain deviates markedly from the lower percentile, or if there is a change in growth velocity, evaluation for potential medical causes can be initiated. Table 24–2 lists as-

---

TABLE 24–2. Specific Low-Frequency Manifestations of Importance in Down Syndrome

Newborn
  Duodenal atresia/esophageal atresia/imperforate anus
  Hirshsprung's disease
  Congenital cataracts
  Congenital leukemia
  Leukemoid reaction
Infancy-Childhood
  Gastroesophageal reflux
  Pulmonary hypoplasia
  Obstructive sleep apnea
  Pulmonary hypertension without cardiac disease
  Infantile spasms
  Leukemia
  Keratoconus
  Diabetes mellitus

---

sociated disorders that are potential causes of growth delay in children with the Down syndrome.

INTERVENTION PROGRAMS

In the late 1970's, early intervention programs for infants with developmental disabilities emerged in most metropolitan areas in the United States. Although research on the effectiveness of these interventions is laden with methodologic problems, there is some empiric evidence available that indicates a "positive" effect in children with Down syndrome.[26,27] However, interpretation of these data is conflicting and controversial.[28] Well-designed investigations that truly sort out variables, such as early vs later entry into the program, home-based vs center-based programs, and long-term outcome or "permanent" effects, are still forthcoming. In addition, potential adverse effects of these programs, as well as the cost and time for the parent, are rarely discussed in the literature. Thus, decision making regarding an infant program is similar to decision making in any clinical problem in which the data necessary for a clear-cut answer are not available. In addition to the possibility of developmental benefit to the child, there are, however, other potential benefits from infant programs that usually are not stated in the evaluative literature. These include parental support provided by professionals and by other parents, development of advocacy roles by the parent, assistance by the program in behavioral management of the child, verbalization of realistic goals for the child, and an opportunity to learn of a child's strengths and weaknesses in an academic setting. In fact, in the last decade, infant programs have established themselves as one of the significant support services for parents of handicapped children in American society. For all of these reasons, there should always be serious consideration given to referral of an infant with Down syndrome to a preschool program.

> Good early intervention programs provide, at a minimum, peer contact for the child, and peer support and respite for the parents—basic services which benefit *all* families with atypical children.
>
> *P. Gorski*

Although infant preschool programs are the most available option, there may be other alternatives for the pediatrician and family in attaining similar goals. These would include:

1. Individual private referral for occupational therapy, physical therapy, and speech therapy
2. Arrangement for therapists to come to the practitioner's office on a periodic basis to work with children in the practice
3. Support groups for parents of children with handicapping conditions, based in a primary care practice
4. Home visits by public health nurses or other trained personnel (In addition, a few tertiary medical centers in the United States provide a multidisciplinary, medically based clinic for children with Down syndrome.)

The practitioner can also provide up-to-date reading material for parents. The most comprehensive works are the books by Pueschel et al. and Rynders and Horrobin. (See Recommended Reading, For Families, at end of chapter.) Referral to a local parent support group should also be offered as an option. (National organizations for support of these families are found in Appendix E.)

OTHER MEDICAL COMPLICATIONS

Besides the more common medical complications mentioned above, there are a number of disorders associated with the syndrome that are of relatively low frequency (less than 10 per cent) but of increased occurrence compared to the general population. Table 24–2 lists the most important of these abnormalities. The primary care practitioner should be aware of their occurrence, so that appropriate testing can be done if specific symptoms suggest any of these disorders.

Pueschel[29] has done a prospective study of infants with Down syndrome to understand the expected natural history. Although a general predisposition for respiratory infections is frequently stated to occur in these infants, they were unable to document this. In addition, the studies on the immune findings in individuals with Down syndrome are conflicting and inconclusive.[9] It may be that the apparent increased occurrence of respiratory infections is due to syndrome-associated structural abnormalities of the craniofacies, respiratory tract, or muscle tone, rather than to a true immune defect. As noted in Tables 24–1 and 24–2, the infant with Down syndrome is at risk for a number of specific problems that could occur as acute or chronic respiratory infections. Thus, when an infant exhibits pneumonia or cyanotic episodes, these manifestations need consideration, as many are treatable. For example, congenital heart disease, obstructive sleep apnea, pulmonary hypoplasia, primary pulmonary hypertension, and gastroesophageal reflux are all potential specific mechanisms for cyanotic spells in a baby with Down syndrome.

OTHER THERAPIES

Facial Surgery. One of the more recent issues in the care of young children with Down syndrome involves the option of reconstructive surgery for the craniofacial defects.[30] Tongue reduction and canthoplasty, which can potentially alter the facial appearance, are being offered in some centers in the United States and Europe. Evidence for actual benefit to the self-image of the child is still to be forthcoming. Because facial appearance is an important value in Western society, and because of the recognized but unfortunate stigmata of the Down syndrome, theoretical benefit from surgery makes discussion of this option appropriate. However, decision making should involve the potential surgical risks, weighed against the unproven benefits.

> Care should be taken to avoid diversion of needed support services and resources away from approaches which enhance the child's self-image to procedures which are painful and may, in fact, damage self-image.
>
> *Editor*

Vitamin Therapy. One of the issues that often surfaces during the care of a child with Down syndrome is the question of the use of certain alternative therapeutic regimens. In recent years, administration of megadoses of vitamins to children with the syndrome has been proposed.[31] In addition, in Europe, an injection therapy, known as Sicca, has been utilized for years in children with Down syndrome and other congenital disorders. The approach to answering parental questions about these unconventional therapies should be the same as in any discussion of a new or unusual therapeutic option. Validation of the parents' questions is crucial, and immediate labeling of these regimens as quackery will not meet the needs of the parents, who are interested in exploring the options in depth. The biologic basis for the regimen and the scientific evidence for efficacy should be reviewed as one would any therapeutic method. In this regard, one can say that there is no biologic basis to indicate that megadoses of vitamins would have any effect on developmental outcome in Down syndrome.

From an epidemiologic standpoint, the use of vitamin regimens has been investigated in two controlled studies, reported in the pediatric literature.[32,33] These investigations did not show any evidence for improvement in developmental outcome after administration of vitamin supplementation. It is important to note that, from a methodologic point of view, these investigations had larger numbers of subjects and controls and more rigorous outcome measures than the original paper that precipitated this discussion.[31] Thus, there is no good biologic or experimental evidence to indicate that megadoses of vitamins improve developmental outcome in school-age children with Down syndrome. In addition, concern about unknown adverse effects of long-term vitamin usage, known toxic effects of fat-soluble vitamins, and cost need to be included in any discussion of risk vs benefit. The issue of the use of Sicca injections and other less conventional therapies has been discussed by Karp[34] and De La Cruz.[35] Once again, as emphasized above, when the benefits have not been proved by scientific study, the finite risks of therapy (e.g., anaphylaxis in Sicca injections) must be weighed against the purported benefits.

GENETIC COUNSELING AND RECURRENCE RISK

The risk for a family who has a child with Down syndrome to have a second affected child depends on the type of chromosome abnormality in the child *and* on maternal age. Whenever a child has a partial trisomy of 21, due to a robertsonian or reciprocal translocation, karyotypes on the parents and referral to a genetic center for consultation are indicated. If the child has the more common situation of complete trisomy 21, the recurrence risk depends on maternal age. Precise data calculated to answer this question

are surprisingly sparse, and the family studies prior to 1982 are summarized in a review by Hook.[12] A more recent study adds more data to the question.[13] These data, along with information from amniocentesis studies, would indicate that the risk when the mother's age is under 30 years is about 1 to 2 per cent. When the mother's age is over 30, the risk of having a second affected child is probably the same as the age-specific risk. Prenatal diagnosis with either chorionic villous sampling or amniocentesis can be offered to the family as an option for future pregnancies. Review of the complexities of reproductive decision making is beyond the scope of this chapter, but has been discussed by Wertz et al.[36]

Doctor Carey's discussion of Down syndrome is so concise and straightforward, that parents could benefit from reading this also.

A. Rosen

Trisomy 18

Trisomy 18, or the Edwards syndrome, is the second most common autosomal chromosome abnormality in man. Approximately 1 in 5000 newborns have this pattern of malformation. Trisomy 18, like trisomy 21, produces a pattern of physical variations and malformations that are consistent enough to allow clinical recognition in the newborn period. However, the implications of the diagnosis of trisomy 18 are more serious with respect to survival, developmental disability, and frequency of medically significant congenital malformations.

MORTALITY AND MEDICAL PROBLEMS

From a relatively recent study of an unselected population, more than 90 per cent of children with trisomy 18 had died by 12 months of age; approximately 50 per cent did not survive past 3 months of age.[37] The reasons for this low survival rate are complex. Certainly the high frequency of congenital heart defect (about 90 per cent), associated central nervous system abnormalities, and a propensity for marked feeding difficulties contribute to the high infant mortality. However, it is often unclear exactly why a baby with trisomy 18 dies; the pathogenesis may be related to the same factors that cause the majority of fetuses with trisomy 18 to die in utero. Obviously this predictive information is overwhelming for the family who learn of the diagnosis of trisomy 18. Usually families are surprised by the seriousness of the disorder, since most babies will not have obvious external abnormalities. Even though many children with trisomy 18 will not leave the newborn nursery, it is important to review with the parents the expected clinical course of children who do go home with their parents and who live past the first few months of life.

Because of the relative infrequency of trisomy 18 and its usual rapid progression to death, most practitioners do not receive much experience with this disorder after the newborn period. Although the problems may seem complex and overwhelming, the primary care practitioner can provide the medical and supportive care needed by these children and their families. Knowledge of the scope of the congenital defects and the developmental disability, along with a willingness to take responsibility for ongoing family support and routine medical care, are the only requirements.

In addition to cardiac defects, the most commonly observed anomalies in trisomy 18 include radial aplasia, omphalocele, ocular malformations, and clubfeet. The frequency of the phenotypic variations and mild malformations that are useful in diagnosis of the syndrome will not be reviewed here. Most infants with trisomy 18 have difficulty in feeding and sucking in the neonatal period and will go home from the nursery requiring gavage feeding. Gastrostomy becomes an option if the child survives the first 12 months. There is also an increased incidence of pulmonary infections.

If an infant is discharged home, a plan of management needs to be outlined. Referral for cardiac evaluation is always appropriate to obtain an idea of the severity of the heart condition. Although there are no data on immunization practices in children with trisomy 18, immunization can be offered as it would in any handicapped infant. Since hearing loss occurs in more than 50 per cent of infants with trisomy 18, referral for audiologic evaluation is recommended before 8 months of age. Other subspecialty referrals, such as ophthalmology and orthopedics, are suggested in any child whose medical situation demands it. Of course, adverse effects of any therapy on the quality of life of the child and its risks need to be weighed against the benefit to the child.

Developmental Disability. The developmental disability that is associated with trisomy 18 is marked. Motor and speech milestones are seriously delayed, and the ability to talk and ambulate has not been reported in older individuals with complete trisomy. In the small number of reports of older children with trisomy 18, the individuals have a degree of mental retardation that is classified as severe or profound. However, all children do progress in their motor milestones to some degree and do smile and recognize their parents. Consideration of the option of early intervention programs is appropriate in infants with trisomy 18, as in any child with a marked motor disability.

Psychosocial Support of Families. The most significant dilemma that the parents and practitioner will have to face together is the uncertainty regarding survival. This particular situation in trisomy 18 is unique, as the parents have to live with both the high mortality rate and the small but finite possibility of survival. Mixed feelings about what is best for the child are a natural occurrence; availability for support by medical professionals is important during this time. Although there are no simple answers and guidelines for helping the families, validation of the dilemma and time for listening to all concerns are necessary. It is important to help the parents cope with the paradox of preparing for both the high probability of dying and the possibility of living. If the child with trisomy 18 lives to 6 months of age, statistics for prediction of survival become less precise. Primary care practitioners then have the challenge (and opportunity) of helping the family face the still existing possibility of death and the preparation for caring for a handicapped child at the same time.

The emotional impact of dealing with the dilemmas presented by trisomy 18 can be overwhelming to both parents and helping professionals. The pamphlet "Trisomy 18: A Book for Families" is available from the University of Nebraska School of Medicine. As in other handicapping conditions, involvement of the family of a child with newly diagnosed trisomy 18 with other families who have a child with this syndrome is an appropriate option. The National Support Organization for Trisomy 18/13 (SOFT), established in Utah in 1980, is a national organization for families with children with the more serious autosomal trisomies. (See Appendix E.)

Trisomy 13

Trisomy 13, or the Patau syndrome, is the third most common autosomal chromosome abnormality in man. This disorder has a frequency of about 1 in 10,000 liveborn infants. Like trisomy 18, more than half of all infants with this condition are stillborn, and mortality figures for liveborn infants with trisomy 13 are similar to those for trisomy 18. Most of the information regarding the family's adaptation and coping in the early months of life for trisomy 18, as stated above, apply equally well to this disorder. However, the pattern of physical abnormalities and malformations as a group are different in trisomy 13, and on a clinical basis, the infants with the individual syndromes can be separated by phenotypic analysis. Infants with trisomy 13 usually have more obvious, major malformations than those with trisomy 18 or trisomy 21. About 60 per cent will have oral facial clefts, with some having the facial malformations of the holoprosencephaly developmental field defect (cyclops malformation, cebocephaly, or premaxillary agenesis). Ocular malformations consisting of anophthalmia, microphthalmia, congenital glaucoma, and colobomas are present in about 50 per cent of infants. Scalp defects (cutis aplasia) and postaxial polydactyly of the hands or feet are distinctive abnormalities that will clue the clinician into this chromosomal disorder. As in trisomy 18, about 90 per cent of infants have congenital heart disease. Feeding problems, propensity to pneumonia, central nervous system malformations, and seizures contribute to the decreased survival in infants with this condition, as in trisomy 18.

A routine plan of management needs to parallel the psychological support. Referral for hearing evaluation and physical therapy are suggested for infants over 6 months of age. Special medical problems that occur in trisomy 13, which may explain unusual symptoms, include gastroesophageal reflux, glaucoma, and hypertension.

The limited number of reports of children older than 1 year indicates that individuals with trisomy 13 have a marked degree of mental retardation. In children with complete trisomy 13 (as opposed to partial trisomy or mosaicism), the degree of disability is such that verbal communication and independent ambulation have not been reported in older children. However, developmental milestones do progress past the newborn level, as the children smile, follow, sit, and communicate to some degree. Referral to SOFT is an appropriate option.

Turner Syndrome

Turner syndrome is due to complete or partial monosomy of the short arm of the X chromosome. Incidence at birth of this disorder is about 1 in 3000 female births. The constellation of abnormalities in the affected individuals is variable and consists of three categories of manifestations: (1) ovarian dysgenesis with associated infertility and amenorrhea, (2) postnatal proportionate short stature, and (3) a variable pattern of physical characteristics and malformations. It is the physical features and/or malformations that allow the diagnosis of the Turner syndrome in the newborn and infancy period. Details of the discussion of the phenotype are beyond the scope of this chapter. However, it is of note that recent investigators have been attempting to tie together some of the diverse phenotypic manifestations to suggest that fetal lymphedema may be a common denominator. Clark[38] has suggested that the left-sided obstructive lesions of the heart (e.g., coarctation of the aorta) are secondary to the primary defect of lymphatic obstruction. Since congenital lymphedema and a webbed neck appear to go together in other syndromes besides the Turner syndrome, it is also reasonable to speculate that the webbed neck may be related pathogenetically to the nuchal blebs seen in fetuses and newborns with the XO Turner syndrome.

When the diagnosis of Turner syndrome is made in infancy, the primary care practitioner can organize the routine management, as in the child with Down syndrome. The natural history of Turner syndrome has been summarized by Hall et al.[39] The two medically significant malformations seen in Turner syndrome are congenital heart disease and structural renal defects. Approximately 10 to 20 per cent of infants with Turner syndrome will have heart defects, most of these being left-sided obstructive lesions: coarctation of the aorta, aortic stenosis, or bicuspid aortic valve. Miller et al.[40] noted that 70 per cent of asymptomatic girls with Turner syndrome had bicuspid aortic valves detected on echocardiography. Thus, even the individuals who have no evidence of congenital heart disease may have a mild left-sided alteration that is of minimal consequence in childhood. A high index of suspicion of heart disease, including routine blood pressure measurement, should be present in visits in infancy and childhood. Complete cardiac evaluation is indicated in all infants with any symptoms or signs suggestive of heart disease or hypertension. Referral for echocardiography is indicated in older asymptomatic children, so that the individual knows whether she is at any risk for later aortic valve problems.

About 30 per cent of individuals with Turner syndrome will have a structural renal malformation. Many of these findings are not of clinical significance and include a horseshoe kidney or unilateral renal agenesis. However, any girl with Turner syndrome who has unusual growth problems, urinary tract infection, or other signs of kidney disease should have radiographic and functional renal studies performed. It is suggested that all newborns or infants with Turner syndrome have a renal ultrasound study, as this is a noninvasive way to document the presence or absence of a renal defect.

Other medical complications that have been noted in the first year of life include chronic serous otitis media and feeding problems. Because of the otitis media, routine audiologic evaluation is recommended in all girls with Turner syndrome before one year of age. Idiopathic hypertension has also been noted in some children with Turner syndrome, and therefore blood pressure should be followed closely in all these children.

Postnatal proportionate growth deficiency is usually present in girls with Turner syndrome before the age of five years. There is some controversy in the literature about the administration of exogenous sex hormones for growth. This controversy is beyond the scope of this chapter, but it has been reviewed by Sybert.[41] Recently, several investigators have reported successful increase in growth with administration of growth hormone to girls with Turner syndrome.[42,43] Referral to an endocrinologist for consideration of administration of any hormonal therapy, including therapy for induction of secondary sex characteristics, is suggested.

The other medical manifestation of note that occurs in older girls with Turner syndrome is an increased occurrence of autoimmune thyroiditis. Because this can often be an asymptomatic manifestation, thyroid studies should be performed routinely in health care maintenance of girls with Turner syndrome after the age of 10 years.

Girls with Turner syndrome usually have normal intelligence; the frequency of mental retardation in individuals with the syndrome who have karyotypic abnormalities limited to the X chromosome appears to be no greater than that of the general population. Some studies in psychomotor evaluation of Turner syndrome have reported a specific learning deficit involving an abnormality in perceptual motor organization that results in a lowering of the performance aspect of an intelligence quotient. Even when present, this learning deficit is compatible with academic success, and most girls with Turner syndrome perform adequately in the school setting.[39]

Other Chromosomal Abnormalities

The phenotypic manifestations and commonly occurring malformations in the rarer chromosomal disorders have been reviewed and summarized by deGrouchy and Turleau [44] and Schinzel in two separate comprehensive catalogues.

CRANIOFACIAL MALFORMATIONS AND SYNDROMES

Malformation of the craniofacies and the associated syndromes account for more than 10 per cent of all serious congenital anomalies in newborns, making the combined incidence of all craniofacial defects about 1 in 400 infants. Thus, as a group, these malformations are more common than either Down syndrome or meningomyelocele. In addition, the social implications of craniofacial defects are unique, and care of children with any craniofacial malformation requires knowledge of associated problems.

Cleft Lip; Cleft Palate

INCIDENCE AND ASSOCIATED PROBLEMS

Cleft lip, with or without cleft palate, is the most common serious craniofacial malformation in man, occurring in about 1 in 800 children. Cleft lip, whether or not it is associated with a cleft of the hard or soft palate, is considered etiologically and genetically distinct from the isolated cleft palate (without cleft lip). This conclusion is based on family studies of cleft lip (with or without cleft palate) and isolated cleft palate. Approximately 10 to 20 per cent of individuals with a cleft lip (with or without cleft palate) have an associated malformation or have it as part of a syndrome. A higher frequency, i.e., 30 per cent of individuals with an isolated cleft palate, have an associated congenital malformation. This would suggest that cleft lip is less often a syndromic malformation than cleft palate. Thus, the first and most crucial question in evaluating any oral-facial cleft in a child is whether or not the abnormality is an isolated one or part of a syndrome. As is mentioned above, this determination is important for predicting the natural history and for recurrence risk information in genetic counseling. In a thorough monograph, Gorlin et al.[45] have summarized the many syndromes in which cleft lip and cleft palate occur. In addition to these disorders, oral-facial clefts occur with increasing frequency in most autosomal chromosomal syndromes. Thus, a karyotype is indicated in an infant with an oral-facial cleft and other malformations that do not fit a recognizable syndrome. Recurrence risk information and anticipatory guidance for development of other medical problems is dependent upon the recognition of a specific syndrome diagnosis.

ISOLATED CLEFT LIP

The care of a child with an isolated cleft lip is fairly straightforward. If there is no cleft of the alveolar ridge, this defect becomes primarily a problem of surgical repair in early infancy. At present, most plastic surgeons repair a cleft lip at about three months of age. Referral to the plastic surgeon in the newborn period is recommended, so that the surgeon can get acquainted with the family and assist them in their process of becoming familiar with the disorder. If an alveolar cleft is present along with the soft tissue defect of the lip, then future orthodontic and dental problems must be anticipated. Some children who have an apparently isolated cleft lip, without an obvious defect of the palate, will have a submucous cleft of the palate that will be detected only after the child is speaking. If a child with an isolated cleft lip has a bifid uvula, the primary care physician's index of suspicion for velopharyngeal insufficiency should be raised.

CLEFT LIP WITH CLEFT PALATE

If a child has a cleft palate or a cleft lip with a cleft palate, then the long-term medical care is even more complicated. Besides the expected referral to the plastic surgeon, referral for impedance testing should be routine in any infant with a cleft palate. Early referral to an otolaryngologist also should be considered in the routine care. These children are at risk for middle-ear effusions and speech problems and commonly have other malformations, making management very complex. For this reason, cleft palate teams and craniofacial panels have been developed in many centers throughout the United States and Canada.

Although the care of most children with a cleft lip with cleft palate that is not part of a syndrome can be coordinated by a primary care practitioner, referral to one of these teams for long-term management is also an option. Some

of the principles outlined in the opening paragraphs of this chapter are exemplified here: audiology, genetics, speech pathology, otolaryngology, dentistry, and orthodontics referrals can be made by the pediatrician, working closely with the plastic surgeon. However, children with complicated clefts or individuals with any other malformations (or syndromes) should always be considered candidates for referral to a multidisciplinary team, because of the number of potential consultants and the complexity of the coordination of their care. The options for long-term care can be re-evaluated on a periodic basis by the pediatrician, working with the plastic surgeon and the family.

PIERRE ROBIN TYPE OF CLEFT PALATE

Infants who have the Pierre Robin type of cleft palate will also have obstructive airway problems in infancy and will require careful management (see Chapter 15). Although the upper airway obstruction in the Robin sequence will improve in some children, many (especially those with syndromes) will have longstanding upper airway difficulties and require referral to a craniofacial or pulmonary center. Pashayan and Lewis[46] have summarized a plan of management of feeding and respiratory distress in infants with the Robin sequence. Proper prone positioning during feeding and rest will improve the status of most babies with the Robin sequence who have no other abnormalities. However, Cozzi and Pierro[47] documented obstructive problems in older infants with the Robin sequence, and their work suggests that many of these infants should have monitoring at home and close follow-up and pulmonary evaluation for determining the need for supplemental oxygen.

The pediatrician should also be aware that the Robin sequence can occur as an isolated set of findings or as one component of several syndromes; therefore, infants with the Robin sequence may need further evaluation.[48] The most common associated syndrome seen in children ascertained as having the Robin sequence is the Stickler syndrome. Because of this frequent association, routine ophthalmologic evaluation is recommended during the first year of life in all children who have the Robin sequence that is not part of an identifiable syndrome. An increased index of suspicion of the Stickler syndrome should always be present in a child with an apparently nonsyndromic form of the Pierre Robin sequence.

INFANT FEEDING

Children who have a cleft palate will often have feeding difficulties in the early weeks of life. The art and science of managing feeding difficulties in a child with cleft palate are not well documented in the pediatric literature. Most hospitals will have a nursing professional who is particularly adept in managing feeding and helping parents with this common difficulty. If such a resource is not available, the pamphlets that are available for parents of children with facial clefts include a discussion of feeding techniques. Recently, Clarren et al.[49] outlined a number of practical suggestions for feeding a baby with cleft palate. Various nipples are available and are listed in the publication entitled, "Feeding the Special Baby." (See Recommended Reading, For Families.) Most children with cleft palate who do not have a Robin defect will master feeding before 1 month of age. If a child is still having serious difficulty by that time, more generalized problems (such as central nervous system abnormalities) need to be considered.

The feeding of a child with a cleft palate has always been a trial and error endeavor. The wide variation in the degree of difficulty makes it totally unpredictable. The parents need lots of support during this very anxious time.

A. Rosen

Because of the known association of oral-facial defects with growth hormone deficiency or hypopituitarism, all children with facial clefts who have linear growth deficiency need to have a complete endocrine evaluation.

Other Craniofacial Syndromes

Reviews by Cohen[50] and Carey[51] summarize the multitude of syndromes that involve alterations of facial morphogenesis. Table 24–3 lists the more important natural history aspects and suggested anticipatory guidance for children with the more common of these disorders. Most of the medical care issues involved in these syndromes require the same disciplines as cleft lip and cleft palate. Each of these craniofacial disorders, especially craniosynostosis syndromes, has its own natural history and its own particular frequency of associated malformations.

Because of the complexity of the plastic surgery involved in these conditions, and because of the frequency of associated malformations, referral of all children with craniofacial syndromes to a center for craniofacial anomalies is recommended. The American Cleft Palate Association publishes a directory of such centers. The most common of these syndromes referred to a craniofacial panel include: Treacher Collins syndrome, hemifacial microsomia, Goldenhar syndrome, frontonasal dysplasia, and the craniosynostosis syndromes (e.g., Apert, Crouzon). In addition to the risk for audiologic, dental, orthodontic, and speech difficulties in children with oral-facial defects, children with some of these disorders are at risk for obstructive sleep apnea, which must be considered in observing them in childhood. Although the frequency of this manifestation is probably low in all of these disorders, except for the Treacher Collins syndrome, a high index of suspicion should be present in routine child care situations.

MENINGOMYELOCELE

Organizing the care of the child with spina bifida is certainly the prototype for the array of issues that surround the medical management of the multihandicapped child. As in craniofacial disorders, multidisciplinary clinics exist in most major medical centers in North America. Two recent papers have reviewed comprehensively the natural history issues and health maintenance of infants and children with meningomyelocele.[52,53] (See also Chapter 19.)

SKELETAL DYSPLASIAS

The skeletal dysplasias are comprised of more than 75 disorders of bone development, almost all of genetic etiology. Among these conditions involving osseous development are the chondrodystrophies, which usually produce disproportionate short stature in the affected individual. These bone dysplasias resulting in short-limbed individuals are sometimes referred to as the dwarfism syndromes. However, because of the stigma associated with the word *dwarf*, avoidance of this label is recommended, and the various conditions are referred to as dysplasias.[54]

The concepts mentioned above regarding knowledge of the individual natural history of a condition apply as well to the skeletal dysplasias. Although almost all of the chondrodystrophies are associated with significant short stature in adulthood, they vary in their specific orthopedic and medical complications. Knowledge of the primary areas of involvement for each condition is necessary in the long-term follow-up of an individual with one of these condi-

TABLE 24–3. Routine Testing for Specific Complications in Selected Malformation Syndromes

DISORDER	AT-RISK MANIFESTATIONS	RECOMMENDATIONS
Beckwith Syndrome	Wilms' tumor/adrenal tumor	Abdominal ultrasound annually until age 5 yr
Craniofacial Malformation		Referral to craniofacial team/plastic surgery
Treacher Collins Syndrome	Conductive hearing loss	Routine audiologic/ENT eval.
	Obstructive sleep apnea	High index of suspicion Consider sleep study
	Hypernasal speech	Speech eval.
Apert Syndrome	Exotropia, optic atrophy	Routine ophthalomology consult.
	Conductive hearing loss	Audiologic/ENT eval.
	Speech problems	Speech eval.
	Craniosynostosis/facial malformations	Refer to craniofacial team; plastic surgery or neurosurgery
Goldenhar Syndrome	Conductive hearing loss	Audiologic/ENT eval.
	Vertebral defects/scoliosis	Spine radiographs
	Congenital heart defects	Cardiac eval.
	Gastroesophageal reflux	Barium swallow, if symptoms
CHARGE Association of Congenital Defects	Congenital heart defect	Cardiac eval.
	Retinal coloboma	Ophthalmology consult.
	Hypopituitarism	If short, endocrinology consult.
	DiGeorge sequence	High index of suspicion; T cell eval. if appropriate
	Hearing loss	Audiologic/ENT consult.
VATER Association of Congenital Defects	Radial defects	Consult., hand surgery
	Renal defects	Renal ultrasound
	Congenital heart defects	Cardiac eval.
	Vertebral defect/scoliosis	Spine films
Ellis–van Creveld Syndrome	Congenital heart disease	Cardiac eval.
	Genu valgum	Orthopedic eval.
	Hypodontia	Dental eval.
Diastrophic Dysplasia	Scoliosis/clubfeet	Orthopedic eval.
Spondyloepiphyseal Dysplasia	Myopia	Ophthalmology eval.
	Odontoid hypoplasia	Routine neck radiographs
	Hearing loss	Audiologic eval. in infancy

tions. For example, individuals with achondroplasia are not at risk for scoliosis or congenital hip dislocation, common findings in other dysplasias, but are at risk for spinal stenosis and tibial bowing (see later). The specific orthopedic complications of the common skeletal dysplasias have been reviewed by Kopitz[55] and Horan and Beighton.[56] In addition, some skeletal dysplasias involve other areas of the body besides the skeleton and typify the concept of a multiple congenital anomaly syndrome (e.g., Ellis–van Creveld syndrome). This presentation will discuss the natural history and health maintenance in children with achondroplasia in detail.

Achondroplasia

Achondroplasia is the most common chondrodystrophy in man. The incidence at birth is estimated to be 1 in 10,000 to 1 in 25,000. Indi-viduals with achondroplasia make up more than one half of all individuals with disproportionate short stature. The condition is inherited in an autosomal dominant fashion, with about 80 per cent representing sporadic de novo mutations. Clinical and radiographic features of achondroplasia have been reviewed extensively by Langer et al.[57] and Scott.[58]

Knowledge of the phenotype and the specific radiographic manifestations is necessary to make a secure diagnosis of achondroplasia in infancy. Prior to the 1960's, when many of the distinct chondrodystrophies were described, most individuals with disproportionate short stature were lumped under this diagnostic label. At present, with the delineation of many of the recently described skeletal dysplasias, phenotype and natural history of achondroplasia have been better defined. Thus, achondroplasia is regarded as a specific entity, rather than a general term. Individuals with achondroplasia are at

TABLE 24–4. Routine Health Maintenance in Children with Achondroplasia

AGE GROUP (YR)	AT-RISK MANIFESTATIONS	RECOMMENDATIONS
Infancy (0–1)	Apparent motor delay	Reassurance; developmental testing
	Hydrocephalus	Follow occipitofrontal head circumference; close follow-up for symptoms; routine CNS ultrasound
	Apnea/foramen magnum compression	Routine sleep study; CT, including foramen magnum
	Serous otitis media	Tympanogram by 8 mo
	Persistent gibbus after weight bearing	Lateral spine radiograph
Childhood (1–10)	Serous otitis media	Audiologic follow-up
	Tibial bowing	Physical examination; if needed, orthopedic consult.
	Spinal canal stenosis	Yearly neurologic exam., high index of suspicion
	Obstructive sleep apnea	High index of suspicion; sleep study

risk for a number of specific complications that occur at different periods in development. Guidelines for long-term care of children with achondroplasia and a review of its manifestations are detailed later and in Table 24–4.

GROWTH AND DEVELOPMENT

Infants with achondroplasia have true macrocephaly and postnatal onset of linear growth deficiency. Standardized growth curves for head circumference and length are available.[59] These curves can be placed in the infant's medical record, in place of the usual growth charts, for well-child care. Monitoring the head circumference is important, as children with achondroplasia are at risk for developing a communicating hydrocephalus. Because of this risk, some investigators have recommended regular ultrasound study of the central nervous system during the first year of life.[60] However, standardized measurements of the ventricles of children with achondroplasia are not available, and it is difficult for the clinician to know what is abnormal, since most children will have mildly enlarged ventricles. Thus, symptoms suggestive of increased intracranial pressure should be especially looked for through the first year of life, because the characteristic time for the development of hydrocephalus is after the newborn period.

Infants with achondroplasia have a moderate degree of joint laxity, especially in the hips and knees. Because of this joint laxity, exaggerated kyphosis of the spine is common until the development of independent ambulation. This finding, as well as the valgus positioning of the feet, is often of concern to the parents; however, both the kyphosis and the foot positioning will change with weight bearing, and the parents can be reassured about these observations. Rarely, the kyphosis will persist past ambulation, and if so, a lateral spine radiograph is indicated to look for wedging of the lumbar bodies. The disproportionately large head and the joint laxity contribute to delayed motor milestones in infants with achondroplasia, compared to the usual standards. However, this apparent delay usually is not a sign for concern, since children who do not have specific neurologic complications are of normal intelligence. A developmental screening test for children with achondroplasia has been adapted from the Denver Developmental Screening Test.[61] This chart can also be placed in the medical record to document developmental progression in early childhood. Children with achondroplasia are also at risk for chronic serous otitis media in the early years of life. For this reason, routine tympanometry is indicated, and referral for hearing screening should occur prior to 12 months of age. Annual hearing evaluation should occur until a normal speech pattern is established in later childhood.

MEDICAL PROBLEMS

The most concerning manifestation in infancy is the potential for respiratory and neurologic complications. These two manifestations are often interrelated, and both are associated with a small foramen magnum. Until recent years, respiratory difficulties in achondroplasia were considered rare. In 1983, Stokes et al.[62] documented that these infants and young children were at risk for a myriad of pulmonary disorders, including obstructive sleep apnea and restrictive lung disease. In 1984, Pauli and colleagues[63] noted the occurrence of sudden, unexpected death in 11 infants. They attributed the events to the small foramen magnum in achondroplasia and to its subsequent effects on upper spinal cord compression. Although the small size of the foramen magnum had been noted as a feature of achondroplasia for many years, its relationship to apnea in infancy in individuals with achondroplasia has only recently been delineated. The frequency of apnea in infancy in individuals with achondroplasia is unknown at the present time. A high index of suspicion by the primary care provider is required when observing the young child with this disorder.

Although most centers are not recommending routine home monitoring of all infants with achondroplasia, screening for central and obstructive apnea by two months of age is indicated for all infants with this disorder. Hecht et al.[64] have provided preliminary data on the size of the foramen magnum in children with achondroplasia. These measurements may be helpful in evaluating respiratory difficulties and apnea in these children.

MANAGEMENT IN INFANCY

Routine health maintenance during the first year of life in infants with achondroplasia should include a high index of suspicion of apnea and respiratory difficulty, regular measurement of the occipitofrontal circumference and chest circumference, detailed history-taking for signs of sleep disturbance and increased intracranial pressure, neurologic examination at all well-child visits, periodic ultrasound study of the central nervous system, and referral for sleep study in early infancy. Some investigators have suggested evaluation with somatic evoked potentials and routine measurement of the foramen magnum by computed tomography.[64] Limited availability of these latter studies and difficulties in interpreting the results make their routine use inappropriate for all infants at the present time. As more natural history data are gathered on size of the foramen magnum and on somatic evoked potentials, these procedures may become routine care for all children with achondroplasia. Consultation with a neurosurgeon experienced in these issues is mandatory when any child has signs or symptoms suggestive of cord compression.

MANAGEMENT IN CHILDHOOD

Tibial Bowing. About 30 per cent of children with achondroplasia will develop significant tibial bowing after ambulation has been established. Most of the remaining children will have straight tibias or mild bowing. The child's lower limbs should be evaluated at rest and during walking at all routine visits during early childhood. The presence of significant tibial bowing can be determined by examining the relationship of the plumb line dropped from the superior iliac crest perpendicular to the floor; if the line drops medial to the knee, or lateral to the ankle, then malalignment of the tibial relationship is present and referral to an orthopedist should be made. Symptomatic malalignment related to the bowing is reason for referral at all ages.

Other problems in childhood include obesity, chronic serous otitis media, and orthodontic difficulties. Examination for these manifestations should be included in routine visits in childhood and appropriate referrals made (see Table 24–4). Scott[65] has reviewed some of the psychosocial and adaptation issues in school-age children with achondroplasia. The stigma of short stature, combined with disproportionate body growth and its perception by our society, has been well documented in the monograph by Ablon.[66] This valuable book is recommended for all practitioners caring for children with achondroplasia.

Routine health maintenance in children with achondroplasia needs to include a neurologic examination for signs of spinal canal compression at all ages. The presence of paresthesias, weakness, asymmetric hyperreflexia, or upper motor neuron signs is reason for referral to a neurosurgeon.

Hall et al.[60] have documented that signs of spinal canal stenosis are present in more than 50 per cent of adults with achondroplasia. Thus, the parents and children need to be informed of the potential for this manifestation in later years.

GENETIC COUNSELING

Referral for genetic counseling is always warranted for any family or individual who has questions about the genetic aspects of achondroplasia. Little People of America (LPA) is a nonprofessional self-help group for individuals with significantly short stature. This group has been a tremendous resource for individuals with achondroplasia, particularly since this disorder is one of the most common causes of severe short stature. Referral to a local chapter of LPA is an option for parents of short children at any age. (See Appendix E.)

Other Skeletal Dysplasias

The other common, nonlethal skeletal dysplasias include hypochondroplasia, the various forms of osteogenesis imperfecta, diastrophic dysplasia, Ellis–van Creveld syndrome, and spondyloepiphyseal dysplasia congenita. The work of Sillence[54] will be helpful to the practitioner following a child with any of these conditions. Table 24–3 includes some of these conditions and their more important manifestations. A brief discussion of osteogenesis imperfecta will be included below, because of its relatively frequent recognition in the newborn period.

OSTEOGENESIS IMPERFECTA

Osteogenesis imperfecta (OI) consists of a heterogeneous group of disorders involving osseous fragility, propensity to fractures, and orthopedic complications. Several different classifications of osteogenesis imperfecta are available, but the one offered by Sillence et al.[67] is the most widely used by clinical geneticists. When an infant is recognized as having some form of OI, the first and most important issue in the newborn period is whether or not the condition is one of the lethal forms. Type II OI (Sillence's classification), also called perinatal OI, can be distinguished from the other forms by examination of the skeletal survey. Biochemical and clinical studies suggest that type II OI is also heterogeneous and includes more than three separable conditions.[68] The genetics of the various forms of type II OI will probably be sorted out in the next decade through molecular studies of collagen protein and through recombinant DNA technology.

A poor prognosis for survival can usually be made with a high degree of certainty in a baby with radiographs consistent with type II OI. The clinical difficulty surrounds prediction of outcome in children in the newborn period with OI that is *not* type II who have a normal family history. In these situations, prediction of outcome is limited. Until the biochemical basis of these conditions has been delineated and correlated with the clinical features, the chances for independent ambulation and orthopedic complications cannot be predicted. If there is a family history of OI, the course in other members of

the family can be used to give the practitioner some feeling for a given infant's progress and outcome. The Osteogenesis Imperfecta Foundation is a resource for families of an individual with OI. (See Appendix E.)

SUMMARY

Assuming primary care of infants with medically complicated congenital defects requires a unique commitment by the practitioner, an understanding of the psychosocial aspects of chronic disorders, and knowledge of current information about the natural history and at-risk complications of the particular disorder. Working with the various consultants, the practitioner can coordinate the comprehensive management of most infants with multiple anomaly syndromes. Knowledge of the various manifestations of a particular disorder enables the care giver to be able to consider specific problems whenever a child has a certain symptom. This chapter has attempted to develop guidelines for routine health maintenance and screening of children with complicated congenital disorders. Recommended Reading, below, includes articles for both the practitioner and families, and resources available to help in the support of these children and their families are listed in Appendix E.

References

1. Holmes LB: Prospective counseling for hereditary malformation in the newborn. In Lubs HA, de la Cruz F (eds.): Genetic Counseling. New York, Raven Press, 1977, pp 241–252.
2. Merlob P, Papier CM, Klingberg MA, et al.: Incidence of congenital malformations in the newborn, particularly minor abnormalities. In Marois M (ed.): Prevention of Physical and Mental Congenital Defects, Part C. New York, Alan R. Liss, 1985, pp 51–56.
3. Stein RE: Caring for children with chronic illness. In Shelov SP, Mezey AP, Edelmann CM (eds.): Primary Care Pediatrics. Norwalk, Appleton-Century-Crofts, 1984.
4. Higuaschi M, Iijimi K, Sujimoto Y, et al.: The birth prevalence of malformation syndromes in Tokyo infants: A survey of 14,430 newborn infants. Am J Med Genet 6:189, 1980.
5. Tugwell PX: How to read clinical journals: To learn the clinical course and prognosis of disease. Can Med Assoc J 124:869, 1981.
6. Ad Hoc Committee on Genetic Counseling: Report to the American Society of Human Genetics. Am J Hum Genet 27:240, 1975.
7. Irvin NA, Kennell JH, Klaus MD: Caring for the parents of an infant with a congenital malformation. In Klaus MH, Kennell JH (eds.): Parent Infant Bonding. St. Louis, C.V. Mosby Company, 1982.

8. Myers BA: The informing interview. Am J Dis Child 137:574, 1983.
9. Pueschel SM: Biomedical aspects in Down syndrome. In Pueschel SM, Rynders JM (eds.): Down Syndrome: Advances in Biomedicine and the Behavior Sciences. Cambridge, Ware Press, 1982, pp 169–303.
10. Carey JC: Chromosomal disorders. In Rudolph AM (ed.): Pediatrics. Norwalk, Appleton-Century-Crofts, 1982, pp 242–247.
11. Thuline HC, Pueschel SM: Cytogenetics in Down syndrome. In Pueschel SM, Rynders JM (eds.): Down Syndrome: Advances in Biomedicine and the Behavior Sciences. Cambridge, Ware Press, 1982, pp 133–167.
12. Hook EB: Epidemiology of Down syndrome. In Pueschel SM, Rynders JM (eds.): Down Syndrome: Advances in Biomedicine and the Behavior Sciences. Cambridge, Ware Press, 1982, pp 11–88.
13. Abuelo D, Barsel-Bowes G, Busch W, et al.: Risk for trisomy 21 in offspring of individuals who have relatives with trisomy 21. Am J Med Genet 25:365, 1986.
14. Mulcahy MT: Down syndrome in Western Australia: Mortality and Survival. Clin Genet 16:103, 1979.
15. Masaki M, Higurashi M, Iijima K, et al.: Mortality and survival for Down syndrome in Japan. Am J Hum Genet 33:629, 1981.
16. Park SC, Mathews RA, Zuberbuhler JR, et al.: Down syndrome with congenital heart malformation. Am J Dis Child 131:29, 1977.
17. Wilson SK, Hutchins GM, Neill CA: Hypertensive pulmonary vascular disease in Down syndrome. J Pediatr 95:722, 1979.
18. Sondheimer HM, Byrum CJ, Blackman MS: Unequal cardiac care for children with Down syndrome. Am J Dis Child 139:68, 1985.
19. Balkany TJ, Downs MP, Jafek EW, et al.: Hearing loss in Down syndrome. Clin Pediatr 18:116, 1979.
20. Fort P, Lifschitz F, Bellisario R, et al.: Abnormalities of thyroid function in infants with Down syndrome. J Pediatr 104:545, 1984.
21. Pueschel SM, Pezzulo JC: Thyroid dysfunction in Down syndrome. Am J Dis Child 139:636, 1985.
22. Cutler AT, Benezra-Oberter R, Bimk SJ: Thyroid function in young children with Down syndrome. Am J Dis Child 140:479, 1986.
23. Pueschel SM, Herndon JH, Gelt MM, et al.: Symptomatic atlantoaxial subluxation in persons with Down syndrome. J Pediatr Orthopsychiatry 4:682, 1984.
24. Committee on Sports Medicine: Atlantoaxial instability in Down syndrome. Pediatrics 74:152, 1984.
25. Cronk CK: Growth of children with Down syndrome: Birth to age 3 years. Pediatrics 61:564, 1978.
26. Bricker D, Carlson L, Schwartz R: A discussion of early intervention for infants with Down syndrome. Pediatrics 67:45, 1981.
27. Connolly B, Morgan S, Russell FF, et al.: Early intervention with Down syndrome children, follow-up report. Phys Ther 60:1405, 1981.
28. Ferry PC: On growing new neurons: Are early intervention programs effective? Pediatrics 67:38, 1981.
29. Pueschel SM: A Study of the Young Child with Down Syndrome. New York, Human Science Press, 1983.
30. Mearig JS, Salyer KE, Witzel MA: Facial surgery for children with Down syndrome: An interdisciplinary perspective. Down Syndrome News 9:77, 1985.
31. Harrell RF, Capp RH, Davis DR, et al.: Can nutritional supplements help mentally retarded children? An exploratory study. Proc Natl Acad Sci USA 78:574, 1981.
32. Bennett FC, McClelland S, Kriegsman EA, et al.: Vitamin and mineral supplementation in Down syndrome. Pediatrics 72:707, 1983.
33. Smith EF, Spiker D, Peterson CP, et al.: Use of megadoses of vitamins with minerals in Down syndrome. J Pediatr 105:228, 1984.
34. Karp LE: New hope for the retarded? Am J Med Genet 16:1, 1983.
35. De La Cruz F: Medical management of mongolism or Down syndrome. In Mittler P (ed.): Research to Practice in Mental Retardation. Biomedical Aspects. 1977, vol 3, pp 221–228.
36. Wertz DC, Sorensen JR, Heeren TC: Genetic counseling and reproductive uncertainty. Am J Med Genet 18:79, 1984.
37. Carter PE, Pearn JH, Bell J, et al.: Survival in trisomy 18. Clin Genet 27:59, 1985.
38. Clark EB: Neck web and congenital heart defects: A pathogenic association in 45,XO Turner syndrome. Teratology 29:355, 1984.
39. Hall JG, Sybert VP, Williamson RA, et al.: Turner's syndrome. West J Med 137:32, 1982.
40. Miller MJ, Geffner ME, Lippe BM, et al.: Echocardiography reveals a high incidence of bicuspid aortic valve in Turner syndrome. J Pediatr 102:47, 1983.
41. Sybert VP: Adult height in Turner syndrome with and without androgen therapy. J Pediatr 104:365, 1984.
42. Rosenfeld RB, Hintz RL, Johanson AJ, et al.: Methionyl human growth and oxandrolone in Turner syndrome: Preliminary results of a prospective randomized trial. J Pediatr 109:936, 1986.
43. Raiti S, Moore WV, Vlict GV, et al.: Growth stimulating effects of human growth hormone therapy in patients with Turner syndrome. J Pediatr 109:944, 1986.
44. deGrouchy J, Turleau C: Clinical Atlas of Human Chromosomes. New York, John Wiley & Sons, 1984.
45. Gorlin RJ, Pindbort J, Cohen MM: Syndromes of the Head and Neck, 2nd ed. New York, McGraw-Hill Book Company, 1976.
46. Pashayan HM, Lewis MB: Clinical experience with the Robin sequence. Cleft Palate J 21:270, 1984.
47. Cozzi F, Pierro A: Glossoptosis-apnea syndrome. Pediatrics 75:836, 1985.
48. Carey JC, Ziter F, Fineman RM: Pierre Robin sequence as a consequence of malformation, dysplasia, and neuromuscular conditions. J Pediatr 101:858, 1982.
49. Clarren SK, Anderson B, Wolf LS: Feeding infants with cleft lip and/or palate. Cleft Palate J. In press.
50. Cohen MM: Craniofacial disorders. In Emery AE, Rimoin DL (eds.): Principles and Practices of Medical Genetics. London, Churchill Livingstone, 1983, pp 575–621.
51. Carey JC: Malformations of the craniofacies. In Rudolph AM (ed.): Pediatrics. Norwalk, Appleton-Century-Crofts, 1982, pp 386–390.
52. McLaughlin JF, Shurtleff DB: Management of the newborn with myelodysplasia. Clin Pediatr 18:463, 1979.
53. Leonard CO: Counseling parents of a child with meningomyelocele. Pediatr Rev 4:317, 1983.
54. Sillence D: The chondrodystrophies. In Emery AE, Rimolin DL (eds.): Principles and Practices of Medical Genetics. London, Churchill Livingstone, 1983, pp 705–735.
55. Kopitz SE: Orthopedic complications of dwarfism. Clin Orthop 114:153, 1976.
56. Horan FT, Beighton P: Orthopedic Problems in Inherited Skeletal Disorders. New York, Springer-Verlag, 1982.

57. Langer LO, Baumann PA, Gorlin RJ: Achondroplasia. Clin Pediatr 7:474, 1968.
58. Scott CI: Achondroplastic and hypochondroplastic dwarfism. Clin Orthop 114:18, 1976.
59. Horton WZ, Lotter JI, Rimoin DL, et al.: Standard growth curves for achondroplasia. J Pediatr 93:435, 1978.
60. Hall JG, Horton W, Kelly T, et al.: Head growth in achondroplasia: Use of ultrasound studies. Am J Med Genet 13:105, 1982.
61. Todorov AB, Scott CI, Warren AE, et al.: Developmental screening in achondroplastic children. Am J Med Genet 9:19, 1981.
62. Stokes DC, Phillips JA, Leonard CO, et al.: Respiratory complications of achondroplasia. J Pediatr 102:534, 1983.
63. Pauli RM, Scott CI, Wassman ER, et al.: Apnea and sudden unexpected death in infants with achondroplasia. J Pediatr 104:342, 1984.
64. Hecht JT, Nelson FW, Butler IJ, et al.: Computerized tomography of the foramen magnum: Achondroplastic values compared to normal standards. Am J Med Genet 20:355, 1985.
65. Scott CI: Medical and social adaptation in dwarfing conditions. Birth Defects 13:(3C):29, 1977.
66. Ablon J: Little People. New York, Praeger, 1980.
67. Sillence DO, Senn AS, Danks DM: Genetic heterogeneity in osteogenesis imperfecta. J Med Genet 16:101, 1979.
68. Sillence DO, Barlow KK, Garbor AP, et al.: Osteogenesis imperfecta type II delineation of phenotype with reference to genetic heterogeneity. Am J Med Genet 17:407, 1984.

Recommended Reading

For Physicians

deGrouchy J, Turleau C: Clinical Atlas of Human Chromosomes. New York, John Wiley & Sons, 1984.

Gorlin RJ, Pindbort J, Cohen MM: Syndromes of the Head and Neck, 2nd ed. New York, McGraw-Hill Book Company, 1976.

Hall BD: Multiple congenital anomaly syndromes. In Rudolph AM (ed.): Pediatrics, 17th ed. Norwalk, Appleton-Century-Crofts, 1984, pp 378–384.

Horan FT, Beighton P: Orthopedic Problems in Inherited Skeletal Disorders. New York, Springer-Verlag, 1982.

Jones KL: Dysmorphology. Curr Probl Pediatr 1, 1978.

Pueschel SM, Rynders JM (eds.): Down Syndrome: Advances in Biomedicine and Biosciences. Cambridge, Ware Press, 1982.

Schinzel A: Catalogue of Unbalanced Chromosome Aberrations. Berlin, de Gruyter, 1984.

Smith DW: Recognizable Patterns of Human Malformation. Philadelphia, W.B. Saunders Company, 1982.

For Families

Aceto T, Ehrhardt AA: Turner's Syndrome. Minneapolis, Human Growth Foundation, 1974.

Novy M, Aduss M: Feeding Your Special Baby. Chicago, University of Illinois, Center for Craniofacial Anomalies, 1982.

Pashayan HM, Lewis MB, Kuehn DP, et al.: The Infant with Cleft Lip, Cleft Palate, or Both. Pittsburgh, American Cleft Palate Association, 1982.

Plumridge D: Good Things Come in Small Packages. Portland, University of Oregon Health Sciences Center, 1976.

Pueschel SM, Canning DC, Murphy A, et al.: Down Syndrome: Growing and Learning. Fairway, KS, Andrews, McMeel, and Parker, 1986.

Rynders JE, Horrobin JM: To Give an Edge. St Paul, Colwell, 1984.

Snyder GB, Berkowitz S, Bzoch KR, et al.: Your Cleft Lip and Palate Child. Evansville, IN, Mead Johnson & Company, 1980.

25

MANAGEMENT OF APNEA IN THE ICN GRADUATE*

RONALD L. ARIAGNO, M.D.

Infants who are discharged from the newborn ICN may not have recovered from all of their problems and may therefore have residual temporary or chronic dysfunction that will require continuing care after they leave the ICN. The purpose of this chapter is to discuss apnea as a potential ongoing problem of the ICN graduate.

DEFINITION OF APNEA

Apnea itself is not a disease; it is more logically regarded as a sign or a symptom. In most instances the infant who has been discharged and now is at home comes to the physician's attention when the parents report what appears to them to be a prolonged pause in breathing and they observe a change in the child's skin color, which appears to be either pale or cyanotic. They may also report that the infant appeared to be limp or stiff. Most preterm infants who have apnea after discharge home from the ICN will have repetitive apnea that can be observed during readmission to the hospital by the medical staff.

* This chapter was supported in part by a grant (RR-81) from the General Clinical Research Centers Program of the Divisions of Research Resources, National Institutes of Health.

However, in the majority of preterm infants apnea of prematurity has resolved prior to discharge (see Appendix B.)

Editor

However, fewer term babies with a similar history will have symptoms observed during a brief hospitalization. As many as 60 to 80 per cent of infants with a history of an apnea episode after discharge home will have recurrent apnea events.[1-3] There may only be a history of "apnea" (symptom) rather than the observation of such an episode (sign) at the time the infant is admitted to the hospital.

Descriptions of apnea have originated from polygraphic recordings and can be categorized by type and duration: *central* (or diaphragmatic) when breathing effort is absent; *obstructive* (or upper airway) when breathing effort is present but air flow is blocked; and *mixed,* an event with a central and an obstructive component. Most mixed events begin as central apneas, but when diaphragmatic movements resume, there is no air flow at the nose or mouth because of an occluded airway. The occlusion may be due to an anatomic or functional obstruction.

An accurate assessment of the duration of the respiratory pause is also important. Brief respiratory pauses are normal and commonly seen during sleep, but pauses longer than 15 to 18 seconds are infrequent during the first six months of life. *Prolonged apnea* is usually defined as a respiratory pause of 20 seconds or longer, or of shorter duration when associated with bradycardia, cyanosis, pallor, or oxygen desaturation. Infants who have ongoing cardiorespiratory dysfunction or limited reserve may have oxygen desaturation with shorter respiratory pauses. Irregular breathing patterns are commonly seen during sleep and are more frequently observed in preterm infants. *Periodic breathing* is that breathing pattern in which there are three or more respiratory pauses of greater than 3 seconds' duration interrupted by periods of respiration 20 seconds or shorter.[4]

It has been difficult to organize the clinical understanding of apnea disorders in infancy, since apnea is a sign or symptom rather than a specific disease. Furthermore, the age and development of the infant and the possibility that the infant's condition may be either a congenital or an acquired problem will alter the presentation as well as the natural history of the problem. Historically, apnea seen in the preterm infant has been collectively considered as apnea of prematurity, an inexact and not necessarily helpful way of directing the treatment of the infant. More recently, it is clear that understanding the pathophysiology of apnea can lead to more effective and logical management.[5-8] Similarly, in the full-term infant, the treatment of conditions or disease processes in which apnea is an associated sign or symptom may lead to resolution of the apnea.[9]

In fact, true respiratory control problems are generally rare, may be present at birth, and are often difficult to diagnose, particularly when the symptoms are intermittent and limited to a specific sleep state (quiet or active rapid eye movement sleep).[10-13] Obstructive sleep apnea problems are more commonly, but not exclusively, seen in the older child. A classification of apnea in infants can be seen in Table 25–1. (See also Appendix B.)

APNEA IN THE ICN INFANT PRIOR TO DISCHARGE

A considerable amount of research has been directed toward apnea as a problem in both the preterm and full-term neonate during the first six months of life.[1,4,5,8,9,21-25] The incidence of apnea and the chronicity during the intensive care period are inversely related to the gesta-

---

TABLE 25–1. CLASSIFICATION OF APNEA IN INFANTS

1. **Apnea in preterm infants (<38 weeks' gestation)**
   a. Secondary to specific cause (immaturity of cardiorespiratory or neurologic function or dysfunction associated with acquired disease).
   b. Idiopathic
2. **Apnea in term neonates and postneonatal infants**
   a. Secondary to specific cause
   b. Idiopathic or apnea of infancy
3. **Respiratory control abnormality**
   a. Congenital
   b. Acquired

---

tional age of the infant (see Fig. 25–1) and are also related to the type of pathophysiologic problems that the baby might have had during the neonatal period.[26,27] The predisposing factors that may lead to apnea problems in the preterm infant have been reviewed by Kattwinkel.[7] If the developmental predisposition and other precipitating factors or associated problems that can lead to apnea are understood, treatment strategies can be based upon an identifiable pathogenesis of apnea in a specific case (Fig. 25–2). In approximately 78 per cent of infants with apnea, a precipitating cause for the apnea can be identified. The apnea or predominant periodic breathing pattern in the remaining 22 per cent is not associated with an obvious disease and therefore is idiopathic.[8] Infants in an ICN are commonly attached to a cardiorespiratory impedance monitor during their entire hospitalization to identify apnea and/or bradycardia events. The extent of the medical evaluation and therapy will depend upon the frequency, duration, and severity of the events observed.

Treatment for the apnea may consist of management of the precipitating cause (e.g., correcting hypoxemia) intervening to limit the severity of the apnea by using tactile and/or vestibular stimulation (e.g., oscillating water bed),[28] the use of continuous positive airway pressure (CPAP) by nasal prongs or mask, the use of respiratory stimulants such as methylxanthines,[29,30] or, in severe apnea, the use of total respiratory support with mechanical ventilation.

Occasionally hypoxemia can be induced by excessive sensory stimuli in the infant's immediate environment. Reversal can then be effected by reducing such peak levels of noise, activity, or handling.

P. Gorski

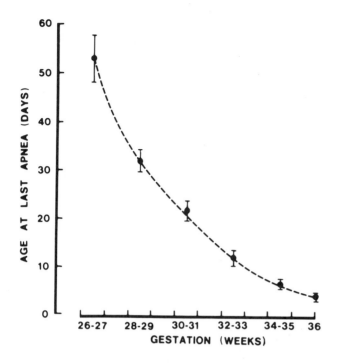

FIGURE 25–1. Mean (± SEM) postnatal age when last apnea was detected vs. gestational age (GA) at birth in 231 preterm babies with recurrent apnea. (Recurrent apnea of > 20 sec duration occurs in the majority of babies < 30 weeks, in approximately 50 per cent of infants at 30 to 32 weeks, and in 7 per cent of infants at 34 to 35 weeks GA.) (Reprinted from Henderson-Smart, DJ: Regulation of breathing in the perinatal period. In Saunders NA, Sullivan CE (eds.): Sleep and Breathing. New York, Marcel Dekker, 1984, pp 423–456.)

RELATIONSHIP BETWEEN NEONATAL APNEA AND LATER APNEA OR SUDDEN INFANT DEATH SYNDROME

In the general population the expected incidence of sudden infant death syndrome (SIDS) is 1 to 2 per 1000 live births (0.15 per cent).[31] High risk for SIDS has been arbitrarily defined as group mortality of 1 per cent or greater. The importance of apnea as a later problem for the ICN graduate, particularly the preterm infant, has received greater attention because of reports indicating that the incidence of SIDS in preterm and low birth weight infants under 2000 grams is increased.[32–37] Yount et al. has reported a SIDS rate of 1 per cent in infants weighing 1500 grams or less at birth.[37]

Other groups have documented a similar disproportionate SIDS rate of 0.6 to 1 per cent in infants weighing 2000 grams or less at birth.[33–35,38] The incidence of SIDS in infants with prolonged exposure to methadone or heroin in utero ranges from 0.5 to 2 per cent.[39,40] There is also some evidence that infants of addicted mothers have a 66 per cent reduction in the ventilation response to carbon dioxide compared to normal infants during the first four days of life.[41] Infants born to teenage mothers may also have an increased incidence of SIDS, which may range from 0.5 to 2.83 per cent.[36,38,42–44] Some of the highest incidence

rates are among surviving preterm infants with bronchopulmonary dysplasia (BPD). Werthammer et al.[45] reported that 11 per cent (6 of 53) of former preterm infants with BPD died from SIDS, in contrast to 1 of 65 infants weighing less than 1000 grams and without BPD. In other words, low birth weight infants discharged from the neonatal ICN appear to be at a significantly higher risk of SIDS than the general population.

However, one must question whether this is truly SIDS or a not totally unexpected complication of hypoxia or other residual illness in a compromised host — requiring appropriate therapy but not shedding light on the pathophysiology of SIDS.

Editor

SIDS refers to an unexplained and unexpected death. The peak incidence occurs in preterm and term infants between 2 and 4 months of age. SIDS represents the leading cause of infant mortality after the neonatal period. It is important to remember that if there are sufficient pathologic findings to explain the cause of death, sudden infant death secondary to that diagnosis would be recorded, and in these cases the mortality would not be considered to be due to SIDS. In 1972, Steinschneider was one of the first to report the relationship between prolonged apnea in infancy and SIDS,[46] and apnea research has accelerated since that report. This initial report described two of five infants with a

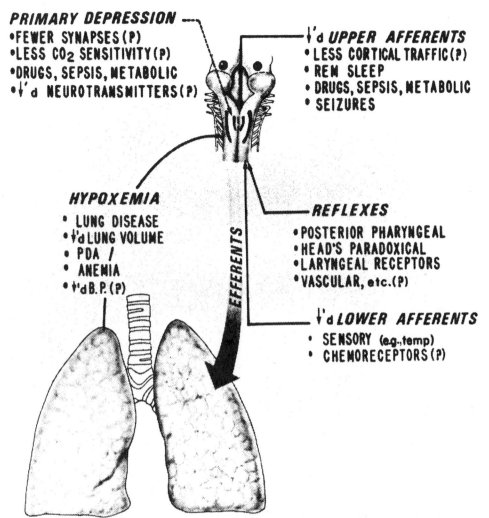

FIGURE 25-2. Proposed pathogenesis for neonatal apnea. (Reprinted from Kelly, DH: Incidence of severe apnea in infants identified at high risk for sudden infant death syndrome. In Tildon JT, Roeder LM, Steinschneider A (eds.): Sudden Infant Death Syndrome. New York, Academic Press, 1983, pp 607-613.)

history of prolonged sleep apnea who later died suddenly and had postmortem findings consistent with SIDS. Since this report, apnea as the possible mechanism for SIDS has captured a great deal of attention from professionals, as well as the public.

Naeye and others have reported pathologic findings (seven tissue markers for hypoxia) that support the hypothesis that there may have been chronic hypoxia in perhaps half of the SIDS victims.[6,47] However, a critical review of these data has been reported by Beckwith, who commented that many more studies are necessary before it can be firmly concluded that most SIDS victims have suffered from chronic hypoxemia prior to death.[48]

If, in fact, chronic recurrent apnea leads to chronic hypoventilation, the surviving infant may theoretically be at risk for the development of pulmonary hypertension and congestive heart failure or cor pulmonale.[49-51] However, this complication is uncommon in the infant and is more frequently seen in the older pediatric patient with obstructive sleep apnea syndrome. The possibility that apnea may be the mechanism for recurrent and chronic hypoxia in some SIDS victims and the possibility that SIDS victims may not be asymptomatic and well prior to death have led to considerable support for clinical investigation and research regarding the apnea hypothesis.

In 1978 and in 1985 the American Academy of Pediatrics Task Force on Prolonged Infant Apnea acknowledged the use of cardiorespiratory home monitors in the management of infants with prolonged apneic episodes.[52] At that time and since, considerable confusion and controversy have surrounded the relationship of SIDS and apnea and what constitutes an appropriate evaluation and management of infants presumed to be at risk.[1-3,5,9,21,25] Although there are normative data regarding the duration and frequency of respiratory pauses or apnea during the first six months of life in preterm and term infants,[4,8,22,23] there is no agreement regarding the significance of prolonged apnea and the long-term risk of SIDS in individual infants.[1,3,25,30,53,54] This confusion, in part, is due to a lack of adequate data to define what the risk of SIDS is in the infant who either has a history of or currently has apnea. It is essential to remember that SIDS and apnea are not synonymous terms. Apnea is one proposed mechanism among many possible causes of SIDS that have been suggested.[31] Apnea itself is not a disease and may therefore represent a symptom of greater or lesser importance in several disease processes.

"Medical research over the last decade has not substantiated the hypothesis that apnea is the major cause of the sudden infant death syndrome. Thus we believe that the National Sudden Infant Death Syndrome Foundation should maintain an open view and support research related to other hypotheses." (Official Statement of the National Sudden Infant Death Syndrome Foundation, April 24, 1985. Pediatrics 76:817, 1985)

M. Abbott

NO SCREENING TEST FOR APNEA OR SIDS "RISK" AVAILABLE

Recently Southall and co-workers prospectively screened for SIDS risk in a population of 1157 preterm and low birth weight infants from six regional neonatal intensive care units in England.[25] A 24-hour recording of respiratory wave form and electrocardiogram was obtained one week prior to discharge in each of these patients. Eight infants (0.7 per cent) who were considered asymptomatic as they entered the study had episodes of apnea greater than 30 seconds in duration. All of these episodes were accompanied by bradycardia, with heart rate less than 100 beats per minute. Twenty-five infants (2.3 per cent) had a total of 36 apneic episodes between 20 and 30 seconds in duration, the majority of which were accompanied by less than 100 heartbeats per minute, and 1.7 per cent had episodes of bradycardia, with heart rate less than 50 beats per minute without prolonged apnea. Five infants had ventricular premature beats,

one of whom had ventricular tachycardia. Eleven infants had supraventricular premature beats, four had supraventricular and ventricular premature beats, and two infants had pre-excitation.

Subsequently there were 11 deaths among the infants who underwent 24-hour recordings, of which 5 were considered SIDS. However, none of the babies who subsequently died of SIDS had had prolonged apnea (greater than 20 seconds); bradycardia, with heart rate less than 50 beats per minute; or cardiac arrhythmias on their 24-hour recordings before discharge.

Indeed, Southall's largest prospective study of respiratory patterns in nearly 10,000 British infants[55] reveals a negative correlation between apnea and SIDS — i.e., infants who had apnea were less likely to die of SIDS than was the general population. Profound apnea is a significant medical problem placing the child at risk for hypoxic/ischemic injury to the central nervous system, but it is not definitely related to SIDS.

P. Gorski

Clearly, apnea as a life-threatening event in the infant must be understood for etiology and prevented. There does *not* appear to be much evidence that symptomatic infant apnea is related to apnea of prematurity, however.

Editor

Unfortunately, "screening" all infants prior to discharge for apnea and bradycardia did not predict which babies would have SIDS. Currently there is *no* test to predict or identify infants at risk for SIDS or apnea, and further research is necessary to explore the possibility that cardiorespiratory monitoring or other polysomnography tests (multichannel recording) may enable detection of infants at risk for SIDS or apnea. There is considerable variation among centers in the methods of evaluation and criteria used to assess "risks." No controlled clinical studies have documented that a specific test or intervention can reduce the risk of SIDS.[56]

EVALUATION OF APNEA IN INFANTS

There are at least two groups of ICN graduates who may have apnea problems: a symptomatic group and an asymptomatic group (see Table 25-2).

SYMPTOMATIC GROUP

The symptomatic group can be further divided into (1) those infants in whom apnea is identified during their ICN hospitalization and

TABLE 25–2. Two Groups of ICN Graduates in Relation to Apnea Problems

SYMPTOMATIC	ASYMPTOMATIC
a. Inpatient—apnea never resolves b. Outpatient—apnea a new problem	a. Never had apnea b. Had symptomatic apnea that resolved

Recommendation for Evaluation

Has Apnea	Never Had Apnea	Had Symptomatic Apnea That Resolved
1. Observation including apnea-cardiac monitor in hospital 2. Trained medical staff available for CPR 3. Medical evaluation directed by history and physical exam 4. Appropriate clinical polygraphic study directed by clinical question and possible therapy	1. Consider appropriate polygraphic studies in infants with significant residual neurologic, cardiac, pulmonary, or other clinical problems that may contribute to apnea problems such as (a) infant with BPD, (b) anemia (Hct < 30) 2. Home apnea–cardiac monitor to observe for apnea problems in a high-risk patient such as (a) infant born to a narcotic addict, (b) surviving twin of SIDS infant	1. None, if no symptomatic apnea for 2 wk prior to discharge during which time infant has not had methylxanthine or other respiratory stimulant treatment 2. History of apnea should be noted in record, since anemia (Hct < 30) or post general anesthesia may increase risk for apnea

Etiology

Disease related or idiopathic	High-risk group; residual dysfunction	None

Treatment

| 1. Treatment of disease alone may be sufficient if apnea resolves.
2. In those infants who continue to have apnea in the hospital, a trial of methylxanthines is worthwhile.
3. Home apnea–cardiac monitor, particularly in those infants in whom apnea does not resolve | 1. Clinical observation only; or
2. Therapy to support residual problem, e.g., supplemental O_2 in BPD infant with suboptimal (PO_2 < 50) oxygenation (home apnea–cardiac monitoring may be helpful in selected cases)
3. Home apnea–cardiac monitor in selected cases
4. Parents trained in CPR; document observations of monitor alarms and interventions daily and review with physician on a regular basis. | None |

BPD = bronchopulmonary dysplasia

who continue to have apnea when they are otherwise ready for discharge home, and (2) those infants who never had apnea problems identified or had apnea problems that resolved, but now return to the hospital after discharge because their parents witnessed a frightening and life-threatening event in which the infant appeared blue, pale, limp, or stiff. The parents may also report intervening with vigorous stimulation, mouth-to-mouth breathing, or cardiopulmonary resuscitation to "revive" the infant. The parents understandably have difficulty reporting objective data about the initial or even later episodes.

It is now suggested that these episodes be referred to as "apparent life-threatening events" (ATLE's), rather than as "near-miss SIDS." (See Appendix B.)

Editor

Infants who have apnea following discharge should be readmitted to the hospital, and cardiorespiratory electronic monitoring should be used. A skilled hospital staff must be available to observe the infant and to perform infant cardiopulmonary resuscitation, should this be required. The purpose of the hospitalization is to provide support if the apnea is immediately "life threatening" and to identify or exclude known disease processes that may explain the frightening apneic cyanotic spell. Many causes of apneic and cyanotic episodes have recently been reviewed by Brooks and others.[7–9] Following a complete history, physical examination, and neurodevelopmental assessment,[30] an appropriate medical evaluation should be planned to identify those disorders most likely to explain the infant's apnea or bradycardia. A general differential diagnostic list that may be considered includes the following:

Congenital problems: congenital heart disease, including conduction abnormalities; cranial, facial, and other anatomic airway or vascular anomalies that may cause airway obstruction.

Infection: such as septicemia, septic and aseptic meningitis, pneumonia, infant botulism, pertussis, and certain viral infections, particularly respiratory syncytial virus.

Toxic-intoxication: sedative overdose, exposure to environmental toxins, electrolyte abnormalities secondary to feeding irregularities or gastrointestinal disturbances, or narcotic addiction.

Trauma: including hypothermia or hyperthermia, or child abuse.

Endocrine and metabolic: hypoglycemia, hypocalcemia, hyperammonemia or other abnormalities due to inborn errors of metabolism.

Neoplasm or tumor: causing intrinsic or extrinsic airway obstruction or lesions in central nervous system that cause abnormalities in respiratory control.

Other: for example, anemia in the preterm infant,[57] seizures, gastroesophageal reflux, with reflex apnea; respiratory control abnormalities; and chronic hypoxia associated with chronic pulmonary diseases, such as bronchopulmonary dysplasia.

In nearly 50 per cent of the patients hospitalized, a specific diagnosis can be made and treatment for that condition started, which may lead to resolution of the apnea problem.[1,3] In general, initial studies that may be helpful are a complete blood count with a differential count and determinations of electrolytes, glucose, calcium, and arterial blood gas (bicarbonate may be decreased after a hypoxic event or there may be a protracted decrease in various metabolic disorders; or an extended elevation may be observed if there has been respiratory acidosis with compensatory metabolic alkalosis). Bacterial and viral cultures may be clinically indicated, and a chest radiograph may be helpful to detect cardiac abnormalities or infiltrates compatible with infection or aspiration. An electrocardiogram may be helpful if there are clinical findings suggesting arrhythmia, heart disease, or pulmonary hypertension. If the description of the event suggests a seizure, an electroencephalogram may be helpful. Other studies may be suggested by the clinical presentation, physical examination, and in-hospital observations. If the cause of apnea is unexplained after completion of the medical evaluation and the infant is asymptomatic during the hospitalization, i.e., no apnea is observed, the remaining concern will be about the risk of recurrence of significant apnea that may be severe and potentially life

threatening. Although several polygraphic tests could be suggested and many are considered routine by some, there is no test to definitively estimate risk of recurrence of apnea or risk of SIDS. Polygraphic studies may be clinically helpful in those patients in the hospital who continue to have symptomatic apnea for which there is no specific cause or therapy or in those infants who continue to have apnea after treatment of their primary problem.

ASYMPTOMATIC GROUP

The asymptomatic group consists of infants who have no history of apnea during their newborn intensive care course or infants who had symptomatic apnea that has resolved. (It is assumed that preterm infants and other critically ill intensive care infants have been observed by means of an apnea cardiac monitor by trained staff during their hospitalization.) There are some infants who have never had apnea who may be considered at higher risk for apnea or sudden, unexplained death, e.g., infants born to mothers with narcotic addiction; the surviving twin of a SIDS victim; infants with significant residual neurologic, cardiopulmonary, or other clinical problems that may predispose to apnea, chronic and recurrent hypoxia, and/or hypoventilation.*

Polygraphic studies to evaluate respiratory control have been suggested for infants born to mothers with narcotic addiction. In those infants who have no apparent clinical or polygraphic abnormality (e.g., surviving twin of a SIDS victim), home apnea-cardiac monitoring can provide observation in the home and an opportunity for the parents or care givers to intervene if the infant has prolonged apnea. Infants who develop symptomatic apnea and then demonstrate increasing frequency and/or severity may require rehospitalization for management and further evaluation.

> Home monitoring causes serious stress on a family, however, and may not be carried out successfully in a setting in which suboptimal coping ability pre-exists, such as the household of a narcotic-addicted mother.
>
> *Editor*

On the other hand, for preterm infants who had apnea in the nursery, but who have had no further symptomatic apnea (without medication) for two weeks prior to discharge, usually no further evaluation or therapy is required. The history of apnea should, however, be clearly

---

* And, indeed, it should be remembered that their risk of SIDS may be unrelated to apnea.

—Ed.

noted in the discharge summary, since some infants who develop anemia (hematocrit less than 30 per cent)[45] or require general anesthesia may have apnea problems.[58] Because of this increased risk of perioperative apnea, some have recommended that surgery in preterm infants be delayed if possible until after 44 weeks' conceptual age and that the infant be monitored electronically for apnea for 24 hours after general anesthesia. Furthermore, these infants should not have surgery in a hospital where infant mechanical ventilation support and staff are not available.[59-61]

CLINICAL POLYGRAPH STUDIES— INDICATIONS AND UTILITY

Physiologic recordings may be accomplished for clinical or research purposes. Although these areas or goals may overlap, the orientations are usually distinct and different. The research protocol may be unrelated to diagnosis or management, whereas the clinical test attempts to address a specific diagnostic or management issue that will determine treatment and disposition for a specific patient.

Polygraphic studies are multiple-channel recordings of several physiologic variables that provide a printout and are usually conducted in a hospital room or a controlled laboratory environment (Table 25 – 3). Pneumograms or pneumocardiograms are magnetic tape recordings of respiratory and/or cardiac rates usually obtained from an impedance respiration – heart rate monitor; they can be obtained in the hospital or home. Polygraphic studies can provide useful clinical information when there is a specific question and the appropriate channels of information to answer that question are recorded. For example, in the infant with symptomatic apnea, the polygraphic study can be used to diagnose the type and severity of apnea: central, obstructive, or mixed, and the amount of periodic breathing.

In Figure 25 – 3, central apnea is seen in which no air movement or breathing movement is detected. In obstructive apnea, chest wall movement is detected, but there is no air flow (Fig. 25 – 4). In mixed apnea, there is a combination of central and obstructive apnea. In most circumstances the central event appears first and is followed by obstructive apnea. The fundamental variables recorded in a basic apnea study are *respiration effort*, detected by impedance, inductance, or strain gauges; *airflow*, detected by thermistor or end-tidal carbon dioxide; *electrocardiogram* or heart rate; and in many studies,

---

TABLE 25 – 3. Polygraphic Evaluations

1. **Basic Apnea Recording Variables**
   Respiration effort
      Impedance or inductance, or
        piezoelectrode or strain gauge
   Airflow
      Nasal thermistor or carbon dioxide
   Heart rate
      ECG or cardiotachometer
   Oxygenation
      Transcutaneous oxygen tension and saturation
   Ventilation
      Transcutaneous carbon dioxide or end-tidal carbon
        dioxide
2. **Gastroesophageal Reflux – Reflex Apnea Recording**
   Variables above, plus:
   Endoesophageal pH
3. **Sleep Apnea Recording**
   Variables above (with or without pH), plus:
   Sleep variables
      Electroencephalogram $C_3/A_2 – C_4/A_1$
      Electro-oculogram
      Electromyelogram, chin
4. **Clinical Multichannel Electroencephalogram Montage and Video Recording**
5. **Continuous Electrocardiogram Recording on Magnetic Tape (Holter)***
6. **Respiratory Control or Arousal Recording**
   Sleep apnea recording (see no. 3), plus:
   Quantitative measure of ventilation response:
      End-tidal carbon dioxide
      Pneumotachygraph or plethysmograph to obtain
        minute ventilation

---

* This is not specifically a polygraph recording technique. However, it is included since it may be done in conjunction with the above recordings or independently in specific patients when ECG changes during sleep and breathing are in question.

---

transcutaneous oxygen, carbon dioxide, and oxygen saturation.

The study can be scored for the number, duration, and type of apnea episodes and the amount of periodic breathing seen over a 12- to 24-hour recording. What is considered adequate duration for the recording is controversial; however, apnea episodes are more frequently observed in the 24-hour study.[62-64]

Other variables that can be added depend upon the clinical information requested:

1. Endoesophageal pH can be measured with a probe at a single level above the gastroesophageal junction, or at multiple levels, to evaluate either a low or high level of gastric reflux. A gastric acid pH below 4 must first be documented. Because milk has a basic pH, it may affect the detection of gastric acid reflux during milk feedings. Feeding the infant apple juice, which is more acidic, may circumvent this problem. The amount of hydrochloric acid production by the gastric mucosa and gastrointesti-

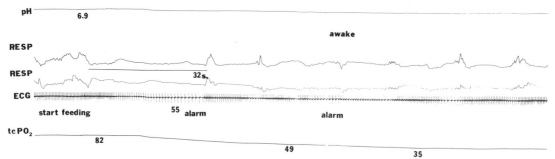

FIGURE 25–3. Recurrent central apneas recorded from a preterm infant during nipple feeding. Respiration was monitored using respiratory inductive plethysmography. RESP, thoracic (channel 2), and abdominal (channel 3) bands. Air flow is not recorded. The RESP signals do not show obstruction, i.e., simultaneous positive and negative deflections (compare with Figure 25–4). No pH decrease or reflux is seen.

A decrease in transcutaneous oxygen tension (tc PO$_2$) is noted from 82 to 35 mm Hg, and repetitive heart rate slowings are seen in the ECG. (Reprinted from Guilleminault C, Coons S: Apnea and bradycardia during feeding in infants weighing <2,000 gm. J Pediatr, 104:932–935, 1984.)

nal transit time may also affect endoesophageal pH monitoring results. Gastroesophageal reflux is detected when there is a precipitous drop in pH to below 4. Reflex apnea is scored when there is a close temporal association between the reflux and apnea events (Fig. 25–5).[65-69] The reflux study results can be compared with published data from normal controls.[70] The frequency, duration, severity, and type of apnea associated with the reflux can be quantified, and

the response to therapy can be documented in a later study.

2. Sleep variables may also be added with or without the pH probe. These additional variables include electromyelogram to detect muscle tone usually in the submental region, electro-oculogram to detect eye movements, and one or two leads for an electroencephalogram (Fig. 25–6).[64] From this recording format, the apnea, bradycardia, or gastroesophageal reflux

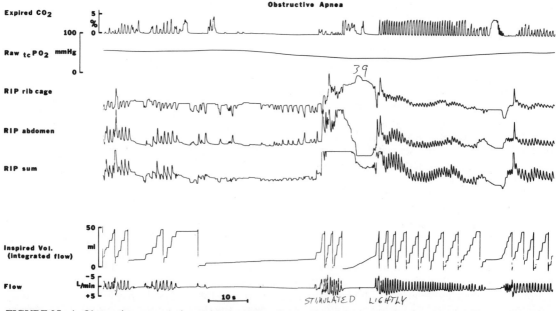

FIGURE 25–4. Obstructive apnea during which the airflow (i.e., expired CO$_2$ signal) is absent. The transcutaneous oxygen tension falls, and the respiratory inductance plethysmography signals from the rib cage and abdominal bands cancel each other so that the sum is zero. No flow is seen from the pneumotachograph (last channel), and therefore no volume is integrated.

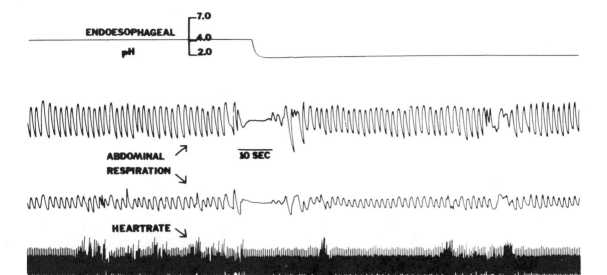

FIGURE 25–5. Short apnea (10 sec.) starting just prior to an acid reflux event. (Reprinted from Ariagno RL: Evaluation and management of infantile apnea. Pediatr Ann 13:210–217, 1984.)

events can be scored for occurrence during a specific sleep state—active rapid eye movement or quiet sleep.

3. Another type of recording is a long-duration multichannel electrocardiogram (the clinical diagnostic montage) with respiratory signals and a simultaneous video recording. This recording may be helpful in evaluating a seizure disorder that has been difficult to diagnose with a routine electroencephalogram. This combination of a continuously recorded electroencephalogram and a video recording allows a more complete survey of cortical electroencephalographic activity and behavior.[71]

4. A Holter recording of a continuous electrocardiogram on magnetic tape can be obtained in the home or the hospital and can be analyzed by a computer program. This test may be helpful in patients who are suspected of having a cardiac arrhythmia or who might have obstructive sleep apnea in which there may be R-R interval variations during the apneic events.[17,18,72]

5. A respiratory control or arousal study includes the apnea study variables, sleep variables, and ventilatory measurements with a hypoxic or hypercarbic challenge. The normal response to a hypoxic or hypercarbic challenge during a specific sleep state is an awakening or arousal and/or a change in ventilation[41,73–76] (Fig. 25–6).

Again it should be emphasized that none of these studies truly constitutes a test for deter-

mining the risk of recurrent severe apnea or SIDS. If results of the study are normal, it does not necessarily mean that the infant is healthy, only that within the limits of the test no further contributory information has been found.

WHAT IS CONSIDERED ABNORMAL IN THE POLYGRAPHIC EVALUATION?

The following are considered abnormal findings: (1) Prolonged apnea of 20 seconds or longer or apnea of shorter duration associated with bradycardia or oxygen desaturation. (2) Obstructive breathing and apnea with oxygen desaturation.[17] (3) Excessive amounts of gastroesophageal reflux and/or reflux temporarily associated with reflex apnea causing oxygen desaturation or obstruction.[67,70,77,78]

Findings of questionable significance are (1) An increase of periodic breathing to greater than 3 per cent of total recording time.[27] (2) Short episodes of apnea (central or obstructive). (3) Variation in arousability.[75,76,79] Although there is general agreement among researchers that periodic breathing occurs in normal infants during sleep, the significance of large amounts of periodic breathing as an indicator of risk remains controversial. Periodic breathing alone may not be a reason for concern; however, its effect on oxygen tension and ventilation should be noted.

Paradoxical breathing, the decoupling of chest wall and abdominal respiratory move-

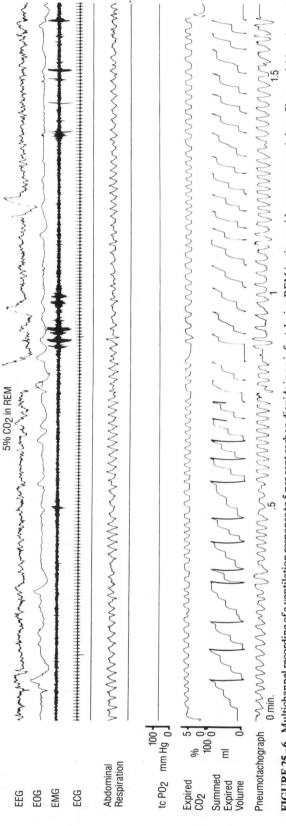

FIGURE 25–6. Multichannel recording of a ventilation response to 5 per cent carbon dioxide in an infant during REM (active rapid eye movement) sleep. Sleep variables, channels 1 to 3 (see Table 25–3). Electrocardiogram (ECG), channel 4. Transcutaneous oxygen tension in mm Hg (tc PO2) channel 6. Abdominal respiration effort recorded with a strain gauge, channel 5. Expired carbon dioxide (CO₂), channel 7. Summed integrated expired volume, channel 8. Flow measured with a pneumotachograph, channel 9. (Reprinted from Ariagno RL, Guilleminault C, Baldwin R, Owen-Boeddiker M: Gastroesophageal reflux and apnea in full term "near miss" SIDS infants. J Pediatr 100:894–897, 1982.)

ments following loss of intercostal muscle activity during active (rapid eye movement) sleep, is a common phenomenon in newborn infants. It does not normally lead to any change in oxygen or carbon dioxide tensions, since diaphragmatic effort and the rate of breathing increase to maintain adequate ventilation.[27] Paradoxical breathing, however, may become pathologic if diaphragmatic fatigue occurs, a phenomenon not yet well documented. It may also be observed with an obstructed airway. Until recently little research had been conducted on respiratory behavior and apnea during nipple feedings in infants who are awake or drowsy. Several authors have detected apnea and bradycardia during wakeful feeding periods in full-term newborn and young infants with normal development and a history of apnea problems.[74,80-82] Therefore, an evaluation of apnea should include study of infants during feeding periods as well as during sleep.

It is difficult to determine whether a patient is absolutely normal when respiratory patterns are not unusual. Apnea symptoms can be intermittent and unpredictable. A "normal" recording does not indicate that the patient will be free of problems. There are, however, significant group differences between infants with apnea of infancy and normal infants in respiratory pauses, episodes of short mixed and obstructive apnea, periodic breathing, and duration of longest apnea.[2,62,77,78]

THERAPY

TREATMENT OF PRIMARY MEDICAL CONDITION

If the primary medical condition causing apnea has been identified, the apnea can be re-evaluated after treatment is instituted. If the apnea is not resolved after treatment, or if the precipitating cause of apnea could not be identified, medical management should be directed toward detecting the occurrence of the apnea and reducing the frequency and severity of episodes. Until the apnea problem has resolved, the parents should be discouraged from taking these infants to mountainous areas (over 5000 ft) or on airplane trips, since a pressurized cabin may be equivalent to 8000 feet of altitude (the equivalent of breathing 15 per cent oxygen) and may cause a significant hypoxic stimulus.

RESPIRATORY STIMULANTS

In preterm and older infants who have recurrent symptomatic apnea, respiratory stimulants such as methylxanthines may be helpful. Theophylline or caffeine is often used in the preterm infant in the hospital to decrease the frequency and severity of apnea without any known long-term deleterious effects on the central nervous system. To decrease the frequency of apnea and periodic breathing, the recommended blood concentration of theophylline is 8 to 12 μg/ml. The usual loading dosage of theophylline is 3 to 4 mg/kg every 8 to 12 hours. Because the recommended dosage to replace the drug clearance in an infant may vary, blood level determinations are needed more frequently in the first week of therapy. Once the maintenance dose is established, determination of levels weekly or less frequently is sufficient if the patient is not having other problems.

> Short-term effects lasting up to four months after treatment may include tremulousness, increased activity and disorganized state regulation (abrupt swings of consciousness levels from sleep to high arousal; "bug-eyed" hyperalertness with concomitant easy tiring). As a result, parents can be challenged by an especially active, fussy infant who is not as visually responsive as expected during wide-eyed alert periods.
>
> *P. Gorski*

> Others, usually neonatologists, have not noted these effects; clearly, careful behavioral follow-up studies are needed.
>
> *Editor*

HOME APNEA-CARDIAC MONITORS

While some investigators have used theophylline as the primary intervention for the management of apnea of infancy, home monitoring for apnea and bradycardia is the most frequently utilized intervention.[1,3,83] Monitors do not prevent apnea symptoms, but they can alert the family to potentially significant apneic episodes. A home monitor should detect both respiration (apnea) and heart rate (bradycardia). Alarm settings are usually placed at a low heart rate of 80 per minute and a respiration pause maximum of 20 seconds. Other alarm settings depend on age-related heart-rate norms and specific clinical circumstances. Apnea-cardiac impedance monitoring is most commonly used for home detection of apnea. While this cannot distinguish shallow breathing or detect obstructive apnea, obstructive apnea may be suspected if unexplained bradycardia is detected.

If a home monitor is prescribed as the primary intervention, it may be started on the basis of a clinical history and diagnosis of apnea of infancy alone. Home monitoring may also be prescribed in addition to other medical management when symptomatic apnea is not resolved. Home monitoring is generally continued until the infant is free of any symptomatic apnea (associated with color change and/or bradycardia) for two months and any episodes requiring vigorous stimulation or resuscitation for three months. Since mild illness such as an upper respiratory tract infection may precipitate apnea symptoms, it is helpful to know that the infant had such an illness and yet did not experience apnea or bradycardia.[84] In infants with recurrent apnea, a home pneumogram or a polygraph recording in the hospital may be helpful in documenting and characterizing a cardiorespiratory abnormality and in distinguishing between real and artifactual alarms. Home apnea-cardiac monitoring has a significant impact on family life and will be most effective for the parents or other caregivers and the physician when everyone involved in the infant's care is thoroughly trained and knowledgeable in the use of the monitor.[55,85-87] Technical support for the family is required 24 hours a day. A daily written record of alarms, observation of the baby during the alarm, and the intervention used are necessary ongoing information that forms the basis for further medical evaluation and treatment. The support of an understanding and knowledgeable primary physician is essential to the family, as is support for the primary physician from the neonatal ICN.

Psychological assessment and support for the family are equally imperative during and following the presence in the home of this constant reminder of SIDS. The potentially harmful effects of bearing this early at-risk label might permanently limit the child's self-image through some form of the syndrome of imagined vulnerability. For a full discussion of this condition, often seen in association with medical risk during infancy, see Chapter 4.

P. Gorski

Many ICN's routinely teach infant cardiopulmonary resuscitation techniques to the parents and caregivers of all graduates. This is absolutely essential for parents whose infant is to be monitored at home. The average duration of monitoring in term infants is 5 months, and the home monitor is discontinued by 9 months of age in approximately 90 per cent of the cases.[1,2] Apnea problems resolve in the majority of preterm infants by 3 to 4 months' postconceptual age.

There have been no controlled clinical studies to determine the efficacy of home monitoring of apnea in decreasing the incidence of SIDS or in decreasing or preventing hypoxic injury.[88]

Such a study is unlikely to occur, since the randomized use or non-use of home apnea cardiac monitoring in infants with a history or finding of prolonged apnea would be unacceptable to many. Furthermore, the ideal control group would require home monitoring in a group of infants without a history or risk for apnea. This would enable the statistical reporting of the incidence of apnea in the general population and the outcome of infants with and without home monitoring.

P. Gorski

Both the physician and the parents should be aware that some infants have, in fact, died despite home monitoring.

OTHER FORMS OF MANAGEMENT

Other forms of management have included use of an oscillating water bed for preterm infants with apnea, a technique used primarily early in the course of treatment in the hospital.[29] Infants with excessive gastroesophageal reflux and reflex apnea should be given a trial of medical management that includes elevating the head of the bed (30 to 45 degrees) and maintaining the infant in a prone position continuously, except when care requires an essential temporary change.[89] If positioning is not helpful, bethanechol[90] or metoclopramide[91] may be tried. A barium swallow and small-bowel follow-through radiographic study are helpful in the initial evaluation to exclude a gastrointestinal abnormality. If medical management is ineffective and the reflux is severe (e.g., cardiopulmonary resuscitation has been required), fundoplication surgery, in spite of its problems, should be seriously considered.[42,67,75]

Those patients who have significant abnormalities of respiratory control frequently need a tracheostomy and mechanical ventilatory support.[10,11,13,92] Cuirass ventilation has been helpful in infants older than 6 months of age who need minimal ventilatory assistance. Such techniques as phrenic nerve electrostimulation have been most helpful in children who are older than 2 years.[93]

FOLLOW-UP OF THE PATIENT REQUIRING THERAPY

The frequency of follow-up outpatient visits is determined by the medical problems of an individual infant. Infants with apnea problems that are infrequent or not severe are usually managed primarily by the family physician or pediatrician. In infants who are undergoing home apnea-cardiac monitoring or receiving methylxanthines, a review of their progress is required—weekly at first and less frequently if the apnea is infrequent or self-limited (i.e., resolves spontaneously or with gentle tactile stimulation), the methylxanthine level is stable with a maintenance dose, and the infant is gaining weight. Rehospitalization and re-evaluation may be required in a minority of infants who are not improving or who have more frequent and severe apnea associated with other illness, such as an upper respiratory tract infection.

In infants who are undergoing home monitoring and receiving theophylline, theophylline administration is usually continued for a minimum of one month. If the apnea has been resolved, the theophylline can be discontinued. Home monitoring is continued for another one or two months and discontinued if the infant has no history of real alarms or apnea events. Further medical evaluation and polygraphic studies are not usually required.*

SUMMARY

Apnea may be an ongoing and unresolved problem or a new problem in the ICN graduate after discharge. Most often, significant apnea can be identified in the infant prior to discharge during apnea–cardiac electronic monitoring and direct nursing observation. After discharge, parents and other care providers report episodes that appear as potentially life threatening, in which the infant appears to stop breathing and the skin becomes pale or cyanotic, and the posture of the infant may be limp or stiff. If the pathophysiology of the apnea can be clarified, therapy that may resolve the apnea can be instituted. In those cases in which the apnea recurs and is significant and the cause is unknown, empiric treatment with respiratory stimulants such as methylxanthine and/or respiration and heart rate monitoring, both for the hospitalized infant and for the infant at home, may be reasonable alternatives.

In the asymptomatic infant there is no test to assess risk for significant apnea or SIDS. Nevertheless, evaluation of residual cardiopulmonary dysfunction may be helpful in clinical management and follow-up. Further research is required to develop a "physiologic profile" evaluation that can improve our understanding of the ongoing problems and needs of many ICN graduates. (See also Appendix B.)

---

* Different centers may approach the use of home monitoring and theophylline in different ways.
—Ed.

References

1. Ariagno RL, Guilleminault C, Korobkin R, et al.: "Near-miss" for sudden infant death syndrome infants: A clinical problem. Pediatrics 71:726, 1983.
2. Kelly DH, Shannon DC, O'Connell K.: Care of infants with near-miss sudden infant death syndrome. Pediatrics 61:511, 1978.
3. Kahn A, Blum D: Home monitoring of infants considered at risk for sudden infant death syndrome. Eur J Pediatr 139:94, 1982.
4. Hoppenbrouwers T, Hodgman JE, Arakawa K, et al.: Respiration during the first six months of life in normal infants: III. Computer identification of breathing pauses. Pediatr Res 14:1230, 1980.
5. Ariagno RL: Evaluation and management of infantile apnea. Pediatr Ann 13:210, 1984.
6. Beckwith JB: Observations of the pathological anatomy of the sudden infant death syndrome. In Bergman AB, Beckwith JB, Ray CG (eds.): Sudden Infant Death Syndrome: Proceedings of the Second International Conference on Causes of Sudden Death in Infants. Seattle, University of Washington Press, 1970, pp 83–102.
7. Kattwinkel J.: Neonatal apnea: Pathogenesis and therapy. J Pediatr 90:342, 1977.
8. Rigatto H: Apnea. Pediatr Clin North Am 29:1105, 1982.
9. Brooks, J: Apnea of infancy and sudden infant death syndrome. Am J Dis Child 136:1012, 1982.
10. Guilleminault C, McQuitty J, Ariagno RL, et al.: Six infants with congenital alveolar hypoventilation syndrome. Pediatrics 70:684, 1982.
11. Haddad GG, Mazza NM, Defendini R, et al.: Congenital failure of autonomic control of ventilation, gastrointestinal motility and heart rate. Medicine 57:517, 1978.
12. Lin HM, Loeu YM, Hunt CE: Congenital central hypoventilation syndrome—A pathologic study of the neuromuscular system. Neurology 28:1013, 1978.
13. Shannon DC, Marsland DW, Gould JB, et al.: Central hypoventilation during quiet sleep in two infants. Pediatrics 57:342, 1976.
14. Brouillette RT, Fernbach SK, Hunt CE: Obstructive sleep apnea in infants and children. J Pediatr 100:31, 1982.
15. Cayler GG, Johnson EL, Lewis BE, et al.: Heart failure due to enlarged tonsils and adenoids. Am J Dis Child 118:708, 717, 1969.
16. Cox MA, Schiebler GL, Taylor WJ, et al.: Reversible pulmonary hypertension in a child with mild respiratory obstruction and cor pulmonale. J Pediatr 67:192, 1965.
17. Guilleminault C, Korobkin R, Winkle R: A review of 50 children with obstructive sleep apnea syndrome. Lung 159:275, 1981.
18. Guilleminault C, Winkle R, Korobkin R, and Simmons B: Children and nocturnal snoring: Evaluation of the effects of sleep related respiratory resistive load and daytime functioning. Eur J Pediatr 139:165, 1982.
19. Kravath RE, Pollak CP, Borowiechi B: Hypoventilation during sleep in children who have lymphoid airway obstruction treated by nasopharyngeal tube and T and A. Pediatrics 59:865, 1977.
20. Tonkin SL, Partridge J, Beach D, Whiteney S: The pharyngeal effect of partial nasal obstruction. Pediatrics 63:261, 1979.
21. Brady JP, Gould JB: Sudden infant death syndrome, the physicians' dilemma. Adv Pediatr 30:635, 1983.

22. Gould JB, Lee AFS, James O, et al.: The sleep state characteristics of apnea during infancy. Pediatrics 59:182, 1976.
23. Hoppenbrouwers T, Hodgman JE, Harper RM, et al.: Polygraphic studies of normal infants during the first six months of life: III. Incidence of apnea and periodic breathing. Pediatrics 60:418, 1977.
24. Shannon DC, Kelly DH: Sudden infant death syndrome. In Saunders NA, Sullivan CE (eds.): Sleep and Breathing. New York, Marcel Dekker, 1984, pp 457–471.
25. Southall DP, Richards JM, Rhoden KJ, et al.: Prolonged apnea and cardiac arrhythmias in infants discharged from neonatal intensive care units: Failure to predict an increased risk for sudden infant death syndrome. Pediatrics 70:844, 1982.
26. Henderson-Smart DJ: The effect of gestational age on the incidence and duration of recurrent apnoea in newborn babies. Aust Pediatr J 17:273, 1981.
27. Henderson-Smart DJ: Regulation of breathing in the perinatal period. In Saunders NA, Sullivan CE (eds.): Sleep and Breathing. New York, Marcel Dekker, 1984, pp 423–456.
28. Korner AF, Guilleminault C, Van den Hoed J, Baldwin RB: Reduction of sleep apnea and bradycardia in preterm infants in oscillating waterbeds: A control and polygraphic study. Pediatrics 61:528, 1978.
29. Aranda JV, Turmen T: Methylxanthines in apnea of prematurity. Clin Perinatol 6:87, 1979.
30. Kelly DH, Shannon DC: Sudden infant death syndrome: A review of the literature, 1964 to 1982. Pediatr Clin North Am 29:1241, 1982.
31. Shannon DC, Kelly DH: SIDS and near SIDS. N Engl J Med 306:959, 1022, 1982.
32. Kulkarni P, Hall RT, Rhodes PG, et al.: Postneonatal infant mortality in infants admitted to a neonatal intensive care unit. Pediatrics 62:178, 1978.
33. Naeye RL, Ladis B, Drage JD: Sudden infant death syndrome: A prospective study. Am J Dis Child 130:1207, 1976.
34. Read A, Stanley F: Postneonatal mortality in Western Australia 1970–1978. Austr Paediatr J 19:18, 1983.
35. Sells CJ, Neff TE, Bennett FC, et al.: Mortality in infants discharged from a neonatal intensive care unit. Am J Dis Child 137:440, 1983.
36. Standfast S, Jereb S, Janerich D: The epidemiology of sudden infant death of upstate, New York: II. Birth characteristics. Am J Pub Health 70:1061, 1980.
37. Yount JE, Flanagan WJ, Dingley EF: Evidence of an exponentially increasing incidence of sudden infant death syndrome (SIDS) with decreasing birth weight (abstract). Pediatr Res 13:510, 1979.
38. Standfast S, Jereb S, Aliferec D, Janerich DT: Epidemiology of SIDS in upstate New York. In Tildon JT, Roeder LM, Steinschneider A (eds.): Sudden Infant Death Syndrome. New York, Academic Press, 1983, pp 59–75.
39. Chavez CJ, Ostrea EM Jr, Stryker JC, et al.: Sudden infant death syndrome among infants of drug-dependent mothers. J Pediatr 95:407, 1979.
40. Finnegan LP: In utero opiate dependence and sudden infant death syndrome. Clin Perinatol 6:163, 1979.
41. Lees MH, Olsen GD, Newcomb JD, Hamel TA: The chemoreceptor response of infants at high risk for SIDS. In Tildon JT, Roeder LM, Steinschneider A (eds.): Sudden Infant Death Syndrome. New York, Academic Press, 1983, pp 681–691.
42. Ashcraft KW, Goodwin CD, Amoury RW, et al.: Thal fundoplication: A simple and safe operative treatment for gastroesophageal reflux. J Pediatr Surg 13:643, 1978.
43. Biering-Sorensen F, Gorgensen T, Hilden J: Sudden infant death in Copenhagen 1956–1971: II. Social factors and morbidity, Acta Paediatr Scand 68:1, 1979.
44. Peterson DR, van Belle G, Chin NM: Sudden infant death syndrome and maternal age. JAMA 247:2250, 1982.
45. Werthammer J, Brown ER, Neff RK, et al.: Sudden infant death syndrome in infants with bronchopulmonary dysplasia. Pediatrics 69:301, 1982.
46. Steinschneider A: Prolonged apnea in the sudden infant death syndrome: Clinical and laboratory observations. Pediatrics 50: 646, 1972.
47. Naeye RL: SIDS: Evidences of antecedent chronic hypoxia and hypoxemia. In Robinson RR, (ed.): SIDS 1972. Toronto, Canadian Foundation for the Study of Infant Deaths, 1974, pp 1–6.
48. Beckwith JB: Chronic hypoxemia in the sudden infant death syndrome: A critical review of the data base. In Tildon JT, Roeder LM, Steinschneider A (eds.): Sudden Infant Death Syndrome. New York, Academic Press, 1983, pp 145–159.
49. Luke MJ, Mehrizi A, Folger GM, Rowe RD: Chronic nasopharyngeal obstruction as a cause of cardiomegaly, cor pulmonale and pulmonary edema. Pediatrics 37:762, 1966.
50. Menashe V, Farrebi C, Miller M: Hypoventilation and cor pulmonale due to chronic upper airway obstruction. J Pediatr 67:198, 1965.
51. Weil JV: Pulmonary hypertension and cor pulmonale in hypoventilating patients. In Weir EK, Reeves JT (eds.): Pulmonary Hypertension. New York, Futura Publishing Company, 1984, pp 321–339.
52. American Academy of Pediatrics: Task Force on Prolonged Infantile Apnea. Pediatrics 76:129, 1985.
53. Kelly DH: Incidence of severe apnea and death in infants identified at high risk for sudden infant death syndrome. In Tildon JT, Roeder LM, Steinschneider A (eds.): Sudden Infant Death Syndrome. New York, Academic Press, 1983, pp 607–613.
54. Mandell F: Cot death among children of nurses. Observations of breathing patterns. Arch Dis Child 58:312, 1981.
55. Silvio KT: SIDS and apnea monitoring: A parent's view. Pediatr Ann 13:229, 1984.
56. Weinstein S, Steinschneider A: The effectiveness of electronic home monitoring programs in preventing SIDS. In Tildon JT, Roeder LM, Steinschneider A (eds.): Sudden Infant Death Syndrome. New York, Academic Press, 1983, pp 719–726.
57. Werthammer J, Kelly DH, Shannon DC: Efficacy of blood transfusion in reducing apnea in anemic preterm infants (abstract). Pediatr Res 17:1529, 1983.
58. Steward DJ: Preterm infants are more prone to complication following minor surgery than are term infants. Anesthesiology 56:304, 1982.
59. Gregory GA, Steward DJ: Life-threatening perioperative apnea in the ex-"premie." Anesthesiology, 59:495–498, 1983.
60. Liu LMP, Cote CJ, Goudsouzian NJ, et al.: Life threatening apnea in infants recovering from anesthesia. Anesthesia 59:506, 1983.
61. Stewart AL, Turcan DM, Rawlings G, et al.: Prognosis for infants weighing 1,000 gm or less at birth. Arch Dis Child 52:97, 104, 1977.

62. Guilleminault C, Ariagno RL, Korobkin R, et al.: Sleep parameters and respiratory variables in "near miss" sudden infant death syndrome in infants. Pediatrics 68:354, 1981.

63. Hoppenbrouwers T, Geidel S, Ruiz ME, et al.: Electronic monitoring in the newborn and young infant: Technical guidelines. In Guilleminault C (ed.): Sleeping and Waking Disorders: Indications and Techniques. Menlo Park, CA, Addison-Wesley Publishing Company, 1982, pp 61–98.

64. Hoppenbrouwers T: Electronic monitoring in the newborn and young infant: Theoretical considerations. In Guilleminault C (ed.): Sleeping and Waking Disorders: Indications and Techniques. Menlo Park, CA, Addison-Wesley Publishing Company, 1983, pp 17–59.

65. Ariagno RL, Guilleminault C, Baldwin R, Owen-Boeddiker M: Gastroesophageal reflux and apnea in full term "near miss" SIDS infants. J Pediatr 100:894, 1982.

66. Downing SE, Lee JC: Laryngeal chemosensitivity. A possible mechanism for sudden infant death. Pediatrics 55:640, 1975.

67. Herbst JJ, Book LS, Bray PT: Gastroesophageal reflux in near miss sudden infant syndrome. J Pediatr 92:73, 1978.

68. Spitzer HR, Boyle JT, Tuchman DN, Fox WW: Awake apnea associated with gastroesophageal reflux: A specific clinical syndrome. J Pediatr 104:200, 1984.

69. Walsh JK, Farrell ML, Keenan WG, et al.: Gastroesophageal reflux in infants: Relation to apnea. J Pediatr 99:197, 1981.

70. Boix-Ochoa JM, Lafuente JM, Gil-Vernet JM: Twenty-four hour esophageal pH monitoring in gastroesophageal reflux. J Pediatr Surg 15:74, 1980.

71. Watanabe K, Hava K, Miyagaki S: Apneic seizures in the newborn. Am J Dis Child 136:980, 1982.

72. Guilleminault C, Ariagno RL, Coons S, et al.: Long-term follow-up of eight near miss SIDS infants with cardiac arrhythmias during sleep. Pediatrics 76:236, 1985.

73. Bower G, Phillipson EA: Arousal responses to respiratory stimuli during sleep. In Saunders NA, Sullivan CE (eds.): Sleep and Breathing. New York, Marcel Dekker, 1984, pp 137–162.

74. Guilleminault C, Coons S: Apnea and bradycardia during feeding in infants weighing 2,000 gm. J Pediatr 104:932, 1984.

75. Johnson DG: Current thinking on the role of surgery in gastroesophageal reflux. Pediatr Clin North Am. 32:1165, 1985.

76. McCullock K, Brouillette RT, Guzzetta AJ, Hunt CE: Arousal responses in near-miss sudden infant death syndrome and in normal infants. J Pediatr 101:911, 1982.

77. Guilleminault C, Ariagno RL, Forno LS, et al.: Obstructive sleep apnea and near miss for SIDS: I. Report of an infant with sudden death. Pediatrics 63:837, 1979.

78. Guilleminault C, Ariagno RL, Korobkin R, et al.: Mixed and obstructive sleep apnea and near miss for sudden infant death syndrome: II. Comparison of near miss and normal control infants by age. Pediatrics 64:882, 1979.

79. Ariagno R, Nagel L, Guilleminault C: Waking and ventilatory responses during sleep in infants near-miss for sudden infant death syndrome. Sleep 3:351, 1980.

80. Johnson P, Salisbury DM: Sucking and breathing during artificial feeding in the human neonate. In Bosma JF, Showacre J (eds.): Symposium on Development of Upper Respiratory Anatomy and Function. U.S. Government Printing Office, 1975, pp 206–209.

81. Steinschneider A, Rabrizzi DD: Apnea and airway obstruction during feeding and sleep. Laryngoscope 86:1359, 1976.

82. Steinschneider A, Weinstein SL, Diamond E: The sudden infant death syndrome and apnea/obstruction during neonatal sleep and feeding. Pediatrics 70:858, 1982.

83. Brown LW: Home monitoring of the high risk infant. Clin Perinatol 11(1):85, 1984.

84. Steinschneider A: Nasopharyngitis and prolonged sleep apnea. Pediatrics 56:967, 1975.

85. Black L, Hersher L, Steinschneider A: Impact of the apnea monitor on family life. Pediatrics 62:681, 1978.

86. Cuin LP, Kelly DH, Shannon DC: Parents' perceptions of the psychological and social impact of home monitoring. Pediatrics 66:37, 1980.

87. Smith J: Psychosocial aspects of infantile apnea and home monitoring. Pediatr Ann 13:219, 1984.

88. Deykin E, Bauman ML, Kelly DH, et al.: Apnea of infancy and subsequent neurologic, cognitive, and behavioral status. Pediatrics 73:638, 1984.

89. Orenstein SR, Whitington PF: Positioning for prevention of infant gastroesophageal reflux. J Pediatr 103:534, 1983.

90. Euler AR: Use of bethanechol for treatment of gastroesophageal reflux. J Pediatr 96:321, 1980.

91. Cohen S, Morris DW, Schoen HJ, DiMarino AJ: The effect of oral and intravenous metoclopramide on human lower esophageal sphincter pressure. Gastroenterology 70:484, 1976.

92. Guilleminault C, Cumiskey J: Progressive improvement of apnea and ventilatory response to CO_2 following tracheotomy in obstructive apnea syndrome. Am Rev Respir Dis 126:14, 1982.

93. Brouillette RT, Ibawi MN, Hunt CE: Phrenic nerve pacing in infants and children: A review of experience and report on the usefulness of phrenic nerve stimulation studies. J Pediatr 102:32, 1983.

Recommended Reading

Ariagno RL: Evaluation and management of infantile apnea. Pediatr Ann 13:210, 1984.

Ariagno RL, Guilleminault C, Korobkin R, et al.: "Near-miss" for sudden infant death syndrome infants: A clinical problem. Pediatrics 71:726, 1983.

Beckwith JB: Observations of the pathological anatomy of the sudden infant death syndrome. In Bergman AB, Beckwith JB, Ray CG (eds.): Sudden Infant Death Syndrome: Proceedings of the Second International Conference on Causes of Sudden Death in Infants. Seattle, University of Washington Press, 1970, pp 83–102.

Brady JP, Gould JB: Sudden infant death syndrome, the physician's dilemma. Adv Pediatr, 30:635, 1983.

Brooks J: Apnea of infancy and sudden infant death syndrome. Am J Dis Child 136:1012, 1982.

Gregory GA, Steward DJ: Life-threatening perioperative apnea in the ex-"premie." Anesthesiology 59:495, 1983.

Johnson DG: Current thinking on the role of surgery in gastroesophageal reflux. Pediatr Clin North Am 32:1165, 1985.

Kattwinkel J: Neonatal apnea: Pathogenesis and therapy. J Pediatr 90:342, 1977.

Rigatto H: Apnea. Pediatr Clin North Am 29:1105, 1982.

Shannon DC, Kelly DH: SIDS and near SIDS. N Engl J Med 306:959, 1022, 1982.

Southall DP, Richards JM, Rhoden KJ, et al.: Prolonged apnea and cardiac arrhythmias in infants discharged from neonatal intensive care units: Failure to predict an increased risk for sudden infant death syndrome. Pediatrics 70:844, 1982.

26

SUPPORT OF THE FAMILY WHOSE INFANT DIES

STEPHANIE A. BERMAN, M.S.W.

One phenomenon that has resulted from the regionalization of perinatal care is that sick or premature babies who die in the newborn period frequently do so in perinatal regional centers. Families are often separated from one another, and parents from each other, from their own extended family supports, and at worst, even from their babies. They are also separated from familiar health care providers. When a baby is transported from a local hospital to a distant center, parents must accommodate themselves not only to the gravity of their child's condition but to a total upheaval in their environment. The death or impending death of a newborn under these circumstances is an incomparable challenge for parents, families, and staff alike.

Drawing from the experience of others (see Recommended Reading), through trial and error, and with the help and ideas of families whose babies have died, we have evolved an approach to neonatal death that helps to provide order, dignity, and some semblance of peace for those who share in the death of a baby.

The following material briefly outlines the ideas that represent the basic approach that has tended to become a standard for ICN's, and one we feel can be adapted easily to working with families experiencing neonatal death in a community hospital. In addition, we will provide the primary physician or pediatrician with a framework from which long-term follow-up and intervention programs can be developed.

SUPPORTIVE APPROACHES IN THE ICN

While it may at first seem obvious, informing parents honestly about the gravity of their child's medical condition is a critical first step in helping parents prepare for death and begin the process of grieving. By and large, parents prefer to be together when they hear this information. The pediatrician who refers a very sick infant to a perinatal care center often has the sensitive task of simultaneously preparing a family for the possibility of death and the hope of survival. This theme is echoed in the ICN.

While the death of a baby is frequently a precipitous event, there are most often clear signs that a baby will not survive and opportunities to prepare families. When possible, involved staff members should meet to share their impressions of the course of the baby's condition and to coordinate efforts to involve the family. We have found it helpful to talk with parents about how their child might die and how they can best provide comfort to themselves, each other, and their dying infant. Although initially apprehensive, parents (with startlingly few exceptions) are grateful to have a chance to be with their babies when they die. For many, it is the only chance they have to be alone with their children. For most, it is a profound parenting experience. For some, it is a time when the death and loss of their infant becomes a reality. It is an opportunity to say goodbye and begin the process of grieving.

Whenever possible, parents need control and choice about how they want to participate in their baby's time of death. Because there are so few role models for such a circumstance, many couples appreciate knowing of others' experiences. Mostly they appreciate knowing that there are no rules or expectations imposed by the staff. There is no universally "appropriate" standard.

Some choices that can be offered and to which parents are most receptive are: Can staff call extended family? Should a priest or clergyman be called before or at the time of the baby's death? Would the parents like to dress the baby in special clothes or take footprints themselves? We routinely obtain photos, footprints, and a lock of hair; along with other mementos (hats, arm bands, even tape with the baby's name); these provide cherished keepsakes and important reminders of their infant's existence.

Parents who are apprehensive about holding their baby at the time of death often need reassurance that the infant will not have a long, agonizing time. Often the presence of an involved team member is reassuring, and in any case, a doctor or nurse should remain in the immediate vicinity. Parents like to know that they (and their extended family, if they choose) can be with their baby for as long as they want. Being asked periodically if they would like more time gives them an opportunity to extricate themselves when they are ready.

Sometimes a child's death comes unexpectedly and quickly. Parents who cannot be with their child at the time of death can nonetheless be offered an opportunity for contact with their deceased infant. Often embarrassed to ask, parents are relieved to know that they may still have a chance to see their baby. For some, it is their only opportunity to see and hold their newborn.

For parents who have observed their infant's struggle for life in the intensive care nursery, seeing and holding the infant after death can provide a surprise blessing. Freed in death from the intravenous lines, endotracheal tube, and monitoring systems, the final image of the baby is often one of relative or restored peace, comfort, and tranquility. This calmer memory lasts forever and possibly helps start the parents' huge long-term effort to cope and eventually to adapt their lives to their loss.

P. Gorski

Once parents are prepared for how their baby will look and feel, they need a quiet place to be with the infant. Finally, parents need to be told about autopsy and disposition options. Some are ready to decide. Some need to know that they can wait to decide if they are uncertain.

The death of a newborn is a time of numbness, pain, and anguish for parents and family. It is helpful when staff are comforting and supportive. When there are family, friends, or others who can be supportive, staff involvement can be more indirect. One or two designated staff members need to remain with or near a family when their baby dies, so they can help guide family and staff through the process. They can provide a buffer between parents and staff as well as extended family. The stress experienced by the staff must also be considered, since a death represents "failure" to them as well. Mutual support for each other will improve the ability of the staff to respond to the family's needs.

When parents leave the hospital, it is often helpful to let them know about available support services. Some pamphlets or brochures or the name of a support parent are welcome, and referral to a parent support group may also be helpful.

FOLLOW-UP NEEDS

Follow-up conferences are of great importance to families. They provide an opportunity to review the particulars of their baby's medical course and the reasons for the baby's death. They are a time to clarify issues and to release parents from the guilt they harbor, often born of misunderstanding. It is a time for parents to reconnect with their child's medical team, a time for them to express gratitude or their anger about things they felt were not right. It is, for many, a chance to talk about their baby with those who knew and cared for him or her. For involved staff members, follow-up conferences are a chance to see the parents again and a time to recognize the resilience of the human spirit. It is a time when community support resources can be reintroduced. It is a chance to assess parents' coping strategies and a window to the grieving process. For everyone involved, it is a time for closure and clarity.

For some families, work demands, family responsibilities, and sheer logistics preclude their return to the perinatal center for follow-up.

Their child's or the siblings' private pediatrician is often the family's choice for providing follow-up. With the aid of autopsy findings and other information from the center where the baby died, important light can be shed on medical specifics. The following is a discussion of the grieving process, when grief has become pathologic in its dimensions, and when the physician has cause to worry.

GRIEVING

Grief and loss are experienced in profoundly individual ways. While many couples are strengthened by this most intimate experience, others are confused and conflictive. Sorting out and accepting individual grieving styles is one of the challenges that confront and confound a couple experiencing the death of an infant. Opportunities for guilt and blame abound.

Many parents isolate themselves from family and friends for various lengths of time. Parents have frequently reported that others do not know what to say or invariably say the wrong thing. For many, the sadness of friends and family seems to exacerbate feelings of guilt. Others are burdened by the sense that they have disappointed their family and that they have turned a joyously expectant event into a time of sadness.

While there is a plethora of literature about death and grieving (see Recommended Reading), there are no real or absolute prescriptions that one can hand to parents to lessen their pain.

Community health care providers are key resource persons to grieving families. Either because they provide care to other children in the family or because of their involvement with the deceased child, local doctors and others provide an important link for parents to the medical specifics and sometimes to the child. A meeting with family members to review the facts surrounding a child's death can be helpful for parents in their efforts to cope.

The process of grieving is not well understood. Because the existing literature focuses mostly on "pathologic" grief, it is helpful to focus here on some of the broad variations of normal grieving patterns exhibited after perinatal loss.

A common misunderstanding is the belief that mourning should last several weeks or, at most, months. Parents are urged by friends and relatives to pull themselves together, put the loss behind them, get on with their lives, and take heart from the expectation of the "next" child.

Parents, and mothers especially, are referred to psychotherapists who seek to exorcise the deep-seated roots of their "inappropriate" grief behaviors.

In fact, grieving is a long-term process of adaptation. It is an adjustment to a fundamental change in the griever's structure of primary relationships. With grieving, parents must come to accept the reality of the loss of their baby and the separation from their child. How parents cope and adapt to their loss is varied and depends in part on mutual support and the support of extended family and community.

The initial period of disequilibrium, depression, and despair, accompanied by forms of somatic distress and persistent images of the baby, lasts six months to a year, or longer. A mother needs to integrate the loss of the baby and the loss of the pregnancy. On the one hand, she has lost the loved object; and on the other, she experiences the loss of physical integrity that affects her sense of trust in her own body and in future pregnancies. Many report a persistent feeling of emptiness. A mother may fear that she did something wrong during her pregnancy or that she harbors a bodily or genetic problem. A father may also express anxiety about something he did that may have caused the baby to die.

These understandable parental feelings of anxiety or guilt can easily get displaced onto parenting surviving or subsequent children. Whether consciously or not, such parents are prone to overprotecting their other children, building within the children a sense of fragility about themselves. The family's physician is in a prime position to help parents realize their children's strengths and avoid creating a chronic syndrome of imagined vulnerability.

P. Gorski

While follow-up conferences help to clarify and provide information about a baby's death, feelings of guilt and responsibility cannot be explained away. They are normal and need to be integrated.

Parents often attempt to memorialize their babies. They make scrapbooks and develop special remembrance times. Parental feelings may include anger toward the baby for abandoning them. Anger is alternatively displaced on obstetricians and pediatricians who become lightning rods for diffused parental rage. It is imperative that the practitioner not take this personally.

A major milestone in the adaptation process is reached when parents attempt to retake control. It is a peer-oriented time and one when support groups are most helpful. Parents can see that they are not alone and that it is possible to endure and even to control their grief. Some parents choose to read about the experience of others and some seek professional care providers to reassure them that they are normal.

Finally, after the integration of events surrounding perinatal loss, parents frequently note a shift in their life values. Philosophic, interpersonal, religious, and even work values change, and parents report a more "present-oriented" set of values. Thus, it appears that neonatal loss is accompanied by a profound and continued effect on parents and siblings.

Practitioners who have strong religious or philosophic faith may be tempted to try to explain what has happened in terms of their personal ideology, but such efforts, however well intended, may not be helpful. Some families may indeed derive comfort and be helped in the necessary integration of grief and its resolution by support that is consistent with their own ideologic framework.

WHEN TO WORRY

It is a common notion that grief is pathologic when it extends for more than several months. Recent studies have demonstrated, however, that the effects may be lasting and profound. The practitioner should expect long-term changes in the couple and in the siblings. Pathologic grief may be defined in two ways (Golenski, personal communication, 1986): First, parents themselves may perceive their responses as distressing. They cannot tolerate the dysfunction that results from their grief. Second, the person who grieves focuses solely on his or her own distress without reference to the baby who died. When there is profound egocentrism about the event, the grieving process has triggered an underlying disorder that should signal referral to a psychotherapist.

> Although no absolute guidelines can be given, in my experience families are usually able to come to grips with the loss of their newborn within 12 months. If the grieving process remains exaggerated after a year, I consider this "pathologic," and recommend that the family seek some additional counseling.
>
> *M. Abbott*

SUMMARY

People in the process of grieving appear unstable for a time. For the most part, this is a normal reaction to integrating loss. Grieving causes disruption of living patterns for individuals, couples, children, and extended family.

While care providers can be helpful in pointing out when physical and emotional problems can be related to a death in the family, parents themselves need to decide when they want or need additional support services to help them cope. While counseling and peer support resources abound, families need assurance that they themselves are the best ones to determine how well their lives are going and whether outside help will lessen their stress. So, bereft of control over the birth and short life of their infant, parents frequently embrace the notion that they can control their process of grieving and the form it takes in their lives.

Parents who seek help and counseling from their primary care provider are not necessarily seeking assertive intervention or referral, but receptivity, comfort, and reassurance that the disequilibrium they are experiencing is normal. By taking the time to do this, the practitioner not only assists the parents to therapeutic verbalization of their feelings but also may prevent the future expression of unresolved feelings as complaints ascribed to siblings or themselves in later months or years.

At best the supportive practitioner can guide parents through a most difficult time and toward successful resolution of their grief.

Recommended Reading

For Health Care Providers

Cavenor JO, Butts NT, Spaulding JG: Grief—Normal or abnormal? N C Med J 39:31, 1978.

Connolly KD: The management of perinatal death. Ir Med J 75:456, 1982.

Dopson CC, et al.: Unresolved grief in one family. Am Fam Physician 27:207, 1983.

Fetus and Newborn Committee, Canadian Pediatric Society: Support for parents experiencing perinatal loss. Can Med Assoc J 129:335, 1983.

Fischoff J, O'Brien N: After the child dies. J Pediatr 88:140, 1976.

Furlong RM, et al.: Grief in the perinatal period. Obstet Gynecol 61:497, 1983.

Kennell J, Klaus M.: Caring for the parents of a stillborn or an infant who dies. In Klaus M, Kennell J (eds.): Parent-Infant Bonding, 2nd ed. St. Louis, C.V. Mosby Company, 1982, pp 159–293.

Lake M, et al.: The role of a grief support team following stillbirth. Am J Gynecol 146:877, 1983.

Mahan CK, et al.: Bibliotherapy: A tool to help parents mourn their infant's death. Health Soc Work 8:126, 1983.

Mulhern RK, et al.: Death of a child at home or in the hospital: Subsequent psychological adjustment of the family. Pediatrics 71:743, 1983.

Support after perinatal death: A study of support and counseling after perinatal bereavement (letter). Br Med J 286:144, 1983.

Videka-Sherman L: Coping with the death of a child: A study over time. Am J Orthopsychiatry 52:688, 1982.

Wessel MA: The primary physician and the death of a child in a specialized hospital setting. Pediatrics 71:443, 1983.

Wilson AL, et al.: The death of a newborn twin: An analysis of parental bereavement. Pediatrics 70:587, 1982.

Zisoff S, et al.: Measuring symptoms of grief and bereavement. Am J Psychiatry 139:1590, 1982.

For Parents

Borg SO, Lasker J: When Pregnancy Fails: Families Coping With Miscarriage, Stillbirth, and Infant Death. Boston, Beacon Press, 1981.

D'Arcy P: Song For Sarah—A Young Mother's Journey Through Grief and Beyond. Wheaton, IL, Shaw Publishers, 1979.

Davidson GW: Understanding Death of the Wished For Child. Springfield, IL, OGR Service Corporation, 1979.

Glick I, et al.: The First Year Of Bereavement. New York, John Wiley & Sons, 1974.

Grollman EA: Explaining Death to Children. Boston, Beacon Press, 1976.

Peppers LG, Knapp RJ: Motherhood and Mourning: Perinatal Death. New York, Praeger, 1980.

Sahler OJZ (ed.): The Child and Death. St. Louis, C.V. Mosby Company, 1978.

Schiff HS: The Bereaved Parent. New York, Crown Publications, 1977.

SECTION V

APPENDICES

APPENDIX A

HOME CARE OF INFANTS WITH CHRONIC LUNG DISEASE

ARNOLD C. G. PLATZKER, M.D., CHERYL D. LEW, M.D., SEYMOUR R. COHEN, M.D., JEROME THOMPSON, M.D., SALLY L. DAVIDSON WARD, M.D., and THOMAS G. KEENS, M.D.

PREPARATIONS FOR DISCHARGE FROM THE ICN

Discharge planning should begin when the diagnosis of airway disability or chronic pulmonary disease is determined. In many circumstances, this planning can be initiated very early in an infant's course in the ICN. Table A–1 is a sample list to be used as a guideline for planning care of infants with complex pulmonary disease.

FOLLOW-UP AFTER DISCHARGE HOME

Regularly scheduled re-evaluations are aimed at minimizing the potential for interval complications, while ensuring that growth and development reach optimal levels. Duplication of services should be avoided. It is therefore desirable that the pediatrician, pulmonologist, and otolaryngologist confer at the outset to plan appropriate division of responsibilities. Assignment of the function of medical coordinator of care should be flexible, depending upon the needs of the specific patient. During the course of each child's lifetime, the medical coordination function may indeed shift among the physicians involved with follow-up, from generalist or pediatrician to specialist and back again.

General Pediatric Care

Comprehensive general pediatric care is intrinsic to the successful management and optimal long-term outcome of infants with significant pulmonary problems. In addition to routine measures of health care maintenance, the pediatrician must become familiar with the rationale and plan of management of the airway or lung problem. Close communication among the primary care physician, pulmonologist, and otolaryngologist is necessary if all aspects of the care plan are to be executed efficiently. During the first several months after discharge from the hospital the child may benefit from frequent evaluation of general status and growth by the primary care physician, perhaps even weekly or biweekly.

> Respite care to free a few hours or even days must be planned at regular intervals for parents who shoulder all the intensive care responsibilities at home. Respite care should be discussed as a routine part of predischarge planning in the hospital, so that parents can anticipate the need for relief and recognize that this is normal.
>
> *P. Gorski*

Pulmonary Home Care

In Chapter 14, the problems to be expected in infants with chronic lung disease have been reviewed in depth. In general, the most demanding schedule adaptable to home care (other than care of ventilator-dependent children) requires routine administration of medications and/or provision of treatments no more frequently than every six hours. Whenever possible, for infants with bronchospasm as well as those with upper airway obstruction, sustained-release forms of medications, such as theophylline granules, should be prescribed. The use of longer-acting agents by aerosol should be reserved for children older than 5 to 6 years. Table A–2 lists the medications, preparations, and dosages generally used. Table A–3 lists equipment that may be needed to provide home care, and Table A–4 gives instructions for administration of bronchodilators.

289

TABLE A–1. ICN Home Care Check List (Children's Hospital of Los Angeles)

Guidelines to Discharge Planning for Complex Infant Care

Generalized Conditions	Conditions requiring this kind of care include chronic lung disease, apneic episodes, congenital heart disease, tracheostomy care, hydrocephalus, requirement for medications and/or treatments no more frequently than every 4 to 6 hr
Lead Time	Two weeks of parental preparation
Training Needs	Parents should spend extensive periods in unit; recommend overnight stay. Training should include:

1. Well-infant care
2. Postural drainage and percussion
3. Suctioning, if applicable
4. Aerosol treatments, if applicable
5. Cardiopulmonary resuscitation
6. Tracheostomy care, if applicable
7. Shunt care; incision care, if applicable
8. Equipment management

Medications/Treatments Parents should be trained to give:
1. Well-infant care
2. Diuretics
3. Bronchodilators, if applicable

Potential Equipment

Diagnosis	Equipment
1. Apnea	a. Apnea-bradycardia monitor with battery pack
2. Simple tracheostomy	a. Portable aspiration suction machine with battery pack
	b. Apnea-bradycardia monitor with battery pack
	c. Infant Laerdol resuscitation bag and tracheostomy tube adapter
	d. Humidifier (when indicated)
3. Simple bronchopulmonary dysplasia with/without tracheostomy	a. Aerosol machine
	b. Portable aspiration suction machine with battery pack
	c. Apnea-bradycardia monitor with battery pack, when indicated
	d. Infant Laerdol resuscitation bag and mask, when indicated
4. Complex bronchopulmonary dysplasia	a. 3 a–d, above, of simple bronchopulmonary dysplasia,
	b. *Oxygen:* one of following two systems:
	(1) Oxygen concentrator with two size E cylinders, one stand, one regulator
	(2) Liquid oxygen with portable reservoir. Must be on a flow of 1 liter

Predischarge Examinations
1. Well-infant examination
2. Arterial blood gases on discharge if infant has lung disease
3. Chest radiograph on discharge
4. Pneumogram if infant has apneic episodes (see also Chapter 25)
5. Laboratory studies as indicated: CBC, electrolytes, creatinine, theophylline level

Home Nursing
Not recommended

Follow-up
1. Neonatology within 2 wk
2. General pediatric visit within 1 to 2 wk
3. Consultant appointments as indicated
4. For apnea patients, provide letters for:
   a. Department of water/power
   b. Fire department/paramedics
   c. Lifeline telephone
5. Community infant program: highly recommended
6. Regional center referral as indicated

TABLE A–2. Pulmonary Medications

THEOPHYLLINE PREPARATIONS

Preparation	How Supplied	Dosage Interval
Short-Acting		
Liquids:		
Accurbron	10 mg/ml	q 6 hr
Slo-Phyllin	80 mg/15 ml (5.33 mg/ml)	q 6 hr
Tablets:		
Quibron	300 mg, scored to provide 100, 150, 200 mg segments	q 6 hr
Intermediate-Acting		
Tablets:		
Theo-Dur	100, 200, 300 mg	q 8–12 hr
Capsules:		
Slo-bid Gyrocap	50, 100, 200 mg	q 8–12 hr
Slo-Phyllin Gyrocap	60, 125, 250 mg	q 8–12 hr
Long-Acting		
Tablets:		
Uniphyl	200, 400 mg	q 24 hr

BETA-ADRENERGIC AGENTS

Preparation	How Supplied	Administration/Dosage

Note: *All beta-adrenergic medications delivered by aerosol should be administered by the 5-breath method.*

Isoproterenol (Isuprel)

Preparation	How Supplied	Administration/Dosage
Liquid	Not available	
Tablets	Not available	
Aerosol	1:200 (0.5%) solution; dilute with normal saline to desired concentration	5 breaths q 6–8 hr For infants 4 mo old, dilute 0.5 ml to 2.5 ml (1:1000 solution) For infants 4–18 mo old, dilute 0.5 ml to 2.0 ml (1:800 solution) For infants 19 mo–4 yr old, dilute 0.5 ml to 1 ml (1:400 solution) or 0.5 ml to 1.5 ml (1:600 solution) For children over 4 years, use 1:200 solution
Metered aerosol (Mistometer)	10 ml, 15 ml, 22.5 ml	75 μg/puff, 1 to 2 puffs inhaled through an Inspirence
Isoetharine (Bronkosol)		
Aerosol	1.0% solution; dilute with normal saline to desired concentration	5 breaths q 6–8 hr For child ≤ 12 mo old, use half-strength solution For child ≥ 13 mo old, use full-strength solution
Metered aerosol (Bronkometer)	1% solution	340 μg/puff, 1 to 2 puffs inhaled through an Inspirence
Metaproterenol (Alupent, Metaprel)		
Liquid	10 mg/5 ml	0.3–0.5 mg/kg, q 6–8 hr
Tablet	10 mg, 20 mg	0.3–0.5 mg/kg, q 6–8 hr
Aerosol	5% solution	0.3 to 0.5 ml diluted with saline to 1 ml, administered as 5–10 breath treatment
Metered aerosol	225 mg/15 ml (650 μg/puff)	q 6–8 hr, 1 to 2 puffs inhaled through an Inspirence
Albuterol (Ventolin, Proventil)		
Liquid	2 mg/5 ml, 16 fl oz	0.1–0.15 mg/kg, q 6–8 hr
Tablets	2 mg	0.1–0.15 mg/kg, q 6–8 hr
Aerosol	17 g cannister	0.2 ml diluted with saline to 1 ml, administered as 5–10 breath treatment, q 6–8 hr, 1 to 2 puffs inhaled through an Inspirence
Metered aerosol	17 g cannister	100 μg/puff, q 6–8 hr

TABLE A–3. Home Care Equipment for Infant with Chronic Lung Disease

Oxygen Delivery Systems
1. Oxygen delivery units
   a. Oxygen cylinders
      E cylinder with stand and regulator
      H cylinder with stand and regulator
   b. Oxygen concentrator (to deliver a specified oxygen concentration)
      Manufacturers' models: Bunn, Oeco, Econo-2, DeVilbiss
2. Humidification apparatus (warmed or cooled)
3. Polyvinyl tubing for connection with patient
4. Face masks or nasal cannulas

Bronchodilator Aerosol Treatment Equipment
1. Small compressor (DeVilbiss Pneumo-Aide)
2. Nebulizer apparatus (Bard-Parker or Lifeline)
   a. For infant less than 6 mo old or for infant or child requiring positive pressure insufflation of bronchodilator aerosol:
      (1) Draeger anesthesia bag (0.5 liter)
      (2) Soft-seal facial mask (Laerdal or Dryden), sizes 1, 2, 3
      (3) 15-mm adapter (connector)

Resuscitation Bag
1. Self-inflating infant resuscitation bag (Laerdal, Hope, Puritan-Bennett)
2. Soft-seal face masks (sizes 0, 1, 2, 3)

INFANTS WITH TRACHEOSTOMIES

Suctioning Equipment. Virtually all infants with airways obstructive disease require devices for removal of respiratory secretions (Table A–5). Electric suction devices are of two types: (1) stationary suction pumps dependent on an AC power source and generally not transportable and (2) portable battery-powered suction devices that are completely self-contained. Since the AC-powered devices are capable of greater suction force, but the battery-powered devices permit the patient to be transported by automobile and to enjoy a reasonable degree of mobility, the ideal plan would provide both types of machines for outpatient use. When a choice must be made, the self-contained unit is preferred, as most patients must be transported out of the home at some time or other. In the event of power failure, contingencies for suctioning of the airway must be developed. Stopgap measures include use of irrigation syringes attached to suction catheter tubing and mouth suctioning (i.e., DeLee type traps).

Humidification. Rarely, a patient who has a tracheostomy will require an increased degree of airways humidification. This is a particular need for patients living in desert conditions or other climates where excessive drying of the air-

TABLE A–4. Home Care Instructions: Bronchodilator Aerosol Treatments

Bronchodilator aerosols work to dilate the narrowed airways and improve the infant's ability to breathe. They may also aid in the clearance of mucus from the lung. These medications are most effective when they are inhaled deeply into the airways. Insufflation by anesthesia bag is most effective when it coincides with a deep breath taken by the infant. If the aerosol is administered when the infant is exhaling, much of the medication may be deposited in the mouth and nose and not in the lung. In this case the infant may experience an unpleasant side effect—a transient increase in heart rate. Older children and adults describe this side effect as palpitations. Thus, it is important to follow these instructions carefully to maximize the benefit of the treatment and to reduce the unnecessary side effects.

The medication ordered for your child is _____.
The concentration of the medication in the bottle is __.
_____ The medication should be diluted before use.
_____ The medication should *not* be diluted before use.
If dilution is required:
   Take __ ml of the medication and add __ ml of saline.
Directions:
1. The treatment is to be administered every __ hours.
2. Count your infant's heart rate.
3. Place __ ml of the medication in the nebulizer.
4. Start the compressor.
5. Administer 5 breaths of the medication.

Newborn to 6 Months of Age (Mask, nebulizer, Draeger bag)
Place mask snugly over infant's face with your left hand. Cover small hole in anesthesia bag with your right thumb (this permits bag to fill with air). At this point, your infant may either hold his or her breath or take a deep breath. Squeeze bag firmly when baby takes a breath. Then take mask off face. Repeat this maneuver 4 more times.

6 Months to 3 Years (Mask, nebulizer, reservoir tail)
With infant-child in a seated position (in an infant seat for baby too small to sit by himself or herself), place mask over face. A child of 2 years or older should be instructed to take a deep breath and then be coached to repeat this maneuver 4 more times. If child is less than 2 years old, it is necessary to time placement of mask over face with end of exhaling a breath and to count 5 breaths before removing face mask.

Infants with a Tracheostomy (tracheostomy adapter, nebulizer, Draeger bag)
Remove inner cannula. Connect tracheostomy adapter to tracheostomy. Occlude small hole in anesthesia bag with your thumb to permit bag to fill with air. When infant begins to inhale, squeeze bag firmly. Repeat this maneuver 4 more times.

Care of Supplies
Supplies used in aerosol treatment must be cleaned carefully *each day* to avoid contaminating apparatus with bacteria or viruses that might cause serious infections.

Before Each Treatment
1. Use clean eye dropper or syringe to measure amount of medication needed for treatment.
2. Replace bottle cap promptly. Fasten cap tightly on container to avoid evaporation and spoiling of medication.
3. Once a new bottle of medication is opened, it should be stored in refrigerator.

Table continued on opposite page

TABLE A–4. Home Care Instructions: Bronchodilator Aerosol Treatments *Continued*

After Each Treatment
1. Discard medication remaining in nebulizer cup.
2. Dry inside of nebulizer with paper towel.
3. Store nebulizer in clean, dry container with paper towel covering apparatus. Do not place apparatus in plastic bag, as it will prevent remaining moisture from evaporating.

Do the Following Every Day
Dishwasher
1. Place each part of aerosol apparatus in top rack of dishwasher.
2. Use your regular detergent and run through normal cleaning cycle.
3. When apparatus is thoroughly dry, it should be stored in clean, dry place.

Sink
1. Soak each part of nebulizer, mouthpiece, mask, and Draeger bag in hot, soapy water. Scrub each part thoroughly with bottle brush.
2. Rinse well with warm water. When all soap is removed, rinse 3 more times under running water.
3. Soak each part for 30 minutes in solution of 2 parts white distilled vinegar and 3 parts water. Stir or agitate frequently.
4. Rinse each part thoroughly in warm water.
5. Drain and dry parts between folds of clean towel. Hang up Draeger bag to permit it to drain adequately and dry.

ways mucosa might take place. Ultrasonic nebulizer devices usually are not necessary, but vaporization devices with adapters (i.e., collars) for administration to the tracheostomy tube should be provided for home use. Such devices might be advisable on a contingency basis in the event of interval airways infections when increased humidification is desirable.

For those requiring airways appliances such as choanal stents and tracheostomy tubes, extra sets of sterilized, ready-to-apply tubes must be provided in the correct sizes for the individual patient. Appliances may be dislodged or removed accidentally. The ability of home care givers or emergency health care personnel to replace the appliance promptly is dependent on the availability of replacement sets at home. Portex endotracheal tubes are already packaged and may be dispensed as needed to the patient's family. We prefer the Hollinger and Jackson type of thin-walled tracheostomy tubes with removable inner cannulas for tracheostomy patients, because of the ability to clean the inner cannulas thoroughly without removing the tracheostomy tube itself. Custom-made, silver tracheostomy tube sets are less readily available, but with planning, extra sets can be dispensed and exchanged against used sets in the posses-

TABLE A–5. Home Care Equipment for Infant with Tracheostomy

Oxygen and bronchodilator equipment, as in Table A–3

Suction Devices
Electric Suction
1. Stationary suction pump (Everset and Jennings or DeVilbiss)
   AC Power
   Nonportable
2. Portable suction pump (Schuco or Laerdal)
   Battery operated
   Portable
Connecting tubing for both of above suction devices: 3/16 in., id × 72 in. long
Manual Suction:
1. DeLee trap
2. Irrigation syringe

Suction Catheters
Individually packaged tracheal suction catheters, sterile, with glove, "airport" adapter, 14 in. long; available in sizes 6, 8, 10 F
Fine-tip tonsil catheters for oropharyngeal suctioning optional

Humidification
1. Vaporizer
2. Ultronic mist device

Tracheostomy Sets
1. Hollinger and Jackson types, or individual matched silver tubes with inner cannulas in various sizes
2. Tracheostomy tape (ties)
3. Tefla surgical dressing pads (optional) for padding tracheostomy ties to avoid or reduce skin breakdown

Choanal Stents
Portex endotracheal tubes, various sizes

Tracheostomy Care Sets
1. Lavage solution: normal saline, 3-ml units, or normal saline, 1-liter bottles
2. Distilled water, 1-liter bottles
3. Hydrogen peroxide, 0.3% solution
4. Pipe cleaners
5. Kelly clamps for handling cannulas
6. Gauze pads, sterile

Medication Nebulizer Device
1. Electric portable devices
2. Nebulizer cup for medication
3. Connecting tubing
4. Adapters for tracheostomy
5. Mouthpiece for older children
6. Face masks for infants
7. Insufflation bag for enhanced delivery in small children

Apnea-Bradycardia Monitor
1. Portable, AC, and battery powered
2. Belt and/or electrodes

Resuscitation Bag
1. Child size
2. Appropriate-size tracheostomy tube adapter
3. Appropriate-size face mask

Notification Letters to Water and Electric Companies
1. Requesting uninterrupted service as medical necessity

sion of the caregivers. A critical part of home care training should be instruction in replacement of these devices on an emergency basis.

Lavage fluids (usually normal saline) and suction catheters with tube-cleaning assessories should also be provided regularly to the caregivers. Standards must be set for routine cleaning techniques and frequency of cleaning.

Some patients are completely dependent on their appliances for airways patency. In these situations, even transient obstruction might result in death. Therefore, use of portable apnea-bradycardia monitoring devices is crucial to provide the caregivers with sufficient warning to permit timely intervention if complete airways obstruction should occur at home. (See Table A–4 for equipment needed.)

ROLE OF THE PEDIATRICIAN

Specific tasks for the pediatrician caring for a child with airways obstructive disease include regular measurement and recording of growth parameters; assessment and quantitation of nutritional intake, with necessary counseling about feedings; administration of routine childhood immunizations on a timely basis*; administration of immunizations specifically indicated for high-risk children, such as influenza A and B virus vaccine (yearly); initial evaluation and management of uncomplicated respiratory tract infections in consultation with the pulmonologist.

HOME VENTILATOR CARE

The special needs of the child discharged home with ventilator are discussed in Chapter 16. Table A–6 lists the criteria to be met by such children prior to discharge, and Table A–7 lists equipment needed for home ventilation.

---

* There are essentially no contraindications to immunization of children with airways obstructive disease. In particular, infants with underlying airways or pulmonary disease are at especially high risk for serious complications of pertussis infection. Our recommendation is that immunizations should be initiated and continued on the usual schedule at the appropriate chronologic age of the child.

TABLE A–6. Criteria for Discharge Home: Ventilator-Assisted Child

1. Child's condition medically stable, permitting relatively constant ventilator settings
2. Family commitment to care for the ventilator-assisted child at home
3. Realistic assessment of medical care requirements and arrangements for family's ability to meet them, including in-home nursing assistance
4. Thorough education of family and other care givers in technical aspects of medical care and equipment operation
5. Selection of respiratory equipment vendor with ability to supply and service needed equipment and with 24-hour availability
6. Selection of local primary pediatrician to provide well-child care, emergency care, and liaison with community resources
7. Information supplied to community's emergency medical systems of ventilator-assisted child and child's needs
8. Notification of telephone and power companies to provide priority service in event of interruption of service
9. Arrange routine and emergency transport from home to medical center responsible for care
10. Arrange other medical, psychosocial, and developmental support (e.g., physical and occupational therapy, respite care, school)

TABLE A–7. Home Respiratory Equipment for the Ventilator-Assisted Child (Positive Pressure Ventilator via Tracheostomy)

1. Electronic, portable positive pressure ventilator with:
   a. 2 cascades and bracket for cascades
   b. 1 cover and jar assembly
   c. 2 circuits (IMV and oxygen)
   d. Flex tubing
   e. Infant manifold
   f. Automobile cigarette lighter adapter for car use
2. Back-up ventilator preferred. Absolutely essential for patients living at long distance from medical and technical support
3. Compatible disconnect or low-pressure alarm
4. Gel cell car battery with case and cables for operation of ventilator
5. E cylinder of oxygen with stand and regulator
6. Aerosol delivery system with 2 aerosol setups, 2 Draeger bags, 2 tracheostomy tube adapters, 2 22/15-cm connectors-adaptors
7. Portable suction machine with battery pack, connecting tubing, appropriate-sized tracheal suction catheters, and fine-tip tonsil catheters
8. Child-size resuscitation bag with appropriate-sized face mask and appropriate-sized tracheostomy tube adapter
9. Infant apnea-bradycardia monitor with portable battery pack, belt, and electrodes

APPENDIX B

INFANTILE APNEA AND HOME MONITORING*

NATIONAL INSTITUTES OF HEALTH CONSENSUS DEVELOPMENT CONFERENCE STATEMENT
VOLUME C, NUMBER 6, OCTOBER 1, 1986

The Consensus Development Conference entitled "Infantile Apnea and Home Monitoring," held September 29 and 30 and October 1, 1986, at the National Institutes of Health led to the following statement, reprinted here, which presents the agreement reached by the panel and participants of the conference. It offers guidelines for decision making with respect to home monitoring at this time and points to areas for further work needed to resolve some of the remaining questions on this subject.

Introduction

Apnea has long been recognized as a clinical problem in infants. Considerable investigative and clinical attention has been directed toward this condition. Although progress has been made and certain categories of apnea have been delineated, etiology remains unclear in many situations. Furthermore, the condition is common in certain populations, such as in infants born prematurely. Whether an apneic event occurs independently or in association with a pathophysiologic process such as sepsis or an environmental factor such as change in temperature, there is concern about possible effects of interrupted breathing.

Measurement of normal and abnormal physiologic processes such as breathing patterns is facilitated by devices. Monitors have emerged in the laboratory and hospital and have contributed to the discovery of new knowledge and management of abnormalities. Monitoring in this document refers to the use of electronic devices. Technical advances, especially in electronics, have resulted in many devices that seem to be accurate, useful, and safe. Others are of questionable value.

Sudden infant death syndrome (SIDS) was recognized before this century but did not receive close attention until relatively recently. Public Law 93-270, the Sudden Infant Death Syndrome Act of 1974, gave the Public Health Service the mandate to stimulate research and administer counseling and information programs.

In 1972, a paper reported that two of five infants with documented prolonged sleep apnea died of SIDS. A great deal of attention during the 1970s was directed toward the relationship of apnea and SIDS. As the 1970s and 1980s unfolded, the use of monitors in the home environment to detect apnea expanded. Research and clinical programs produced many reports about the merits of this activity, and controversy emerged.

In an effort to resolve this controversy, the Consensus Development Program at the National Institutes of Health has now directed its attention to this subject, and the panel for this Consensus Development Conference on Infantile Apnea and Home Monitoring was asked to focus on the following questions:

1. What is known about the relation of neonatal and infant apnea to each other and to mortality (especially SIDS) and morbidity in infancy?

2. What are the efficacy and safety of currently available home devices for detecting infant apnea?

3. What evidence exists regarding the effectiveness of home monitoring in reducing infant mortality (especially SIDS) and morbidity?

4. Based on the above, what recommendations can be made at present regarding the circumstances for use of home apnea monitoring in infancy?

5. What further research is needed on home apnea monitoring for infants?

Definitions

Expression of concepts and terminology has been difficult. Continued intense efforts di-

---

* U.S. Department of Health and Human Services, Public Health Service, Office of Medical Applications of Research, Building 1, Room 216, Bethesda, Maryland 20892

rected toward definitions are important. The following definitions are used in this document.

Apnea—Cessation of respiratory air flow. The respiratory pause may be central or diaphragmatic (i.e., no respiratory effort), obstructive (usually due to upper airway obstruction), or mixed. Short (15 seconds), central apnea can be normal at all ages.

Pathologic Apnea—A respiratory pause is abnormal if it is prolonged (20 seconds) or associated with cyanosis; abrupt, marked pallor or hypotonia; or bradycardia.

Periodic Breathing—A breathing pattern in which there are three or more respiratory pauses of greater than 3 seconds duration with less than 20 seconds of respiration between pauses. Periodic breathing can be a normal event.

Apnea of Prematurity (AOP)—Periodic breathing with pathologic apnea in a premature infant. Apnea of prematurity usually ceases by 37 weeks gestation (menstrual dating) but occasionally persists to several weeks past term.

Asymptomatic Premature Infants—Preterm infants who either never had AOP or whose AOP has resolved.

Symptomatic Premature Infants—Preterm infants who continue to have pathologic apnea at the time when they otherwise would be ready for discharge.

Apparent Life-Threatening Event (ALTE)—An episode that is frightening to the observer and that is characterized by some combination of apnea (central or occasionally obstructive), color change (usually cyanotic or pallid but occasionally erythematous or plethoric), marked change in muscle tone (usually marked limpness), choking, or gagging. In some cases, the observer fears that the infant has died. Previously used terminology such as "aborted crib death" or "near-miss SIDS" should be abandoned because it implies a possibly misleadingly close association between this type of spell and SIDS.

Apnea of Infancy (AOI)—An unexplained episode of cessation of breathing for 20 seconds or longer, or a shorter respiratory pause associated with bradycardia, cyanosis, pallor, and/or marked hypotonia. The terminology "apnea of infancy" generally refers to infants who are greater than 37 weeks gestational age at onset of pathologic apnea. AOI should be reserved for those infants for whom no specific cause of ALTE can be identified. In other words, these are infants whose ALTE was idiopathic and believed to be related to apnea.

Sudden Infant Death Syndrome (SIDS)—The sudden death of any infant or young child, which is unexplained by history and in which a thorough post mortem examination fails to demonstrate an adequate explanation of cause of death.

A pediatrician commentator at the public meeting stated: "We need to be taken out of confusion of regional opinions, the pressures of public perceptions, and unfounded technological claims and be given guidance on what we do while we await data."

It is hoped that this consensus statement and the final report that follows will serve as helpful educational tools and provide guidance while stimulating the research process leading to new knowledge.

1.

What is known about the relation of neonatal and infant apnea to each other and to mortality (especially SIDS) and morbidity in infancy?

There is no evidence that apnea of prematurity is an independent risk factor for infant apnea.

Apnea of prematurity, a developmental phenomenon, usually resolves by the time the infant is 34 to 36 weeks gestational age. In many infants, a pattern of periodic breathing may persist until several weeks past term; in fact, some periodic breathing is probably normal at any age.

There is evidence that apnea of prematurity is NOT a risk factor for SIDS.

Although preterm infants make up a disproportionate share of all infants with SIDS (18 percent), there is evidence that apnea of prematurity is not an independent risk factor for SIDS. In the NICHD Cooperative Epidemiological Study of SIDS Risk Factors, there was no difference in the incidence of reported (hospital record) apnea in the infants dying of SIDS compared with a control group matched for birth weight and ethnicity. This observation was true for all birth-weight-specific groups.

An apparent life-threatening event is a risk factor for sudden death (including SIDS).

The term ALTE describes a clinical syndrome. A variety of identifiable diseases or conditions can cause such episodes (e.g., ALTE secondary to gastroesophageal reflux or ALTE secondary to seizures), but in approximately one-half of the cases, despite extensive workup, no cause can be identified. These episodes can occur during sleep, wakefulness, or feeding and are in infants who are generally of greater than 37 weeks gestational age at the time of onset.

The reported mortality of patients with apnea of infancy (AOI), some of whom have been electronically monitored at home, varies from 0 to 6 percent. This variability is due to differences in terminology and the inherent heterogeneity of the population.

The mortality of other ALTE subgroups is unknown. It must not always be assumed, however, that once a specific cause of ALTE has been identified, the infant is no longer at increased risk of sudden unexpected death. Certain subgroups of infants with ALTE may be at higher risk.

There are data to suggest that infants presenting with an apneic spell during sleep who were perceived to require resuscitation may have a mortality as high as 10 percent despite the use of home monitors. Infants with this ominous history are rare. Infants with two or more such episodes may have up to a threefold further increase in risk of death.

There is no evidence that apnea of prematurity per se causes subsequent morbidity.

Although early studies suggested an increased incidence of spastic diplegia in preterm infants with a history of apnea and bradycardia, many of these infants may have had other conditions that may have caused the apnea and could confound studies of developmental outcome.

ALTE may be associated with an increased morbidity.

Rarely, infants who experience severe ALTE also develop serious neurodevelopmental sequelae (e.g., vegetative state). Some ALTE survivors demonstrate behavioral and neurodevelopmental abnormalities, but there is no proof that this is a result of ALTE.

Infants with a history of ALTE or apnea of prematurity comprise only a very small proportion of total SIDS cases.

The NICHD Cooperative Epidemiological Study of SIDS cases found only 2 to 4 percent had a hospital record of apnea of prematurity and less than 7 percent had a history of ALTE.

2.

___

What are the efficacy and safety of currently available home devices for detecting infant apnea?

Essential Features

An infant cardiorespiratory monitor must meet essential criteria to be of clinical value. Primary among these is the ability to recognize central, obstructive, or mixed apneas and/or bradycardia as they occur. Alarms that accurately reflect the predisposing condition must consistently alert and be understandable to the care giver. In other words, the monitor must be efficacious in recognizing apnea and triggering its alarm for prolonged apnea. In addition, the monitor must be capable of monitoring its own internal essential functions to assure proper operation. It must be noninvasive and easy to use and understand.

The best of the currently available impedance-based cardiorespiratory monitors meet many but not all of the essential criteria.

Although there are several methods that can be used for sensing breathing, only a few of these have been applied in currently available home cardiorespiratory monitors. Of these, the transthoracic electrical impedance monitors are by far the most frequently applied and have the widest availability in the United States. These monitors are generally efficacious in identifying and alarming on central apneas; however, there are some situations where "breaths" are detected during apparent apneas (false negative) and other cases where apneas are indicated even though the infant is breathing (false positive). The former often is related to cardiogenic artifact, a significant problem with impedance monitors, or to motion artifact resulting from active or passive infant movement. The latter is associated with low amplitude respiration signals that can occur with impedance monitors even though other sensors of ventilation simultaneously monitoring the infant do not show significant hypoventilation. False positive alarms also can be seen in some rare cases as a result of the signal processing in the monitor to reduce false negative apnea detection. Obstructive and mixed apneas, on the other hand, are not directly detected by presently available impedance monitors.

Some noninvasive methods of sensing breathing other than transthoracic impedance might be more efficacious than impedance.

Cardiogenic artifact can be significant with transthoracic impedance monitors, and it also is seen to a lesser extent in other sensors of breathing. These other methods also may have reduced sensitivity to some infant motion. Primary among these sensors are the abdominal strain gauge, inductance plethysmograph, and nasal thermistor. The latter two also may be able to detect obstructive apnea.

Cardiac monitors may be sufficient for monitoring some infants.

Cardiac monitors, or the cardiac monitor portion of a cardiorespiratory monitor, that utilize the electrocardiogram have fewer false positive or negative alarms than the respiration monitors. Although these devices do not meet the essential criteria listed above and are affected by motion artifact, they can, for the most part, reliably recognize conditions of tachycardia and bradycardia. In some cases, it may be sufficient to monitor heart rate alone for infants at home. Heart rate monitors are less expensive than cardiorespiratory monitors, which makes this alternative attractive. Future work is needed to determine whether this is a valid approach.

Desirable Features

Other features of monitors for home use might be desirable, even though no documented evidence exists to that effect at the present time. These features include the capability of capturing and storing patterns surrounding significant events for later analysis, detection of hypoxemia secondary to hypoventilation or apnea as well as the detection of the hypoventilation itself, estimation of tidal volume, and the identification of heart rate patterns and variability as well as cardiac arrhythmias. No presently available home monitor meets all these criteria. Thus, new instruments should be developed so that monitors with these features can be made available for research purposes.

It is important to note that the development of hard copy monitors alone is not sufficient to identify false alarms. It is essential that these devices provide sufficient information to fully characterize "alarm conditions." Even so, it will not be possible to use this technique to document false negative apnea detection.

The pulse oximeter offers opportunities to monitor blood hemoglobin oxygen saturation as a means of detecting hypoxemia secondary to apnea and hypoventilation. This instrument should be evaluated further in this application, with special attention paid to the effect of signal processing on the measured signal and methods of minimizing motion artifact.

Other Considerations

A set of minimal standards for monitors is needed.

An important issue in considering monitor efficacy is the development of appropriate standards and test methods. The development of such standards with clinical as well as technical input to the process needs to be encouraged. Testing procedures must be relevant to the clinical application of the devices if they are to be meaningful. Manufacturers should publish performance characteristics of monitors for use by physicians when prescribing. The need for mandatory standards may be necessary if voluntary standards cannot be developed and followed within a reasonable time (1 to 2 years). The reporting of problems of efficacy and safety with monitors must be mandatory.

The marketing of "over the counter" monitors should be strongly discouraged.

Monitoring devices should not be made available to consumers without professional recommendation and supervision. Because it is unlikely that the efficacy of such devices would be markedly improved over present monitors, such widespread availability of monitors might lead to a significant increase in the number of infants referred to apnea centers due to false alarms of the instrument. Furthermore, the support systems available to parents who purchase such machines would be nonexistent or not uniform. In addition, the care giver needs to be specially trained in the use of the monitor, including knowing how to operate and apply the instrument and knowing what actions to take when the alarm sounds. This training is essential for monitors to be effective.

With the exception of a few isolated incidents, home cardiorespiratory monitors appear to be safe.

A few isolated problems have been reported, and these problems subsequently have been largely corrected.

3.
_____

What evidence exists regarding the effectiveness of home monitoring in reducing infant mortality (especially SIDS) and morbidity?

Effectiveness of Home Monitoring

For the purpose of this statement, effectiveness means the ability to assist in preventing death of infants for whom home monitors are prescribed. This implies a proper choice of home monitoring instruments, adequate training, and continuous logistic and professional support of care takers and their acceptance and persistence with recommended management. In addition, effectiveness implies the ability of care takers to abort an apneic episode by techniques they have learned, including resuscitation.

Home Monitoring for ALTE

There are no reports of scientifically designed studies of the effectiveness of home monitoring for ALTE. There are, however, several case studies from apnea programs that suggest that home monitoring may be an appropriate intervention for some infants. These include infants with ALTE who present with an initial episode requiring vigorous stimulation or resuscitation.

Home Monitoring for Subsequent Siblings of SIDS Victims

There are no reports of scientifically designed studies of the effectiveness of home monitoring for subsequent siblings of SIDS victims. While this is an emotionally charged issue, the decision to monitor subsequent siblings in families with a single SIDS loss cannot be substantiated from existing clinical reports. No clinical studies have adequately investigated home monitoring of siblings of SIDS or the survivor of a twin pair.

Home Monitoring for Premature Infants

There are no reports of scientifically designed studies of the effectiveness of home monitoring of premature infants. Reports from some neonatal intensive care units indicate that for some symptomatic premature infants home monitoring may be a successful alternative to prolonged hospitalization after the infants meet all other criteria for hospital discharge.

Home Monitoring for Other Pathologic Conditions

There are no reports of scientifically designed studies of the effectiveness of home monitoring for other pathologic conditions. Clinical evidence may support the decision to monitor infants with tracheostomies at home. Other conditions with high postneonatal mortality such as severe bronchopulmonary dysplasia may warrant home monitoring, although supportive data are lacking.

SIDS Mortality Trends and Home Monitoring

Evidence from several communities in which SIDS surveillance has been maintained for a decade or more indicates that annual SIDS rates vary from year to year but have not declined perceptibly since the introduction of home monitoring. The proportion of SIDS victims with a history of apnea is too small for the impact of home monitoring of this group to be perceived. Mortality from all other causes of death during infancy has fallen dramatically over the corresponding timespan. It is, therefore, unlikely that an increase in deaths from some other cause has been offset by benefits from the use of home monitors in the community.

Home Monitoring and Morbidity

There are no studies of long-term morbidity associated with apnea or the use of home monitors, but clinical evidence suggests that research on this question might be fruitful. No evidence exists to support the contention that home monitoring prevents development of seizures, intellectual deficits, or developmental disorders.

Problems in Dealing with Studies of Effectiveness

No randomized studies of adequate size have addressed effectiveness of home monitoring for any category of patients. There have been several published clinical reports purporting to assess mortality among monitored infants. The data from these studies are invariably presented without appropriate comparison groups. They address (1) apnea with "successful intervention," (2) deaths following apnea where compliance has been questionable, and (3) deaths in spite of appropriate parental response to monitor alarms. Without data on all infants monitored (survivors as well as decedents), these studies are inconclusive and potentially misleading.

The ability of care takers to consistently determine the true nature of an alarm from a home monitor is questionable. This poses a problem in assessing effectiveness. Some studies have used parental reports as a means of evaluation.

However, one study reported that most alarms reported by parents as truly life-threatening were not.

4.

Based on the above, what recommendations can be made at present regarding the circumstances for use of home apnea monitoring in infancy?

Experience suggests that cardiorespiratory monitoring is effective in preventing death due to apnea for certain selected infants but is clearly inappropriate for others. For some infants, the appropriateness of home monitoring is uncertain. In deciding to monitor or not to monitor, the primary objective is to serve the best interest of the infant and therefore the decision should primarily be based on the infant's history. For example, has the infant had recurrent, severe apnea? For all groups, it should be clearly understood that monitoring cannot guarantee survival. As summarized below, monitoring creates its own risks for infants.

Cardiorespiratory monitoring or an alternative therapy is medically indicated for certain groups of infants at high risk for sudden death.

These groups include infants with one or more severe ALTE's requiring mouth-to-mouth resuscitation or vigorous stimulation, symptomatic preterm infants, siblings of two or more SIDS victims, and infants with certain diseases or conditions such as central hypoventilation. Although no controlled clinical trials have rigorously proved monitoring to be effective in these groups, evidence indicates that these infants are at an extraordinarily high risk for dying and that lives can be saved. Alternative or ancillary treatments such as methylxanthines and/or hospitalization may be considered for specific infants.

Cardiorespiratory monitoring is not medically indicated for normal infants.

SIDS occurs at a rate of approximately 2 per 1,000 live births in the United States. For the normal newborn, the risks, disadvantages, and costs of monitoring outweigh the possible benefit of preventing SIDS.

Routine monitoring of asymptomatic preterm infants, as a group, is not warranted.

Individual preterm infants such as those with certain residual diseases may be considered for monitoring.

For several groups, currently available evidence on the benefits and risks of monitoring and alternative treatment is inconclusive.

These groups include siblings of SIDS infants, infants with less severe ALTE episodes, infants with tracheostomies, and infants of opiate- or cocaine-abusing mothers. For each of these groups, the risk of death is elevated to some degree. For infants in this category, the decision to monitor must be made by the family after a full discussion with the physician of the potential benefits as well as the psychosocial burdens. The decision reached will be specific to the infant, and there are no hard and fast guidelines that will apply to all cases. No family in this category should be made to feel that monitoring is necessary.

The pneumogram should not be used as a screening tool.

Pneumograms have been widely used as *screening tests* to predict SIDS or life-threatening apnea in asymptomatic preterm and term infants. However, no prospective controlled study has confirmed that these 12- to 24-hour recordings of heart rate and thoracic impedance are predictive of SIDS or life-threatening apnea. In fact, in one study, similar cardiorespiratory recordings on over 9,000 infants have not demonstrated differences between subsequent SIDS victims and surviving infants. In premature infants, SIDS siblings, or ALTE infants, no studies to date have proved that the pneumogram has *predictive value* that distinguishes infants who will survive from those who will die. However, pneumograms occasionally may be helpful in *clinical management.* For instance, pneumograms may be used to distinguish false from true apnea monitor alarms.

Decisions to discontinue home monitoring should be based on clinical criteria.

The criteria for monitor discontinuation should be based on the infant's clinical condition. Clinical experience and the literature support monitor discontinuation when ALTE infants have had 2 to 3 months free of significant alarms or apnea (vigorous stimulation or resuscitation was not needed). Additionally, assessing the infant's ability to tolerate stress (e.g., immunizations, illnesses) during this time is advisable. Requiring one or more normal pneumograms before discontinuing the monitor may prolong needlessly the monitoring period.

Decision making about home monitoring is a collaborative enterprise.

When a clinician has determined that clinical indications justify the use of a home monitor, the clinician must seek the cooperation and permission of the parent or guardian of the infant to be monitored. Parents, acting as proxies for their infant, and clinicians should attempt to reach a joint decision on whether home monitoring should be undertaken. The physician should disclose the available information on alternative treatments, benefits, and limitations of the monitors. Understanding the impact of monitoring on the family should be a central consideration in the decision. The literature on the effects of monitoring in families has serious flaws, but it suggests that monitoring can be *both* a source of stress and a source of support and reassurance for parents. Some of the stresses parents report are related to monitor equipment problems, isolation, the extra demands and responsibility of caring for a monitored infant, the cost of monitoring, difficulty in finding child care, sibling rivalry, depression, and marital strains. Parents also report that home monitoring can be reassuring for those whose infants are judged to be at medical risk.

In discussing these substantive matters with parents, a good faith effort should be made to take into account the values and the social and economic circumstances of the parents insofar as they are relevant to the alternative selected.

The possibility of economic benefit to providers should not materially affect decisions to test or monitor infants. Individuals and institutions should be aware of potential financial conflicts of interest and make appropriate disclosures.

Finally, institutions and clinicians might find it useful to relay the information in writing after the discussion of these matters to ensure understanding of and consistency in the information conveyed.

Ordinarily, parents and clinicians will agree about whether to use the monitor. However, there will be some instances of disagreement.

When the clinician concludes that cardiorespiratory monitoring is medically indicated and the parents disagree, the clinician has several options. The clinician may defer to parental preferences, continue hospitalization, seek suitable assistance and support to facilitate monitoring, and, in the rare case, initiate procedures to remove the infant from the home. Such decisions should be reached on a case-by-case basis,

taking into account factors specific to the situation, including the medical needs of the infant, the home environment, and the expectation that, on balance, a better outcome is likely in another care-giving environment.

When cardiorespiratory monitoring is not indicated (see above), clinicians are encouraged not to prescribe monitors when they are requested by parents. When evidence on the benefits and risks of monitoring or alternative treatments is inconclusive and there is disagreement, the decision whether to use a monitor should be left to the parents. Deferring to parental choice is appropriate because the parents are the ones who have to implement the decision and take primary responsibility for its consequences.

An adequate monitoring support system encompasses medical, technical, psychosocial, and community support services.

This coordinated, multidisciplinary approach can include hospital-based monitoring programs, community-based physicians, health care agencies, durable medical equipment vendors, local public health and social service agencies, and peer or voluntary support groups. In the hospital, the support system includes: (1) an informed consent process; (2) an assessment of the family's strengths, weaknesses, and support resources; (3) anticipatory guidance to help prepare the family for the demands of home monitoring; (4) a thorough explanation of monitor operation, trouble-shooting, and a written monitor service contract; (5) training and demonstrated proficiency in infant CPR and resuscitation methods; (6) written guidelines on home monitoring; and (7) discharge planning, including discussion of followup services and procedures for discontinuation. After discharge, formal and regular followup contact with the family should be maintained. Consultant and primary care physicians must coordinate their activities. There should be 24-hour availability of monitor program support staff and monitor repair or replacement. Access to psychosocial support mechanisms, including community social services such as public health nurses and social workers, peer support, and respite care, should be provided. Extra assistance at the time of monitor termination should be available.

Effective monitor use is dependent on the technical support network outside the home. A formal support system for users includes mechanisms for quality assurance, maintenance service and replacement, and education and users manuals for parents and physicians on monitor operation and maintenance. In addition, means for communication about machine problems among manufacturers, parents, physicians, and vendors are essential to ensure the safety of the apnea monitor in the home. It is important to emphasize that home monitoring is not one but a cluster of interrelated services.

5.

What further research is needed on home apnea monitoring for infants?

There should be definitive prospective studies involving randomization and concurrent control populations of issues involved in home monitoring for apnea. Unless studies are conducted soon, we may lose the opportunity and pay a price in unforeseen and untoward outcomes.

The fact that controversy exists regarding home apnea monitoring reflects an inadequate fund of knowledge. This was constantly brought up in testimony at the conference as well as in the deliberations of the panel.

From the perspective of advancing SIDS research, it is important to focus on those infants dying of SIDS. For clinicians, however, it is important to look carefully at all of these infants who die suddenly and unexpectedly of any cause (e.g., from aspiration pneumonia, upper airway obstruction, chronic lung disease). Many such deaths are potentially preventable, although they should not be called SIDS.

Sudden death, including SIDS, is a major part of all postneonatal infant deaths. Furthermore, there may be multiple causes of SIDS. Therefore, the panel makes the following general recommendation:

- All sudden death in infants, not only sudden infant death syndrome, should receive high priority in future research initiatives.

The hypothesis that apnea is the major cause of sudden death has not been substantiated, yet many clinical and research efforts are proceeding with acceptance of this hypothesis. These efforts should proceed with the realization that causality is unclear. In addition:

- The apnea hypothesis should be further tested.
- Causal hypotheses for SIDS other than apnea should receive more attention.

Research related to five substantive areas considered by the panel might include the following:

Apnea

- A prospective controlled study of the use of monitoring in specific populations that may be at risk, including infants with apnea of prematurity, apnea of infancy, and other conditions such as bronchopulmonary dysplasia and maternal exposure to drugs, is indicated. The following questions should be addressed:
    - Are there clinical markers for infants at high risk for ALTE and sudden death (including SIDS)?
    - Will monitoring reduce the incidence of mortality in these infants?
    - Will monitoring influence morbidity of these infants?
    - Are there adverse consequences of monitoring?
- Continued efforts to elucidate basic pathophysiology of apnea of prematurity and apnea of infancy are important.
- Identification of risk assessment methods and pharmacologic treatments and their use in conjunction with monitors should be pursued.

Monitoring: Technical

- New methods of sensing infant breathing need to be developed and evaluated. Particular attention needs to be paid to nonimpedance types of sensors that are suitable for home use, the simultaneous recording of several sensors, and signal processing that makes apnea detection more efficacious.
- The use of heart rate monitors needs further investigation. Studies must be designed to determine if heart rate monitors are adequate for detecting and alarming on life-threatening events.
- The use of pulse oximetry for infant apnea monitoring needs further investigation. Reliable, less expensive instrumentation appropriate for home use should be developed, and the usefulness of this measurement for hypoxemia detection needs to be determined. The use of hard copy recordings of this variable along with respiration and heart rate must also be evaluated.
- Infant monitors, no matter what type, need to be more reliable. Monitors with improved self-testing algorithms must be developed, and standards and methods of signal simulation and testing must be established. Studies that determine the optimal means of quality assurance, trouble-shooting, and service (i.e., support) for home apnea monitors are needed.

Monitoring: Psychosocial

- Research to identify the psychosocial characteristics and apnea program operational procedures that help families adapt, cope with, and use home monitors effectively needs to be undertaken.
- Short- and long-term effects of monitoring on infants, parents, siblings, parent-child interactions, and families should be investigated.
- The hypothesis of a relationship between monitoring and child abuse needs further study.
- Studies to establish the rates, causes, and consequences of noncompliance and premature termination of monitoring should receive high priority.
- Research to identify factors related to and interventions promoting the ability of families to terminate monitoring would be of benefit.

Apnea Program: Health Services

- Identification of ways of assuring access to assessment, monitoring, and coordinated medical, technical, psychosocial, and community support services for infants at risk should be a priority of regional, state, and Federal authorities.
- Development and coordination of appropriate regional patterns of care, including the identification of the role of the referral center, community hospital, primary care physician, community agencies, and informal supports, should be pursued further.
- The components, organizations, and relative value of community supports that are necessary to minimize family stress and promote effective monitoring should be better delineated.

Sudden Death, Including SIDS

- Comparative epidemiologic studies of apnea of infancy, ALTE, and sudden death should receive high priority.
- New and improved technologies or markers with predictive value for prospective identification of infants destined to develop ALTE (including apnea of infancy) and SIDS need to be identified.
- The possibility that tissue specimens can be utilized to identify subsets of the SIDS group and that a national SIDS tissue bank would be worthwhile should be evaluated.
- The possibility that methodologies such as intense psychosocial support and other interventions might be more effective than monitoring in mortality prevention needs further study.

Conclusion

This statement summarizes a consensus process devoted to questions focusing on infantile apnea and home monitoring. The level of concern is high, the need for definition and knowledge helpful to the clinician is evident, and the overall fund of knowledge is inadequate.

The relation of neonatal and infant apnea is that of two apparently separate problems, each with an unclear relationship to mortality and morbidity in infancy. Presently available devices appear to be safe, but their efficacy needs additional study, and technology needs to be advanced. Beneficial and adverse effects of monitoring are evident but need further study.

The need for adequate support systems is apparent. The effectiveness of home monitoring in reducing infant mortality and morbidity is not yet established. Additional studies need to be done. A recommendation to monitor selected high-risk infants is made. Routine monitoring or screening of normal term or preterm infants is not recommended. There are certain patients for whom evidence is inconclusive and decisions will have to be individualized. Recommendations for future research of a general and specific nature are made.

Members of the Consensus Development Panel Were:

GEORGE A. LITTLE, M.D.
Panel Chairman
Professor and Chairman
Department of Maternal and Child Health
Dartmouth-Hitchcock Medical Center
Hanover, New Hampshire

ROBERTA A. BALLARD, M.D.
Director
Maternal and Child Health Services
Mount Zion Hospital and Medical Center
Adjunct Associate Professor of Pediatrics
University of California at San Francisco
San Francisco, California

JOHN G. BROOKS, M.D.
Associate Professor of Pediatrics
University of Rochester
School of Medicine and Dentistry
Rochester, New York

ROBERT T. BROUILLETTE, M.D.
Associate Professor of Pediatrics
Northwestern University Medical School

Associate Director
Sleep Laboratory
Attending Neonatologist
Children's Memorial Hospital
Chicago, Illinois

LARRY CULPEPPER, M.D.
Associate Professor of Family Medicine
Brown University
The Memorial Hospital of Rhode Island
Pawtucket, Rhode Island

HERMAN B. GRAY, JR., M.D.
Medical Director
Apnea Identification Program
Wayne County SIDS Center
Children's Hospital of Michigan
Detroit, Michigan

PATRICIA KING, J.D.
Associate Professor
Georgetown University Law Center
Washington, D.C.

MARVIN O. KOLB, M.D., F.A.A.P.
Department of Pediatrics
Fargo Clinic, Ltd.
Fargo, North Dakota

ANN NEALE, PH.D.
Vice President
Bon Secours Health System
Columbia, Maryland

MICHAEL R. NEUMAN, M.D., PH.D.
Associate Professor of Biomedical
   Engineering in Reproductive Biology
Case Western Reserve University
Cleveland, Ohio

DONALD R. PETERSON, M.D., M.P.H.
Professor Emeritus
University of Washington
Seattle, Washington

STUART O. SCHWEITZER, PH.D.
Professor
University of California at Los Angeles
School of Public Health
Los Angeles, California

HEATHER WEISS, ED.D.
Director
Harvard Family Research Project
Harvard University Graduate
   School of Education
Cambridge, Massachusetts

Members of the Planning Committee Were:

DUANE ALEXANDER, M.D.
Planning Committee Chairperson
Director

National Institute of Child Health
   and Human Development
National Institutes of Health
Bethesda, Maryland

HEINZ W. BERENDES, M.D., M.H.S.
Director
Epidemiology and Biometry Research
   Program
National Institute of Child Health
   and Human Development
National Institutes of Health
Bethesda, Maryland

CHARLOTTE CATZ, M.D.
Chief
Pregnancy and Perinatology Branch
National Institute of Child Health
   and Human Development
National Institutes of Health
Bethesda, Maryland

SUSAN M. CLARK
Social Science Analyst
Office of Medical Applications
   of Research
National Institutes of Health
Bethesda, Maryland

MARLENE E. HAFFNER, M.D.
Director
Office of Health Affairs
Department of Health and Human Services
Food and Drug Administration
Silver Spring, Maryland

JAMES G. HILL
Chief
Office of Planning and Evaluation
National Institute of Child Health
   and Human Development
National Institutes of Health
Bethesda, Maryland

ITZHAK JACOBY, PH.D.
Acting Director
Office of Medical Applications of Research
National Institutes of Health
Bethesda, Maryland

SAMUEL KESSEL, M.D.
Chief
Research and Training Branch
Division of Maternal and Child Health
Department of Health and Human Services
Rockville, Maryland

JAMES KILEY, PH.D.
Health Scientist Administrator
Division of Lung Diseases
National Heart, Lung, and Blood Institute
National Institutes of Health
Bethesda, Maryland

GEORGE A. LITTLE, M.D.
Consensus Panel Chairman
Professor and Chairman
Department of Maternal and Child Health
Dartmouth Medical School
Hanover, New Hampshire

COL. JOHN R. PIERCE, M.D.
Assistant Chief
Department of Pediatrics
Walter Reed Army Medical Hospital
Washington, D.C.

JONELLE C. ROWE, M.D.
Associate Professor
Department of Pediatrics
Division of Neonatology
University of Connecticut Health Center
Farmington, Connecticut

SUMNER J. YAFFE, M.D.
Director
Center for Research for
    Mothers and Children
National Institute of Child Health
    and Human Development
National Institutes of Health
Bethesda, Maryland

MICHAEL J. BERNSTEIN
Director of Communications
Office of Medical Applications of Research
National Institutes of Health
Bethesda, Maryland

MICHAELA P. RICHARDSON
Chief
Office of Research Reporting
National Institute of Child Health
    and Human Development
National Institutes of Health
Bethesda, Maryland

The Conference Was Sponsored By:

National Institute of Child Health
    and Human Development
Duane Alexander, M.D.
Director

National Heart, Lung, and Blood Institute
Claude Lenfant, M.D.
Director

Division of Maternal and Child Health, Health
    Resources and Services Administration
Vince Hutchins, M.D.
Director

Food and Drug Administration
Frank E. Young, M.D.
Commissioner

NIH Office of Medical Applications of Research
Itzhak Jacoby, Ph.D.
Acting Director

APPENDIX C

HOME OSTOMY CARE

LORI J. HOWELL R.N., M.S.

The procedures described in this appendix are guidelines for parents used by the pediatric surgery division at the University of California, San Francisco.

ILEOSTOMY CARE

Ileostomy is the surgical formation of an opening into the ileum. The opening, or stoma, so created is also known as an ileostomy. Management of an ileostomy is described below.

Supplies

1. Appropriate sized pouch (Greer or Bongart bag)
2. Stomahesive paste
3. Skin Barrier
4. Scissors (fingernail scissors work best)
5. Indelible marking pen

Procedure

1. Remove plastic backing from Skin Barrier and hold it over ileostomy.
2. Trace stoma and surrounding skin with marking pen to make pattern. Opening should be close to but not touching stoma.
3. Place pattern on Skin Barrier, cut out and round edges.
4. Place pattern on pouch and cut out with opening slightly larger than Skin Barrier opening.
5. Attach barrier and pouch together.
6. Remove old pouch and cleanse the skin with warm water. A tub bath will be soothing to the skin and not harm the stoma.
7. If your child has a stoma that is not at skin level, is recessed, or has uneven surrounding skin, apply a thin layer of paste with your finger moistened in water. (Water will allow you to spread the paste more evenly.) Wait until dry. A hair dryer on cool to warm setting is helpful to speed this process.
8. Remove the barrier backing and center the pouch and barrier over stoma.
9. Place your hand over the pouch and bar-

rier for several minutes, since heat will help seal the barrier to the skin.
10. Fanfold the bottom of the bag and fold up; secure with a rubber band.
11. Empty pouch when one-third to one-half full of stool or when full of gas.
12. Change pouch if it leaks, or every three days.

If the surrounding skin has broken down, apply Stomahesive powder before applying the paste and pouch as above. Another alternative is to apply a thick layer of Orabase to the peristomal skin; keep your infant prone as much as possible and give him or her frequent tub baths.

If a large amount of skin breakdown has occurred or leakage continues, notify the pediatric surgeon or the clinical nurse specialist for help.

COLOSTOMY CARE

A colostomy is a surgically created opening, called a stoma, between the large bowel, or colon, and the abdominal wall. Since the function of the colon is to absorb water and store stool, the type of stool drainage will depend upon where the stoma is created.

Right-Sided or Ascending Colostomy. Because most of the colon is bypassed in this type of colostomy, stool output will be liquid to semiformed, and an appliance will be necessary.

Transverse Colostomy. A transverse colostomy is created from the transverse portion of the large intestine. There are a variety of surgical techniques used that will result in one or two stomas. The double-barreled colostomy has two separate stomas, while the loop colostomy contains two openings in one stoma. The stoma with the portion of the colon still attached to the small intestine will drain semiformed stool, while the remaining stoma will drain mucus. An appliance may be necessary if the stools are loose and watery.

Sigmoid Colostomy. A sigmoid colostomy is created in the last portion of the colon. Because the majority of the colon is still in use to absorb water, the stool output will be soft and formed. The diaper method should be used unless the output becomes watery or until the child is older and stool output is increased. Generally the stomas are created so low on the abdomen that an appliance cannot be fitted.

DIAPER METHOD

This method is to be used when stools have a fairly solid consistency.

Supplies

1. Stomahesive powder
2. Desitin ointment. (Buy the large 1-pound size.)
3. Bounty or Top Job paper towels in white. (They are among the softest towels available, do not break down as tissue does when wet, and are less expensive than 4 × 4s.)
4. Masking tape, which costs less than surgical tape and works just as well as long as it is on top of the Skin Barrier
5. Skin Barrier in 4 × 4 squares

Procedure

1. Mix 4 to 6 ounces of Stomahesive powder per 1-pound jar of Desitin. It is not very hard to mix; it just takes a long time. Add the powder a little at a time. The final mixture should be the consistency of natural peanut butter.
2. Clean around stoma well with warm water. A tub bath is very soothing to the skin and will not harm the stoma.
3. Cover the area surrounding the stoma with a $\frac{1}{8}$- to $\frac{1}{4}$-in.–thick layer of the Desitin-Stomahesive mixture.

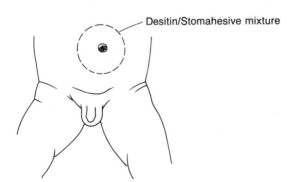

Desitin/Stomahesive mixture

4. Cut 2 strips $\frac{3}{4}$-in. wide × 3 in. long of the Skin Barrier to fit on either side of the pasty area.

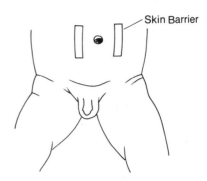

Skin Barrier

5. Cut one section of paper towels in quarters and apply one to the stoma-pasty area. Tape towel to Skin Barrier with masking tape.
6. Change the paper towel when soiled and reapply the Desitin-Stomahesive mixture and the new paper towel.
7. Diaper as usual. Sometimes the stool will leak upward onto tee shirts and other clothing. Rubber pants work well to prevent leakage.

BAG METHOD

This method is often used with larger and more frequent bowel movements as your child gets older (after 9 or 10 months), if stools are loose and watery, if skin breakdown is occurring, or if you prefer this method.

Supplies

1. Appropriate-sized bags (Hollister Pediatric Pouch or Bongart bags)
2. Stomahesive paste
3. Skin Barrier
4. Scissors (fingernail scissors work best)
5. Indelible marking pen

Procedure

1. Remove plastic backing from Skin Barrier and hold it over colostomy.
2. Trace pattern of stoma and surrounding skin with marking pen. The opening should be close to but not touching stoma.
3. Place pattern on Skin Barrier, cut out and round edges.
4. Place pattern on pouch and cut out with an opening slightly larger than Skin Barrier opening.
5. Attach barrier and pouch together.
6. Remove old pouch and cleanse skin with warm water. A tub bath will be soothing and not harm the stoma.
7. If your child's stoma is not at skin level, is recessed, or has uneven surrounding skin, apply

a thin layer of paste with your finger moistened in water. (Water will allow you to spread the paste more evenly.) Wait until dry. A hair dryer on cool to warm setting is helpful to speed this process.

8. Remove the barrier backing and center pouch and barrier over stoma.

9. Place your hand over the pouch and barrier for several minutes, since the heat will help seal the barrier to the skin.

10. Fanfold the bottom of the bag and fold up; secure with a rubber band.

11. Open the end of the bag to empty out stool whenever necessary, usually two or three times a day.

12. Change the bag whenever stool is leaking, or every 3 days.

The stoma itself has no feeling, but will frequently bleed to the touch. Your child may be receiving iron to compensate for this blood loss.

If the skin around the stoma does start to break down, removal of the bag at night when there is less stool output and returning to the Desitin-Stomahesive mixture may protect the skin, while still allowing it to breathe.

GASTROSTOMY CARE

Definition. A gastrostomy tube is a soft rubber tube inserted into the stomach through the skin and stomach wall to feed your child.

Types of Gastrostomy. STAMM. While your child is asleep in the operating room, an opening is made into the stomach through the skin and a tube is inserted. A stitch will hold the tube in place. If the tube falls out, the hole will close in two to three hours.

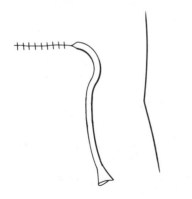

JANEWAY. While your child is asleep in the operating room, an opening is made into the

skin, and a portion of the stomach is used to make a tunnel.

A hole is made from the skin to this tunnel. The rubber tube runs through this tunnel into the stomach. The tunnel will not close when the rubber tube is removed, and the tube can be inserted for each feeding.

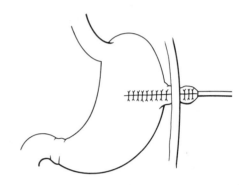

Tubes. The tube initially placed is called a Malecot. This tube has a flared end that prevents the tube from slipping out and prevents stomach acid juices from getting on the skin. For a Stamm gastrostomy, sutures are kept in for 10 days to prevent the tube from slipping and to promote healing and tunnel formation. For a Janeway gastrostomy, the sutures and the tube are left in for a longer time to prevent breakdown of the sutures and narrowing of the tube. Once the tube is removed, you will be shown how to insert a red tube for feedings. When the Malecot tube falls out, it is replaced with a *Foley* tube. A Foley tube is easier to replace. The tube has a balloon at the end to prevent it from slipping out.

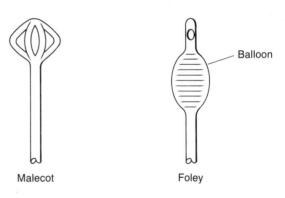

Malecot   Foley

Skin Care. The sutures are removed after 10 days.

The dressing is changed once a day or more often if wet. Remove the dressing before bath time. Inspect the site. A tub bath is permissible 2 weeks after surgery.

Cleaning

1. Materials
   Half-strength hydrogen peroxide—new wounds
   Soap and water—healed wounds
   Q-tips
   Roll of 1-in. tape
   Hollister Skin Barrier
   Skin preparation—1 package
2. Wash hands; inspect site.
3. Cleanse around site, using Q-tips.
4. Dry site well.
5. Apply skin preparation around site.

Dressing

1. The purpose of the dressing is to stabilize the tube to prevent skin breakdown from leakage of stomach acid onto the skin.
2. If the tube is not stabilized against the stomach wall, it can "float" further into the stomach and possibly cause blockage. Your child may feel nauseated or vomit if this happens.
3. The dressing is changed every day. The Skin Barrier need only be changed when loose, usually every 3 days.

Procedure

1. Cut the tape and set aside what you will need.
   a. two 1-in. pieces

   b. three 6-in. strips

   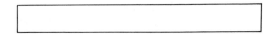

2. Fold under the ends of the long pieces to make small tabs.

   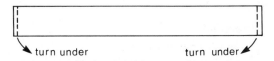
   turn under   turn under

3. Cut two of the long pieces halfway up the length.

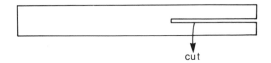
cut

4. Open a package of 4 × 4s; open both pieces all the way. Place the two pieces on top of each other and fold in thirds.
5. Using the 1-in. piece of tape, tape the ends to hold the folded dressing together.
6. Wipe the skin around the site with skin preparation.
7. Cut two pieces of skin barrier 1 in. × 2 in.

8. Place one piece on one side of the tube and the other piece on the opposite side.

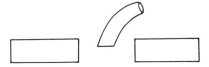

9. Gently pull on the tube until resistance is met.
10. Wrap the folded 4 × 4 around the edge of the tube and fasten it with the short piece of tape.

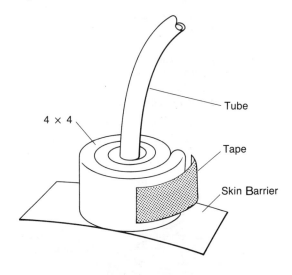
Tube
4 × 4
Tape
Skin Barrier

11. Take one of the split pieces of tape and place one of the tails over the top of the 4 × 4 (see figure at top of this column).
12. Run the unsplit end down the side of the 4 × 4 and attach to the Skin Barrier.

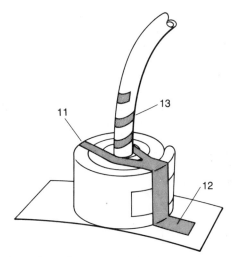

13. Using the other tail, wrap it up and around the tube.

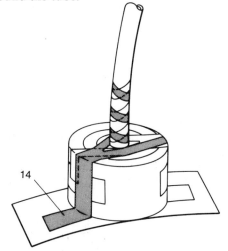

14. Using the other split tape, repeat the above steps from the opposite side.

15. Using the last piece of tape, wrap the outside of the dressing. This is the most important

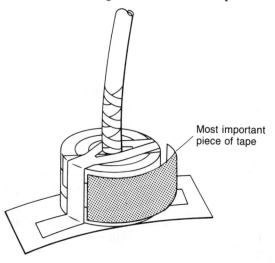

Most important piece of tape

piece of tape, since it prevents the tube from moving back and forth.

WHAT IF THE TUBE FALLS OUT?

Sometimes the baby will accidentally pull the tube out, or the balloon will leak and deflate.

You will be instructed how to place a new tube should it come out while you are at home.

Supplies

1. Appropriate-sized Foley tube
2. 3 cc syringe
3. Tap water
4. K.Y. jelly. *Do not use petroleum jelly.*

Procedure

1. Wash your hands.
2. Remove the dressing.
3. Check the skin.
4. Draw up 3 cc of water into syringe.
5. Check the balloon of the new tube before inserting by injecting 3 cc of water into the plastic-tipped side port.
6. Remove the water to deflate the balloon.
7. Dip the end of the tube into lubricating jelly.
8. Gently insert the tube into the opening in the hole—about 2 in.
9. Inject 3 cc of water and remove the syringe.
10. Gently pull tube back to check that the balloon is against the stomach wall; you will feel resistance.
11. Clean around the site with soap and water and redress.

WHEN SHOULD I CHANGE THE TUBE?

If leakage continues despite redressing:

1. Call your doctor or clinical nurse specialist.
2. If instructed, remove the tube and replace with a new one.
3. You may be told to use a larger tube *or* to leave the tube out for a while to allow the hole to become smaller.

Procedure

1. Wash your hands.
2. Withdraw 3 cc of water from the balloon port.
3. Gently pull the old tube out.
4. Follow the procedure to insert a new tube, then clean and redress.

WHAT SHOULD I DO IF I SEE:

Redness Around the Site

Slight red—Some stomach juices may be leaking out. Clean area and redness, using traction to secure the tube against the stomach wall.

Very red—Call doctor or clinical nurse specialist.

Crusting

Crust should be removed; it can trap bacteria and cause an infection.

Loosen with warm water or half-strength hydrogen peroxide to remove crust.

Bleeding

Some bleeding may occur because of rubbing, irritation, and the like. If it persists, notify the doctor.

Pus

Distinguish from formula. Notify the doctor; note color, amount, and smell; cleanse per protocol.

Note surrounding area for redness or if child has a fever.

Formula Leakage

Caused by not enough traction to the tube. Cleanse and redress, pulling tube taut.

Persistent Leakage

The hole is getting too large. Call your doctor or clinical nurse specialist.

Increasing Tissue at Site

Notify surgeon. The tissue will either be left alone, or cut off, or you might be asked to apply a silver nitrate stick daily to gradually remove this extra tissue. This tissue is called granulation tissue and is a common reaction of the body to an ostomy.

PHONE NUMBERS

Your pediatrician:
Your surgeon:
Emergency room:
Your hospital:
Clinical nurse specialist:

TRACHEOSTOMY CARE

Preparation for Discharge

To safely care for your child at home, it is necessary for you *and at least one other family member* to learn (feel confident and give a return demonstration of) the following techniques.

CLEANING AROUND THE STOMA

1. At least two times a day and every 8 hours if an odor is present, clean around stoma with half-strength hydrogen peroxide (equal parts peroxide and water) and Q-tips (use two to four Q-tips).
2. Roll Q-tip over the skin to remove crusted mucus. Then rinse area with Q-tip dipped in water and dry.
3. If child's skin has areas of redness, open areas, or excessive tracheal secretions, cleanse more frequently and apply a Sorbit gauze sponge between the skin and tracheostomy tube. Do not let gauze flop over the tracheostomy tube opening and block child's airway.
4. Change gauze when it becomes wet.
5. Foul odors and green-yellow drainage from the tracheostomy may indicate an infection, and you should contact your doctor.
6. Do not use powders like talc or cornstarch anywhere on the infant's skin. Lotion may be used if not applied near tracheostomy tube.

Additional equipment needed:

1. Pipe cleaners
2. 2 × 2 gauze dressing sponges (optional)

CLEANING THE TRACHEOSTOMY TUBE

1. Wash hands.
2. Twist the inner cannula to bring the flat portion to 12 o'clock, pointing toward the chin.
3. Remove the inner cannula and place in half-strength hydrogen peroxide.
4. Hold the inner cannula by the outer rim and insert a pipe cleaner into the upper end and pull through the lower end. It helps to hold the cannula under the hot water tap.
5. Use as many pipe cleaners as necessary to thoroughly clean the inner cannula, because secretions accumulate here.
6. Rinse the inner cannula well with hot tap water; shake off excess water.

After cleaning and suctioning the outer cannula, replace the inner cannula, inserting the inner cannula gently into the outer cannula while supporting the outer cannula with the other hand. Insert with the flat portion up, then twist to hold firmly in place.

CHANGING TRACHEOSTOMY TIES

1. It is best to change tracheostomy ties every day to prevent skin irritation from wet, soiled ties.

2. Change ties with a bath if possible.

3. Use two people if possible; otherwise you may have to wrap your baby-child mummy style in a blanket to prevent wiggling.

4. Slip the old ties up to top of hole on tracheostomy tube.

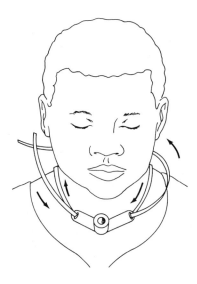

5. Attach new ties as shown in picture.

6. Secure with a bow first; check the ties for snugness and tie a square knot. Ties should be snug enough to allow your little finger to get underneath.

7. Examine back of neck every day for sores, redness. Rotate the knot to prevent sores on the skin.

SUCTIONING TRACHEOSTOMY TUBE

Suctioning your child's tracheostomy tube is an important part of caring for the child with a tracheostomy. Suctioning removes the mucus from your child's tube and trachea. With the tube clear of secretions, it is easier for your child to breathe.

1. Suction only as needed—usually early morning (after awakening), before meals, and before bedtime. Signs that indicate your child needs suctioning:

> May be anxious, restless, unable to be calmed
> May breathe faster and harder
> May have frightened look

> May have mucus bubbling from tracheostomy
> The color around the mouth or lips may be pale, bluish, dark.
> The nostrils may flare.
> May have retractions. (The hollow in the neck and skin between the ribs may pull inward.)
> May sound "gurgly"
> May have difficulty eating or sucking

2. If your infant is able to cough secretions up to the opening of the tracheostomy, place the bulb syringe or olive-tip catheter at the tracheostomy opening for *surface* suctioning.

3. Be careful not to suction too frequently. The more you suction, the more secretions are produced.

4. Always suction *before* a feeding (and before changing diapers).

5. Blood-tinged secretions may mean there is too much suctioning or that suction machine is turned on too high.

Procedure

1. Wash hands well; this is the best way to prevent an infection.

2. Open the sterile glove and suction catheter package without touching the contents.

3. Have the suction tubing nearby; open sterile water container for rinsing catheter.

4. Put on sterile glove, touching only the cuff. Remove the sterile catheter from the package with your gloved hand.

Note: To keep the catheter sterile, you must not touch anything with it or your gloved hand before suctioning.

5. Attach catheter to suction tubing.

6. Dip the end of the catheter into the container of sterile water to allow it to pass easily through the tracheostomy.

7. Turn on the suction machine.

8. Using nongloved hand, place several drops of saline into the tracheostomy tube to stimulate a cough and loosen secretions. Without applying suction (with your thumb off), gently insert the catheter into the tracheostomy tube until resistance is met, then pull it back about $\frac{1}{2}$ in. Never forcibly insert the catheter, as this may cause bleeding and possible damage to the trachea. As you withdraw it, gently rotate the catheter between your thumb and forefinger, applying suction intermittently. Suction for 10 to 15 seconds.

9. Let the infant relax after each pass with the suction catheter. *Remember, suctioning removes oxygen as well as the secretions.* Usually the infant's crying will be enough to let him or

her inhale deeply several times. If you can still hear mucus gurgling, allow the infant to rest several minutes before suctioning one more time.

10. Rinse connecting tubing with water.

11. Throw away catheter, glove, and sterile water.

12. Check your supplies. Make sure you have enough catheters and gloves to get you through weekends and nights.

CHANGING THE TRACHEOSTOMY TUBE

Always make sure that the new tube is fully prepared and ready for insertion before removing the old, dirty tube. Never change a tracheostomy tube without adequate assistance unless it is an emergency. Change the tracheostomy tube if:

a. It becomes plugged and suctioning does not remove secretions.

b. It is very soiled or accidentally falls out.

c. If it is plastic, use once and then throw it away.

Procedure

1. Attach new ties to clean tracheostomy tube and insert guide (obturator) into tube; do not touch the part to be inserted into the trachea.

2. Place a roll under the shoulders to expose insertion site, or have another person expose the area by holding the infant.

3. While holding onto the cannula with one hand, cut old ties with scissors, then remove the tube.

4. Insert new tube in a backward and downward motion, holding onto the "wings" of the tube.

5. Remove obturator (guide) and secure tie according to previous directions, making sure that you hold the tracheostomy tube in place with one hand. Observe that child is breathing adequately.

6. Suction if necessary.

If you are unable to insert the tracheostomy tube:

1. Reposition the head and try again.

2. If tube will not enter, try to insert the old tube. If you are unable to insert this tube, take a suction catheter and put it into the stoma, hold it in place, and cut it off about 6 in. from the stoma. Do not let go of the catheter. This will prevent the hole from closing completely while allowing your child to breathe through the hole.

3. Have someone call 911, or take your child to the emergency room.

4. *Do not leave your child alone.*

Changing the Hollinger Tube.* The procedure for changing the Hollinger tube is the same as for the Shiley tube, except that you need to remove the *inner cannula* of the new tracheostomy tube and insert the obturator before inserting the tube into the stoma.

HUMIDITY

When a child breathes through a tracheostomy tube, air is not warmed, moisturized, or filtered. It is therefore necessary for some form of humidification to keep your child's secretions loose; thick secretions make it harder to breathe and can cause blockage as well as respiratory infections. With a new tracheostomy, continuous humidification is necessary. However, usually after 10 days the infant-child may need the humidity only during naps and sleep. Humidification during these times is necessary to prevent mucus from plugging the tube. Certain climates and seasons may require you to use more or less mist.

1. Humidification is produced by a "trach collar" attached to a nebulizer.

2. During a power failure, or if you are traveling where there is no access to electricity, one drop of saline (special sterile salt water) instilled hourly into the tracheostomy tube will keep airway moist. Do not suction afterward.

3. Clean nebulizer, trach collar, and suction bottle daily in hot soapy water and rinse well.

Emergencies and Cardiopulmonary Resuscitation (CPR)

If an emergency occurs, you must be ready to act immediately. If you know what to do and how to do it, you can remain calm and be prepared.

1. Place a list of emergency phone numbers next to the phone.

2. If tracheostomy tube becomes plugged, or the child stops breathing, instill saline and attempt to suction. If unable to clear tube, remove it and insert a new one. (Always keep nearby, ready for use, a tube with ties attached.)

3. If these measures do not enable your child to begin breathing, begin CPR as instructed.

---

* Your doctor will let you know if you should change your child's Hollinger tracheostomy tube.

4. If you are alone after several minutes of CPR, stop momentarily to call for emergency help (911). Continue CPR until help arrives or child responds by breathing or his or her heart begins to beat on its own.

Home Care

FEEDING SCHEDULE

The child with a tracheostomy can usually eat normally. A few considerations are necessary, however.

1. Burp baby well and never prop the bottle.
2. Do not let food, formula, or objects get into the tracheostomy.
3. The child should always be supervised when eating.
4. If choking and, possibly, aspiration (when "choked" contents are inhaled into the lungs) occur, immediately suction the tube well.
5. Always do routine suctioning *before* feeding (doing it after feeding can cause the child to gag and vomit).

BATHING

1. You may bathe your child in a bathtub, as long as the water is shallow.
2. Do not allow any water to get into tracheostomy. If it does, suction immediately.
3. Wearing the trach collar in the tub is a good way of helping to prevent water from entering the tracheostomy.
4. Never leave your child alone in bathtub.
5. Older children should not shower.

CLOTHING AND BEDDING

No special clothing is required; however, you need to make sure that your child's clothing does not cover the tracheostomy opening (no clothes with turtlenecks). Any type of fuzzy clothing, blankets, or stuffed animals, as well as necklaces and beads, should be avoided. These fibers or particles can enter the tracheostomy tube and make it difficult for your child to breathe. Ask your nurse about special bibs made of material that allows air to pass through.

EQUIPMENT CARE

The nebulizer collar and suction machine can be cared for in the following manner.

1. Humidifier and nebulizer collar
   a. Wash in hot, soapy water and rinse thoroughly every day (prevents bacterial growth)
2. Suction machine
   a. Instructions on how to operate and care for the machine are usually given by the company renting or selling it or by the person delivering it.
   b. Empty the bottle and wash and rinse thoroughly at least once a day. The bottle should be sterilized at least once a week (by boiling).
   c. Clean the suction tubing with hot water. Soap every day and rinse well.

APNEA MONITOR

An apnea monitor is a small electric device attached to your child with a Velcro belt or chest "leads" that "counts" your child's heartbeats and breaths. It is necessary for your infant to wear this device whenever he or she is unattended (when napping or sleeping) to ensure his or her safety. If your child has difficulty breathing, or stops breathing, an alarm will sound to alert you that there may be a problem. You should always respond immediately to the alarm and look at your child first. Your child may have pulled off the leads or may be restless or crying.

1. Fasten belt securely over the child's rib cage (middle of chest) under clothing.
2. Make sure alarm limits are set appropriately and turn on monitor.
3. Always make sure that the machine is functioning properly before leaving room.
4. An intercom is ideal in this situation to monitor your child and hear the alarm, but if it is not possible, make sure that child's room is within hearing range and the door is open at all times.

PLAY

Normal play activity for your child should be encouraged; water sports should be avoided. No swimming is allowed until the tracheostomy tube has been permanently removed and the stoma has closed. When your child plays or travels outdoors, you should cover the tracheostomy with a gauze bandage or loosely tied scarf to prevent dust, cold air, and sand from entering the tracheostomy tube. A crocheted bib for infants works well. Always keep small objects out of reach. Children have been known to put them into their tracheostomy tubes!

BABY SITTERS

Children with a tracheostomy must always be watched by someone who knows how to suction, change the tracheostomy tube, and administer CPR. One or two additional adults (other than parents) should learn tracheostomy care so that you can get adequate rest and an occasional night out. If you know any parents of other children with a tracheostomy, perhaps you could take turns baby-sitting.

COMMUNICATION

At first, most children with a tracheostomy cannot make noise when they try to talk, because air cannot pass around the tracheostomy tube and through the vocal cords. Because your child cannot communicate in the usual way, you need to be alert to detect any breathing problems. You should continue to talk to your child normally. Read stories and show pictures —your child needs to *hear* talking to learn to talk. Your child may begin to talk or make sounds when the swelling around the tracheostomy decreases. Supply an older child with a bell or keep a pad of paper and pencil nearby so written messages can be shared. Some older children can talk by taking a deep breath, placing a finger or thumb over the tracheostomy tube, and then speaking. Not all children, however, can talk around the tube. Consult your nurse or doctor if your child has difficulty. If the tube will remain in place for several years, learning sign language is important for your child's ability to communicate and social development.

GENERAL GUIDELINES AND SAFETY TIPS

1. Always take at least one complete tracheostomy set, saline drops, and portable suction machine and catheters or De Lee suction catheters when leaving home. Suction tracheostomy before you leave the house.

2. Do not keep pets with fine hair in your home, because hair can enter the tracheostomy tube and cause an obstruction.

3. Keep home as free from lint and dust as possible.

4. Do not use powders or aerosol sprays near your child. Fumes or particles can enter the tracheostomy tube and cause breathing problems.

5. Smoking should be avoided near a child with a tracheostomy because the smoke can irritate the child's lungs.

6. Do not let water enter the tracheostomy tube.

7. Keep small objects (that could plug tracheostomy) away from the child.

SAMPLE LETTERS TO UTILITY COMPANIES FOR SPECIAL CONSIDERATION IN EMERGENCY

Telephone Company

ATTENTION: _____

Our child, _____, is under a physician's care for a tracheostomy. While the tracheostomy is in place, the child requires constant monitoring.

Therefore, while the infant is sleeping at home, breathing and/or heart rate is monitored with a device to detect a decrease in breathing and/or heart rate. If an obstruction of the tracheostomy tube occurs, this will be recognized by monitoring and corrected.

If we need to resuscitate our baby, we will call for help. Therefore, *telephone contact with emergency services must be available at all times.*

The telephone company's support is urgently needed. We ask that our home be placed on a priority list for restoration of service in the event of an interruption of service. If there is a forewarning of temporary phone disconnection, please notify us so that proper arrangements can be made for emergencies.

Sincerely,

_____

Electric Company

ATTENTION: _____

Our child, _____, is under a physician's care for a tracheostomy. While the tracheostomy is in place, the child requires constant monitoring.

Therefore, while the infant is sleeping at home, breathing and/or heart rate is monitored with a device to detect a decrease in breathing and/or heart rate. This monitor requires AC current and can be operated from a battery source for a limited period. If an obstruction of the tracheostomy tube occurs, this will be recognized by monitoring and corrected.

In addition to the monitor, each parent is provided with a power failure alarm that will sound when electricity has been discontinued.

The electric company's support is urgently needed. We ask that our home be placed on a priority list for restoration of electricity in the event there is a power failure. Also, if there is a forewarning of a power discontinuation, please notify us so that we can make arrangements for emergency generator power.

Sincerely,

_____

OUTCOME AFTER NEONATAL INTENSIVE CARE

JOAN GROBSTEIN, M.D., and ROBERTA A. BALLARD, M.D.

with

CHRONIC LUNG DISEASE

by

CHERYL D. LEW, M.D., and THOMAS G. KEENS, M.D.

EVALUATING FOLLOW-UP STUDIES

Follow-up studies are inevitably plagued with methodologic and tactical difficulties, not the least of which is the high cost of frequent, comprehensive evaluations of children's physical, neurologic, developmental, auditory, and visual status. Various follow-up groups have differing capacities for making frequent evaluations. Some studies report on a single evaluation within the first two or three years of life, whereas others do serial evaluations up to and including school age. It is impossible to compare these two types of studies directly for several reasons:

Neonatal intensive care is not uniform. Although certain practices are fairly universal, details of routine care vary considerably from nursery to nursery. It is quite possible that these details may have important influences on infants' long-term outcome.

Neonatal management, even in a given unit, may vary, and prenatal care and timing of an infant's delivery may be as important as postnatal care. Some studies have shown significant differences in the outcome of "inborn" vs "outborn" infants. This, too, seems to be changing as more and more physicians are becoming proficient in the resuscitation, stabilization, and transport of sick neonates. It has been pointed out that only studies of outcome of all infants in a given geographic area allow control for differences between transported and inborn infants in a given tertiary care center.

Neonatal intensive care is not static. Evaluations made in children at school age show that they may not be at the same risk as infants who are leaving ICN now. There certainly has been a decrease in mortality over the past 10 years in many categories of infants; the decline in mor-

bidity has not been as impressive, but this too is difficult to evaluate, since the types of morbidity may be changing.

Morbidity and mortality may be affected by philosophic stance. The philosophy of the attending staff of any given neonatal intensive care unit regarding withdrawal of support from infants thought to have sustained irreversible neurologic damage will affect both the morbidity and mortality experience of the unit. This, too, may change over the years, with changing attitudes of staff and parents, as well as with changes in the legal climate.

Environmental influences are important. Children obviously do not all grow up in similar environments. Outcome at school age is much more affected by social, economic, and psychological factors than is outcome at earlier ages. Indeed, one study suggests that the IQ among children of lower socioeconomic status tends to decrease between the ages of 2 and 6 years, while the IQ of infants of higher socioeconomic status tends to increase. Some studies have attempted to control for these factors by making evaluations in siblings of ICN graduates, but this approach greatly increases the cost of the studies.

Demographic differences among infants may influence outcome. Black female premature infants have a lower incidence of respiratory distress syndrome than black male infants or infants of other ethnic groups. If there is a preponderance of a given group of infants in a particular study, overall outcome data may be affected.

Developmental outcome in ICN graduates is not static. Some studies indicate that infants who appear normal at 2 years of age may have significant difficulties in school at 6 to 8 years of age. Conversely, other studies show that infants who may appear to have cerebral palsy at 6 months of age may seem normal at 2 years.

Long-term outcome of early developmental delay is difficult to predict. Many follow-up programs refer children for intervention (such as speech therapy or physical therapy) when delays are detected. The effect of some of these interventions on outcome, especially long-term outcome, is not clear. In fact, most studies do not mention whether interventions were made by the follow-up group itself, a family physician, or other concerned parties, such as schools. Intervention efforts presumably explain some of the differences seen in socioeconomic groups.

Compliance with follow-up appointments influences data. From a statistical point of view, if more than 20 per cent of infants in a given study are lost to follow-up, the outcome results may not be valid; not all studies have been able to achieve an 80 per cent level of compliance, and this must be kept in mind in interpreting the information.

OUTCOME OF LOW BIRTH WEIGHT INFANTS

In 1981, Stewart, Reynolds, and Lipscomb[1] reviewed the world literature of outcome studies in small preterm infants (Figs. D–1 to D–3, below). They pointed out that from 1960 to 1977 the proportion of healthy survivors among infants weighing less than 1500 grams at birth tripled, and the proportion of handicapped children remained low (6 to 8 per cent). They noted that some of the same trends were also emerging for infants weighing less than 1000 grams. The references below include studies published through 1987 of outcome of low birth weight and very low birth weight infants. As infants of lower and lower birth weight survive, there will be a lag in determining what their eventual outcome at school age will be. However, there are some emerging concerns about outcome of very low birth weight infants at school age. Some of these infants have shown specific problems with spatial relationships and are having difficulty with perceptual and visual motor tasks at age 7

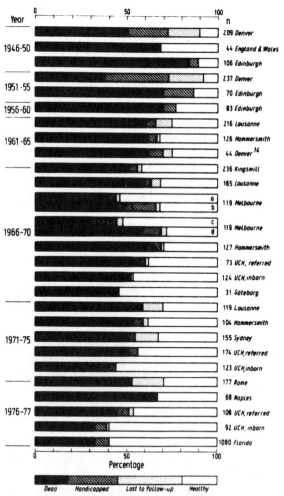

FIGURE D–1. Percentage of VLBW infants (<1500 grams) who died, survived handicapped, were lost to follow-up, or survived healthy. (From Stewart AL, Reynolds EOR, Lipscomb AP: Outcome for infants of very low birthweight: Survey of world literature. Lancet 1:1038–1041, 1981. Reprinted with permission. Reference numbers refer to original article.)

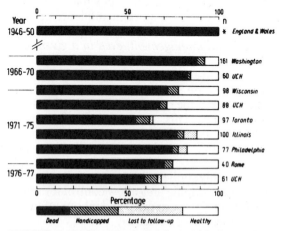

FIGURE D–2. Percentage of infants weighing <1000 grams who died, survived handicapped, were lost to follow-up, or survived healthy. (From Stewart AL, Reynolds EOR, Lipscomb AP: Outcome for infants of very low birthweight: Survey of world literature. Lancet 1:1038–1041, 1981. Reprinted with permission. Reference numbers refer to original article.)

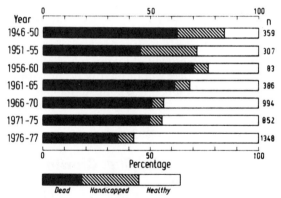

FIGURE D-3. Data from Figure D-1 pooled by quinquennium to show percentage of VLBW infants (<1500 grams) who died, survived handicapped, were lost to follow-up, or survived healthy. (From Stewart AL, Reynolds EOR, Lipscomb AP: Outcome for infants of very low birthweight: Survey of world literature. Lancet 1:1038–1041, 1981. Reprinted with permission. Reference numbers refer to original article.)

years.[2] It is also clear that, as infants with more complicated neonatal courses are surviving, chronic illness may also interfere with eventual outcome. (See Recommended Reading, Growth, Neurodevelopmental Outcome.)

References

1. Stewart AL, Reynolds EOR, Lipscomb AP: Outcome for infants of very low birth weight: Survey of world literature. Lancet 1:1038, 1981.
2. Klein N, Hack M, Gallagher J, et al.: Preschool performance of children with normal intelligence who were very low-birth-weight infants. Pediatrics 75:531, 1985.

Recommended Reading: Low Birth Weight Infants

NEURODEVELOPMENTAL OUTCOME

Bennett FC, Robinson NM, Sells CJ: Growth and development of infants weighing less than 800 grams at birth. Pediatrics 71:319, 1983.
Brann AW, Volpe JJ (eds.): Neonatal Neurological Assessment and Outcome. Report of 77th Ross Conference on Pediatric Research. Columbus, Ross Laboratories, 1980.
Britton SB, Fitzhardinge PM, Ashby S: Is intensive care justified for infants weighing less than 801 gm at birth? J Pediatr 99: 937, 1981.
Brothwood M, Wolke P, Gamsu H, et al.: Prognosis of the very low birthweight baby in relation to gender. Arch Dis Child 61:559, 1986.
Buckwald S, Zorn WA, Egan EA: Mortality and follow-up data for neonates weighing 500 to 800 g at birth. Am J Dis Child 138:779, 1984.
Cohen I, Altaras M, Jaffe R, et al.: Perinatal factors influencing outcome of very-low-birth weight infants. Isr J Med Sci 22:430, 1986.

Cohen RS, Stevenson DK, Malachowski N, et al.: Favorable results of neonatal intensive care for very low-birth-weight infants. Pediatrics 69:621, 1982.
Crombie SV, Darlow BA: Neurodevelopmental outcome for infants of very low-birthweight admitted to a regional neonatal unit, 1979–1983.
Doyle LW, Richards AL, Ford GW, et al.: Outcome for the very low birth-weight (500-1,499 g) singleton breech: Benefit of cesarean section. Aust NZ J Obstet Gynaecol 25:259, 1986.
Driscoll JM, Driscoll YT, Steir ME, et al.: Mortality and morbidity in infants less than 1,001 grams birth weight. Pediatrics 69:21, 1982.
Eilers BL, Desai NS, Wilson MA, et al.: Classroom performance and social factors of children with birth weights of 1,250 grams or less: Follow-up at 5 to 8 years of age. Pediatrics 77:203, 1986.
Haas G, Buchwald-Saal M, Leidig E, et al.: Improved outcome in very low birthweight infants from 1977 to 1983. Eur J Pediatr 145:337, 1986.
Hirata T, Epcar JT, Walsh A, et al.: Survival and outcome of infants 501 to 750 gm: A six-year experience. J Pediatr 102:741, 1983.
Kitchen WH, Ford GW, Rickards AL, et al.: Children of birthweight less than 1000 g: Changing outcome between ages 2 and 5 years. J Pediatr 110:283, 1987.
Kitchen WH, Rickards A, Ryan MM, et al.: A longitudinal study of very low birthweight infants: II. Dev Med Child Neurol 21:582, 1979.
Kitchen WH, Rickards AL, Ryan MM, et al.: Improved outcome to two years of very low-birthweight infants: Fact or artifact? Dev Med Child Neurol 28:579, 1986.
Knobloch H, Malone A, Ellison PH, et al.: Considerations in evaluating changes in outcome for infants weighing less than 1,501 grams. Pediatrics 69:285, 1982.
Kumar SP, Anday EK, Sacks LM, et al.: Follow-up studies of very low birthweight infants (1,250 grams or less) born and treated within a perinatal center. Pediatrics 66:438, 1980.
Lasky RE, Tyson JE, Rosenfeld CR, et al.: Disappointing follow-up findings for indigent high-risk newborns. Am J Dis Child 141:100, 1987.
Lee, K-S, Paneth N, Gartner LM, et al.: Neonatal mortality: An analysis of the recent improvement in the United States. Am J Public Health 70:15, 1980.
Levi S, Taylor W, Robinson LE, et al.: Analysis of morbidity and outcome of infants weighing less than 800 g at birth. South Med J 77:975, 1984.
Lipper E, Kwant-sun L, Gartner LM, et al.: Determinants of neurobehavioral outcome in low-birth-weight infants. Pediatrics 67:502, 1981.
Lubchenko LO, Bard H, Goldman AL, et al.: Newborn intensive care and long-term prognosis. Dev Med Child Neurol 16:421, 1974.
Lubchenko LO, Delivoria-Papadopoulos M, Butterfield LJ, et al.: Long-term follow-up studies of prematurely born infants. J Pediatr 80:501, 1972.
Michelsson K, Lindahl E, Parre M, et al.: Nine-year follow-up of infants weighing 1500 g or less at birth. Acta Paediatr Scand 73:835, 1984.
Nickel RE, Bennett FC, Lamson FN: School performance of children with birth weights of 1,000 g or less. Am J Dis Child 136:105, 1982.
Ross G, Lipper E, Auld PA: Early predictors of neurodevelopmental outcome of very low-birthweight infants at three years. Dev Med Child Neurol 28:171, 1986.
Rothberg AD, Maisels MJ, Bagnato S, et al.: Outcome for survivors of mechanical ventilation weighing less than 1,250 gm at birth. J Pediatr 98:106, 1981.

Rothberg AD, Maisels MJ, Bagnato S, et al.: Infants weighing 1,000 grams or less at birth: Developmental outcome for ventilated and nonventilated infants. Pediatrics 71:599, 1983.

Ruiz MPD, LeFever JA, Hakason DO, et al.: Early development of infants of birth weight less than 1,000 grams with reference to mechanical ventilation in newborn period. Pediatrics 68:330, 1981.

Saigal S, Rosenbaum P, Stoskopf B, et al.: Outcome in infants 501–1000 gm birth weight delivered to residents of the McMaster Health Region. J Pediatr 105:969, 1984.

Sell, EJ: Outcome of very very low birth weight infants. Clin Perinatol 13(2):451, 1986.

Steiner ES, Sanders EM, Phillips ECK, et al.: Very low birth weight children at school age: Comparison of neonatal management methods. Br Med J 281:1237, 1980.

Stewart AL, Reynolds EOR: Improved prognosis for infants of very low birthweight. Pediatrics 54:724, 1974.

Stewart AL, Reynolds EOR, Lipscomb AP: Outcome for infants of very low birth weight: Survey of world literature. Lancet 1:1038, 1981.

Stewart AL, Turcan DM, Rawlings G, et al.: Prognosis for infants weighing 1000 grams or less at birth. Arch Dis Child 52:97, 1977.

Tudehope DI, Rogers YM, Buens YR, et al.: Apnoea in very low birthweight infants: Outcome at 2 years. Cust Paediatr J 22:131, 1986.

Vohr BR, Garcia Coll CT: Neurodevelopmental and school performance of very low-birth-weight infants: A seven-year longitudinal study. Pediatrics 76:345, 1985.

Voyer M: What is the prognosis of preterm infants? III. Follow-up at school age. Arch Fr Pediatr 43:741, 1986.

Wright FH, Blough RR, Chamberlin A, et al.: A controlled follow-up study of small prematures born from 1952 through 1956. Am J Dis Child 124:506, 1972.

Yu VYH, Hollingsworth E: Improving prognosis for infants weighing 1,000 grams or less at birth. Arch Dis Child 55:422, 1980.

Yu VY, Loke HL, Bajuk B, et al.: Prognosis for infants born at 23 to 28 weeks' gestation. Br Med J [Clin Res] 293:1200, 1986.

Yu VY, Wong PY, Bajuk B, et al.: Outcome of extremely-low-birthweight infants. Br J Obstet Gynecol 93:162, 1986.

GROWTH: INFLUENCE ON OUTCOME

As discussed in Chapter 5, both intrauterine and extrauterine growth may have a very powerful impact on eventual neurodevelopmental outcome of high-risk infants. The following general statements can be made about growth and its impact on neurodevelopment.

1. The infant with symmetric growth retardation that occurs early in gestation is at the highest risk for poor neurodevelopmental outcome.

2. The combination of very low birth weight with small size for gestational age is more likely to be associated with poor outcome than that expected for very low birth weight alone.

3. In any graduate from an ICN who is of low birth weight, head circumference at age 8 months is a powerful predictor of eventual neurodevelopmental outcome.

4. Catch-up growth of infants who are small for gestational age will ordinarily occur within the first year of life, if it is going to happen.

5. In very low birth weight infants who are not small for gestational age, catch-up growth may occur up until age $2\frac{1}{2}$ to 3 years.

Recommended Reading: Growth in ICN Graduates

Babson SG, Benda GI: Growth graphs for the clinical assessment of infants at varying gestational age. J Pediatr 89:814, 1976.

Brann AW, Volpe JJ (eds.): Neonatal Neurological Assessment and Outcome. Report of 77th Ross Conference on Pediatric Research. Columbus, Ross Laboratories, 1980.

Davies DP: Growth of "small for dates" babies. Early Hum Dev 5:95, 1981.

Davies DP, Platts P, Pritchard JM: Nutritional status of light-for-date infants at birth and its influence on early postnatal growth. Arch Dis Child 54:707, 1979.

Desmond MM, Williamson WD, Wilson GS: School failure in prematurely born children: Can it be prevented? J Perinatol 6:309,

Fancourt R, Campbell S, Harvey D, et al.: Follow-up study of small-for-dates babies. Br Med J 1:1435, 1976.

Fitzhardinge PM, Steven EM: The small-for-date infant: I. Later growth patterns. Pediatrics 49:671, 1972.

Fitzhardinge PM, Steven EM: The small-for-date infant: II. Neurological and intellectual sequelae. Pediatrics 50:50, 1972.

Georgieff MK, Hoffman JS, Pereira GR, et al.: Effect of neonatal caloric deprivation on head growth and 1-year developmental status in preterm infants. J Pediatr 107:581, 1985.

Greer FR, McCormick A: Bone mineral content and growth in very-low-birth-weight premature infants. Does bronchopulmonary dysplasia make a difference? Am J Dis Child 141:179, 1987.

Hack M, Breslau N: Very low birth weight infants: Effects of brain growth during infancy on intelligence quotient at 3 years of age. Pediatrics 77:196, 1986.

Hack M, Merkatz IR, Gordon D, et al.: The prognostic significance of postnatal growth in very low birthweight infants. Am J Obstet Gynecol 43:693, 1982.

Hack M, Merkatz IR, McGrath SK, et al.: Catch-up growth in very-low-birthweight infants. Am J Dis Child 38:370–375, 1984.

Hack M, Rivers A, Fanaroff AA: The very low birthweight infant: The broader spectrum of morbidity during infancy and early childhood. J Dev Behav Pediatr 4:343, 1983.

Harvey D, Prince J, Bunton J, et al.: Abilities of children who were small-for-gestational-age babies. Pediatrics 69:296, 1982.

Hurt H (ed.): Continuing Care of the High-Risk Infant. Clin Perinatol, Vol 11, 1984.

Karniski W, Blair C, Vitucci JS: The illusion of catch-up growth in premature infants. Am J Dis Child 141:520, 1987.

Kitchen WH, Richards A, Ryan MM, et al.: A longitudinal study of very low birth weight infants: II. Dev Med Child Neurol 21:582, 1979.

Kimble KJ, Ariagno RL, Stevenson DK, et al.: Growth to age 3 years among very low-birth-weight sequelae-free survivors of modern neonatal intensive care. J Pediatr 100:622, 1982.

Kumar SP, Anday EK, Sacks LM, et al.: Follow-up studies of very low birth weight infants (1,250 grams or less) born and treated within a perinatal center. Pediatrics 66:438, 1980.

Low JA, Gailbraith RS, Muir D, et al.: Intrauterine growth retardation: A preliminary report of long-term morbidity. Am J Obstet Gynecol 130:534, 1978.

Lubchenko LO, Bard H, Goldman AL, et al.: Newborn intensive care and long-term prognosis. Dev Med Child Neurol 16:421, 1974.

Parkinson C, Wallis S, Harvey D: School achievement and behavior of children who were small-for-dates at birth. Dev Med Child Neurol 23:41, 1981.

Roche AF, Mukherjee D, Gus S: Head circumference growth pattern: Birth to 18 years. Hum Biol 58:893, 1986.

Ross G, Krauss AN, Auld PAM: Growth achievement in low-birth-weight premature infants: Relationship to neurobehavioral outcome at one year. J Pediatr 103:105, 1983.

Sann L, Darre E, Lasne U, et al.: Effects of prematurity and dysmaturity on growth at age 5 years. J Pediatr 109:681, 1986.

Steiner ES, Sanders EM, Phillips ECK, et al.: Very low birth weight children at school age: Comparison of neonatal management methods. Br Med J 281:1237, 1980.

Stewart AL, Reynolds EOR: Improved prognosis for infants of very low birth weight. Pediatrics 54:724, 1974.

Stewart AL, Reynolds EOR, Lipscomb AP: Outcome for infants of very low birth weight: Survey of world literature. Lancet 1:1038, 1981.

Stewart AL, Turcan DM, Rawlings G, et al.: Prognosis for infants weighing 1000 g or less at birth. Arch Dis Child 52:97, 1977.

Usher R, McLean F: Intrauterine growth of live born caucasian infants at sea level. J Pediatr 74:901, 1974.

Villar J, Belizan JM: The relative contribution of prematurity and fetal growth retardation to low birth weight in developing and developed societies. Am J Obstet Gynecol 143:793, 1982.

Villar J, Smeriglio V, Martorell R, et al.: Heterogeneous growth and mental development of intrauterine growth-retarded infants during the first 3 years of life. Pediatrics 74:783, 1984.

Vohr BR, Oh W, Rosenfield AG, et al.: Preterm small-for-gestational-age infants: Two-year follow-up study. Am J Obstet Gynecol 133:425, 1979.

Westwood M, Kramer MS, Munz D, et al.: Growth and development of full-term nonasphyxiated small-for-gestational-age newborns: Follow-up through adolescence. Pediatrics 71:376, 1983.

Wright FH, Blough RR, Chamberlin A, et al.: A controlled follow-up study of small prematures born 1952 through 1956. Am J Dis Child 124:506, 1972.

Yu VYH, Hollingsworth E: Improving prognosis for infants weighing 1000 g or less at birth. Arch Dis Child 55:422, 1980.

RESPIRATORY DISTRESS SYNDROME

The incidence of respiratory distress syndrome in infants weighing less than 2.5 kg at birth is approximately 14 per cent. Therefore it can be estimated that about 35,000 infants per year (U.S.) will suffer from respiratory distress syndrome. Of these, approximately one third will be treated with mechanical ventilation, and of those, 15 per cent may develop chronic lung disease, i.e., about 1300 infants per year. It is difficult to separate the neurodevelopmental impact of respiratory distress syndrome alone, since it occurs in infants of low birth weight who may suffer from other problems. A number of investigators, however, have attempted to look at the effect of respiratory distress syndrome on both neurodevelopmental and pulmonary outcome of these infants.

Recommended Reading: Respiratory Distress Syndrome

NEURODEVELOPMENTAL OUTCOME

Ambrus C, Weintraub D, Niswander K, et al.: Evaluation of survivors of the respiratory distress syndrome. J Pediatr 120:296, 1970.

Bozynski ME, Nelson MN, Matalon TAS, et al.: Prolonged mechanical ventilation and intracranial hemorrhage: Impact on developmental progress through 18 months in infants weighing 1200 grams or less at birth. Pediatrics 79:670, 1987.

Field T, Dempsey J, Shuman HH: Developmental assessments of infants surviving the respiratory distress syndrome. In Field T, Sostek S, Goldberg S, et al. (eds.): Infants Born At Risk. New York, Spectrum Publications, 1979.

Field TM, Dempsey JR, Shuman HH: Developmental follow-up of pre- and post-term infants. In Friedman SF, Sigman M (eds.): Preterm Birth and Psychological Development. New York, Academic Press, 1981.

Fisch R, Bilek M, Miller L, Engel R: Physical and mental status at 4 years of age of survivors of the respiratory distress syndrome. J Pediatr 86:497, 1975.

Fisch RO, Graven HJ, Engel RR: Neurological status of survivors of neonatal respiratory distress syndrome. J Pediatr 73:395, 1968.

Fitzhardinge PM, Pape K, Arstikaitis M, et al.: Mechanical ventilation of infants of less than 1,501 grams birth weight: Health, growth and neurological sequelae. J Pediatr 88:531, 1976.

Harrod JR, L'Heureaux P, Wangensteen DO, et al.: Long-term follow-up of severe respiratory distress syndrome treated with IPPV. J Pediatr 84:277, 1974.

Hunt JV, Predicting intellectual disorders in childhood for preterm infants with birth weights below 1,502 gm. In Friedman SF, Sigman M (eds.): Preterm Birth and Psychological Development. New York, Academic Press, 1981, pp 329–349.

Johnson JD, Malachowski NC, Grobstein R, et al.: Prognosis of children surviving with the aid of mechanical ventilation in the newborn period. J Pediatr 84:171, 1974.

Ludman WL, Halperin JM, Driscoll JM Jr: Birth weight, respiratory distress syndrome, and cognitive development. Am J Dis Child 141:79, 1987.

Outerbridge EW, Stern L: Developmental follow-up of artificially ventilated infants with neonatal respiratory failure. Pediatr Res 6:412, 1972.

Piekkala P, Kero P, Sillanpää M, et al.: Growth and development of infants surviving respiratory distress syndrome: a 2-year follow-up. Pediatrics 79:529, 1987.

Rothberg AD, Maisels MS, Bagnato S, et al.: Infants weighing 1,000 grams or less at birth: Developmental outcome for ventilated and nonventilated infants. Pediatrics 71:599, 1983.

Ruiz MPD, LeFever JA, Hakason DO, et al.: Early development of infants of birth weight less than 1,000 grams with reference to mechanical ventilation in the newborn period. Pediatrics 68:330, 1981.

Stahlman M, Hedwall G, Dolanski E, et al.: A six-year follow-up of clinical hyaline membrane disease. Pediatr Clin North Am 20:433, 1973.

Stewart AL, Reynolds EOR, Lipscomb AP: Outcome for infants of very low birth weight: Survey of world literature. Lancet 1:1038, 1981.

PULMONARY OUTCOME

Coates AL, Bergsteinsson H, Desmond K, et al.: Long-term pulmonary sequelae of premature birth with and without idiopathic respiratory distress syndrome. J Pediatr 90:611, 1977.

Heldt GP, McIlroy MB, Hansen TN, et al.: Exercise performance of the survivors of hyaline membrane disease. J Pediatr 96:995, 1980.

Maclusky IB, Zarfin J, Pape K, et al.: Bronchial hyperreactivity in long-term survivors of the neonatal respiratory distress syndrome. Pediatr Res 18:396A, 1984.

Stocks J, Godfrey S, Reynolds EOR: Airway resistance in infants after various treatments for hyaline membrane disease: Special emphasis on prolonged high levels of inspired oxygen. Pediatrics 61:178, 1978.

(See also Recommended Reading: Outcome in Infants with Chronic Lung Disease.)

CHRONIC LUNG DISEASE

Pulmonary Function Findings

The variable degrees of chronic lung disability among groups of infants after neonatal lung injury, under apparently equivalent circumstances, make a cohesive summary of long-term outcome difficult. Rapidly changing techniques of neonatal respiratory care, longer-term medical interventions, and the complexity of the various medical sequelae, all of which may affect recovery from infantile chronic lung disease, further confuse evaluation of patient outcome.

The lack of widely available quantitative methods for assessing lung mechanics and airways function at the bedside during the course of acute respiratory disease during early infancy makes it difficult to correlate pulmonary function parameters obtained later in childhood and adolescence with objectively measured severity of the early disease. In addition, the still rudimentary understanding of the neonatal lung's responses to injury is associated with an equally rudimentary understanding of healing and repair processes that are influenced by age at time of injury and by subsequent growth and development.

This section summarizes the findings of available studies of early and long-term pulmonary function findings following neonatal lung injury.

REVIEW OF THE LITERATURE

A selection of papers from the literature is summarized below. It should be noted that infantile chronic lung disease is generally reported to consist of either or both episodes of recurrent respiratory infection and episodes of airways hyperreactivity. Observations of the presence and severity of defects in pulmonary function vary, perhaps reflecting changes in the numbers and types of survivors, as well as changing practices in neonatal respiratory care. A major criticism of all the studies presented is that, in general, they examine outcome in children who experienced injury 5 to 10 years previously. The earliest studies, therefore, are of children born about 1960, in the very earliest era of neonatal intensive care. The patient populations of these early studies are not comparable to children born more recently, who may be younger in gestational age at birth and who are managed with more aggressive techniques of ventilatory support. The prevailing conclusion, however, is that pulmonary function, if initially abnormal, appears to improve with age and somatic growth. Growth may be slowed early, however, in relation to the increased caloric requirements seen in some of the patients due to increased work of breathing.

CONCLUSIONS

1. Lung disability can be expected to improve with time.

2. Certain medical interventions (continuing oxygen therapy, diuretics, bronchodilators) can be expected to ameliorate the course of chronic lung disability, although whether healing can be hastened is uncertain at this time.

3. Lung healing appears to be related closely to somatic growth and nutritional status.

4. The ultimate outcome in these few infants who remain ventilator or oxygen dependent or significantly hypoxic indefinitely is still unclear.

5. Theoretically, outcome for all survivors of neonatal or infantile lung injury depends on po-

TABLE D–1. Chronic Lung Disease in Infancy: Literature Summary

AUTHORS AND TYPE OF STUDY	CLINICAL OUTCOME	PULMONARY FUNCTION FINDINGS
Stahlman et al. Pediatrics (1982) Survivors born 1961–1970. Long-term study	Wheezing, rales; recurrent pneumonia; eventual complete resolution except for those with family history of asthma after 4 yr of age.	"Mildly" abnormal with progressive improvement with time
Lamarre et al. Am Rev Respir Dis (1973) Survivors born 1963–1966. Long-term study	No incidence of recurrent respiratory infections	Mild, sporadic changes in lung volumes, flow rates, gas exchange; most patients normal
Coates et al. J Pediatr (1977) Survivors born 1967–1971. Long-term study		Airways obstruction; hyperinflation
Heldt et al. J Pediatr (1980) Survivors born 1968–1974. Long-term study	Wheezing, recurrent respiratory infections	Most had normal ventilation during exercise; 5% of study population had CO_2 retention during exercise
Bryan et al. Pediatrics (1973) Survivors born 1970–1971. Short-term study	Recurrent pneumonia	PCO_2 elevated; hypoxemia (BPD > RDS only); hyperinflation; airways obstruction
Smyth et al. Pediatrics (1981) Survivors born 1970–1972. Long-term study	Recurrent bronchial reactivity with improvement over time	Mild hypoxemia; hyperinflation and airways obstruction
Bertrand et al. N Engl J Med (1985) Survivors born 1973–1978. Long-term study		Hyperinflation; airways obstruction; airways hyperreactivity
Mansell et al. Am Rev Respir Dis (1985) Survivors born 1975–1978. Long-term study		Airways obstruction in both RDS patients and "normal" prematures
Morray et al. Pediatr Res (1982) Survivors born 1979–1980. Short-term study	Clinical "turning point" around 7 mo of age with slowing of respiratory rate and improved $PaCO_2$ levels	Minute ventilation increased; airways obstruction that improves with age
Weinstein, OH. J Pediatr (1981) Survivors born 1980–1981. Short-term study		Increased oxygen consumption, consistent with elevated caloric requirements
Kao et al. Pediatrics (1984) Lung Mechanics Survivors born 1982–1983. Short-term study		Airways obstruction; hyperinflation
Bader et al. J Pediatr (1987) Survivors born 1974–1977. Long-term study	Recurrent respiratory infections; wheezing	Airways obstruction; hyperinflation; normal exercise tolerance
Berman et al. J Pediatr (1986) Survivors of severe BPD with pulmonary hypertension. Long-term study	4 of 10 still in oxygen at 5.5 yr of age; poor growth	Hypoxia, airways obstruction; elevated pulmonary artery pressure and pulmonary vascular resistance at cardiac catheterization in 4 of 10

tential for lung growth and remodeling of damaged airways and parenchyma.

6. It is likely that survivors are left with residual pulmonary function abnormalities, generally indicating airways obstruction, hyperinflation, and, perhaps, airways hyperreactivity. The significance of these findings is unclear, since many of these infants are asymptomatic. However, there is a real possibility that these infants and children will be more likely to develop chronic obstructive pulmonary disease as adults if they are exposed to air pollutants (such as cigarette smoke).

Recommended Reading: Outcome in Infants with Chronic Lung Disease

PULMONARY OUTCOME

Bader D, Ramos AD, Lew CD, et al.: Persistent exercise and pulmonary dysfunction in late childhood following bronchopulmonary dysplasia. Clin Res 35:240A, 1987.

Bader D, Ramos AD, Lew CD, et al.: Childhood sequelae of infant lung disease: Exercise and pulmonary function abnormalities after bronchopulmonary dysplasia. J Pediatr 110:693, 1987.

Berman W Jr, Katz R, Yabek, et al.: Long-term follow-up of bronchopulmonary dysplasia. J Pediatr 109:45, 1986.

Bertrand J-M, Riley SP, Popkin J, et al.: The long-term pulmonary sequelae of prematurity: The role of familial airway hyperreactivity and the respiratory distress syndrome. N Engl J Med 312:742, 1985.

Bryan MH, Hardie MJ, Reilly BJ, et al.: Pulmonary function studies during the first year of life in infants recovering from the respiratory distress syndrome. Pediatrics 52:169, 1973.

Coates AL, Bergsteinsson H, Desmond K, et al.: Long-term pulmonary sequelae of premature birth with and without idiopathic respiratory distress syndrome. J Pediatr 90:611, 1980.

Durand M, Rigatto H: Control of tidal volume and respiratory frequency in infants with bronchopulmonary dysplasia (BPD). Pediatr Res 13: 533A, 1979.

Gerhardt, Hehre D, Feller R, et al.: Serial determination of pulmonary function in infants with chronic lung disease. J Pediatr 110:448, 1987.

Kao GP, McIlroy MB, Hansen TN, et al.: Exercise performance of the survivors of hyaline membrane disease. J Pediatr 96:995, 1980.

Kao LC, Warburton D, Cheng MH, et al.: Effect of isoproterenol inhalation on airway resistance in chronic bronchopulmonary dysplasia: Results of a double-blind cross-over sequential trial. Pediatrics 74:37, 1984.

Koops BL, Abman SH, Accurso FJ: Outpatient management and follow-up of bronchopulmonary dysplasia. Clin Perinatol 11:101, 1984.

Lamarre A, Linsao L, Reilly BJ, et al.: Residual pulmonary abnormalities in survivors of idiopathic respiratory distress syndrome. Am Rev Resp Dis 108:56, 1973.

Mansell AL, Driscoll JM, James LS: Pulmonary follow-up of moderately low birth weight infants with and without respiratory distress syndrome. Am Rev Respir Dis 131:A249, 1985.

Meisels SJ, Plunkett JW, Roloff DW, et al.: Growth and development of preterm infants with respiratory distress syndrome and bronchopulmonary dysplasia. Pediatrics 77:345, 1986.

Morray JP, Fox WW, Kettrick RG, et al.: Improvement in lung mechanics as a function of age in the infant with severe bronchopulmonary dysplasia. Pediatr Res 16:290, 1982.

Nickerson BG: Bronchopulmonary dysplasia—Chronic pulmonary disease following neonatal respiratory failure. Chest 87:528, 1985.

Northway WH, Rosan RD, Porter DY: Pulmonary disease following respirator therapy of hyaline membrane disease. N Engl J Med 276:357, 1967.

Sauve RS, Singhal N: Long-term morbidity of infants with bronchopulmonary dysplasia. Pediatrics 76:725, 1985.

Shepard FM, Johnson RB, Klatte EC, et al.: Residual pulmonary findings in clinical hyaline membrane disease. N Engl J Med 279:1063, 1968.

Smyth JA, Tabachnik E, Duncan WJ, et al.: Pulmonary function and bronchial hyperreactivity in long-term survivors of bronchopulmonary dysplasia. Pediatrics 68:336, 1981.

Stahlman M, Hedvall G, Lindstrom D, et al.: Role of hyaline membrane disease in production of later childhood lung abnormalities. Pediatrics 69:572, 1982.

Stocks J, Godfrey S: The role of artificial ventilation, oxygen and CPAP in the pathogenesis of lung damage in neonates: Assessment by serial measurements of lung function. Pediatrics 571:352, 1976.

Stocks J, Godfrey S, Reynolds EOR: Airway resistance in infants after various treatments for hyaline membrane disease: Special emphasis on prolonged high levels of inspired oxygen. Pediatrics 61:178, 1968.

Taussig LM: Long-term management and pulmonary prognosis of bronchopulmonary dysplasia. Report of 90th Ross Conference on Pediatric Research. Columbus, Ross Laboratories, 1986, pp 126–133.

Watts JL, Ariagno RL, Brady JP: Chronic pulmonary disease in neonates after artificial ventilation: Distribution of ventilation and pulmonary interstitial emphysema. Pediatrics 60:273, 1977.

Weinstein MR, Oh W: Oxygen consumption in infants with bronchopulmonary dysplasia. J Pediatr 99:958, 1981.

NEURODEVELOPMENTAL OUTCOME

Goldson E: Bronchopulmonary dysplasia: Its relation to 2-year developmental functioning in the very low birth-weight infant. In Field T, Sostek S, Goldberg S, et al. (eds.): Infants Born at Risk. New York, Spectrum Publications, 1979.

Markestad T, Fitzhardinge P: Growth and development in children recovering from bronchopulmonary dysplasia. J Pediatr 98:597, 1981.

Vohr BR, Bell EF, Oh N: Infants with bronchopulmonary dysplasia—Growth pattern and developmental outcome. Am J Dis Child 136:443, 1982.

INTRACRANIAL HEMORRHAGE

IMPACT OF INTRACRANIAL HEMORRHAGE ON NEURODEVELOPMENTAL OUTCOME

Many investigators have attempted to evaluate the long-term impact of intracranial hemorrhage (ICH) on outcome. In general, it can be said for those infants with uncomplicated hemorrhages (Papile grade I or II), that the outcome is no different from that expected for other low birth weight infants without ICH. For infants who have complicated ICH (Papile grade III or IV), which includes ventricular dilatation or parenchymal involvement, the outcome is significantly worse than for those with smaller hemorrhages. It has been estimated that significant deficit occurs in approximately 50 per cent of infants with grade III or IV hemorrhages. Current efforts are attempting to refine the ability to review cranial ultrasound studies in these small infants, and there is some suggestion that periventricular intraparenchymal echodensities and cystic changes may enable better prediction of eventual neurodevelopmental outcome.

Recommended Reading: ICH and Other Indicators of CNS Abnormalities

Ahmann PA, Lazzara A, Dykes FD, et al.: Intraventricular hemorrhage in the high-risk preterm infant: Incidence and outcome. Ann Neurol 7:118, 1980.

Allan WC, Dransfield DA, Tito AM: Ventricular dilation following periventricular-intraventricular hemorrhage: Outcome at age 1 year. Pediatrics 73:158, 1984.

Allan WC, Hold PJ, Sawyer LR, et al.: Ventricular dilation after neonatal periventricular-intraventricular hemorrhage. Am J Dis Child 136:589, 1982.

Amato M, Howald H, von Muralt G: Neurological prognosis of high-risk preterm infants with peri-intraventricular hemorrhage and ventricular dilatation. Eur Neurol 25:241, 1986.

Boynton BR, Boynton CA, Merritt TA, et al.: Ventriculoperitoneal shunts in low birth weight infants with intracranial hemorrhage: Neurodevelopmental outcome. Neurosurgery 18:141, 1986.

Bozynski ME, Nelson MN, Genaze D, et al.: Intracranial hemorrhage and neurodevelopmental outcome at one year in infants weighing 1200 grams or less. Prognostic significance of ventriculomegaly at term gestational age. Am J Perinatol 1:325, 1984.

Calvert SA, Hoskins EM, Fong KW, et al.: Periventricular leucomalacia: Ultrasonic diagnosis and neurological outcome. Acta Paediatr Scand 75:489, 1986.

Catto-Smith AG, Yu VY, Bajuk B, et al.: Effect of neonatal periventricular hemorrhage on neurodevelopmental outcome. Arch Dis Child 60:8, 1985.

Clark C, Clyman RI, Roth RR, et al.: Risk factor analysis of intraventricular hemorrhage in low-birth-weight infants. J Pediatr 99:625, 1981.

Cohen RS, Stevenson DK, Malachowski N, et al.: Favorable results of neonatal intensive care for very low-birthweight infants. Pediatrics 69:621, 1982.

Fawer CL, Calame A, Furrer MI: Neurodevelopmental outcome at 12 months of age related to cerebral ultrasound appearances of high risk preterm infants. Early Hum Dev 11:123, 1985.

Fawer CL, Diebold P, Calame A: Periventricular leucomalacia and neurodevelopmental outcome in preterm infants. Arch Dis Child 62:30, 1987.

Gaiter JL: The effects of intraventricular hemorrhage on Bayley developmental performance in preterm infants. Semin Perinatol 6:305, 1982.

Griesen G, Petersen MB, Pedersen SA, et al.: Status at two years in 121 very low birth weight survivors related to neonatal intraventricular hemorrhage and mode of delivery. Acta Paediatr Scand 75:24, 1986.

Guzzetta F, Shackelford GD, Volpe S, et al.: Periventricular intraparenchymal echodensities in the premature newborn: Critical determinant of neurologic outcome. Pediatrics 78:995, 1986.

Hawgood S, Spong J, Yu VYH: Intraventricular hemorrhage: Incidence and outcome in a population of very-low-birth-weight infants. Am J Dis Child 138:136, 1984.

Horwood SP, Boyel MJ, Torrance GW, et al.: Mortality and morbidity of 500 to 1499-gm birth weight infants liveborn to residents of a defined geographic region before and after neonatal intensive care. Pediatrics 69:613, 1982.

Knobloch H, Malone A, Ellison PH, et al.: Considerations in evaluating changes in outcome for infants weighing less than 1501 grams. Pediatrics 69:285, 1982.

Kosmetains M, Dinter C, Williams ML, et al.: Predictive factors and outcome of intracranial hemorrhage in the premature. Am J Dis Child 134:855, 1980.

Lacey DJ, Topper WH, Buckwald S, et al.: Preterm very-low-birth-weight neonates: Relationship of EEG to intracranial hemorrhage, perinatal complications, and developmental outcome. Neurology 36:1084, 1986.

Leonard C, Clyman R, Behle M, et al.: Late outcome of social and neonatal risk factors in the VLBW infant. Clin Res 35:201A, 1987.

Leonard CH, Miller CA, Piecuch RE, et al.: Neurodevelopmental outcome and intraventricular hemorrhage (IVH) in infants 1,250 gm. Clin Res 31:100A, 1983.

McMenamin JB, Shackelford GD, Volpe JJ: Outcome of neonatal intraventricular hemorrhage with periventricular echodense lesions. Ann Neurol 15:285, 1984.

Ment LR, Scott DT, Ehrenkranz RA, et al.: Neonates of 1250-gm birthweight: Prospective neurodevelopmental evaluation during the first year post-term. Pediatrics 70:292, 1982.

Pape K, Wigglesworth JS: Haemorrhage, Ischemia and the Perinatal Brain. Philadelphia, J.B. Lippincott Company, 1979.

Papile L, Burnstein J, Burnstein R, et al.: Incidence and evolution of subependymal and intraventricular hemorrhage: A study of infants with birthweights less than 1,500 g. J Pediatr 92:529, 1978.

Papile LA, Munsick-Bruno G, Schaefer A: The relationship of cerebral intraventricular hemorrhage and early childhood neurologic handicaps.

Partridge JC, Babcock DS, Steichen JJ, et al.: Optimal timing for cranial ultrasound in low-birthweight infants. Detection of intracranial hemorrhage and ventricular dilation. J Pediatr 102:281, 287, 1983.

Piecuch R, Clyman R, Ballard R: Risk factors associated with infant death after discharge from an ICN. Clin Res 35:214A, 1987.

Scott DT, Ment LR, Ehrenkranz, et al.: Prognostic significance of neonatal intraventricular hemorrhage: Follow-up results from discordant twins. Pediatr Res 19:363A, 1985.

Scott DT, Ment LR, Ehrenkranz, et al.: Evidence for late developmental deficit in very low birth weight infants surviving intraventricular hemorrhage. Childs Brain 11:261, 1984.

Seigal S, Rosenbaum P, Stoskopf B, et al.: Follow-up of infants 501 to 1500-gm birth weight delivered to residents of a geographically defined region with perinatal intensive care facilities. J Pediatr 100:606, 1982.

Shankaran S, Slovis TL, Bedard MP, et al.: Sonographic classification of intracranial hemorrhage: A prognostic indicator of mortality, morbidity and short-term neurologic outcome. J Pediatr 100:469, 1982.

Speer ME, Blifeld C, Rudolph AJ, et al.: Intraventricular hemorrhage and vitamin E in the very-low-birth-weight infant: Evidence for efficacy of early intramuscular vitamin E administration. Pediatrics 74:1107, 1984.

Stewart AL, Thornburn RJ, Hope PL, et al.: Relation between ultrasound appearance of the brain in very preterm infant and neurodevelopmental outcome at 18 months of age. The 2nd Special Ross Laboratories Conference on Perinatal Intracranial Hemorrhage. Columbus, Ross Laboratories, 1982, pp 1090–1116.

Szymonowicz W, Yu VY: Periventricular haemorrhage and leukomalacia in extremely low birthweight infants. Aust Paediatr J 22:207, 1986.

Szymonowicz W, Yu VY, Bajuk B, et al.: Neurodevelopmental outcome of periventricular haemorrhage and leukomalacia in infants 1250 g or less at birth. Early Hum Dev 14:1, 1986.

Thornburn RJ, Stewart AL, Hope PL, et al.: Prediction of death and major handicap in very preterm infants by brain ultrasound. Lancet 1:1119, 1981.

Volpe JJ: Neurology of the Newborn, 2nd ed. Philadelphia, W.B. Saunders Company, 1986, pp 311–361.

Williamson WD, Desmond MM, Wilson GS, et al.: Low-birthweight infants surviving neonatal intraventricular hemorrhage: Outcome in the preschool years. The 2nd Special Ross Laboratories Conference on Perinatal Intracranial Hemorrhage. Columbus, Ross Laboratories, 1982, pp 1266–1281.

Williamson WD, Desmond MM, Wilson GS, et al.: Survival of low-birth-weight infants with neonatal intraventricular hemorrhage. Outcome in the preschool years. Am J Dis Child 137:1181, 1983.

PERINATAL ASPHYXIA

The outcome after perinatal asphyxia can best be predicted by careful staging of the clinical evidence that severe hypoxia has occurred. The important findings are presence of seizures and of posthypoxic encephalopathy of severe degree. In general, the outcome at age 3 to 5 years for infants who have had severe hypoxic ischemic encephalopathy[1] is 100 per cent for death or handicap. For infants who have experienced moderate degrees of encephalopathy, approximately 25 per cent will have been expected to die or have severe handicaps at 3 to 5 years of age. It has recently been noted[2] that in infants with clinical signs of asphyxia, a careful neurodevelopmental discharge examination[3] will allow prediction of approximately 90 per cent of those infants who can be expected to go on to have severe handicaps.

References

1. Sarnat HB, Sarnat MS: Neonatal encephalopathy following fetal distress. Arch Neurol 33:696, 1975.
2. Piecuch R, Leonard C, Clyman R, et al.: Predicting neurodevelopmental outcome in infants with severe perinatal asphyxia. Pediatr Res 21:401A, 1987.

Recommended Reading: Perinatal Asphyxia

Amiel-Tison C: Neurologic disorders in neonates associated with abnormalities of pregnancy and birth. Curr Probl Pediatr 3:1, 1973.

Apgar VA: A proposal for a new method of evaluation of the newborn infant. Curr Res Anesth Analg 40:340, 1953.

Barbas G, Taft LTL: The early signs and differential diagnosis of cerebral palsy. Pediatr Ann 15:230, 1986.

Brann AW Jr, Dykes FD: The effects of intrauterine asphyxia in the term neonate. Clin Perinatol 4:149, 1977.

Broman S: Perinatal anoxia and cognitive development in early childhood. In Field T, Sostek AM, Goldberg S, et al. (eds.): Infants Born at Risk. New York, Spectrum Publications, 1979.

Brown JK, Purvis RJ, Foffar JO, et al.: Neurological aspects of perinatal asphyxia. Dev Med Child Neurol 16:567, 1974.

Chi G, Dooling EC, Gilles FH: Gyral development of the human brain. Ann Neurol 1:86, 1977.

Clancy R, Malin S, Laraque D, et al.: Focal motor seizures heralding stroke in full-term neonates. Am J Dis Child 139:601, 1985.

DeSouza SW, Richards B: Neurological sequelae in newborn babies after perinatal asphyxia. Arch Dis Child 53:564, 1978.

Dorini-Zis K, Dolman CL: Gestational development of the brain. Arch Pathol Lab Med 101:192, 1977.

Dweck HS, Huggins W, Dorman D, et al.: Developmental sequelae in infants having suffered severe perinatal asphyxia. Am J Obstet Gynecol 119:811, 1974.

Ellenberg JH, Nelson KB: Birth weight and gestational age in children with cerebral palsy or seizure disorders. Am J Dis Child 133:1044, 1979.

Finer NN, Richards RT, Peters KL: Hypoxic-ischemic encephalopathy in term neonates: Perinatal factors and outcome. J Pediatr 98:112, 1981.

Fitzhardinge PM, Flodmark O, Fritz CR, et al.: The prognostic value of computed tomography as an adjunct to assessment of the term infant with postasphyxial encephalopathy. J Pediatr 99:777, 1981.

Friede RL: Developmental Neuropathology. New York, Springer-Verlag, 1975.

Gilles FH, Leviton A, Dooling EC: The Developing Human Brain. Boston, John Wright Company, 1983.

Gluck L (ed.): Intrauterine Asphyxia and the Developing Brain. Chicago, Year Book Medical Publishers, 1977.

Gottfried AW: Intellectual consequences of perinatal anoxia. Psychol Bull 80:231, 1973.

Hagberg B, Hagberg G, Lewerth A, et al.: Mild mental retardation in Swedish school children. Acta Paediatr Scand 70:441, 1981.

Hagberg G, Hagberg B, Olow I: The changing panorama of cerebral palsy in Sweden 1954–1970: III. The importance of foetal deprivation of supply. Acta Paediatr Scand 65:403, 1976.

Hill A, Martin DJ, Daneman A, et al.: Focal ischemic cerebral injury in the newborn: Diagnosis by ultrasound and correlation with computed tomographic scan. Pediatrics 71:790, 1983.

Holm VA: The causes of cerebral palsy. JAMA 247:1473, 1983.

Illingworth RS: A paediatrician asks — Why is it called brain injury? JAMA 25:1843, 1984.

James LS, Weisbrot IM, Prince CE, et al.: The acid-base status of human infants in relation to birth asphyxia and the onset of respiration. J Pediatr 52:379, 1958.

Kim MS, Elyaderani MK: Sonographic diagnosis of cerebroventricular hemorrhage in utero. Radiology 142:479, 1982.

Larroche JC: The development of the central nervous system during intrauterine life. In Falkner F (ed.): Human Development. Philadelphia, W.B. Saunders Company, 1966, pp 257–276.

Levene MI, Grindulis H, Sands C, et al.: Comparison of two methods of predicting outcome in perinatal asphyxia. Lancet 1:67, 1986.

Levene MI, Kornberg J, Williams THC: The incidence and severity of postasphyxial encephalopathy in full-term infants. Early Hum Dev 11:21, 1985.

Little WJ: On the influence of abnormal parturition, difficult labours, premature birth and asphyxia neonatorum on the mental and physical condition of the child, especially in relation to deformities. Trans Obstet Soc Lond 3:293, 1861–1862.

Low JA, Gailbraith RS, Muir DW, et al.: The relationship between perinatal hypoxia and newborn encephalopathy. Am J Obstet Gynecol 152:256, 1985.

Low JA, Galbraith RS, Muir D, et al.: Intrapartum fetal asphyxia: A preliminary report in regard to long-term morbidity. Am J Obstet Gynecol 130:525, 1978.

MacDonald HM, Mulligan JC, Allen AC, et al.: Neonatal asphyxia: I. Relationship of obstetric and neonatal complications to neonatal mortality in 38,405 consecutive deliveries. J Pediatr 898, 1980.

McGahan JP, Haesslein HC, Meyer M, et al.: Sonographic recognition of in utero intraventricular hemorrhage. AJR 142:171, 1984.

Mellits ED, Holden KR, Freeman JM: Neonatal seizures: II. A multivariate analysis of factors associated with outcome. Pediatrics 70:177, 1982.

Milstein JM, Rennick J, Goetzman BW: Computerized axial tomography of the brain in neonates and young infants. Surg Neurol 8:59, 1977.

Naeye RL, Chez R: Effects of maternal acetonuria and low pregnancy weight gain on children's psychomotor development. Am J Obstet Gynecol 139:189, 1981.

Neligan G, Purdham D, Steiner H: The Formative Years: Birth, Family and Development in Newcastle-upon-Tyne. London, Oxford University Press, 1974.

Nelson KB, Ellenberg JH: Epidemiology of cerebral palsy. Adv Neurol 19:421, 1978.

Nelson KB, Ellenberg JH: Apgar scores as predictors of chronic neurologic disability. Pediatrics 68:36, 1981.

Niswander KR: Asphyxia in the fetus and cerebral palsy. In Yearbook of Obstetrics and Gynecology. Chicago, Year Book Medical Publishers, 1983, p 107.

Niswander KR, Gordon M (eds.): The Collaborative Perinatal Study of the National Institute of Neurological Diseases and Stroke: The Women and Their Pregnancies. Philadelphia, W.B. Saunders Company, 1972.

Niswander KR, Gordon M, Drage JS: The effect of intrauterine hypoxia on the child surviving to 4 years. Am J Obstet Gynecol 121:892, 1975.

Painter MJ, Depp R, O'Donoghue PD: Fetal heart rate patterns and development in the first year of life. Am J Obstet Gynecol 132: 271, 1978.

Paneth I: Etiologic factors in cerebral palsy. Pediatr Ann 15:191, 1986.

Paneth W, Fox HE: The relationship of Apgar score to neurologic handicap: A survey of clinicians. Obstet Gynecol 61:547, 1983.

Paneth N, Start RI: Cerebral palsy and mental retardation in relation to indicators in perinatal asphyxia. Am J Obstet Gynecol 61:547, 1983.

Peckham GJ: Risk-benefit relationships of current therapeutic approaches. In Peckham GJ, Heyman MA (eds.): Cardiovascular Sequelae of Asphyxia in the Newborn. Report of the 83rd Ross Conference on Pediatric Research. Columbus, 1982, pp 110–116.

Pryse-Davies J, Beard RW: A necropsy study of brain swelling in the newborn with special reference to cerebellar herniation. J Pathol 109:51, 1973.

Robertson C, Finer N: Term infants with hypoxic-ischemic encephalopathy: Outcome at 3–5 years. Dev Med Child Neurol 27:473, 1985.

Rosen MG: Factors during labor and delivery that influence brain disorders. In Freeman JM (ed.): Prenatal and Perinatal Factors Associated with Brain Disorders. Bethesda, National Institutes of Health, Publication no 85-1149, 1985, pp 237–261.

Scott H: Outcome of very severe birth asphyxia. Arch Dis Child 51:712, 1976.

Sims ME, Turke SG, Halterman PAC, et al.: Brain injury and intrauterine death. Am J Obstet Gynecol 151:721, 1985.

Skov H, Lou H, Pederson H: Perinatal brain ischaemia impact at 4 years of age. Dev Med Child Neurol 26:353, 1984.

Slovis TL, Shankaran S: Ultrasound in the evaluation of hypoxic-ischemic injury and intracranial hemorrhage in neonates: The state of the art. Pediatr Radiol 14:67, 1984.

Stein ZA, Susser MW: Mental retardation. In Last JM (ed.): Public Health and Preventive Medicine, 11th ed. New York, Appleton-Century-Crofts, 1980.

Steiner H, Neligan G: Perinatal cardiac arrest. Quality of the survivors. Arch Dis Child 50:696, 1975.

Sykes GS, Molloy PM, Johnson P, et al.: Do Apgar scores indicate asphyxia? Lancet 1:494, 1982.

Thomson AJ, Searle M, Russell G: Quality of survival after severe birth asphyxia. Arch Dis Child 52:620, 1977.

Towbin A: Central nervous system damage in the human fetus and newborn infant. Am J Dis Child 119:529, 1970.

TABLE D–2. Persistent Pulmonary Hypertension of the Newborn: Early Outcome*

STUDY	N	NEUROLOGIC OUTCOME Mean Age and Range at Follow-up	Outcome	N	COGNITIVE OUTCOME Mean Age and Range at Follow-up	Mean Age and Range
Brett et al. (1981)	9	21.5 mo (6–48)	9 normal	4	17 mo (12–18)	Bayley MDI = 107.5 (89–130)
				4	31.5 mo (25–35)	Stanford Binet IQ = 108 (96–119)
Bernbaum et al. (1981)	12	29 mo (6–48)	9 normal; 2 slightly increased tone in lower extremity; 1 moderate unilateral hypotonia	12	29 mo (6–48)	9 infants in DQ or IQ range 87–105 2 infants in DQ or IQ range 70–90 1 infant DQ = 50
Ferrara et al. (1983)	15	11 mo (5–13)	14 normal; 1 mild right hemiparesis	10	12 mo (10–13)	Bayley MDI = 106.5 (84–131) Bayley PDI = 94.7 (80–115)
Sell et al. (1984)	37	(1–4 yr)	3 "severely" damaged; 5 infants with hearing loss			Bayley MDI 101–108 Bayley PDI 89–94 McCarthy GCI 101–116

* Modified from Ballard RA, Leonard CH: Clin Perinatol 11:737, 1984.

PERSISTENT PULMONARY HYPERTENSION OF THE NEWBORN

Recent studies of outcome of persistent pulmonary hypertension of the newborn are reviewed in Table D-2. It is currently fair to say that, again, outcome in these infants reflects other aspects of their perinatal course, particularly the degree of perinatal asphyxia sustained. The majority of these infants have a good neurodevelopmental outcome; however, Sell et al.[1] have noted that, in their group of 37 infants, 5 had hearing loss, which was severe in 3. This clearly needs further investigation.

Reference

1. Sell E, Gluckman C, Williams E: Hearing problems in children who had persistent fetal circulation as neonates. Clin Res 32:92A, 1984.

Recommended Reading: Outcome in Infants with PPHN

Bayley N: Bayley Scales of Infant Development. New York, Psychological Corporation, 1969.

Bernbaum J, Russell P, Gewitz M, et al.: Neurodevelopmental (ND) and cardiorespiratory (CR) follow-up of infants with persistent pulmonary hypertension of the newborn (PPHN). Pediatr Res 15:651A, 1981.

Bifano EM, Pfannenstiel A: Outcome for survivors of persistent pulmonary hypertension. Pediatr Res 18:101A, 1984.

Brett C, Dekle M, Leonard CH, et al.: Developmental follow-up of hyperventilated neonates: Preliminary observations. Pediatrics 68: 588, 1981.

Cohen RS, Stevenson DK, Malachowski N, et al.: Late morbidity among survivors of respiratory failure treated with tolazoline. J Pediatr 97:644, 1980.

Ferrara B, Johnson DE, Chang PN, et al.: Efficacy and neurologic outcome of profound hypocapneic alkalosis for the treatment of persistent pulmonary hypertension in infancy. J Pediatr 105:457, 1984.

Ferrara TB, Johnson DE, Thompson TR: Hypocapneic alkalosis for treatment of persistent pulmonary hypertension (PPH) in infants with severe pulmonary pathology. Pediatr Res 17:312A, 1983.

Fox WW, Duara S: Persistent pulmonary hypertension in the neonate: Diagnosis and management. J Pediatr 103:505, 1983.

Holden RH: Prediction of mental retardation in infancy. Ment Retard 10:28, 1972.

McBride DC, Wilson JL, Pettett G: Hyperventilation in the treatment of persistent fetal circulation. J Pediatr 96:174, 1980.

McCarthy D: McCarthy Scales of Children's Abilities. New York, Psychological Corporation, 1972.

Rubin RA, Balow B: Measures of infant development and socioeconomic status as predictors of later intelligence and school achievement. Dev Psychol 15:225, 1979.

APPENDIX E

COMMUNITY AND AGENCY RESOURCES

JOSEPH HEADLEE, M.S.W.

CHILDREN'S SERVICES

The Maternal-Child Health Division of most states' Department of Health and Human Services (DHHS) provides financial assistance for follow-up of certain infants whose families meet state-established financial criteria. These services are variously named, e.g., Crippled Children's Services (CCS), California Children's Services (CCS). Services vary from state to state, but usually include diagnostic and treatment services, laboratory tests, appliances, equipment, and others if a family's insurance will not pay for needed services. Some CCS programs also provide or will contract for services such as physical or occupational therapy. Inquires can be made by calling the state or local Maternal and Child Health Division of the Department of Health and Human Services.

EASTER SEALS SOCIETY

Each community served by the Easter Seals Society defines what services are needed for that community. Physical and occupational therapy programs are common. The cost of services is based on ability to pay, and no one is denied services because of financial limitations. The national office address is: National Easter Seals Society, 2023 West Ogden Avenue, Chicago, IL 60612.

HOME CARE AGENCIES

Many communities have local home care agencies that offer services, such as oxygen and stoma care, for infants with special needs. Some are privately operated, while others contract with local county health or social service departments. Fees vary with location and services. When an infant with special medical home care needs is to be discharged, the local health department is the best place to begin to locate such an agency.

INFANT PROGRAMS

Most areas have specialized infant programs that provide services to infants and their families until age 3 years. These programs may be state, locally, or privately funded and provide a range of services. Infant programs are a good resource for conferring with infant specialists from various disciplines.

MARCH OF DIMES BIRTH DEFECTS FOUNDATION

There are 650 March of Dimes chapters nationally, with the goal of achieving healthy babies, born free of handicapping-fatal problems caused by birth defects or prematurity. Their focus is on preventing birth defects, and the Foundation funds scientific research, medical services, and professional and public health education. Some chapters provide specialized services, such as special day care programs for children with cerebral palsy or other handicapping conditions.

SUPPORT GROUPS FOR PARENTS OF CHILDREN WITH DOWN AND OTHER SYNDROMES

Numerous support groups exist for parents of children with Down and other genetic syndromes or congenital anomalies. Information for the respective groups can be obtained by writing or calling:

American Cleft Palate Association, 331 Salk Hall, University of Pittsburgh, Pittsburgh, PA 15261

Down Syndrome Congress, 1640 W Roosevelt Road, Chicago, IL 60808

National Down Syndrome Society, 70 West 40th Street, New York, NY 10018

Little People of America, PO Box 633, San Bruno, CA 94066

Osteogenesis Imperfecta Foundation, Box 838, Manchester, NH 03105

Turner Syndrome Support Group, PO Box 9082, Morristown NJ 07960

The support organization for trisomy 18/13 (SOFT), established in Utah in 1980, is a national organization for families who have a child with the more serious autosomal trisomies:

Support Organization for Trisomy 18/13, c/o Debbie Stutz, 3646 West Valley West Drive, West Jordan, Utah 84084 or 478 Terrace Lane, Todele, Utah 84074

PARENTS OF PREMATURES AND HIGH-RISK INFANTS (PPHRI)

This is a nationwide clearinghouse for parents of premature infants. Listings are maintained for local parent support groups, reading materials, clothing, and breast-feeding information related to premature and high-risk infants. This information is published in *The Resource Directory,* which can be obtained by calling PPHRI (212-869-2818).

PUBLIC HEALTH NURSES

Every county has a public health department. For premature and high-risk infants, a home visit by a public health nurse before discharge is encouraged to assess the parents' readiness for the homecoming and the home situation. Public health nursing home visits are free of charge, and some health departments also provide home care services for at-risk infants. Usually the public health nurse will visit once a week until the family and nurse mutually agree the visits are no longer necessary. The teaching done by the nurses should be coordinated with the pediatrician or family physician; therefore an ongoing dialogue between the nurse and the physician is encouraged. Finally, local health departments also provide immunization and well-child clinics at no or very low cost.

REGIONAL CENTERS

Most state health departments also provide regional centers, which offer services to children up to 3 years of age. These state-funded programs usually serve children who are developmentally delayed or have cerebral palsy, epilepsy, autism, or other long-term handicapping disabilities. The centers usually provide comprehensive assessment, referral to local programs most appropriate to a child's needs, and case management services.

SCHOOL DISTRICTS

Every school district is required to provide special educational services to children with severe learning disabilities or significant handicap at 3 years of age. A parent can request an Individualized Education Plan (IEP) conference, which will assess the child's learning needs and if a special classroom environment is required. These IEP conferences are free; however, long waiting periods may occur. The local school district administrative office can provide specific guidelines for scheduling an IEP conference.

WOMEN INFANTS AND CHILDREN (WIC) PROGRAM

This is a federal supplemental food program, funded through the United States Department of Agriculture and administered by local health departments. WIC offers nutrition education and supplemental food to financially eligible pregnant women and children up to 5 years of age who are assessed as being at risk.

PARENTERAL NUTRITION

The Lifeline Foundation provides education concerning parenteral or enteral nutrition and publishes a free newsletter for patients on home nutrition programs. For information write to:

The Lifeline Foundation, 2 Osprey Road, Sharon, MA 02067

INDEX

Note: Page numbers in *italics* represent illustrations;
t indicates tables.